FIVE-LIPOXYGENASE PRODUCTS IN ASTHMA

LUNG BIOLOGY IN HEALTH AND DISEASE

Executive Editor

Claude Lenfant
Director, National Heart, Lung and Blood Institute
National Institutes of Health
Bethesda, Maryland

1. Immunologic and Infectious Reactions in the Lung, *edited by Charles H. Kirkpatrick and Herbert Y. Reynolds*
2. The Biochemical Basis of Pulmonary Function, *edited by Ronald G. Crystal*
3. Bioengineering Aspects of the Lung, *edited by John B. West*
4. Metabolic Functions of the Lung, *edited by Y. S. Bakhle and John R. Vane*
5. Respiratory Defense Mechanisms (in two parts), *edited by Joseph D. Brain, Donald F. Proctor, and Lynne M. Reid*
6. Development of the Lung, *edited by W. Alan Hodson*
7. Lung Water and Solute Exchange, *edited by Norman C. Staub*
8. Extrapulmonary Manifestations of Respiratory Disease, *edited by Eugene Debs Robin*
9. Chronic Obstructive Pulmonary Disease, *edited by Thomas L. Petty*
10. Pathogenesis and Therapy of Lung Cancer, *edited by Curtis C. Harris*
11. Genetic Determinants of Pulmonary Disease, *edited by Stephen D. Litwin*
12. The Lung in the Transition Between Health and Disease, *edited by Peter T. Macklem and Solbert Permutt*
13. Evolution of Respiratory Processes: A Comparative Approach, *edited by Stephen C. Wood and Claude Lenfant*
14. Pulmonary Vascular Diseases, *edited by Kenneth M. Moser*
15. Physiology and Pharmacology of the Airways, *edited by Jay A. Nadel*
16. Diagnostic Techniques in Pulmonary Disease (in two parts), *edited by Marvin A. Sackner*
17. Regulation of Breathing (in two parts), *edited by Thomas F. Hornbein*
18. Occupational Lung Diseases: Research Approaches and Methods, *edited by Hans Weill and Margaret Turner-Warwick*
19. Immunopharmacology of the Lung, *edited by Harold H. Newball*
20. Sarcoidosis and Other Granulomatous Diseases of the Lung, *edited by Barry L. Fanburg*

21. Sleep and Breathing, *edited by Nicholas A. Saunders and Colin E. Sullivan*
22. *Pneumocystis carinii* Pneumonia: Pathogenesis, Diagnosis, and Treatment, *edited by Lowell S. Young*
23. Pulmonary Nuclear Medicine: Techniques in Diagnosis of Lung Disease, *edited by Harold L. Atkins*
24. Acute Respiratory Failure, *edited by Warren M. Zapol and Konrad J. Falke*
25. Gas Mixing and Distribution in the Lung, *edited by Ludwig A. Engel and Manuel Paiva*
26. High-Frequency Ventilation in Intensive Care and During Surgery, *edited by Graziano Carlon and William S. Howland*
27. Pulmonary Development: Transition from Intrauterine to Extrauterine Life, *edited by George H. Nelson*
28. Chronic Obstructive Pulmonary Disease: Second Edition, Revised and Expanded, *edited by Thomas L. Petty*
29. The Thorax (in two parts), *edited by Charis Roussos and Peter T. Macklem*
30. The Pleura in Health and Disease, *edited by Jacques Chrétien, Jean Bignon, and Albert Hirsch*
31. Drug Therapy for Asthma: Research and Clinical Practice, *edited by John W. Jenne and Shirley Murphy*
32. Pulmonary Endothelium in Health and Disease, *edited by Una S. Ryan*
33. The Airways: Neural Control in Health and Disease, *edited by Michael A. Kaliner and Peter J. Barnes*
34. Pathophysiology and Treatment of Inhalation Injuries, *edited by Jacob Loke*
35. Respiratory Function of the Upper Airway, *edited by Oommen P. Mathew and Giuseppe Sant'Ambrogio*
36. Chronic Obstructive Pulmonary Disease: A Behavioral Perspective, *edited by A. John McSweeny and Igor Grant*
37. Biology of Lung Cancer: Diagnosis and Treatment, *edited by Steven T. Rosen, James L. Mulshine, Frank Cuttitta, and Paul G. Abrams*
38. Pulmonary Vascular Physiology and Pathophysiology, *edited by E. Kenneth Weir and John T. Reeves*
39. Comparative Pulmonary Physiology: Current Concepts, *edited by Stephen C. Wood*
40. Respiratory Physiology: An Analytical Approach, *edited by H. K. Chang and Manuel Paiva*
41. Lung Cell Biology, *edited by Donald Massaro*
42. Heart–Lung Interactions in Health and Disease, *edited by Steven M. Scharf and Sharon S. Cassidy*
43. Clinical Epidemiology of Chronic Obstructive Pulmonary Disease, *edited by Michael J. Hensley and Nicholas A. Saunders*
44. Surgical Pathology of Lung Neoplasms, *edited by Alberto M. Marchevsky*
45. The Lung in Rheumatic Diseases, *edited by Grant W. Cannon and Guy A. Zimmerman*

46. Diagnostic Imaging of the Lung, *edited by Charles E. Putman*
47. Models of Lung Disease: Microscopy and Structural Methods, *edited by Joan Gil*
48. Electron Microscopy of the Lung, *edited by Dean E. Schraufnagel*
49. Asthma: Its Pathology and Treatment, *edited by Michael A. Kaliner, Peter J. Barnes, and Carl G. A. Persson*
50. Acute Respiratory Failure: Second Edition, *edited by Warren M. Zapol and Francois Lemaire*
51. Lung Disease in the Tropics, *edited by Om P. Sharma*
52. Exercise: Pulmonary Physiology and Pathophysiology, *edited by Brian J. Whipp and Karlman Wasserman*
53. Developmental Neurobiology of Breathing, *edited by Gabriel G. Haddad and Jay P. Farber*
54. Mediators of Pulmonary Inflammation, *edited by Michael A. Bray and Wayne H. Anderson*
55. The Airway Epithelium, *edited by Stephen G. Farmer and Douglas Hay*
56. Physiological Adaptations in Vertebrates: Respiration, Circulation, and Metabolism, *edited by Stephen C. Wood, Roy E. Weber, Alan R. Hargens, and Ronald W. Millard*
57. The Bronchial Circulation, *edited by John Butler*
58. Lung Cancer Differentiation: Implications for Diagnosis and Treatment, *edited by Samuel D. Bernal and Paul J. Hesketh*
59. Pulmonary Complications of Systemic Disease, *edited by John F. Murray*
60. Lung Vascular Injury: Molecular and Cellular Response, *edited by Arnold Johnson and Thomas J. Ferro*
61. Cytokines of the Lung, *edited by Jason Kelley*
62. The Mast Cell in Health and Disease, *edited by Michael A. Kaliner and Dean D. Metcalfe*
63. Pulmonary Disease in the Elderly Patient, *edited by Donald A. Mahler*
64. Cystic Fibrosis, *edited by Pamela B. Davis*
65. Signal Transduction in Lung Cells, *edited by Jerome S. Brody, David M. Center, and Vsevolod A. Tkachuk*
66. Tuberculosis: A Comprehensive International Approach, *edited by Lee B. Reichman and Earl S. Hershfield*
67. Pharmacology of the Respiratory Tract: Experimental and Clinical Research, *edited by K. Fan Chung and Peter J. Barnes*
68. Prevention of Respiratory Diseases, *edited by Albert Hirsch, Marcel Goldberg, Jean-Pierre Martin, and Roland Masse*
69. *Pneumocystis carinii* Pneumonia: Second Edition, Revised and Expanded, *edited by Peter D. Walzer*
70. Fluid and Solute Transport in the Airspaces of the Lungs, *edited by Richard M. Effros and H. K. Chang*
71. Sleep and Breathing: Second Edition, Revised and Expanded, *edited by Nicholas A. Saunders and Colin E. Sullivan*
72. Airway Secretion: Physiological Bases for the Control of Mucous Hypersecretion, *edited by Tamotsu Takishima and Sanae Shimura*

73. Sarcoidosis and Other Granulomatous Disorders, *edited by D. Geraint James*
74. Epidemiology of Lung Cancer, *edited by Jonathan M. Samet*
75. Pulmonary Embolism, *edited by Mario Morpurgo*
76. Sports and Exercise Medicine, *edited by Stephen C. Wood and Robert C. Roach*
77. Endotoxin and the Lungs, *edited by Kenneth L. Brigham*
78. The Mesothelial Cell and Mesothelioma, *edited by Marie-Claude Jaurand and Jean Bignon*
79. Regulation of Breathing: Second Edition, Revised and Expanded, *edited by Jerome A. Dempsey and Allan I. Pack*
80. Pulmonary Fibrosis, *edited by Sem Hin Phan and Roger S. Thrall*
81. Long-Term Oxygen Therapy: Scientific Basis and Clinical Application, *edited by Walter J. O'Donohue, Jr.*
82. Ventral Brainstem Mechanisms and Control of Respiration and Blood Pressure, *edited by C. Ovid Trouth, Richard M. Millis, Heidrun F. Kiwull-Schöne, and Marianne E. Schläfke*
83. A History of Breathing Physiology, *edited by Donald F. Proctor*
84. Surfactant Therapy for Lung Disease, *edited by Bengt Robertson and H. William Taeusch*
85. The Thorax: Second Edition, Revised and Expanded (in three parts), *edited by Charis Roussos*
86. Severe Asthma: Pathogenesis and Clinical Management, *edited by Stanley J. Szefler and Donald Y. M. Leung*
87. *Mycobacterium avium*–Complex Infection: Progress in Research and Treatment, *edited by Joyce A. Korvick and Constance A. Benson*
88. Alpha 1–Antitrypsin Deficiency: Biology • Pathogenesis • Clinical Manifestations • Therapy, *edited by Ronald G. Crystal*
89. Adhesion Molecules and the Lung, *edited by Peter A. Ward and Joseph C. Fantone*
90. Respiratory Sensation, *edited by Lewis Adams and Abraham Guz*
91. Pulmonary Rehabilitation, *edited by Alfred P. Fishman*
92. Acute Respiratory Failure in Chronic Obstructive Pulmonary Disease, *edited by Jean-Philippe Derenne, William A. Whitelaw, and Thomas Similowski*
93. Environmental Impact on the Airways: From Injury to Repair, *edited by Jacques Chrétien and Daniel Dusser*
94. Inhalation Aerosols: Physical and Biological Basis for Therapy, *edited by Anthony J. Hickey*
95. Tissue Oxygen Deprivation: From Molecular to Integrated Function, *edited by Gabriel G. Haddad and George Lister*
96. The Genetics of Asthma, *edited by Stephen B. Liggett and Deborah A. Meyers*
97. Inhaled Glucocorticoids in Asthma: Mechanisms and Clinical Actions, *edited by Robert P. Schleimer, William W. Busse, and Paul M. O'Byrne*
98. Nitric Oxide and the Lung, *edited by Warren M. Zapol and Kenneth D. Bloch*

99. Primary Pulmonary Hypertension, *edited by Lewis J. Rubin and Stuart Rich*
100. Lung Growth and Development, *edited by John A. McDonald*
101. Parasitic Lung Diseases, *edited by Adel A. F. Mahmoud*
102. Lung Macrophages and Dendritic Cells in Health and Disease, *edited by Mary F. Lipscomb and Stephen W. Russell*
103. Pulmonary and Cardiac Imaging, *edited by Caroline Chiles and Charles E. Putman*
104. Gene Therapy for Diseases of the Lung, *edited by Kenneth L. Brigham*
105. Oxygen, Gene Expression, and Cellular Function, *edited by Linda Biadasz Clerch and Donald J. Massaro*
106. $Beta_2$-Agonists in Asthma Treatment, *edited by Romain Pauwels and Paul M. O'Byrne*
107. Inhalation Delivery of Therapeutic Peptides and Proteins, *edited by Akwete Lex Adjei and Pramod K. Gupta*
108. Asthma in the Elderly, *edited by Robert A. Barbee and John W. Bloom*
109. Treatment of the Hospitalized Cystic Fibrosis Patient, *edited by David M. Orenstein and Robert C. Stern*
110. Asthma and Immunological Diseases in Pregnancy and Early Infancy, *edited by Michael Schatz, Robert S. Zeiger, and Henry N. Claman*
111. Dyspnea, *edited by Donald A. Mahler*
112. Proinflammatory and Antiinflammatory Peptides, *edited by Sami I. Said*
113. Self-Management of Asthma, *edited by Harry Kotses and Andrew Harver*
114. Eicosanoids, Aspirin, and Asthma, *edited by Andrew Szczeklik, Ryszard J. Gryglewski, and John R. Vane*
115. Fatal Asthma, *edited by Albert L. Sheffer*
116. Pulmonary Edema, *edited by Michael A. Matthay and David H. Ingbar*
117. Inflammatory Mechanisms in Asthma, *edited by Stephen T. Holgate and William W. Busse*
118. Physiological Basis of Ventilatory Support, *edited by John J. Marini and Arthur S. Slutsky*
119. Human Immunodeficiency Virus and the Lung, *edited by Mark J. Rosen and James M. Beck*
120. Five-Lipoxygenase Products in Asthma, *edited by Jeffrey M. Drazen, Sven-Erik Dahlén, and Tak H. Lee*
121. Complexity in Structure and Function of the Lung, *edited by Michael P. Hlastala and H. Thomas Robertson*
122. Biology of Lung Cancer, *edited by Madeleine A. Kane and Paul A. Bunn, Jr.*

ADDITIONAL VOLUMES IN PREPARATION

The Lung at Depth, *edited by Claes Lundgren and John N. Miller*

Lung Tumors, *edited by Christian Brambilla and Elisabeth Brambilla*

Diagnostic Pulmonary Pathology, *edited by Philip Cagle*

Immunotherapy of Asthma, *edited by Jean Bousquet and Hans Yssel*

Rhinitis, *edited by Robert M. Naclerio, Stephen R. Durham, and Niels Mygind*

Interleukin-5: From Molecule to Drug Target for Asthma, *edited by Colin Sanderson*

Viral Infections of the Lung, *edited by Raphael Dolin and Peter F. Wright*

Pediatric Asthma, *edited by Shirley J. Murphy, H. William Kelly, and Bennie C. McWilliams*

LAM and Other Diseases Characterized by Smooth Muscle Proliferation, *edited by Joel Moss*

Gastroesophageal Reflux and Airway Disease, *edited by Mark R. Stein*

Control of Breathing in Health and Disease, *edited by Murray D. Altose and Yoshikazu Kawakami*

Neurobiology of Sleep and Circadian Rhythms, *edited by Fred Turek and Phyllis Zee*

Multimodality Treatment of Lung Cancer, *edited by Arthur T. Skarin*

Cytokines in Pulmonary Infectious Disease, *edited by Steven Nelson and Thomas Martin*

Air Pollutants and the Respiratory Tract, *edited by David L. Swift*

Exercise-Induced Asthma, *edited by E. Regis McFadden, Jr.*

Asthma's Impact on Society: The Social and Economic Burden, *edited by Kevin B. Weiss, A. Sonia Buist, and Sean D. Sullivan*

FIVE-LIPOXYGENASE PRODUCTS IN ASTHMA

Edited by

Jeffrey M. Drazen

Harvard Medical School and
Brigham and Women's Hospital
Boston, Massachusetts

Sven-Erik Dahlén

Karolinska Institutet
Stockholm, Sweden

Tak H. Lee

United Medical and Dental Schools,
Guy's Hospital
London, England

MARCEL DEKKER, INC. NEW YORK • BASEL • HONG KONG

ISBN: 0-8247-0167-4

This book is printed on acid-free paper.

Headquarters
Marcel Dekker, Inc.
270 Madison Avenue, New York, New York 10016
tel: 212-696-9000; fax: 212-685-4540

Eastern Hemisphere Distribution
Marcel Dekker AG
Hutgasse 4, Postfach 812, CH-4001 Basel, Switzerland
tel: 44-61-261-8482; fax: 44-61-261-8896

World Wide Web
http://www.dekker.com

The publisher offers discounts on this book when ordered in bulk quantities. For more information, write to Special Sales/Professional Marketing at the headquarters address above.

Current printing (last digit):
10 9 8 7 6 5 4 3 2 1

PRINTED IN THE UNITED STATES OF AMERICA

INTRODUCTION

The discovery of slow-reacting substances (SRS) and their smooth muscle contracting action during anaphylaxis was a landmark event in the search for an understanding of allergy, asthma, and inflammation. Although that occurred in the first half of this century, years had to pass before SRSs were characterized and identified as leukotrienes by Bengt Samuelsson. The further description of the pathway of the formation of leukotrienes from arachidonic acid opened the door to many avenues of research that are today transforming our understanding of the inflammatory process that dominates asthma. It was soon to be discovered that the enzyme 5-lipoxygenase (5-LO) is a key player in the pathway leading to the leukotrienes. In fact, it was clearly established that when 5-LO was absent, or was inhibited, leukotrienes were not formed and bronchoconstriction could not happen. The obvious resulted: the search for 5-LO inhibitors and/or leukotriene receptor antagonists was actively pursued. Today, synthesized compounds are available and are part of the therapeutic armament available to physicians.

This volume, edited by Drs. Drazen, Dahlén, and Lee, describes the 25- to 30-year voyage of 5-LO from its role in a biochemical pathway to the development of novel and very specific therapeutic agents for the management of asthma. The editors called on international experts to report their experience in this emerging field. All together, this volume is unique: in a way, it can be cited as a paradigm of how basic research leads to clinical application, to patient benefits, and to improvement of public health. The voyage has certainly not ended, as more work needs to be done to fully establish when, and how, the 5-LO and leukotriene inhibitors will give the greatest benefits.

I am grateful to the editors and authors for their major contribution to the Lung Biology in Health and Disease series. It is safe to predict that this volume and its up-to-date, state-of-the-art scientific contributions will pave the way to important additional discoveries.

Claude Lenfant, M.D.
Bethesda, Maryland

PREFACE

In 1938, Kellaway and Trethewey, working in Australia, identified a material in the effluent of anaphylactic guinea pig lungs, which they termed "slow-reacting substance" (SRS) because it elicited constriction of isolated guinea pig ileum in a manner that was slower and harder to reverse than that induced by histamine. Almost two decades later, Brockelhurst provided very clear evidence that SRS was *not* histamine since the newly discovered antihistamines did not inhibit its action. More importantly, over the period from 1956 to 1979, it was demonstrated that slow-reacting substance, derived from anaphylactic exudates, was an extremely potent and unique airway smooth muscle contractile material. This material was called "slow-reacting substance of anaphylaxis" (SRS-A).

In 1979, Robert Murphy, working in Bengt Samuelsson's laboratory, described the chemical structure of SRS-A as the leukotrienes and defined the major arms of the 5-lipoxygenase pathway. Over the ensuing 18 years, a worldwide research effort was launched to (1) define the molecular biology, cell biology, and physiology of the leukotrienes; (2) find agents that inhibited the synthesis or action of the leukotrienes; and (3) show that such agents were able to provide a salutary therapeutic effect in patients with asthma.

This book provides a state-of-the-art review of our understanding of the 5-lipoxygenase pathway and, more importantly, of how it can be specifically interrupted to provide a therapeutic effect in asthma. Part I reviews in detail the basic science of the 5-lipoxygenase pathway and its cell and molecular biology. In Part II, clinical applications with respect to inhibiting the 5-lipoxygenase pathway are reviewed. A unique feature of this volume is that it provides concise and comprehensive reviews of each of the available pharmacological agents acting on the 5-LO pathway used in the treatment of asthma.

This book will be of value to researchers who need to obtain the most current information on the 5-lipoxygenase pathway, as well as to clinicians who wish to use these products to provide the most up-to-date asthma therapy.

Jeffrey M. Drazen
Sven-Erik Dahlén
Tak H. Lee

CONTRIBUTORS

K. Frank Austen, M.D. Professor, Division of Rheumatology, Immunology, and Allergy, Department of Medicine, Harvard Medical School and Brigham and Women's Hospital, Boston, Massachusetts

Walid M. Awni, Ph.D. Manager, Department of Pharmacokinetics and Biopharmaceutics, Abbott Laboratories, Abbott Park, Illinois

Neil C. Barnes, F.R.C.P. Consultant, Department of Respiratory Medicine, London Chest Hospital, London, England

Randy L. Bell, Ph.D. Immunological Disease Research, Abbott Laboratories, Abbott Park, Illinois

Timothy D. Bigby Department of Medicine, University of California, and Chief, Department of Veterans Affairs Medical Center, San Diego, California

Catherine M. Bonuccelli, M.D. Medical Director, Medical Research and Communications Group, Zeneca Pharmaceuticals, Wilmington, Delaware

George W. Carter, Ph.D. Divisional Vice-President, Immunological Disease Research, Abbott Laboratories, Abbott Park, Illinois

Sven-Erik Dahlén, M.D., Ph.D. Experimental Asthma and Allergy Research, Institute of Environmental Medicine, Karolinska Institutet, Stockholm, Sweden

Jeffrey M. Drazen, M.D. Professor, Department of Medicine, Harvard Medical School and Chief, Department of Pulmonary and Critical Care Medicine, Brigham and Women's Hospital, Boston, Massachusetts

Jeffrey W. Dubb Pulmonary/Diabetes Therapeutic Unit, SmithKline Beecham Pharmaceuticals, Collegeville, Pennsylvania

Louise M. Dubé, Ph.D. Director, Immunoscience Venture, Abbott Laboratories, Abbott Park, Illinois

Jilly F. Evans, Ph.D. Director, Department of Biochemistry and Molecular Biology, Merck Frosst Canada, Inc., Pointe-Claire-Dorval, Quebec, Canada

Jesper Z. Haeggström, M.D., Ph.D. Associate Professor, Department of Medical Biochemistry and Biophysics, Division of Chemistry II, Karolinska Institutet, Stockholm, Sweden

Trevor J. C. Higgins, Ph.D. Product Information Manager, Medical Research and Communications Group, Zeneca Pharmaceuticals, Cheshire, England

Elliot Israel, M.D. Associate Professor of Medicine, Harvard Medical School and Director, Clinical Research, Department of Pulmonary and Critical Care Medicine, Brigham and Women's Hospital, Boston, Massachusetts

Bing K. Lam Assistant Professor, Division of Rheumatology, Allergy, and Immunology, Department of Medicine, Harvard Medical School and Brigham and Women's Hospital, Boston, Massachusetts

Tak H. Lee, M.D., Sc.D., F.R.C.Path., F.R.C.P. Professor, Department of Allergy and Respiratory Medicine, United Medical and Dental Schools, Guy's Hospital, London, England

Bruce D. Levy, M.D. Instructor in Medicine, Harvard Medical School, and Department of Pulmonary and Critical Care Medicine, Brigham and Women's Hospital, Boston, Massachusetts

Robert C. Murphy, Ph.D. Department of Pediatrics, National Jewish Medical and Research Center, Denver, Colorado

S. M. Shuaib Nasser, M.B.B.S., M.R.C.P. Department of Respiratory Medicine, Allergy, and Clinical Immunology, Addenbrooke's Hospital, Cambridge, England

Paul M. O'Byrne, M.B., B.Ch., F.R.C.P.I., F.R.C.P.(C). Professor, Department of Medicine, McMaster University, Hamilton, Ontario, Canada

Rachel F. Ochs, M.D., J.D. Adjunct Associate Professor, Department of Neurology, Northwestern University Medical School, Chicago, Illinois

John F. Penrose, M.D. Assistant Professor, Division of Rheumatology, Immunology, and Allergy, Department of Medicine, Harvard Medical School and Brigham and Women's Hospital, Boston, Massachusetts

Anthony S. Rebuck, M.B., B.S., M.D., F.R.C.P.(C) Vice President and Director, Department of Research, Development, and Medical Affairs, SmithKline Beecham Pharmaceuticals, Collegeville, Pennsylvania

Theodore F. Reiss, M.D. Merck & Co., Inc., Rahway, New Jersey

Bengt Samuelsson, M.D. Professor, Department of Medical Biochemistry and Biophysics, Division of Chemistry II, Karolinska Institutet, Stockholm, Sweden

Beth C. Seidenberg, M.D. Merck & Co., Inc., Rahway, New Jersey

Charles N. Serhan, Ph.D. Professor of Anesthesia, Harvard Medical School, and Director, Center for Experimental Therapeutics and Reperfusion Injury, Brigham and Women's Hospital, Boston, Massachusetts

Lewis J. Smith, M.D. Professor, Department of Pulmonary and Critical Care Medicine, Northwestern University Medical School, Chicago, Illinois

Linda J. Swanson, Ph.D. Associate Director, Department of Immunoscience Venture, Abbott Laboratories, Abbott Park, Illinois

Graham W. Taylor, Ph.D. Section of Clinical Pharmacology, Division of Medicine, Imperial College School of Medicine, Hammersmith Hospital, London, England

Ian K. Taylor, B.Sc., M.B.B.S., F.R.C.P. Department of Respiratory Medicine, Sunderland Royal Hospital, Sunderland, England

Jay Y. Westcott, Ph.D. Department of Medicine, National Jewish Medical and Research Center, Denver, Colorado

Pat Wheelan, Ph.D. Department of Pediatrics, National Jewish Medical and Research Center, Denver, Colorado

CONTENTS

IV. PHYSIOLOGICAL ACTIONS OF THE LEUKOTRIENES

1

Overview of the 5-Lipoxygenase Pathway

JESPER Z. HAEGGSTRÖM and BENGT SAMUELSSON

Karolinska Institutet
Stockholm, Sweden

Lipoxygenases are enzymes that catalyze a stereospecific dehydrogenation and subsequent dioxygenation of polyunsaturated fatty acids with a 1,4-*cis*-pentadiene structure. The reaction leads to formation of a hydroperoxide, containing a 1-hydroperoxy-2-*trans*-4-*cis*-pentadiene fragment. Considering the substrate arachidonic acid, oxygen may consequently be introduced at six different positions, yielding 5-, 8-, 9-, 11-, 12-, and 15-hydroperoxy-eicosatetraenoic acid (HPETE), in which the number indicates the position of the respective hydroperoxy group (1). In most biological systems, the hydroperoxide undergoes reduction into the corresponding monohydroxy acid (HETE) either nonenzymatically or by a peroxidase-catalyzed reaction. The stereospecificity exhibited by mammalian lipoxygenases leads to oxygenated derivatives in which the resulting substituent is in the *S* configuration.

Of special interest among mammals is the arachidonate 5-lipoxygenase, which was originally identified in rabbit and human polymorphonuclear leukocytes (PMNL) (2,3). Via the formation of 5(S)-HPETE, this enzyme generates an unstable epoxide intermediate, leukotriene A_4 (LTA_4), which is the most important precursor molecule in the biosynthesis of the biologically active leukotrienes (Fig. 1).

Arachidonic acid may be dioxygenated twice by the cooperative action of two lipoxygenases with different positional specificities. Reduction of the hydroperoxide groups results in the formation of dihydroxy eicosatetraenoic acids (DHETE:s). Thus, 5(S),12(S)-DHETE is formed in mixtures of neutrophils and platelets (4,5), whereas 5(S),15(S)-DHETE has been isolated from human neutrophils as well as eosinophils (6). Both compounds are closely related to leukotrienes in their structures. In addition, 5- and 15-lipoxygenase activities are in-

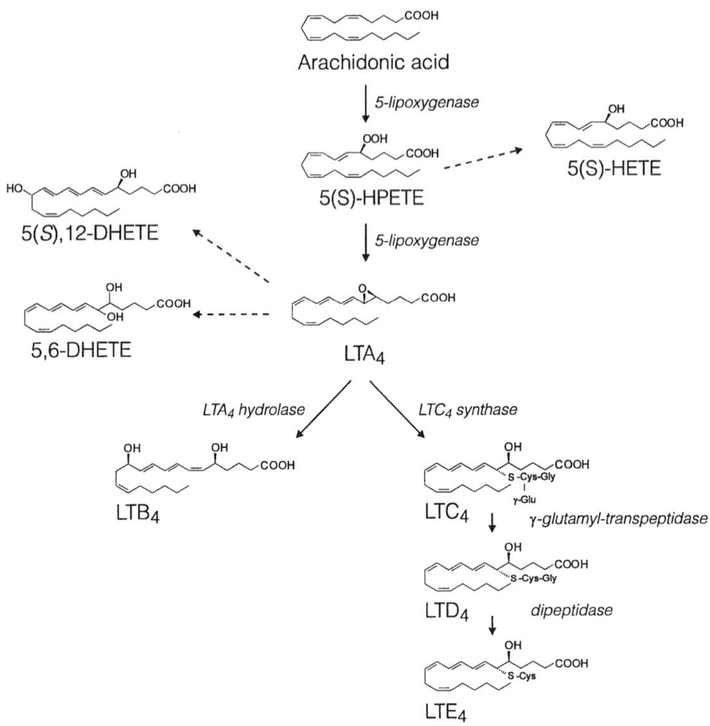

Figure 1 Overview of the 5-lipoxygenase pathway.

volved in the formation of lipoxins, trihydroxylated compounds containing a conjugated tetraene moiety, which constitute the most recent family of potent lipid mediators derived from arachidonic acid (7).

I. Leukotrienes A_4 and B_4

The first evidence for the presence of the 5-lipoxygenase pathway was the discovery of 5-HETE in rabbit PMNL (2). Further studies revealed the production of a more polar compound, structurally identified as 5(S),12(R)-dihydroxy-6,14-*cis*-8,10-*trans*-eicosatetraenoic acid (8). In addition, two epimeric 5(S),12-dihydroxy acids and small amounts of two diastereoisomeric 5,6-dihydroxy acids were isolated (9). Studies with $^{18}O_2$ gas and $H_2{}^{18}O$ demonstrated that the hydroxyl groups at C5 and C6/C12 originated from molecular oxygen and water, respectively. These results led to the postulation of an epoxide intermediate in the biosynthesis of these dihydroxy acids. Trapping experiments with ethanol or methanol, yielding 12-O-alkyl-derivatives of the 5,12-dihydroxy acids, confirmed this hypothesis (10). Nonenzymatic hydrolysis of the epoxide afforded two pairs of epimeric 5,12- and 5,6-dihydroxy acids, whereas an enzyme activity, today known as LTA_4 hydrolase, catalyzed the hydrolysis into the third isomer of 5,12-dihydroxy acid. Due to their cellular origin and typical conjugated triene chromophore with a triplet peak in UV spectroscopy, the epoxide intermediate [5(S)-*trans*-5,6-oxido-7,9-*trans*-11,14-*cis*-eicosatetraenoic acid] and its enzymatic hydrolysis product were named leukotrienes A_4 and B_4 (LTA_4 and LTB_4), respectively, where the subscript denotes the number of double bonds in the molecule (11). The proof for the existence and absolute structure of LTA_4 was obtained by isolation of intact epoxide from human polymorphonuclear leukocytes and by conversion of chemically synthesized material with known stereochemistry into LTB_4 (12,13).

The biosynthesis of LTA_4 is initiated by stereospecific abstraction of hydrogen at C7 of arachidonic acid and dioxygenation at C5 leading to 5(S)-HPETE. The reaction sequence proceeds from 5(S)-HPETE by a second stereospecific removal of the pro-R hydrogen at C10 (14,15) followed by radical migration and epoxide formation. The enzyme activities catalyzing the formation of the hydroperoxide and its subsequent dehydration into the epoxide moiety of LTA_4, respectively, were shown to reside in one single protein, namely, 5-lipoxygenase (16–20). For full activity, 5-lipoxygenase requires Ca^{2+}, ATP, and arachidonate hydroperoxides, as well as several soluble and membrane-bound factors (21–23). In this context it should be noted that formation of LTA_4 from 5-HPETE may occur nonenzymatically in the presence of various hemeproteins such as hemoglobin and cytochromes (24).

II. Leukotrienes C_4, D_4, and E_4 (Cysteinyl Leukotrienes)

In 1953, Brocklehurst demonstrated that the anaphylactic guinea pig lung released a factor distinct from histamine or other contractile agents and introduced the term "slow-reacting substance of anaphylaxis" (SRS-A), referring to its immunological origin, in analogy with earlier work by Feldberg and Kellaway. Lung fragments of human asthmatics were shown to produce this biologically potent entity (25), and a role for SRS as a mediator in the pathophysiology of asthma and other immediate hypersensitivity reactions was proposed.

The chemical nature of SRS was intriguing and the subsequent structural elucidation proved to be complicated. That arylsulfatases were found to inactivate SRS, whereas thiols stimulated its formation, suggested the presence of sulfur in the molecule (26,27). A biosynthetic link to fatty acid metabolism was suggested when incorporation of arachidonic acid in the bioactive material was demonstrated (28). Release of SRS from human polymorphonuclear leukocytes could be provoked by the ionophore A23187 (29,30), and pharmacological evidence indicated the involvement of a lipoxygenase reaction in its formation (31). In 1979, the first structure of an SRS, isolated from mouse mastocytoma cells, was announced by Murphy and coworkers. The material was identified as 5(S)-hydroxy-7,9-*trans*-11,14-*cis*-eicosatetraenoic acid with a cysteine-containing moiety in thioether linkage at C6. The compound was named leukotriene C_4 (LTC_4), and subsequent work revealed that the substituent at C6 was the common tripeptide glutathione (32). The absolute structure of LTC_4 was deduced from comparison with material obtained by total organic synthesis (33), and the precursor role of LTA_4 was established by trapping of intact epoxide from SRS-producing cells (rat basophilic leukemia cells and mouse mastocytoma cells) and by conversion of synthetic LTA_4 into LTC_4 in similar cell systems (34). The enzyme responsible for the addition of glutathione to the epoxide function of LTA_4 is a microsomal enzyme, referred to as LTC_4 synthase. It is specific for the reaction and distinct from other forms of soluble or membrane-bound glutathione S-transferases (35–37).

Glutamic acid and glycine may be successively cleaved off the peptide moiety of LTC_4 by γ-glutamyl transpeptidase and dipeptidase to yield leukotrienes D_4 and E_4 (LTD_4 and LTE_4), respectively (38–43). Leukotrienes C_4, D_4, and E_4 have similar biological properties, and different preparations of SRS are comprised of varying proportions of the respective leukotriene depending upon the source and experimental conditions. The earlier distinction between SRS and SRS-A has become obsolete since leukotriene formation is elicited by both immunological and nonimmunological stimuli.

III. Enzymology and Molecular Biology

Since the early discoveries and structural characterization of metabolites in the 5-lipoxygenase pathway, the further elucidation of the corresponding enzymology, cell and molecular biology, have developed very quickly. Although each of the enzymes involved in leukotriene biosynthesis is discussed by other authors of this volume, a few points may be worth mentioning. For instance, a major breakthrough was achieved more than a decade ago when 5-lipoxygenase was purified from human polymorphonuclear leukocytes and characterized (21). Soon thereafter, a cDNA encoding human 5-lipoxygenase was isolated and sequenced, which in turn made it possible to isolate the human gene and characterize its promoter (44,45).

An 18 kDa microsomal protein termed FLAP (five lipoxygenase activating protein) was found to be required for cellular leukotriene biosynthesis and the corresponding cDNA and gene was characterized (46,47). Unexpectedly, this protein was found to be located at the nuclear membrane, and recent work has

Table 1 Molecular Properties of the 5-Lipoxygenase Pathway[a]

Protein	Protein size (no. of amino acids)[b]	Prosthetic group[c]	Gene size (kb)	Exon no.	Putative *cis*-elements of promoter regions	Chromosomal location
5-Lipoxygenase	673	Fe	>82	14	Sp1, AP-2, NF-kB	10
LTA_4 hydrolase	610	Zn	>35	19	XRE, AP-2	12
LTC_4 synthase	149	—	2.5	5	Sp1, AP-1, AP-2	5
FLAP	160	—	>31	5	TATA, AP-2, GRE	13
BLT receptor	351	—	—	—	—	14
$CysLT_1$/$CysLT_2$ receptor	—	—	—	—	—	—

[a]Data refers to human proteins.
[b]Initial methionine excluded.
[c]1 mol metal per mol protein.
Source: Refs. 49, 55–60.

revealed that upon cell activation, 5-lipoxygenase will translocate to the same compartment (48). Thus, essentially all components of the 5-lipoxygenase pathway, except LTA_4 hydrolase, reside at the nuclear membrane, which in turn suggests that metabolites or enzymes of this pathway may have intranuclear functions yet to be identified.

Another intriguing finding was that LTA_4 hydrolase, which catalyzes the committed step in the biosynthesis of LTB_4, is a zinc metalloenzyme with a previously unknown peptide-cleaving activity (49–51). Although several synthetic peptides are hydrolyzed by the enzyme, the endogenous substrate(s) remain to be identified. Considering the high levels of enzyme in epithelial cells of the intestine and respiratory tract, the peptidase activity of LTA_4 hydrolase may well play a role in an early host-defense reaction.

For a long time, the notoriously unstable LTC_4 synthase escaped purification and characterization and was not successfully isolated and cloned until very recently (52,53). This microsomal enzyme turned out to be related to FLAP, and together with a newly discovered microsomal GSH transferase that displays LTC_4 synthase activity, they can be regarded as a new family of enzymes/proteins (54). The precise role of each of these proteins in leukotriene biosynthesis remains to be delineated.

If the effector cells and the molecules that transduce the biological responses are included in the 5-lipoxygenase pathway, one may note that very little is still known about the receptors for LTB_4 and the cysteinyl leukotrienes. It seems, however, as if LTB_4 may be a ligand for the nuclear receptor PPARα, in line with a nuclear function for this metabolite. In addition, a cDNA encoding a G-protein coupled cell-surface receptor for LTB_4 was recently isolated and ligand-mediated activation could elicit chemotaxis (55). Some molecular aspects of the 5-lipoxygenase pathway are summarized in Table 1.

Acknowledgments

This work was financially supported by The Swedish Medical Research Council (O3X-217, O3X-10350) and The European Union (BMH4-CT960229).

References

1. Bailey DM, Chakrin LW. Arachidonate lipoxygenase. Ann Rep Med Chem 1981; 16:213–227.
2. Borgeat P, Hamberg M, Samuelsson B. Transformation of arachidonic acid and homo-γ-linolenic acid by rabbit polymorphonuclear leukocytes. Monohydroxy acids from novel lipoxygenases. J Biol Chem 1976; 251:7816–7820 (published erratum in J Biol Chem 1977; 252:8772).

3. Borgeat P, Samuelsson B. Arachidonic acid metabolism in polymorphonuclear leukocytes: unstable intermediate in formation of dihydroxy acids. Proc Natl Acad Sci USA 1979; 76:3213–3217.
4. Lindgren J-Å, Hansson G, Samuelsson B. Formation of novel hydroxylated eicosatetraenoic acids in preparations of human polymorphonuclear leukocytes. FEBS Lett 1981; 128:329–335.
5. Borgeat P, Picard S, Vallerand P, Sirois P. Transformation of arachidonic acid in leukocytes. Isolation and structural analysis of a novel dihydroxy derivative. Prostaglandins Med 1981; 6:557–570.
6. Maas RL, Turk J, Oates JA, Brash AR. Formation of a novel dihydroxy acid from arachidonic acid by lipoxygenase-catalyzed double oxygenation in rat mononuclear cells and human leukocytes. J Biol Chem 1982; 257:7056–7067.
7. Serhan CN. Lipoxins: Eicosanoids carrying intra- and intercellular messages. J Bioenerg Biomembr 1991; 23:105–122.
8. Borgeat P, Samuelsson B. Transformation of arachidonic acid by rabbit polymorphonuclear leukocytes. Formation of a novel dihydroxyeicosatetraenoic acid. J Biol Chem 1979; 254:2643–2646.
9. Borgeat P, Samuelsson B. Metabolism of arachidonic acid in polymorphonuclear leukocytes. Structural analysis of novel hydroxylated compounds. J Biol Chem 1979; 254:7865–7869.
10. Borgeat P, Samuelsson B. Arachidonic acid metabolism in polymorphonuclear leukocytes: effects of ionophore A23187. Proc Natl Acad Sci USA 1979; 76:2148–2152.
11. Samuelsson B, Borgeat P, Hammarström S, Murphy RC. Introduction of a nomenclature: leukotrienes. Prostaglandins 1979; 17:785–787.
12. Rådmark O, Malmsten C, Samuelsson B, Goto G, Marfat A, Corey EJ. Leukotriene A: isolation from human polymorphonuclear leukocytes. J Biol Chem 1980; 255: 11828–11831.
13. Rådmark O, Malmsten C, Samuelsson B, et al. Leukotriene A: stereochemistry and enzymatic conversion to leukotriene B. Biochem Biophys Res Commun 1980; 92: 954–961.
14. Panossian A, Hamberg M, Samuelsson B. On the mechanism of biosynthesis of leukotrienes and related compounds. FEBS Lett 1982; 150:511–513.
15. Maas RL, Ingram CD, Taber DF, Oates JA, Brash AR. Stereospecific removal of the D_R hydrogen atom at the 10-carbon of arachidonic acid in the biosynthesis of leukotriene A_4 by human leukocytes. J Biol Chem 1982; 257:13515–13519.
16. Shimizu T, Rådmark O, Samuelsson B. Enzyme with dual lipoxygenase activities catalyzes leukotriene A_4 synthesis from arachidonic acid. Proc Natl Acad Sci USA 1984; 81:689–693.
17. Shimizu T, Izumi T, Seyama Y, Tadokoro K, Rådmark O, Samuelsson B. Characterization of leukotriene A_4 synthase from murine mast cells: evidence for its identity to arachidonate 5-lipoxygenase. Proc Natl Acad Sci USA 1986; 83:4175–4179.
18. Rouzer CA, Matsumoto T, Samuelsson B. Single protein from human leukocytes possesses 5-lipoxygenase and leukotriene A_4 synthase activities. Proc Natl Acad Sci USA 1986; 83:857–861.

19. Ueda N, Kaneko S, Yoshimoto T, Yamamoto S. Purification of arachidonate 5-lipoxygenase from porcine leukocytes and its reactivity with hydroperoxyeicosatetraenoic acids. J Biol Chem 1986; 261:7982–7988.
20. Hogaboom GK, Cook M, Newton JF, et al. Purification, characterization, and structural properties of a single protein from rat basophilic leukemia (RBL-1) cells possessing 5-lipoxygenase and leukotriene A_4 synthetase activities. Mol Pharmacol 1986; 30:510–519.
21. Rouzer CA, Samuelsson B. On the nature of the 5-lipoxygenase reaction in human leukocytes: enzyme purification and requirement for multiple stimulatory factors. Proc Natl Acad Sci USA 1985; 82:6040–6044.
22. Rouzer CA, Samuelsson B. The importance of hydroperoxide activation for the detection and assay of mammalian 5-lipoxygenase. FEBS Lett 1986; 204:293–296.
23. Rouzer CA, Shimizu T, Samuelsson B. On the nature of the 5-lipoxygenase reaction in human leukocytes: characterization of a membrane-associated stimulatory factor. Proc Natl Acad Sci USA 1985; 82:7505–7509.
24. Rådmark O, Shimizu T, Fitzpatrick F, Samuelsson B. Hemoprotein catalysis of leukotriene formation. Biochim Biophys Acta 1984; 792:324–329.
25. Brocklehurst WE. The release of histamine and formation of a slow-reacting substance (SRS-A) during anaphylactic shock. J Physiol 1960; 151:416–435.
26. Orange RP, Murphy RC, Austen KF. Inactivation of slow reacting substance of anaphylaxis (SRS-A) by arylsulfatases. J Immunol 1974; 113:316.
27. Orange RP, Chang P-L. The effects of thiols on immunologic release of slow reacting substance of anaphylaxis. J Immunol 1975; 115:1072–1077.
28. Jakschik BA, Falkenhein S, Parker CW. Precursor role of arachidonic acid in release of slow reacting substance from rat basophilic leukemia cells. Proc Natl Acad Sci USA 1977; 74:4577–81.
29. Bach MK, Brashler JR. In vivo and in vitro production of slow reacting substance in the rat upon treatment with calcium ionophores. J Immunol 1974; 113:2040–2044.
30. Conroy MC, Orange RP, Lichtenstein LM. Release of slow-reacting substance of anaphylaxis (SRS-A) from human leukocytes by the calcium ionophore A23187. J Immunol 1976; 116:1677.
31. Piper PJ, Tippins JR, Morris HR, Taylor GW. Arachidonic acid metabolism and SRS-A. Agents Actions 1979(suppl); 6:37–48.
32. Hammarström S, Murphy RC, Samuelsson B, Clark DA, Mioskowski C, Corey EJ. Structure of leukotriene C: identification of the amino acid part. Biochem Biophys Res Commun 1979; 91:1266–1272.
33. Hammarström S, Samuelsson B, Clark DA, et al. Stereochemistry of leukotriene Cl. Biochem Biophys Res Commun 1980; 92:946–953.
34. Rådmark O, Malmsten C, Samuelsson B. Leukotriene A_4: enzymatic conversion to leukotriene C_4. Biochem Biophys Res Commun 1980; 96:1679–1687.
35. Bach MK, Brashler JR, Hammarström S, Samuelsson B. Identification of a component of rat mononuclear cell SRS as leukotriene D. Biochem. Biophys Res Commun 1980; 93:1121–1126.
36. Mannervik B, Jensson H, Ålin P, Örning L, Hammarström S. Transformation of

leukotriene A_4 methyl ester to leukotriene C_4 monomethyl ester by cytosolic rat glutathione tranferases. FEBS Lett 1984; 174:289–293.
37. Bach MK, Brashler JR. A comparison of the leukotriene synthesizing ability of subfractions of rat liver glutathione S-transferases. Prostaglandins Leuk Med 1985; 17: 125–136.
38. Örning L, Hammarström S, Samuelsson B. Leukotriene D: a slow reacting substance from rat basophilic leukemia cells. Proc Natl Acad Sci USA 1980; 77:2014–2017.
39. Morris HR, Taylor GW, Piper PJ, Samhoun MN, Tippins JR. Slow reacting substances (SRSs): the structure identification of SRSs from rat basophilic leukaemia (RBL-1) cells. Prostaglandins 1980; 19:185–201.
40. Parker CW, Falkenhein SF, Huber MM. Sequential conversion of the glutathionyl side chain of slow reacting substance (SRS) to cysteinyl-glycine and cysteine in rat basophilic leukemia cells stimulated with A-23187. Prostaglandins 1980; 20:863–886.
41. Houglum J, Pai J-K, Atrache V, Sok D-E, Sih CJ. Identification of the slow reacting substances from cat paws. Proc Natl Acad Sci USA 1980; 77:5688–92.
42. Lewis RA, Drazen JM, Austen KF, Clark DA, Corey EJ. Identification of the C(6)-*S*-conjugate of leukotriene A with cysteine as a naturally occurring slow reacting substance of anaphylaxis (SRS-A). Importance of the 11-*cis*-geometry for biological activity. Biochem Biophys Res Commun 1980; 96:271–277.
43. Bernström K, Hammarström S. Metabolism of leukotriene D by porcine kidney. J Biol Chem 1981; 256:9579–9582.
44. Matsumoto T, Funk CD, Rådmark O, Höög J-O, Jörnvall H, Samuelsson B. Molecular cloning and amino acid sequence of human 5-lipoxygenase. Proc Natl Acad Sci USA 1988; 85:26–30 (published erratum in Proc Natl Acad Sci USA 85:3406).
45. Dixon RAF, Jones RE, Diehl RE, Bennett CD, Kargman S, Rouzer CA. Cloning of the cDNA for human 5-lipoxygenase. Proc Natl Acad Sci USA 1988; 85:416–420.
46. Miller DK, Gillard JW, Vickers PJ, et al. Identification and isolation of a membrane protein necessary for leukotriene production. Nature 1990; 343:278–281.
47. Dixon RAF, Diehl RE, Opas E, et al. Requirement of a 5-lipoxygenase-activating protein for leukotriene synthesis. Nature 1990; 343:282–284.
48. Woods JW, Evans JF, Ethier D, et al. 5-lipoxygenase and 5-lipoxygenase activating protein are localized in the nuclear envelope of activated human leukocytes. J Exp Med 1993; 178:1935–1946.
49. Haeggström JZ, Wetterholm A, Shapiro R, Vallee BL, Samuelsson B. Leukotriene A_4 hydrolase: a zinc metalloenzyme. Biochem Biophys Res Commun 1990; 172: 965–970.
50. Haeggström JZ, Wetterholm A, Vallee BL, Samuelsson B. Leukotriene A_4 hydrolase: an epoxide hydrolase with peptidase activity. Biochem Biophys Res Commun 1990; 173:431–437.
51. Minami M, Ohishi N, Mutoh H, et al. Leukotriene A_4 hydrolase is a zinc-containing aminopeptidase. Biochem Biophys Res Commun 1990; 173:620–626.
52. Nicholson DW, Klemba MW, Rasper DM, Metters KM, Zamboni RJ, Ford-Hutchinson AW. Purification of human leukotriene C_4 synthase from dimethylsulfoxide-differentiated U937 cells. Eur J Biochem 1992; 209:725–734.
53. Lam BK, Penrose JF, Freeman GJ, Austen KF. Expression cloning of a cDNA for

human leukotriene C_4 synthase, an integral membrane protein conjugating reduced glutathione to leukotriene A_4. Proc Natl Acad Sci USA 1994; 91:7663–7.

54. Jakobsson PJ, Mancini JA, Fordhutchinson AW. Identification and characterization of a novel human microsomal glutathione S-transferase with leukotriene C_4 synthase activity and significant sequence identity to 5-lipoxygenase-activating protein and leukotriene C_4 synthase. J Biol Chem 1996; 271:22203–22210.
55. Yokomizo T, Izumi T, Chang K, Takuwa Y, Shimizu T. A G-protein-coupled receptor for leukotriene B_4 that mediates chemotaxis. Nature 1997; 387:620–624.
56. Funk CD. Molecular biology in the eicosanoid field (review). Prog Nucl Acid Res Mol Biol 1993; 45:67–98.
57. Ford-Hutchinson AW, Gresser M, Young RN. 5-Lipoxygenase (review). Annu Rev Biochem 1994; 63:383–417.
58. Mancini JA, Evans JF. Cloning and characterization of the human leukotriene A_4 hydrolase gene. Eur J Biochem 1995; 231:65–71.
59. Penrose JF, Spector J, Baldasaro M, et al. Molecular cloning of the gene for human leukotriene C_4 synthase—organization, nucleotide sequence, and chromosomal localization to 5q35. J Biol Chem 1996; 271:11356–11361.
60. Owman C, Nilsson C, Lolait, SJ. Cloning of cDNA encoding a putative chemoattractant receptor. Genomics 1996; 37:187–194.

2

5-Lipoxygenase and 5-Lipoxygenase–Activating Protein

JILLY F. EVANS

Merck Frosst Canada, Inc.
Pointe-Claire-Dorval, Quebec, Canada

I. Introduction

The first committed step in the biological production of leukotrienes is the reaction catalyzed by the 78 kDa enzyme 5-lipoxygenase (5-LO), which results in the formation of the unstable epoxide leukotriene A_4 (LTA_4). LTA_4 is the precursor for the leukocyte activator leukotriene B_4 and for the bronchoconstrictive and proinflammatory cysteinyl leukotrienes, leukotriene C_4, D_4, and E_4. In cells, an essential activator of the 5-LO reaction is the 18 kDa membrane-bound protein, 5-lipoxygenase–activating protein (FLAP). This chapter begins with a discussion of the mechanism and expression of 5-LO followed by the genetic knockout and chemical inhibition of 5-LO. The subsequent section discusses the discovery, expression, and inhibition of FLAP.

A number of excellent papers have covered, in more detail than is possible here, the historical aspects of the discovery of leukotrienes and lipoxygenase catalysis in general (1–3). Although this chapter is divided into sections that individually discuss 5-LO and FLAP, it is clear that the cellular synthesis of (LTA_4) requires their concerted action. A simplified cellular view of leukotriene synthesis, leukotriene receptor activation, and 5-LO and FLAP localization is shown in Figure 1.

II. 5-Lipoxygenase

A. Enzyme Catalytic Reactions

5-LO is a member of the lipoxygenase family of enzymes, which are widely distributed in the plant and animal kingdoms and catalyze the oxidative metabo-

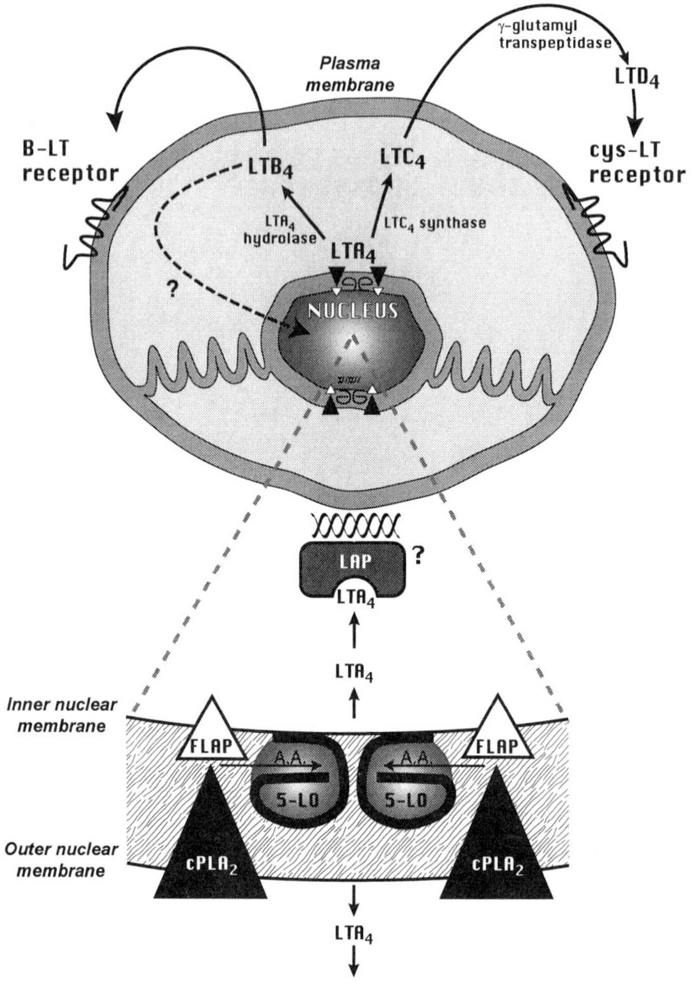

Figure 1 Cellular view of leukotriene synthesis and leukotriene receptor activation. Activation of a leukocyte by invading bacteria or other stimuli causes an increase in intracellular calcium. 5-Lipoxygenase (5-LO) and cytosolic PLA_2 ($cPLA_2$) move to the nuclear membrane. $cPLA_2$ cleaves arachidonic acid (AA) from membrane phospholipids and 5-lipoxygenase–activating protein (FLAP) holds the 5-LO in an activated conformation and selectively channels the fatty acid to its active site. The two-step oxygenation and dehydration reactions of 5-LO produce LTA_4, which can either exit the cell or be converted in the cell to LTB_4 or LTC_4 (by LTA_4 hydrolase or LTC_4 synthase, respectively) or enter the nucleus. In the nucleus, LTA_4 may interact with a putative leukotriene-activated protein (LAP) enhancing or repressing transcription of specific genes. LTB_4 or LTC_4, LTD_4 or LTE_4 can interact with specific G-protein coupled receptors either on the same cell or on other cells to signal-specific activation processes.

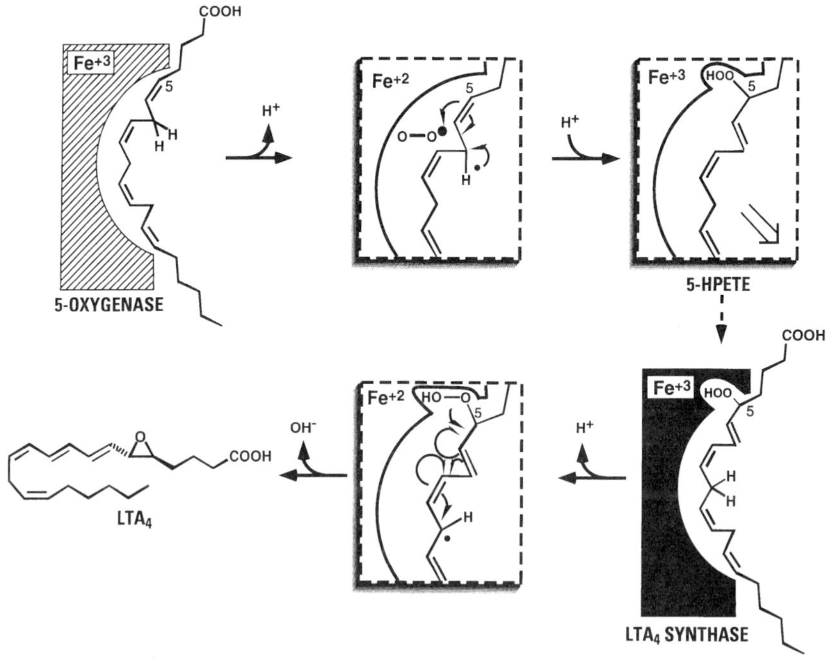

Figure 2 Concerted 5-oxygenase and LTA_4 synthase reactions of 5-lipoxygenase.

lism of unsaturated fatty acids. All lipoxygenases catalyze the addition of molecular oxygen to a 1-4-*cis,cis*-pentadiene moiety to produce a 1-hydroperoxy-2,4-*trans,cis* pentadiene unit (2). In animal cells the predominant substrate for the lipoxygenases is arachidonic acid (C20:4), and the lipoxygenases are classified according to the position at which the enzyme oxidizes arachidonic acid (2). The most common lipoxygenases are the 5, 12, and 15-lipoxygenases (5-LO, 12-LO, and 15-LO). 5-LO catalyzes the oxygenation of arachidonic acid at C5 to produce 5(*S*)-hydroperoxy-6,8,11,14(E,Z,Z,Z)-eicosatetraenoic acid (5-HPETE), and also the dehydration of this hydroperoxide intermediate to produce the epoxide, 5(*S*),6(*S*),-oxido-7,9,11,15(E,E,Z,Z)-eicosatetraenoic acid or LTA_4. All fatty acid substrates of 5-LO contain one or more pentadiene moieties and can be partially oxidized fatty acids as in the cases of 12- or 15-HPETE. The latter substrate can be converted to the conjugated tetraene compound lipoxin A by the action of 5-LO (4). The 5-oxygenase activity of 5-LO removes the pro S hydrogen atom from C7 of arachidonic acid by a redox mechanism, involving reduction of the nonheme iron of the enzyme, forming a radical intermediate (Fig. 2). The iron is then reoxidized and oxygen reacts with the arachidonic acid radical complex to form the hydroperoxide intermediate, 5-HPETE (Fig. 2). The LTA_4 synthase activity of 5-LO then catalyzes the second stereospecific removal of a hydrogen atom, this time from the pro R hydrogen at C10, and through this second redox cycle dehydrates 5-HPETE to LTA_4 (Fig. 2). The inactive 5-LO is in the ferrous state and must be oxidized to the ferric state for oxygenation of arachidonic acid (3). The addition of glutathione peroxidase and glutathione can completely inhibit 5-LO and 15-LO activities in human leukocyte homogenates (5). Conditions that reduce glutathione concentrations in intact human leukocytes or B cells result in increased leukotriene synthesis (6,7). Therefore, in cells, 5-LO appears to be active in the oxidized ferric state.

Detailed kinetic studies with 5-LO are difficult to interpret because of the presence of activity lags and rapid turnover inactivation with half-times of less than 1 minute with the fully activated enzyme (3). The mechanism of the turnover-dependent inactivation is not known, but the half-times for this inactivation are longer in the presence of low Ca^{2+} concentrations (8) and some classes of non–redox inhibitors (9,10). Redox inhibitors that act as alternate substrates do not increase the half-times for turnover-dependent inactivation (9). Inactivation of 5-LO in phospholipid vesicles is dependent on the structure of the unsaturated fatty acid substrate for the reaction, on the concentration of oxygen, and on a turnover-independent oxidation at the active site leading to the sequential loss of the oxygenase and pseudoperoxidase activities of the enzyme (10). The irreversible inactivation of 5-LO that occurs in aerobic buffers has been shown to be due mainly to hydrogen peroxide, since the inactivation rate can be reduced by addition of catalase (8).

Under anaerobic conditions human 5-LO has also been shown to catalyze the arachidonate-dependent decomposition of fatty acid hydroperoxides, such as 13-HPODE (11). This activity is referred to as a pseudoperoxidase activity, since the reaction involves a one-electron reduction of the fatty acid hydroperoxide, rather than a two-electron reduction as with peroxidases. 5-LO inhibitors that are reducing agents inhibit the enzyme due to their activity as pseudoperoxidase agents and may produce reactive species which covalently couple to proteins (12).

Prior to the complete purification of 5-LO, several factors had been shown to be activators of the oxygenase and LTA_4 synthase activities of the enzyme. These factors included ATP, Ca^{2+}, phosphatidylcholine, and lipids and leukocyte factors (2,13).

B. Protein Purification and Cloning of cDNA

5-LO has been purified to homogeneity from human (14,15), pig (16), rat (17), and guinea pig (18) leukocytes. The human 5-LO cDNA was cloned at about the same time by several groups (19,20). The complete cDNA sequence from the

DMSO-differentiated HL-60 library and the placenta-derived library were identical, encoding a mature protein of 674 amino acids (including the initiator methionine) with a molecular weight of about 78,000 (19,20). There was no defined ATP binding motif in the cDNA sequence and no obvious Ca^{2+}-binding domains. However, human 5-LO is nearly identical to rat 5-LO (21) and significantly related to other lipoxygenases, such as 12-LO, 15-LO (approximately 40% identity), and less so to plant lipoxygenases such as soybean lipoxygenase isozymes 1, 2, and 3 and pea seed lipoxygenase (26–28% identity) (22). Another significant homology region to other proteins is a short sequence in lipoprotein and hepatic lipases within the interface binding domain. In all the lipoxygenase sequences there is a central core motif His-X4-His-X4-His-X17-His-X8-His that is highly conserved at the putative iron-binding site (22). Mutagenesis studies with human 5-LO have shown that His-368 and His-373 are essential for enzyme activity and may be required for coordination of the iron atom (23–25). Human 5-LO has been expressed in osteosarcoma cells, COS-M6 cells, baculovirus-infected Sf9 insect cells, yeast, and *Escherichia coli* (26–30). The recombinant enzyme appears to be equivalent to the human leukocyte enzyme in all these systems, maintaining the dual oxygenase and LTA_4 synthase activities and dependence on Ca^{2+} and ATP for activity. Recombinant human 5-LO purified from baculovirus-infected Sf9 insect cells has shown 1.1 mole of iron per mole of enzyme, which is tightly bound and released after exposure of the enzyme to oxygen (31). The specific activity of purified recombinant human 5-LO has been shown to correlate linearly with the iron to protein stoichiometry (11,31). EPR studies showed that one mole of fatty acid hydroperoxide per mole of Fe^{2+} in the native enzyme could convert all Fe^{2+} to Fe^{3+}. The ferric ion could be completely reduced to the ferrous ion by one mole equivalent of an *N*-hydroxyurea (32). Microsomal and cytosolic factors are not required for maximal enzyme activity as previously reported, but rather appear to enhance the stability of the enzyme in dilute concentrations (28).

A number of consensus phosphorylation sequences have been found in the 5-LO sequence, and tyrosine phosphorylated 5-LO can be found in DNA associated precipitates from HL-60 cells following stimulation with calcium ionophore (33). In addition, 5-LO contains a proline-rich motif that may interact with the Src homology 3 (SH3) domain of Grb-2 as well as cytoskeletal proteins (34). A model has been proposed whereby interaction of unactivated cytosolic 5-LO with the SH3 domain of a protein that contained an SH2 domain could result in a complex of 5-LO and the SH3:SH2 domain protein attached to phosphorylated tyrosine residues of cytoskeletal units (33).

C. Expression, Gene Structure, and Gene Knockout

5-LO expression at both the mRNA and protein level is restricted to a specific subset of myeloid cells, including neutrophils, granulocytes, monocytes/macrophages, mast cells, eosinophils, and B lymphocytes (35). However, no 5-LO mRNA or protein is detected in T cells, erythrocytes, platelets, or endothelial cells (35). The induction of 5-LO has been shown in a number of myeloid cell lines with various stimuli including dimethylsulfoxide (DMSO) and cytokines such as granulocyte macrophage colony stimulating factor (GMCSF) (36,37). One case of 5-LO expression in a nonmyeloid cell is in the porcine pancreatic acinar cell (38). The specific role of leukotrienes in this cell type is not clear.

The gene for human 5-LO has been isolated from bacteriophage genomic libraries and a genomic cosmid library (39). The gene spans more than 82 kilobases and consists of 14 exons, varying in size from 82 to 613 base pairs. The exact size of the gene is unclear since there was a gap in the very large (>26 kilobase) third intron. The 5-LO gene is located on human chromosome 10. All lipoxygenase genes appear to be organized in the same exon/intron format but the 5-LO gene is much larger (22). It is interesting to speculate that the larger intron size in the 5-LO gene may reflect evolutionary sophistication in the transcriptional control of the gene. A major transcription initiation site in leukocytes was mapped 65 base pairs upstream of the ATG initiation codon. The putative promoter region contains multiple GC boxes within a (G + C)-rich region, which have been shown to be essential for transcription but no TATA or CCAAT sequences upstream of the initiation site (39). In addition, myeloid-derived HL-60 nuclear extracts contained specific nuclear factors binding to 5-lipoxygenase promoter DNA, which could not be detected in HeLa cell nuclear extracts (40). It has been reported that there are human polymorphisms in the number of GGGCGG repeat units in the 5-LO promoter, and these are being mapped to determine if there is a correlation with any phenotype (J. Drazen, unpublished data).

Two groups have reported the genetic knockout of the 5-LO gene (41,42). 5-LO–deficient mice are unable to produce leukotrienes but develop normally and are healthy. Although these mice show similar endotoxin-induced mortality to wild-type mice, the 5-LO knockouts are resistant to platelet-activating factor-induced death. In addition, 5-LO knockout mice showed a normal response to phorbol ester-induced ear edema but demonstrated less arachidonic acid-induced ear edema (42). Peritoneal macrophages from 5-LO knockout mice showed enhanced production of cyclooxygenase metabolites. Arachidonic-induced ear edema in the 5-LO knockout mice could be lowered by the cyclooxygenase inhibitor Indomethacin to a greater extent than in controls. 5-LO knockout mice have also been shown to exhibit lower hyperreactivity to antigen challenge, to show reduced eosinophil accumulation in bronchial lavage fluids and less ovalbumin specific lgG and lgE antibodies in ovalbumin sensitized animals after antigen challenge (43).

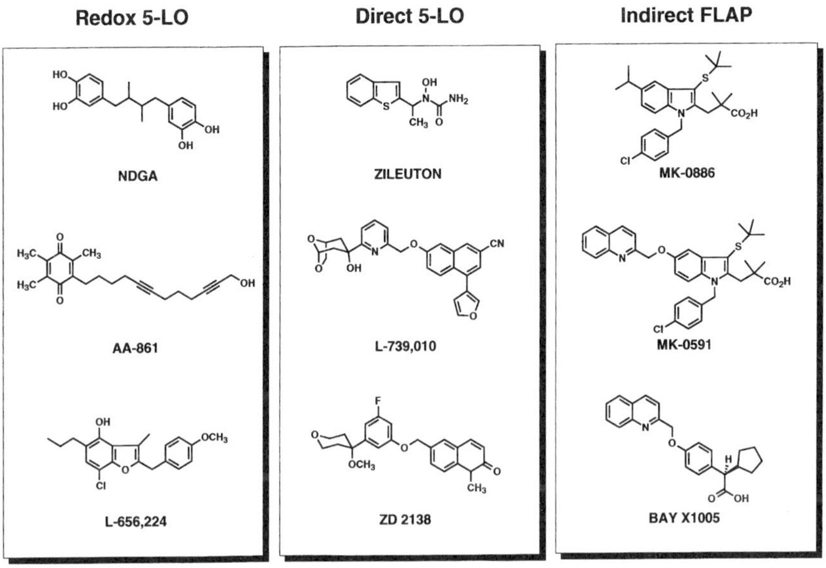

Figure 3 Inhibitors of leukotriene synthesis. The redox 5-LO inhibitors, nordihydroguaiaretic acid (NDGA), AA-861, and L-656,224 maintain the enzyme in the ferrous state unable to catalyze oxygenation of the substrate. Direct inhibitors of 5-LO work either through iron chelation, such as zileuton, or through competition with substrate, such as L-739,010 and ZD 2138. Indirect inhibitors of leukotriene synthesis act by binding to FLAP. Examples of indirect inhibitors are the Merck compounds MK-886 and MK-591 and the Bayer compound BAY X1005.

D. Enzyme Inhibition

A number of excellent reviews have been written on inhibitors of 5-lipoxygenase (44–46). Many of the inhibitors of 5-LO developed in the 1970s and early 1980s, such as NDGA, AA-861, and L-656,224, had antioxidant properties that maintained the enzyme in the ferrous state and thus prevented catalytic activity (Fig. 3). Scientists at Abbott Laboratories developed a series of *N*-hydroxyureas, including zileuton, whose inhibition of the enzyme involved iron chelation (47, Fig. 3). Zileuton advanced through clinical trials in asthma to FDA approval in 1996 (48). In addition, Abbott developed several more potent *N*-hydroxyurea inhibitors of 5-LO, including A-78773 as backups to zileuton (49). Direct inhibitors of 5-LO that have the characteristics of competitive inhibitors include the Merck Frosst compound L-739,010 and methoxyalkyl thiazoles, such as ICI 211965, and methoxytetrahydropyrans such as ZD 2138 (50–52, Fig. 3). Another type of highly selective inhibitor of 5-LO which does not involve reduction of the nonheme iron are the thiopyrano[2,3,4-*c*,*d*]indoles (53). In contrast to the redox type of inhibitors these compounds do not function as pseudoperoxidase substrates but rather inhibit this activity (54). In addition, these inhibitors slow the turnover-dependent irreversible inactivation of 5-LO and act as reversible dead end inhibitors of the enzyme (3,54). Competition of a thiopyranoindole photoaffinity labeled inhibitor to 5-LO was shown to be correlated to the affinity of 5-LO activity inhibition for thiopyranoindoles, ZD-2138 and zileuton (55). This suggests that these inhibitors all interact with the arachidonic acid binding site of 5-LO (55).

III. 5-Lipoxygenase–Activating Protein

A. Discovery and FLAP Inhibitors

FLAP was discovered as the protein target of two potent classes of leukotriene synthesis inhibitors that were inactive or weakly active as inhibitors of 5-LO and had no effect on other lipoxygenases (56,57). The discovery of FLAP was an interdisciplinary team effort of medicinal chemists, biochemists, and molecular biologists at Merck. One of the indole class of compounds, namely, MK-886, was shown to be a potent leukotriene synthesis inhibitor in a variety of myeloid cells and to inhibit bronchoconstriction in the rat and squirrel monkey (58; Fig. 3). In order for Merck to take this compound into clinical development for anti-asthmatic indications, it was necessary to identify the protein target. The medicinal chemists at Merck Frosst synthesized a radioiodinated azido photoaffinity analog of MK-886, namely, L-669,083, and an MK-886 affinity gel via coupling the carboxyl group to Affigel 10 (56; Fig. 4). An 18 kDa protein was identified in rat and human leukocyte membrane fractions that selectively bound both the radioidinated probe and the MK-886 analog affinity gel (56). MK-886 was subsequently shown to inhibit the translocation of 5-LO to human neutrophil membranes in activated cells (59). Further characterization of the protein that was selectively radioiodinated by the MK-886 photoaffinity probe and bound to the MK-886 affinity gel demonstrated that a second structural class of leukotriene synthesis inhibitors inhibited photoaffinity labeling and selectively eluted the 18 kDa protein from the MK-886 affinity gel (60; Fig. 5). The 18 kDa protein from rat neutrophil CHAPS solubilized membranes was selectively eluted from the affinity column by MK-886 and purified to homogeneity by chromatography on Superose-12 and TSK3000 columns (56). Amino acid sequence information was obtained from the whole protein and from cyanogen bromide and tryptic cleavage fragments (56).

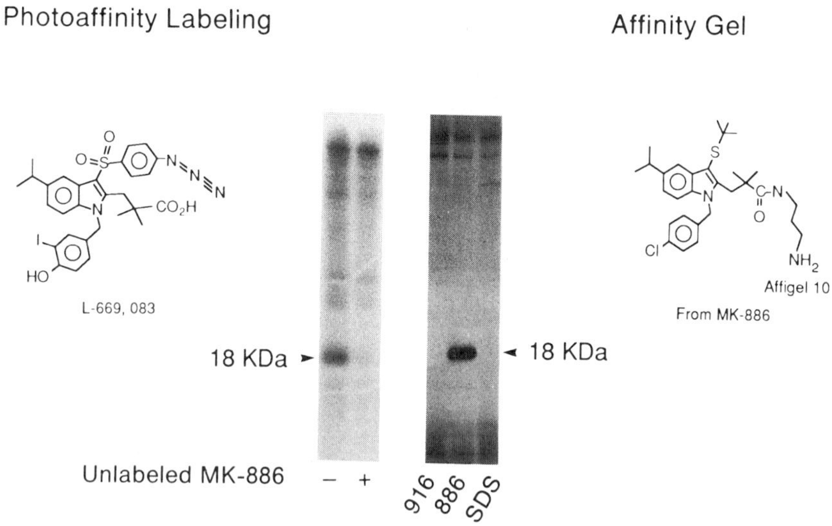

Figure 4 Identification of 5-lipoxygenase–activating protein (FLAP) as an 18 kDa protein in neutrophil membranes by photoaffinity labeling and affinity gel chromatography. A photoaffinity analog [^{125}I]-L-669,083, of the MK-886 class of leukotriene synthesis inhibitors selectively bound to an 18 kDa protein in CHAPS-solubilized rat neutrophil membranes as identified by autoradiography of SDS-polyacrylamide gel separated proteins. This binding could be prevented by preincubation with 1 μM MK-886. The 18 kDa protein from CHAPS-solubilized rat neutrophil membranes also bound selectively to an MK-886 affinity gel (as shown by silver-stained gel on the right). The protein was unable to be eluted by an inactive analog L-583,916, and no protein remained after MK-886 elution as shown by SDS lane.

B. Cloning of cDNA, Mutants, and Inhibitor Binding Site

Complimentary oligonucleotide probes to the amino acid sequences obtained from the 18 kDa protein purification were used to screen a rat basophilic leukemic cell cDNA library and a cDNA obtained that coded for a unique 161-amino-acid protein (including the initiator methionine) (57). This cDNA was used to screen a DMSO-differentiated HL-60 cDNA library and the corresponding human protein was obtained, which was 92% identical to the rat protein (57). Immunoprecipitation experiments using polyclonal peptide and fusion protein antisera demonstrated that the cloned protein was the same protein that had been selectively labeled with the photoaffinity probe (57). The structure contained three strongly

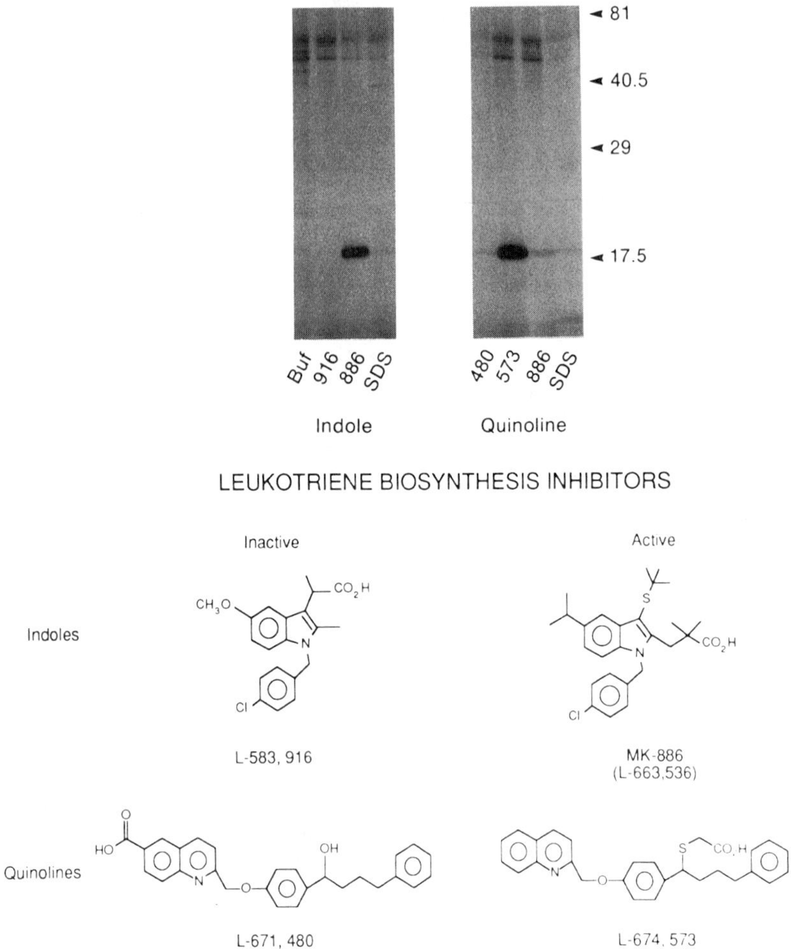

Figure 5 Interaction of FLAP with two different structural classes of leukotriene synthesis inhibitors. CHAPS-solubilized rat neutrophil membrane protein elution profiles (silver-stained) show selective elution of an 18 kDa protein from the MK-886 affinity gel by active indole and quinoline leukotriene synthesis inhibitors, MK-886 and L-674,573, respectively, but not by inactive analogs, L-583,916 and L-671,480, respectively.

hydrophobic segments with two hydrophilic intervening loops (57). In an elegant series of experiments in osteosarcoma cells that do not express 5-LO or FLAP it was shown that transfection of both cDNAs was essential for cellular leukotriene synthesis (57). There were no strong homologies to any other protein in the database in 1990, although an EGF-like domain was observed in the second hydrophilic loop.

In order to assess the potency of FLAP-binding inhibitors, a sensitive FLAP-binding assay was set up using human leukocyte membranes as source of FLAP, and a radioiodinated leukotriene synthesis inhibitor as ligand (61). This assay was used to show an excellent correlation between potency for inhibition of FLAP binding with potency for inhibition of leukotriene synthesis in cells (61). A hybrid class of indole-quinoline leukotriene synthesis inhibitors exemplified by MK-591 were shown to bind with high affinity to FLAP (62,63). The inhibitors' binding site to FLAP was investigated initially by photoaffinity labeling the protein and cleaving specifically at the single tryptophan residue or the two internal methionine residues and immunoprecipitation of the resulting products (64). Inhibitors were shown to bind N-terminal to Trp72 (64). By creation of a series of site-specific and deletion mutants, it was determined that a negative charge associated with the residue Asp62 was critical for inhibitor binding and that mutants in this highly conserved region of the protein (residues 42–61) do not bind indole or quinoline or hybrid inhibitors (65). This acidic residue is in the first hydrophilic loop of FLAP located at the putative interface of the membrane. The exact membrane topology of FLAP has not been elucidated, and although the protein is traditionally represented as having three transmembrane domains, it is entirely possible that one or more transmembrane domains exist with the remaining hydrophobic regions being embedded in one monolayer of the lipid bilayer (as is the case for the hydrophobic domain in the cyclooxygenases) (Fig. 6).

A breakthrough in the understanding of the role of FLAP in cellular leukotriene synthesis came when Mancini et al. demonstrated high affinity binding of an arachidonic acid photoaffinity analog to FLAP (66). This binding was inhibited by MK-886 but not by the indole analog L-685,079, which was relatively inactive as a leukotriene synthesis inhibitor (66). It was shown in studies in Sf9 baculovirus-infected 5-LO and FLAP cells that the presence of FLAP enhanced the two-step oxygenation-dehydration reactions of 5-LO (67). Further insight into the role of FLAP in cells came from studies by Hill et al. that showed accumulation of active membrane-associated 5-LO following ionophore stimulation of human leukocytes in the presence of zileuton (68). In the absence of zileuton, cellular activation and translocation of 5-LO to membrane fractions resulted in a totally inactive enzyme. The accumulation of zileuton-protected active 5-LO could be prevented and reversed by incubation with the FLAP inhibitor MK-886 (68). The membrane-associated 5-LO was two times more efficient in the second step

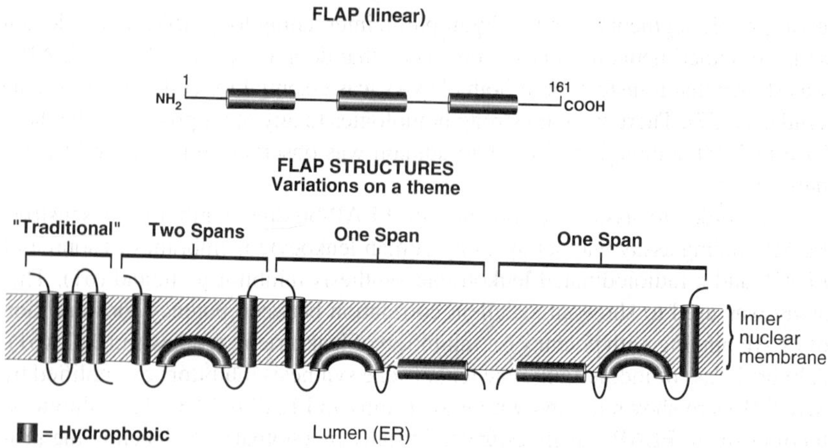

Figure 6 Potential FLAP membrane insertion modes. The three highly hydrophobic regions of FLAP have traditionally been drawn as forming three transmembrane spanning domains. Alternative structural possibilities include a single or two transmembrane spanning domains, with two or one hydrophobic domains, respectively, inserted into one leaflet of the membrane bilayer. The first hydrophilic loop of FLAP in human neutrophils has been localized to the lumenal face of the inner nuclear membrane (89).

dehydration reaction than cytosolic 5-LO, and in contrast to the cytosolic enzyme, the membrane-bound enzyme could oxygenate 12(S)- and 15(S)-HETE to 5(S),12(S)- and 5(S),15(S)-dihydroxyeicosatetraenoic acid, respectively (68). This suggests that in the presence of membrane containing FLAP, 5-LO has a somewhat different conformation and hence different substrate specificity. Another class of 5-LO inhibitors, the thiopyranoindoles, which was able to be modified to also inhibit FLAP and LTC_4 synthase, both promoted the translocation of 5-LO and allowed active 5-LO to be found on membrane fractions of leukocytes after ionophore challenge (69). It was hypothesized that these inhibitors may mimic arachidonic acid and upon binding to 5-LO may induce and stabilize a hydrophobic conformation of the enzyme at the same time binding to FLAP and preventing arachidonic acid transfer to 5-LO (69). The Bayer compound BAY X1005 and other quinoline leukotriene synthesis inhibitors developed at Wyeth-Ayerst were also shown to act as a leukotriene synthesis inhibitor by binding to FLAP (70,71). Kreft et al. propose an interesting model overlapping the binding of arachidonic acid with the binding of MK-591 to FLAP (71). In this model top and bottom hydrophobic lipid binding pockets hold the fatty acid or hydrophobic portions of the drug in position with a left-hand quinoline-binding pocket and a right-hand carboxylic acid–binding pocket (71). However, Charleson et al. have shown that the presence of a free carboxyl group on fatty acids or leukotriene synthesis inhibitors is not required for specific binding to FLAP (72). In this study the compound anandamide (arachidonylethanolamide) competed with a radioiodinated analog of MK-591 slightly more effectively than arachidonic acid (72). Saturated fatty acids with alkyl chains from C12 to C24 were inactive in the FLAP-binding assay, while fatty acids with two to six double bonds were all as effective as arachidonic acid (72). It is clear that FLAP may selectively transfer arachidonic acid and other saturated long-chain fatty acids to 5-LO depending on their availability in the cell. It is difficult to visualize the unsaturated fatty acid–binding site on FLAP, although some of the key residues have been identified in mutagenesis studies as just outside of the putative second transmembrane domain (64). X-ray crystallographic studies of cyclooxygenases demonstrate a hydrophobic pocket for a hairpin-looped arachidonic acid structure. This pocket is in a portion of the enzyme just beyond the membrane-binding motif that binds to one leaflet of the lipid bilayer of the lumen of the endoplasmic reticulum (73). The x-ray crystal structure of mammalian 15-LO shows that the substrate-binding site is also a hydrophobic pocket; however, arachidonic acid would be predicted to bind in an extended conformation. By comparison of the amino acid sequences of 15-LO and 5-LO, Browner et al. suggest that the arachidonic acid may be more deeply embedded in 5-LO (unpublished data). It is interesting to speculate why 5-LO (but not 12-LO or 15-LO) requires FLAP to enable selective transfer of unsaturated fatty acids. Perhaps 5-LO binds to the membrane in a nonproductive conformation. FLAP both channels substrate to the active site and stabilizes a conformation favoring the two-step oxygenation and dehydration. This would be a membrane interfacial activation system somewhat analogous to the situation for pancreatic lipase and its small activating protein colipase (74).

C. Expression, Gene Structure, Gene Knockout, and FLAP Homologs

FLAP is expressed in a very defined subset of myeloid cells, most of which are capable of leukotriene synthesis (35,36,56,75). In HL-60 cells induced to differentiate into a granulocyte lineage by DMSO, coinduction of 5-LO and FLAP and leukotriene synthesis capacity were observed (36). A number of other stimuli have been shown to increase the expression of 5-LO and FLAP in human neutrophils, including GMCSF (37). However, discordant induction of 5-LO and FLAP were reported in HL-60 cells in response to treatment with 1,25-dihydroxyvitamin D_3 and phorbol ester (75). Differentiation of human peripheral blood monocytes by 1,25-dihydroxyvitamin D_3 increases 5-LO metabolism and expression of FLAP, but not 5-LO (76). In addition, alveolar macrophages from 1,25-dihydroxyvitamin D_3–deficient rates had reduced 5-LO metabolism, reduced FLAP expression, but no change in 5-LO expression (76). The human monocytic U937 cell line expresses FLAP and not 5-LO (77). When 5-LO was introduced into the undifferentiated U937 cells even though FLAP was present, there was no leukotriene synthesis (77). Differentiation with DMSO resulted in increased FLAP and 5-LO protein and leukotriene synthesis. This system has some similarity to human B cells, where there is expression of 5-LO and FLAP but, unless glutathione is depleted, leukotrienes are not produced (7). It is clear that the regulation of leukotriene synthesis in cells is complex and subject to factors such as peroxide tone and perhaps inhibitory proteins.

The FLAP gene is a very large gene (>31 kilobases) consisting of five small exons and four large introns (78). The exon/intron sites do not match the sites of the putative three transmembrane binding domains. Southern blot analysis of human genomic DNA suggests a single FLAP gene per haploid genome (78). The transcription start site was mapped to 74 base pairs upstream of the ATG initiation codon, and the promoter region of the FLAP gene contained a possible TATA box and AP-2 and glucocorticoid receptor–binding sites. Functional analysis of the FLAP gene promoter in a mouse macrophage cell line revealed enhancer-like activities that were missing in a hepatoma cell line (78). The FLAP gene has been mapped to human chromosome 13 (B. Kennedy, unpublished data). The FLAP gene has been knocked out in an embryonic cell line from DBA/1 mice that is an arthritis-susceptible background (79). The FLAP (-/-) mice are fertile, healthy, and have no developmental problems. Leukotriene production was abolished and plasma protein extravasation diminished by 60% in FLAP knockout mice injected with zymosan. In addition, the severity of collagen-induced arthritis was reduced by 73% in the FLAP knockout mice (79).

The first homolog of FLAP to be cloned was LTC_4 synthase, showing 31% amino acid identity to FLAP with a highly conserved region in the putative arachidonic acid–binding site (80,81). LTC_4 synthase was shown to be weakly inhibited by the FLAP inhibitor MK-886 (80). LTC_4 synthase is localized to human chromosome 5q35, and the synthase gene exon structure is identical to FLAP but has much smaller introns spanning a total of only 2.5 kilobases (82). The second FLAP homolog is microsomal GST-II, a 16,600 dalton protein with a calculated pl of 10.4 with both LTC_4 synthase and glutathione S-transferase activity (83). GST-II shows 33% amino acid identity to FLAP and a 44% amino acid identity to LTC_4 synthase and has a similar hydrophobicity pattern to both FLAP and LTC_4 synthase (83). GST-II was localized to human chromosome 4q28-31, but the gene has not yet been cloned (83).

IV. Cellular Activation of 5-LO

Cellular synthesis of leukotrienes only occurs following a stimulus that significantly raises intracellular calcium. The first evidence that 5-LO activation in human leukocytes was associated with movement of the enzyme from the cytosol to a membrane fraction was shown by Rouzer and Kargman (84). In calcium ionophore A23187–challenged leukocytes that were subsequently sonicated and fractionated, about 50% of the 5-LO activity was lost from the 100,000 × *g* supernatant fraction and inactive 5-LO protein detected in the 100,000 × *g* membrane fraction (84). At the time a membrane-bound 18 kDa protein (i.e., FLAP) that selectively bound MK-886 analogs was being characterized, it was shown that MK-886 could prevent this membrane movement in a concentration-dependent fashion, which correlated with its ability to inhibit LTB_4 synthesis (59). There was a correlation between some compounds that inhibited leukotriene synthesis and prevention of 5-LO translocation (59). Subsequent studies showed inhibition of A23187 or *N*-formyl-methionyl-leucyl-phenylalanine–induced translocation of HL-60 cell 5-LO by indole and quinoline FLAP-binding leukotriene synthesis inhibitors (85). After the cloning of the 18 kDa protein (and its christening as FLAP), osteosarcoma cells (that do not normally express 5-LO or FLAP) were transfected with 5-LO and FLAP and translocation to a membrane fraction was observed that could be inhibited by MK-886 (86). In the osteosarcoma cells transfected with 5-LO alone, translocation of 5-LO in response to ionophore was also observed. However, in the latter case no leukotriene synthesis occurred and the translocation was not inhibited by MK-886 (86). Other studies demonstrated a separation between the inhibition of 5-LO translocation and leukotriene synthesis (87,88). A lack of 5-LO translocation inhibition and inhibition of leukotriene synthesis was observed with a series of quinoline-based inhibitors (87). In unstimulated alveolar macrophages 5-LO appeared to be in a membrane compartment, and although following stimulation MK-886 inhibited leukotriene synthesis, it did not affect membrane association (88). These results suggest that 5-LO translocation can occur in the absence of FLAP but a FLAP-dependent activation step is required in cells for leukotrienes to be synthesized. As suggested above, perhaps FLAP is required not only to channel substrate to 5-LO but also to promote an active conformation, which enhances the concerted two-step reaction to make LTA_4.

Electron micrographic studies utilizing 5-LO and FLAP-specific antisera demonstrated that in human leukocytes the membrane to which 5-LO translocates is the lumenal face of the inner nuclear membrane (89). This is the compartment in which FLAP is found in both unstimulated and stimulated cells (89). In retrospect, the sonication procedures used to prepare 100,000 × *g* fractions in the translocation experiments would have dispersed the nuclear membranes into this pellet. Pouliot et al. studied the distribution of cytosolic phospholipase A_2 ($cPLA_2$), 5-LO, and FLAP in subcellular fractions of human neutrophils disrupted by sonication and cavitation (90). Both techniques found $cPLA_2$ and 5-LO to be mainly in the cytosol prior to stimulation. Following calcium ionophore A23187 activation, both proteins were found mainly in nuclear membranes. As previously observed in the electron micrographic studies of Woods et al., FLAP was found in the nuclear membranes of both resting and stimulated cells (90). A23187 stimulation enhanced 5-LO activity in the nuclear membrane fraction. 5-LO was protected during cellular activation from suicide inactivation by the presence of a 5-LO inhibitor (90). Neutrophil activation caused an increase in phosphorylation of $cPLA_2$, a process that is known to enhance phospholipase catalytic activity (90). The cellular enzymes responsible for conversion of the 5-LO product LTA_4 to LTB_4 and LTC_4 are cytosolic and membrane bound (possibly nuclear), respectively. In rat leukocytes, activated by the calcium ionophore A23187, LTA_4 hydrolase did not move to any membrane (J. Evans and S. Kargman, unpublished data).

5-LO is not found in the cytosol of all cells. In human alveolar macrophages and rat basophil leukemia cells, 5-LO was shown to be present in the nucleus in the unactivated state and moved to nuclear fractions following stimulation (91). Electron micrographic studies showed that the unstimulated location of 5-LO in these cells was in the nucleus and translocation was to the inner nuclear membrane (92). A question is posed by these cellular localization studies: Why make leukotrienes on the nuclear membrane? This question is unanswerable at the moment, but may reflect the change from an ancient detoxification system to a more sophisticated second messenger signaling system. The timing of the evolution of seven transmembrane domain G-protein coupled receptors may postdate an early more primitive nuclear transcriptional control function through as yet undiscovered LAPs (leukotriene-activated proteins) (Fig. 1). A great deal of exciting research remains to be performed into both the structural activation of 5-LO by FLAP and the cellular functional consequences.

Acknowledgments

The author would like to thank Douglas Miller (Merck Research Laboratories) for his pivotal role in the discovery of FLAP and for supplying two of the FLAP figures. Sincere thanks also to Denis Riendeau, Michael Gresser, Joe Mancini, and Per-Johann Jakobsson for stimulating discussions, to Kevin Clark for his wonderful artistry, and to S. Kargman, B. Kennedy, J. Drazen, M. Browner, and S. Gillmor for allowing me to quote unpublished data.

References

1. Samuelsson B. Leukotrienes: mediators of hypersensitivity reactions and inflammation. Science 1983; 220:568–575.
2. Yamamoto S. Mammalian lipoxygenases: molecular structures and functions. Biochim Biophys Acta 1992; 1128:117–131.
3. Ford-Hutchinson AW, Gresser M, Young RN. 5-Lipoxygenase. Annu Rev Biochem 1994; 63:383–417.
4. Serhan CN, Hamberg M, Samuelsson B. Trihydroxytetraenes: a novel series of com-

pounds formed from arachidonic acid in human leukocytes. Biochem Biophys Res Commun 1984; 118:943–949.

5. Hatzelmann A, Ullrich V. Regulation of 5-lipoxygenase activity by the glutathione status in human polymorphonuclear leukocytes. Eur J Biochem 1987; 169:175–184.
6. Hatzelmann A, Schatz M, Ullrich V. Involvement of glutathione peroxidase activity in the stimulation of 5-lipoxygenase activity by glutathione-depleting agents in human polymorphonuclear leukocytes. Eur J Biochem 1989; 180:527–533.
7. Jakobsson P-J, Odlander B, Steinhilber D, Rosen A, Claesson H-E. Human B lymphocytes possess 5-lipoxygenase activity and convert arachidonic acid to leukotriene B_4. Biochem Biophys Res Commun 1991; 178:302–308.
8. Percival MD, Denis D, Riendeau D, Gresser MJ. Investigation of the mechanism of non-turnover-dependent inactivation of purified human 5-lipoxygenase. Eur J Biochem 1992; 210:109–117.
9. Falgueret J-P, Hutchinson JH, Riendeau D. Criteria for the identification of non-redox inhibitors of 5-lipoxygenase. Biochem Pharmacol 1993; 45:978–981.
10. De Carolis E, Denis D, Riendeau D. Oxidative inactivation of human 5-lipoxygenase in phosphatidylcholine vesicles. Eur J Biochem 1996; 235:416–423.
11. Percival MD, Ouellet M. The characterization of 5 histidine-serine mutants of human 5-lipoxygenase. Biochem Biophys Res Commun 1992; 186:1265–1270.
12. Rouzer CA, Riendeau D, Falgueyret J-P, Lau CK, Gresser MJ. Inhibition of human leukocyte 5-lipoxygenase by 4-hydroxybenzofuran, L-656,224. Evidence for enzyme reduction and inhibitor degradation. Biochem Pharmacol 1991; 41:1354–1373.
13. Riendeau D, Falgueyret J-P, Nathaniel DJ, Rokach J, Ueda N, Yamamoto S. Sensitivity of immunoaffinity-purified porcine 5-lipoxygenase to inhibitors and activating lipid hydroperoxides. Biochem Pharmacol 1989; 38:2313–2321.
14. Rouzer CA, Samuelsson B. On the nature of the 5-lipoxygenase reaction in human leukocytes: enzyme purification and requirement for multiple stimulatory factors. Proc Natl Acad Sci USA 1985; 82:6040–6044.
15. Rouzer CA, Matsumoto T, Samuelsson B. Single protein from human leukocytes possesses 5-lipoxygenase and leukotriene A_4 synthase activities. Proc Natl Acad Sci USA 1986; 83:857–861.
16. Ueda N, Kaneko S, Yoshimoto T, Yamamoto S. Purification of arachidonate 5-lipoxygenase from porcine leukocytes and its reactivity with hydroperoxyeicosatetraenoic acids. J Biol Chem 1986; 261:7982–7988.
17. Skoog MT, Nichols JS, Wiseman JS. 5-Lipoxygenase from rat PMN lysate. Prostaglandins 1986; 31:561–576.
18. Aharony D, Stein RL. Kinetic mechanism of guinea pig neutrophil 5-lipoxygenase. J Biol Chem 1986; 261:11512–11519.
19. Dixon RAF, Jones RE, Diehl RE, Bennett CD, Kargman S, Rouzer CA. Cloning of the cDNA for human 5-lipoxygenase. Proc Natl Acad Sci USA 1988; 85:416–420.
20. Matsumoto T, Funk CD, Radmark O, Hoog J-O, Jornvall H, Samuelsson B. Molecular cloning and amino acid sequence of human 5-lipoxygenase. Proc Natl Acad Sci USA 1988; 85:26–30.
21. Balcarek JM, Theisen TW, Cook MN, Varrichio A, Huang S-M, Strohsacker MW, Crooke ST. Isolation and characterization of a cDNA clone encoding rat 5-lipoxygenase. J Biol Chem 1988; 263:13937–13941.

22. Funk CD. Molecular biology in the eicosanoid field. Prog Nucleic Acid Res 1993; 45:67–98.
23. Nguyen T, Falgueyret J-P, Abramovitz M, Riendeau D. Evaluation of the role of conserved His and Met residues among lipoxygenases by site-directed mutagenesis of recombinant human 5-lipoxygenase. J Biol Chem 1991; 266:22057–22062.
24. Zhang YY, Radmark O, Samuelsson B. Mutagenesis of some conserved residues in human 5-lipoxygenase. Proc Natl Acad Sci USA 1992; 89:485–489.
25. Ishii S, Noguchi M, Miyano M, Matsumoto T, Noma M. Mutagenesis studies on the amino acid residues involved in the iron-binding and the activity of human 5-lipoxygenase. Biochem Biophys Res Commun 1992; 182:1482–1490.
26. Rouzer CA, Rands E, Kargman S, Jones ER, Register RB, Dixon RAF. Characterization of cloned human leukocyte 5-lipoxygenase expressed in mammalian cells. J Biol Chem 1988; 263:10135–10140.
27. Funk CD, Gunne H, Steiner H, Izumi T, Samuelsson B. Native and mutant 5-lipoxygenase expression in a baculovirus/insect cell system. Proc Natl Acad Sci USA 1989; 86:2592–2596.
28. Denis D, Falgueyret J-P, Riendeau D, Abramovitz M. Characterization of the activity of purified recombinant human 5-lipoxygenase in the absence and presence of leukocyte factors. J Biol Chem 1991; 266:5072–5079.
29. Nakamura M, Matsumoto T, Noguchi M, Noma M. Expression of a cDNA encoding human 5-lipoxygenase under control of the STA1 promoter in *Saccharomyces cerevisiae*. Gene (Amst) 1990; 89:231–237.
30. Noguchi M, Matsumoto T, Nakamura M, Noma M. Expression of human 5-lipoxygenase in *Escherichia coli*. FEBS Lett 1989; 247:267–270.
31. Percival MD. Human 5-lipoxygenase contains an essential iron. J Biol Chem 1991; 266:10058–10061.
32. Chasteen ND, Grady JK, Skorey KI, Neden KJ, Riendeau D, Percival MD. Characterization of the non-heme iron center of human 5-lipoxygenase by electron paramagnetic resonance, fluorescence, and ultraviolet-visible spectroscopy: redox cycling between ferrous and ferric states. Biochemistry 1993; 32:9763–9771.
33. Lepley RA, Muskardin DT, Fizpatrick FA. Tyrosine kinase activity modulates catalysis and translocation of cellular 5-lipoxygenase. J Biol Chem 1996; 271:6179–6184.
34. Lepley RA, Fitzpatrick FA. 5-Lipoxygenase contains a functional Src homology 3-binding motif that interacts with the Src homology 3 domain of Grb2 and cytoskeletal proteins. J Biol Chem 1994; 269:24163–24168.
35. Jakobsson P-J, Steinhilber D, Odlander B, Radmark O, Claesson H-E, Samuelsson B. On the expression and regulation of 5-lipoxygenase in human lymphocytes. Proc Natl Acad Sci USA 1992; 89:3521–3525.
36. Reid GK, Kargman S, Vickers PJ, Mancini JA, Leveille C, Ethier D, Miller DK, Gillard JW, Dixon RAF, Evans JF. Correlation between expression of 5-lipoxygenase-activating protein, 5-lipoxygenase, and cellular leukotriene synthesis. J Biol Chem 1990; 265:19818–19823.
37. Pouliot M, McDonald PP, Khaminza L, Borgeat P, McColl SR. Granulocyte-macrophage colony-stimulating factor enhances 5-lipoxygenase levels in human polymorphonuclear leukocytes. J Immunol 1994; 152:851–858.
38. Natsui K, Ueda N, Yamamoto S, Komatsu N, Watanabe K. Arachidonate 5-lipoxy-

genase of porcine pancreas: its localization in acinar cells. Biochem Biophys Acta 1991; 1085:241–247.

39. Funk CD, Hoshiko S, Matsumoto T, Radmark O, Samuelsson B. Characterization of the human 5-lipoxygenase gene. Proc Natl Acad Sci USA 1989; 86:2587–2591.
40. Hoshiko S, Radmark O, Samuelsson B. Characterization of the human 5-lipoxygenase gene promoter. Proc Natl Acad Sci USA 1990; 87:9073–9077.
41. Chen X-S, Sheller JR, Johnson EN, Funk CD. Role of leukotrienes revealed by targeted disruption of the 5-lipoxygenase gene. Nature 1994; 372:179–182.
42. Goulet JL, Snouwaert JN, Latour AM, Coffman TM, Koller BH. Altered inflammatory responses in leukotriene-deficient mice. Proc Natl Acad Sci USA 1994; 91: 12852–12856.
43. Irvin CG, Tu Y-P, Sheller JR, Funk CD. 5-Lipoxygenase products are necessary for ovalbumin-induced airway responses in mice. Am J Physiol, in press.
44. Fitzsimmons BJ, Rokach J. Enzyme inhibitors and leukotriene receptor antagonists. In: Rokach J, ed. Leukotrienes and Lipoxygenases. New York: Elsevier, 1989:427–502.
45. Musser JH, Kreft AF. 5-Lipoxygenase: properties, pharmacology, and the quinolinyl(bridged)aryl class of inhibitors. J Med Chem 1990; 35:2501–2524.
46. McMillan RM, Walker ERH. Designing therapeutically effective 5-lipoxygenase inhibitors. TIPS 1992; 13:323–330.
47. Carter GW, Young PR, Albert DH et al. 5-Lipoxygenase inhibitory action of zileuton. J Pharmacol Exp Ther 1991; 256:929–937.
48. Israel E, Drazen JM, Pearlman H, Cohn J, Rubin P. A double-blind multicenter study of zileuton, a potent 5-lipoxygenase (5-LO) inhibitor versus placebo in the treatment of spontaneous asthma in adults. J Allergy Clin 1992; 89:236.
49. Bell RL, Brooks DW, Young PR, Lanni C, Stewart AO, Bouska J, Malo PE. A-78773: a selective, potent 5-lipoxygenase inhibitor. J Lipid Mediators 1993; 6:259–264.
50. Bird TG, Bruneau P, Crawley GC, Edwards MP, Foster SJ, Girodeau J-M, Kingston JF, McMillan RM. (Methoxyalkyl)thiazoles: a new series of potent, selective, and orally active 5-lipoxygenase inhibitors displaying high enantioselectivity. J Med Chem 1991; 34:2176–2186.
51. Crawley GC, Dowell RI, Edwards PN, Foster SJ, McMillan RM, Walker ERH, Waterston D. Methoxytetrahydropyrans. A new series of selective and orally potent 5-lipoxygenase inhibitors. J Med Chem 1992; 35:2600–2609.
52. Ducharme Y, Brideau C, Dube D, Chan C, Falgueyret J-P, Gillard JW, Guay J, Hutchinson JH, McFarlane CS, Riendeau D, Scheigetz J, Girard Y. Naphthalenic lignan lactones as selective, nonredox 5-lipoxygenase inhibitors. Synthesis and biological activity of (methoxyalkyl)-thiazole and methoxytetrahydropyran hybrids. J Med Chem 1994; 37:512–518.
53. Hutchinson JH, Riendeau D, Brideau C, Chan C, Delorme D, Denis D, Falgueyret J-P, Fortin R, Guay J, Hamel P, Jones TR, Macdonald D, McFarlane CS, Piechuta H, Scheigetz J, Tagari P, Therien M, Girard Y. Substituted thiopyrano[2,3,4-*c,d*]indoles as potent, selective and orally active inhibitors of 5-lipoxygenase. Synthesis and biological evaluation of L-691,816. J Med Chem 1993; 36:2771–2787.
54. Falgueyret J-P, Hutchinson JH, Riendeau D. Criteria for the determination of nonredox inhibitors of 5-lipoxygenase. Biochem Pharmacol 1993; 45:978–981.
55. Falgueyret J-P, Denis D, Macdonald D, Hutchinson JH, Riendeau D. Char-

acterization of the arachidonate and ATP binding sites of human 5-lipoxygenase using photoaffinity labeling and enzyme immobilization. Biochemistry 1995; 34: 13603–13611.

56. Miller DK, Gillard JW, Vickers PJ, Sadowski S, Leveille C, Mancini JA, Charleson P, Dixon RAF, Ford-Hutchinson AW, Fortin R, Gauthier J-Y, Rodkey J, Rosen R, Rouzer CA, Sigal IS, Strader C, Evans JF. Identification and isolation of a membrane protein necessary for leukotriene production. Nature (Lond) 1990; 343:278–281.
57. Dixon RAF, Diehl RE, Opas E, Rands E, Vickers PJ, Evans JF, Gillard JW, Miller DK. Requirement of a 5-lipoxygenase-activating protein for leukotriene synthesis. Nature (Lond) 1990; 343:282–284.
58. Gillard J, Ford-Hutchinson AW, Chan C, Charleson S, Denis D, Foster A, Fortin R, Leger S, McFarlane CS, Morton H, Piechuta H, Riendeau D, Rouzer CA, Rokach J, Young RN, Maclntyre DE, Peterson L, Bach T, Eirmann G, Hopple S, Humes J, Luell S, Metzger J, Meuer R, Miller DK, Opas E, Pacholok SL. L-663,536 (MK-886) (3-[1-(4-chlorobenzyl)-3-t-butyl-thio-5-isopropylindol-2-yl]-2,2-dimethylpropanoic acid), a novel, orally active leukotriene biosynthesis inhibitor. Can J Physiol Pharmacol 1989; 67:456–464.
59. Rouzer CA, Ford-Hutchinson AW, Morton HE, Gillard JW. MK886, a potent and specific leukotriene biosynthesis inhibitor, blocks and reverses membrane association of 5-lipoxygenase in ionophore-challenged leukocytes. J Biol Chem 1990; 265: 1436–1442.
60. Evans JF, Leveille C, Mancini JA, Prasit P, Therien M, Zamboni R, Gauthier J-Y, Fortin R, Charleson P, Maclntyre DE, Luell S, Bach TJ, Meurer R, Vickers PJ, Rouzer CA, Gillard JW, Miller DK. 5-Lipoxygenase-activating protein is the target of a quinoline class of leukotriene synthesis inhibitor. Mol Pharmacol 1991; 40:22–27.
61. Charleson S, Prasit P, Léger S, Gillard JW, Vickers PJ, Mancini JA, Charleson P, Guay J, Ford-Hutchinson AW, Evans JF. Characterization of a 5-lipoxygenase-activating protein binding assay: correlation with leukotriene synthesis inhibition. Mol Pharmacol 1992; 41:873–879.
62. Brideau C, Chan C, Charleson S, Denis D, Evans JF, Ford-Hutchinson AW, Fortin R, Gillard JW, Guay J, Guevremont D, Hutchinson JH, Jones TR, Leger S, Mancini JA, McFarlane CS, Picket C, Piechuta H, Prasit P, Riendeau D, Rouzer CA, Tagari P, Vickers PJ, Young RN, Abraham WM. Pharmacology of MK-0591 (3-[1-(4-chlorobenzyl)-3-(t-butylthio)-5-(quinolin-2-yl-methoxy)-indol-2-yl]-2,2-dimethylpropanoic acid), a potent, orally active leukotriene biosynthesis inhibitor. Can J Physiol Pharmacol 1992; 70:799–807.
63. Mancini JA, Prasit P, Coppolino MG, Charleson P, Leger S, Evans JF, Gillard JW, Vickers PJ. 5-Lipoxygenase-activating protein is the target of a novel hybrid of two classes of leukotriene biosynthesis inhibitor. Mol Pharmacol 1992; 41:873–879.
64. Vickers PJ, Adam M, Charleson S, Coppolino MG, Evans JF, Mancini JA. Identification of amino acid residues of 5-lipoxygenase-activating protein essential for the binding of leukotriene biosynthesis inhibitors. Mol Pharmacol 1992; 42:94–102.
65. Mancini JA, Coppolino M, Klassen JH, Charleson S, Vickers PJ. The binding of leukotriene biosynthesis inhibitors to site-directed mutants of human 5-lipoxygenase-activating protein. Life Sci 1994; 54:137–142.

66. Mancini JA, Abramovitz M, Cox ME, Wong E, Charleson S, Perrier H, Wang Z, Prasit P, Vickers PJ. 5-Lipoxygenase-activating protein is an arachidonate binding protein. FEBS Lett 1993; 3:277–281.
67. Abramovitz M, Wong E, Cox ME, Richardson CD, Li C, Vickers PJ. 5-Lipoxygenase-activating protein stimulates the utilization of arachidonic acid by 5-lipoxygenase. Eur J Biochem 1993; 215:105–111.
68. Hill E, Maclouf J, Murphy RC, Henson PM. Reversible membrane association of neutrophil 5-lipoxygenase is accompanied by retention of activity and a change in substrate specificity. J Biol Chem 1992; 267:22048–22053.
69. Hutchinson JH, Charleson S, Evans JF, Falgueyret J-P, Hoogsteen K, Jones TR, Kargman S, Mcdonald D, McFarlane CS, Nicholson DW, Piechuta H, Riendeau D, Scheigetz J, Therien M, Girard Y. Thiopyranol[2,3,4-*c,d*]indoles as inhibitors of 5-lipoxygenase, 5-lipoxygenase-activating protein, and leukotriene C_4 synthase. J Med Chem 1995; 38:4538–4547.
70. Hatzelmann A, Fruchmann R, Mohrs KH, Raddatz S, Müller-Peddinghaus R. Mode of action of the new selective leukotriene synthesis inhibitor BAY X1005 ((R)-2-[4-(quinolin-2-yl-methoxy)phenyl]-2-cyclopentyl acetic acid) and structurally related compounds. Biochem Pharmacol 1993; 45:101–111.
71. Kreft AF, Marshall LA, Wong A. Structure-activity relationships in the quinoline-containing class of inhibitors of 5-lipoxygenase (5-LO) enzyme translocation and activation. Drugs Future 1994; 19(3):255–264.
72. Charleson S, Evans JF, Leger S, Perrier H, Prasit P, Wang Z, Vickers PJ. Structural requirements for the binding of fatty acids to 5-lipoxygenase-activating protein. Eur J Pharmacol 1994; 267:275–280.
73. Picot D, Loll PJ, Garavito M. The x-ray crystal structure of the membrane protein prostaglandin H_2 synthase. Nature 1994; 367:243–249.
74. van Tilbeurgh H, Egloff M-P, Martinez C, Rugani N, Verger R, Cambillau C. Interfacial activation of the lipase-colipase complex by mixed micelles revealed by x-ray crystallography. Nature 1993; 362:814–820.
75. Bennett CF, Chiang M, Monia BP, Crooke ST. Regulation of 5-lipoxygenase and 5-lipoxygenase-activating protein expression in HL-60 cells. Biochem J 1993; 289: 33–39.
76. Coffey M, Gyeto M, Peters-Golden M. 1,25-Dihydroxyvitamin D_3 upregulates 5-lipoxygenase metabolism and 5-lipoxygenase-activating protein in peripheral blood monocytes as they differentiate into mature macrophages. J Lipid Mediators 1993; 6:43–51.
77. Kargman S, Rousseau P, Reid GK, Rouzer CA, Mancini JA, Rands E, Dixon RAF, Diehl RE, Leveille C, Nathaniel D, Vickers PJ, Evans JF. Leukotriene synthesis in U937 cells expressing recombinant 5-lipoxygenase. J Lipid Mediators 1993; 7:31–45.
78. Kennedy BP, Diehl RE, Boie Y, Adam M, Dixon RAF. Gene characterization and promoter analysis of the human 5-lipoxygenase-activating protein (FLAP). J Biol Chem 1991; 13:8511–8516.
79. Griffiths RJ, Smith MA, Roach ML, Stam EJ, Milici AJ, Scampoli DN, Byrum RS, Koller BH, McNeish JD. Diminished inflammatory responses in FLAP-deficient mice. J Exp Med, in press.
80. Lam BK, Penrose JF, Freeman GJ, Austen KF. Expression cloning of a cDNA for

human leukotriene C_4 synthase, an integral membrane protein conjugating reduced glutathione to leukotriene A_4. Proc Natl Acad Sci USA 1994; 91:7663–7667.

81. Welsch DJ, Creely DP, Hauser SD, Mathis KJ, Krivi GG, Isakson PC. Molecular cloning and expression of human leukotriene C_4 synthase. Proc Natl Acad Sci USA 1994; 91:9745–9749.
82. Penrose JF, Spector J, Baldasaro M, Xu K, Boyce J, Arm JP, Austen FK, Lam BK. Molecular cloning of the gene for human leukotriene C_4 synthase. Organization, nucleotide sequence, and chromosomal localization to 5q35. J Biol Chem 1996; 271: 11356–11361.
83. Jakobsson P-J, Mancini JA, Ford-Hutchinson AW. Identification and characterization of a novel human microsomal glutathione S-transferase with leukotriene C_4 synthase activity and significant sequence identity to 5-lipoxygenase-activating protein and leukotriene C_4 synthase. J Biol Chem 1996; 271:2203–2210.
84. Rouzer CA, Kargman S. Translocation of 5-lipoxygenase to the membrane in human leukocytes challenged with ionophore A23187. J Biol Chem 1988; 263:10980–10988.
85. Kargman S, Prasit P, Evans JF. Translocation of HL-60 cell 5-lipoxygenase Inhibition of A23187-or N-formyl-leucyl-phenylalanine-induced translocation by indole and quinoline leukotriene synthesis inhibitors. J Biol Chem 1991; 266:23745–23752.
86. Kargman S, Vickers PJ, Evans JF. A23187-induced translocation of 5-lipoxygenase in osteosarcoma cells. J Cell Biol 1992; 119:1701–1709.
87. Hatzelmann A, Goosens J, Fruchtmann R, Mohrs K-H, Raddatz S, Muller-Peddinghaus R. Inversely correlated inhibition of human 5-lipoxygenase activity by BAY X1005 and other quinoline derivatives in intact cells and a cell-free system—implications for the function of 5-lipoxygenase-activating protein. Biochem Pharmacol 1994; 47:2259–2268.
88. Coffey M, Peters-Golden M, Fantone JC, Sporn PHS. Membrane association of active 5-lipoxygenase in resting cells. Evidence for novel regulation of the enzyme in the rat alveolar macrophage. J Biol Chem 1992; 267:570–576.
89. Woods JW, Evans JF, Ethier D, Scott S, Vickers PJ, Hearn L, Heibein JA, Charleson S, Singer II. 5-Lipoxygenase and 5-lipoxygenase-activating protein are localized in the nuclear envelope of activated human leukocytes. J Exp Med 1993;178:1935–1946.
90. Pouliot M, McDonald PP, Krump E, Mancini JA, McColl SR, Weech PK, Borgeat P. Colocalization of cytosolic phospholipase A_2. 5-lipoxygenase, and 5-lipoxygenase-activating protein at the nuclear membrane of A23187-stimulated human neutrophils. Eur J Biochem 1996; 238:250–258.
91. Peters-Golden M, Mcnish RW. Redistribution of 5-lipoxygenase and cytosolic phospholipase A_2 to the nuclear fraction upon macrophage activation. Biochem Biophys Res Commun 1993; 196:147–153.
92. Woods JW, Coffey MJ, Brock TJ, Singer II, Peters-Golden M. 5-Lipoxygenase is located in the euchromatin of the nucleus in resting human alveolar macrophages and translocates to the nuclear envelope upon cell activation. J Clin Invest 1995; 95:2035–2046.

3

Leukotriene C_4 Synthase

A Pivotal Enzyme in the Biosynthesis of Cysteinyl Leukotrienes

JOHN F. PENROSE and K. FRANK AUSTEN

Harvard Medical School
and Brigham and Women's Hospital
Boston, Massachusetts

I. Introduction and Background

The cysteinyl leukotrienes are a family of proinflammatory lipid mediators consisting of the parent compound, LTC_4, and it biologically receptor-active metabolites, LTD_4 and LTE_4. These compounds, formerly known as slow-reacting substance of anaphylaxis (SRS-A), were first identified in the perfusates from isolated guinea pig lungs subjected to an anaphylactic reaction in vitro (1). The biological activity of these perfusates was measured by contraction of the smooth muscle of guinea pig ileum. More than a decade passed before the use of the histamine antagonist mepyramine allowed the effects of SRS-A to be separated from those of histamine (2,3). After the recognition that a latent period existed between the biosynthesis of SRS-A and its subsequent release (4), the chemical structure of SRS-A was defined. The chemical structure of the parent compound, LTC_4, was determined in 1979 (5), followed by elucidation of the other family members, LTD_4 and LTE_4, in the next 2 years (6,7). The definition of the cysteinyl leukotriene structures then allowed their chemical synthesis, which was followed by studies of their pharmacological effects. Cysteinyl leukotrienes administered in vivo were found to cause tissue edema as a result of post–capillary venule dilatation (8,9), bronchial smooth muscle contraction (10), and mucus secretion in tracheal epithelial cells (11).

After these seminal observations, abundant research yielded evidence that the cysteinyl leukotrienes are pathophysiological mediators of asthma. Eosinophils and mast cells, both found in high numbers in airways of individuals with asthma, can synthesize the cysteinyl leukotrienes (12,13), and the in vivo manifestation of this finding is the recovery of cysteinyl leukotrienes in biological fluids during induced and spontaneous asthma (14,15). The cysteinyl leukotrienes have a spectrum of biological effects consistent with the mediation of abnormalities in asthma (8–11), and agents that block the action of the cysteinyl leukotrienes at their receptors or inhibit their biosynthesis ameliorate induced and spontaneous asthma (16–19). Having briefly emphasized the integral role of the cysteinyl leukotrienes in bronchial asthma, we will review the biosynthesis of leukotrienes with specific attention to the pivotal role of LTC_4 synthase as the only committed enzyme in the formation of the cysteinyl leukotrienes.

II. Biosynthetic Pathway of Cysteinyl Leukotriene Formation

The series of biochemical reactions leading to the formation of cysteinyl leukotrienes is initiated by a cellular activation signal that causes the release of arachidonic acid from membrane phospholipids by the action of cytosolic phospholipase A_2 (20), which translocates from the cytosol to the perinuclear membrane. Indeed, within the restricted group of hematopoietic cell populations that generate LTC_4, all the enzymes/proteins involved in LTC_4 biosynthesis are located at, or translocated to, the perinuclear membrane. When released, arachidonic acid binds to an 18 kDa integral perinuclear membrane protein, 5-lipoxygenase–activating protein (FLAP), which presents the arachidonic acid to 5-lipoxygenase (5-LO) (21,22). This step allows the enzymatic function of 5-LO, which, depending on the cell source examined, translocates to the perinuclear membrane from either the cytosol or the nucleoplasm (23,24). 5-LO catalyzes arachidonic acid in two sequential steps to form 5-hydroperoxyeicosatetraenoic acid and then the unstable epoxide intermediate, LTA_4 (24). LTA_4 is acted on by the integral membrane protein, LTC_4 synthase, which conjugates LTA_4 with reduced glutathione (GSH) to form the intracellular product, LTC_4 (25).

LTC_4 is exported from the cell by a carrier-mediated mechanism (26,27) and is processed extracellularly by the sequential cleavage of glutamic acid and glycine residues. These reactions are catalyzed by gamma-glutamyl transpeptidase (28) and dipeptidases (29), respectively, and respectively yield LTD_4 and LTE_4, the receptor-active derivatives.

Thus, the generation of the pathophysiologically important cysteinyl leukotrienes depends on LTC_4 synthase. The characterization of this enzyme, in terms of function and gene regulation, will likely contribute to the understanding of the severity and/or susceptibility to phenotypes of bronchial asthma.

III. Biochemical Characterization of LTC_4 Synthase

Despite the glutathione-conjugating function of authentic LTC_4 synthase, this enzyme clearly differs from any of the known cytosolic, mitochondrial, or microsomal GSH S-transferases. Two observations have made this distinction important. First, authentic LTC_4 synthase is present in cells that contain the complement of enzymes/proteins necessary to generate LTA_4. Second, a cytosolic GSH S-transferase in brain tissue and a recently described microsomal GSH S-transferase II catalyze the conjugation of GSH to LTA_4 as well as to xenobiotics (30,31). Neither of these enzymes is distributed to cells capable of generating LTA_4. The presence of an authentic LTC_4 synthase was originally inferred from its restricted cellular distribution and its restricted substrate specificity for LTA_4 and its analogs while being specifically inactive in the detoxification of xenobiotics (32). Further evidence supporting LTC_4 synthase as a member of a separate family, perhaps within a GSH S-transferase superfamily, was provided by its nucleotide and protein sequences, gene structure, and chromosomal localization.

A. Restricted Cellular Distribution of Authentic LTC_4 Synthase

LTC_4 synthase activity has been identified, in many cases with partial biochemical characterization, in human eosinophils (12), human and mouse mast cells (13,33), human platelets (34), and human monocytes/macrophages (35). Leukemic cell lines such as RBL-1 (25,36), KG-1 (37), human erythroleukemia cells (38), U-937 (39), THP-1 (40), and HL-60 (41) have LTC_4 synthase activity. Tissues of guinea pig lung (32,42), human lung (43), and rat kidney (44) contain the enzymatic function and in the case of human lung tissue, the immunoreactive protein (43). The function of this enzyme has also been found in cells that lack 5-LO, including platelets (34), endothelial cells (45), vascular smooth muscle cells (46), and synoviocytes (47). For these cells, a transcellular mechanism for LTC_4 generation has been proposed in which LTA_4 is supplied by vicinal cells.

B. Substrate Specificity, Kinetic Data, and Biochemical and Inhibitor Studies of LTC_4 Synthase

Further evidence that LTC_4 synthase differs from cytosolic and microsomal GSH S-transferases was based on a narrow substrate specificity, inability to conjugate GSH to xenobiotics, and differential susceptibility to inhibitors. The first report of a distinct bioactivity conjugating GSH to LTA_4 was a crude separation of particulate and soluble cellular fractions in which the particulate activity was more specific for LTA_4 than for 2,4-dinitrochlorobenzene and 2,3-dichloronitrobenzene (25). Subsequently, a highly substrate-specific LTC_4 synthase was partially purified from guinea pig lung (32,42) (Table 1). Furthermore, *N*-ethyl maleimide, which stimulates microsomal GSH S-transferase activity, inhibited the activity of LTC_4 synthase (25). Finally, specific non–cross-reacting antibodies to GSH S-transferases supported the separation of LTC_4 synthase from microsomal and cytosolic GSH S-transferases in various cells and tissues (39,40).

Initial kinetic studies with crude and partially purified preparations of LTC_4

Table 1 Substrate Specificities of LTC_4 Synthase and Cytosolic GSH S-Transferase

	LTC_4 synthase (guinea pig lung)		Cytosolic GSH S-transferase (rat liver)	
Substrate	V_{max} (nmol/min/mg)	K_m (μM)	V_{max} (nmol/min/mg)	K_m (μM)
LTA_3	16	4.3	n.d.	n.d.
LTA_4	36	3	270	280
LTA_5	18	2.6	n.d.	n.d.
LTA_4-methyl ester	140	16	570	31
14, 15-LTA_4	68	77	180	58
Chlorodinitrobenzene	0	Not functional as a substrate	620	n.d

Source: Ref. 32, 42.
n.d., not done.

synthase from guinea pig lung (32,42), platelets (34), and RBL-1 cells (36) yielded similar data, with K_m values of 7–36 μM for LTA_4 and 1.2–6 mM for GSH. Subsequent kinetic studies with LTC_4 synthase purified >10,000-fold from dimethyl sulfoxide (DMSO)-differentiated U-937 cells yielded K_m values for LTA_4 and GSH of 19.6 μM and 1.83 mM, respectively, with a V_{max} value of 2–4 μmol/min/mg (39). LTC_4 synthase purified to homogeneity from THP-1 cells provided K_m values for LTA_4 and GSH of 9.9 μM and 1.7 mM, respectively, with a V_{max} value of 4.1 μmol/min/mg (40). Crude human microsomal GSH S-transferase has a K_m of 41 μM for LTA_4 and most likely has a transcellular dependent disposal function for excess LTA_4 (31), which may be incidental to its central role as a detoxifying GSH S-transferase for xenobiotic-type substrates.

Because of the extreme lability of the function of the enzyme, especially in its purified form, many activity-preserving features were identified. The addition of up to 10 mM GSH to buffers containing LTC_4 synthase stabilized bioactivity during isolation and freeze-thawing cycles (39,42). Moreover, certain cations, such as Ca^{2+} and Mg^{2+}, stimulated LTC_4 synthase bioactivity, whereas Co^{2+} reduced activity (39).

C. Purification and N-Terminal Amino Acid Sequence of the LTC_4 Synthase Polypeptide

The purification of LTC_4 synthase was hindered because of the requirements of detergent extraction, its low abundance in cell lines, and its lability, especially in the purified state. Because the protein did not bind efficiently to polyvinylidene difluoride (PVDF) by electrophoretic transfer, LTC_4 synthase had to be purified to homogeneity for N-terminal amino acid sequencing, and then PVDF was immersed in the purified protein solution for passive adherence (40,43). Homogeneously purified human LTC_4 synthase was identified as an 18 kDa protein after isolation from 6×10^{10} human myelocytic KG-1 cells (37). This initial purification was performed with probenecid as a novel elution reagent for S-hexyl glutathione chromatography followed by native gel electrophoresis (37). An 18 kDa protein identified as LTC_4 synthase was also obtained by anion exchange chromatography, modified LTC_2 affinity chromatography, and gel-filtration chromatography of the solubilized microsomes from 2×10^{11} THP-1 cells (40).

Gel-filtration chromatography revealed that LTC_4 synthase appears to function as a homodimer. Enzymatic function was limited to column fractions filtering at a molecular mass of 36 kDa and exhibiting an 18 kDa protein by SDS-PAGE; fractions filtering at a predicted molecular mass of 18 kDa had no LTC_4 synthase bioactivity (40). Nicholson et al. (40) also obtained the first sequence of the N-terminal 35 amino acid residues of the LTC_4 synthase from THP-1 cells. LTC_4 synthase purified from human lung tissue or from KG-1 cells confirmed 19 of 20 residues from the N-terminal amino acid sequence and provided additional amino acid sequence in the KG-1 cell for 14 internal amino acid residues positioned at residues 35–48 (43).

D. Immunochemical Identity of LTC_4 Synthase

In support of the immunological identity of authentic LTC_4 synthase, the functional 18 kDa protein isolated from THP-1 cells and from DMSO-differentiated U-937 cells did not cross-react with antibodies against human microsomal GSH S-transferase and against human α, μ, and Pi class GSH S-transferases (40). A rabbit polyclonal LTC_4 synthase antibody raised against fully purified human lung LTC_4 synthase recognized an 18 kDa protein in immunoblot analysis of LTC_4 synthase purified from KG-1 cells, human lung tissue, and COS cells transfected with LTC_4 synthase cDNA, as well as from a platelet extract, indicating immunological identity (43). An 18 kDa protein was also identified in mouse bone marrow–derived mast cells and human cord blood–derived eosinophils during their cytokine regulation in culture (33,48). Immunohistochemical examination of sections of human lung tissue revealed the subcellular localization of human LTC_4 synthase in alveolar macrophages to be perinuclear (43). Subsequently, an antipeptide antibody developed against amino acid residues 37–51 of LTC_4 synthase was used to examine the appearance of LTC_4 synthase during the eosinophilic differentiation of HL-60 cells (49).

IV. Expression Cloning of the LTC_4 Synthase cDNA

The techniques of traditional molecular cloning were difficult to apply to LTC_4 synthase in light of the degeneracy of the nucleotides encoding the available N-

```
mGST II        MAGNSILLAAVSILSACQQSYFALQVGKARLKYKVTPPAVTGSPEF
LTC4 SYN   ----MKDEVALLAAVTLLGVLLQAYFSLQVISARRAFRVSPPLTTGPPEF
FLAP       MDQETVGNVVLLAIVTLISVVQNGFFAHKVEHESRTQNGRSFQRTGTLAF

mGST II    ERVFRAQQNCVEFYPIFIITLWMAGWYFNQVFATCLGLVYIYGRHLYFWG
LTC4 SYN   ERVYRAQVNCSEYFPLFLATLWVAGIFFHEGAAALCGLVYLFARLRYFQG
FLAP       ERVYTANQNCVDAYPTFLAVLWSAGLLCSQVPAAFAGLMYLFVRQKYFVG

mGST II    YSEAAKKRITGFRLSLGILALLTLLGALGIANSFLDEYLDLNIAKKLRRQ
LTC4 SYN   YARSAQLRLAPLYASARALWLLVALAALGLLAHFLPAALRAALLGRLRTL
FLAP       YLGERTQSTPGYIFGKRIILFLFLMSVAGIFNYYLIFFFGSDFENYIKTI

mGST II    F
LTC4 SYN   LPWA-------
FLAP       STTISPLLLIP
```

Figure 1 Comparison of the deduced amino acid sequences of human microsomal GSH S-transferase II (mGST II), LTC_4 synthase (LTC_4 SYN), and FLAP. The sequences of mGSH S-transferase II that are identical to those of LTC_4 synthase are in bold letters, and the sequences of FLAP that are identical to those of LTC_4 synthase are in bold italics.

terminal amino acid sequence. Thus, expression cloning was undertaken to provide a functional readout for isolation of the appropriate cDNA. The success of this approach required the development of a highly sensitive screening step with rapid throughput to assess the COS cells transfected with a KG-1 expression library. The initial screening employed a novel fluorescent-linked competitive immunoassay, sensitive to 2.5 pg of LTC_4, to identify clones conjugating added LTA_4 free acid (50). HPLC quantitation and identification of the enzymatic product LTC_4-methyl ester from LTA_4 methyl ester substrate detected positive transfectants in subsequent rounds of purification screening (50).

A positive clone was selected that contained a 694-bp cDNA insert. This cDNA had a 450-bp open reading frame; a 54-bp 5′ UTR; and within the 3′ UTR, an ATTAAA polyadenylylation signal (50). The deduced 150-amino-acid polypeptide sequence of LTC_4 synthase contains two potential protein kinase C phosphorylation sites (SAR sequences beginning with serine residues 28 and 111), a potential N-glycosylation site at asparagine 55, and two cysteine residues (C56 and C82)(50).

The nucleotide sequence of the cDNA and the deduced amino acid sequence of human LTC_4 synthase were not homologous with the corresponding sequences of any members of the families of the cytosolic, mitochondrial, or microsomal GSH S-transferases. The only significant homology identified in the analysis of the protein sequence was with FLAP (31% overall amino acid identity) (Fig. 1). The identity at the N-terminal two thirds of these proteins is 44% and includes the putative binding site for FLAP inhibitors (51). When the secondary structure analysis of deduced LTC_4 synthase polypeptide (Fig. 2) was compared to that of FLAP, the overlap was nearly identical for their three respective

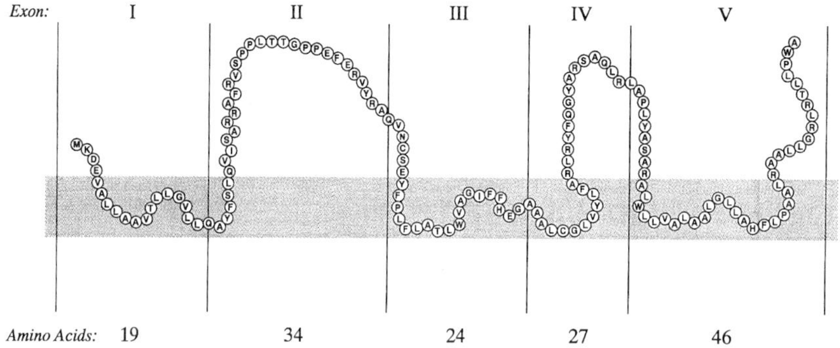

Figure 2 Schematic representation of the predicted secondary structure of LTC_4 synthase. The deduced 150-amino acid structure of LTC_4 synthase is shown with the hydrophobic domains putatively within a cellular membrane and interspersed with the two hydrophilic loops. The exon encoding for the respective amino acid residues is shown at the top. The number of amino acid residues per exon is shown at the bottom.

hydrophobic domains and two similar hydrophilic loops. A noteworthy difference is that LTC_4 synthase has more arginine residues in the hydrophilic loops. Because of the high degree of homology between LTC_4 synthase and FLAP, the effect of the FLAP inhibitor MK-886 was examined against human LTC_4 synthase. When incubated with COS cell microsomes from LTC_4 synthase transfectants, MK-886 exhibited an IC_{50} of 3 μM for LTC_4 synthase.

The cDNA for LTC_4 synthase was independently obtained by molecular cloning from a THP-1 cell library using a PCR product generated from primers deduced from the N-terminal and most C-terminal amino acid sequences available, with inosine in the positions with maximal degeneracy (52).

Recently, a third member of this novel gene family containing LTC_4 synthase and FLAP has been proposed, termed microsomal GSH S-transferase II. Microsomal GSH S-transferase II, also an 18 kDa integral membrane protein, shares 44% amino acid homology with LTC_4 synthase and 33% homology with FLAP (Fig. 1), but only 11% homology with human microsomal GSH S-transferase I (31). Microsomal GSH S-transferase II displays a unique dual function in conjugating reduced GSH to the xenobiotic 1-chloro-2,4-dinitrobenzene, as well as to LTA_4. Microsomal GSH S-transferase II also acts nonstereospecifically with LTA_4 to produce an isomer of LTC_4 and is not inhibited by N-ethylmaleimide, unlike authentic LTC_4 synthase (31). Hydropathy plotting of the sequence of microsomal GSH S-transferase II demonstrates secondary structural characteristics similar to those of LTC_4 synthase and FLAP, and the three hydropathy plots essentially overlap (31). The distribution of the mRNA for microsomal GSH

S-transferase II is not restricted to cells relevant to the inflammatory response as is that of LTC_4 synthase; but instead the transcript is predominant in the liver, suggesting a primary role as a detoxifying GSH S-transferase (31).

Molecular cloning of the cDNA for mouse LTC_4 synthase allowed assessment of the degree of conservation in a second species. A cDNA was isolated from a mouse expression library after screening with oligonucleotides based on the human LTC_4 synthase cDNA (53). The mouse cDNA encodes for a 150-amino-acid residue polypeptide and is 88% identical to the human sequence. There are 18 amino acid residue differences, of which half are located in the carboxyl terminus. The potential protein kinase C phosphorylation sites, an N-glycosylation site, and the two cysteine residues are completely conserved when compared to the human sequence (53). To investigate the implications of the conserved regions of the two species of LTC_4 synthase, kinetic studies were undertaken with fully purified recombinant enzyme from both sources.

V. Biochemical Properties of Purified Human and Mouse Recombinant LTC_4 Synthase

The data from the kinetic analyses of fully purified recombinant human and mouse LTC_4 synthases were essentially the same (Table 2) (53). These results show that the 13% difference in amino acid residues does not significantly affect enzymatic function. Furthermore, as 9 of the 18 amino acid substitutions occur in the carboxyl tail, this portion of LTC_4 synthase may not be important for enzymatic function.

In both the human and the mouse, the region of LTC_4 synthase that contains

Table 2 Comparison of Kinetic Data for Purified Recombinant Mouse and Human LTC_4 Synthases

		Recombinant LTC_4 synthase	
		Mouse	Human
K_m (μM)	LTA_4 free acid	2.5	3.6
	LTA_4 methyl ester	10.3	7.6
	GSH	1900.0	1600.0
V_{max} (μmol/min/mg protein)	LTA_4 free acid	1.2	1.3
	LTA_4 methyl ester	2.3	2.5
	GSH	2.2	2.7
IC_{50} (μM)	(for MK-886)	2.7	3.1

Source: Ref. 53.

the putative FLAP-like inhibitor binding domain (amino acid residues 41–62) is located in the carboxyl terminus of the first hydrophilic loop. There were only two modifications in this domain in mouse LTC_4 synthase: substitutions of a serine for threonine at position 41 and a phenylalanine for tyrosine at position 50. To determine whether these differences alter the effect of the FLAP inhibitor, microsomes of COS cells transfected with either human or mouse LTC_4 synthase cDNA were assayed for LTC_4 synthase in the presence of various concentrations of MK-886 (Table 2). MK-886 displayed similar levels of inhibition in a dose-related manner with both recombinant human and mouse LTC_4, thereby further excluding T41 and Y50 as critical residues involved in enzymatic function.

VI. Genomic Organization, Regulatory Elements, and Chromosomal Localization of the Human LTC_4 Synthase Gene

The regulation of LTC_4 synthase activity had been examined before the probes necessary to actually study the expression of the gene in terms of transcript and protein became available. The first of these studies in human erythroleukemia (HEL) cells revealed up to 10-fold induction of LTC_4 synthase activity in response to a variety of agonists including TPA, retinoic acid, vitamin D_3, and to a lesser degree DMSO (38). The LTC_4 synthase activity of RBL-1 cells has also been induced 5- to 10-fold with retinoic acid (54). The activation of protein kinase C by phorbol 12-myristate 13-acetate (PMA) treatment of HEL cells (38), platelets (55), and HL-60 and U-937 cells (56) induces LTC_4 synthase activity.

To examine the regulatory mechanisms more specifically and to seek polymorphisms, the gene for human LTC_4 synthase was cloned and its organization and chromosomal localization were determined. With oligonucleotides specific for the human LTC_4 synthase cDNA sequence, a P1 library was screened and a clone was identified that contained the human LTC_4 synthase gene (57). Restriction digests of this fragment probed with the 5′ and 3′ ends of the cDNA for LTC_4 synthase revealed that a 5.5 kb Sac I fragment contained the entire gene. Sequencing of the Sac I-digested fragment revealed a 2.51 kb gene containing 5 exons and 4 introns. The exon sizes are small (71–257 nucleotides) and are interspersed with relatively small introns (Fig. 3). This structure contrasts greatly with the gene size of the nearest homologous family member, FLAP, which is >31 kb (58). Despite the size discrepancy, the exons of the gene for LTC_4 synthase are identical in size to those of FLAP with the exception of the 5′ and 3′ untranslated regions of the first and fifth exons (Fig. 3). Thus, the exons of LTC_4 synthase and FLAP align identically with regard to the amino acids that they encode. The identical intron/exon organization of LTC_4 synthase and FLAP sug-

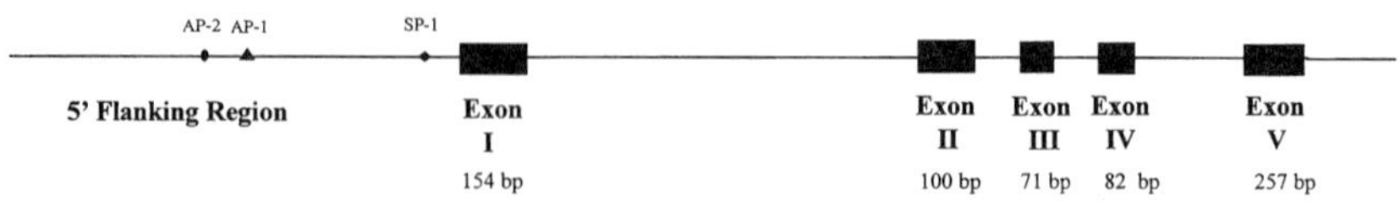

Figure 3 The intron/exon gene structure for LTC_4 synthase. 1.44 kb of the 5′ flanking region is shown with the location of the consensus sequences for AP-2, AP-1, and SP-1 sites. The exons are shown in boxes with exact exon sizes indicated.

gests the evolution of these two molecules from a process termed gene duplication (59).

5′ Extension analysis of the mRNA from KG-1 cells or from in vitro–derived eosinophils revealed three putative transcription initiation sites for the human LTC_4 synthase gene located 66, 69, and 96 nucleotides upstream of the ATG translation start site (57). When THP-1 cell RNA was examined by the same method, a single transcription initiation site was found 78 nucleotides upstream of the ATG translation start site (60).

The nucleotide sequence of 1.44 kb of 5′ flanking region of the human LTC_4 synthase gene contains the typical features of genes with multiple transcription initiation sites: a high G/C content and at least one consensus sequence (GGGCGG) for SP-1 binding, of which the first is located 24 nucleotides upstream of the first transcription start site. SP-1 is a ubiquitous transcription factor identified in many housekeeping genes (61). In addition, consensus sequences for an AP-1 site (TGAFTCAG) (62) and an AP-2 site (TCCCCCTCCC) (63) were identified 807 and 877 nucleotides 5′ of the first transcription initiation site (57,60) (Fig. 3). The presence of these elements is consistent with reports that LTC_4 synthase activity is upregulated in RBL-1 cells, HEL cells, platelets, and HL-60 cells by treatment with phorbol myristate acetate (38,55,56).

In the human FLAP gene, single a transcription initiation site resides in an A residue 74 nucleotides upstream from the ATG start codon, and a modified TATA box sequence has been identified (58). The human microsomal GSH S-transferase II genomic structure has not been characterized, nor have any regulatory agonists been defined.

Fluorescent in situ hybridization with the P1 plasmid containing LTC_4 synthase revealed that the gene is located on chromosome 5. Specific measurements demonstrated that this clone is localized at a position 98–99% of the distance from the centromere of chromosome arm 5q, corresponding to band 5q35 (57,60). In contrast to the human LTC_4 synthase gene, fluorescence in situ hybridization for the FLAP gene revealed its localization to the long arm of chromosome 13. The human microsomal GSH S-transferase II resides on chromosome 4 (31).

The long arm of the fifth chromosome is the site at which many of the

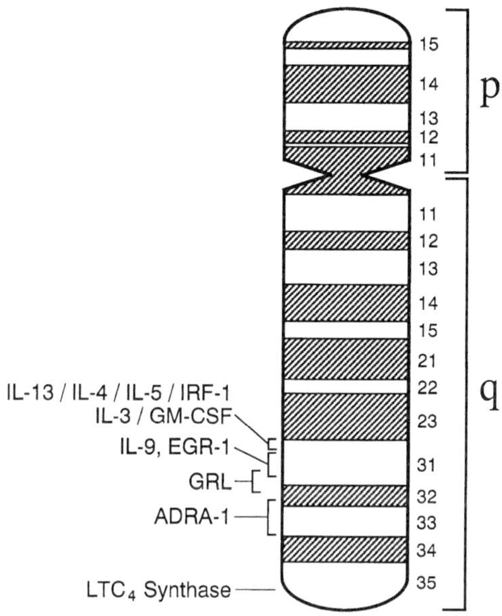

Figure 4 Partial map of human chromosome 5. The regions of the chromosome that encode molecules relevant to asthmatic inflammation are noted. IRF-1, Interferon regulatory factor-1; GM-CSF, granulocyte/macrophage colony-stimulating factor; EGR-1, early growth response-1; GRL, glucocorticoid receptor; ADRB-2, β_2-adrenergic receptor.

genes encoding growth factors, cytokines, and receptors (64–67) relating to the asthmatic phenotype are localized (Fig. 4). A portion of the inflammatory response in bronchial asthma originates with activated TH2 cells. The profile of cytokines produced by the TH2 phenotype includes IL-4, which is essential to the switch of B-cell immunoglobulin production to isotype IgE. Additional cytokines encoded from the cluster of genes on 5q include IL-3, IL-5, and granulocyte/macrophage colony-stimulating factor, which regulate eosinophilopoiesis and convert eosinophils to an aggressive phenotype associated with increased survival and augmented function including LTC_4 generation (68–70). In addition to the chromosomal localization of these cytokine genes, which amplify and perpetuate allergic inflammation, there is also genetic linkage evidence of these regions of human chromosome 5 to atopy and asthmatic states (71,72).

VII. Summary

Leukotriene C_4 synthase is the pivotal, committed enzyme involved in the formation of cysteinyl leukotrienes. Authentic LTC_4 synthase is an 18 kDa integral perinuclear membrane enzyme that conjugates reduced glutathione only with LTA_4. This protein is found in a hematopoietically restricted cellular distribution, with the complete biosynthetic pathway for cysteinyl leukotrienes appearing limited to mast cells, eosinophils, basophils, and monocytes. The kinetics of LTC_4 synthase have been determined for the isolated natural or recombinant proteins, and the protein is functional as a homodimer. The cDNA encodes a 150-amino-acid polypeptide monomer with three hydrophobic domains interspersed with two hydrophilic loops. The deduced amino acid sequence of LTC_4 synthase contains two potential protein kinase C phosphorylation sites, a potential N-glycosylation site, and two cysteine residues. The 2.51 kb gene for LTC_4 contains five small exons and four introns. The 5′ UTR contains consensus sequences for an AP-1 and AP-2 site as well as an SP-1 site. The gene for LTC_4 synthase is located on band q35 of chromosome 5, distal to that of cytokine, growth factor, and receptor genes that are relevant to the development of allergic inflammation, including those controlling and representing the TH2 phenotype.

The chromosomal positioning of the LTC_4 synthase gene and its pivotal biosynthetic function in the formation of the cysteinyl leukotrienes make the gene for human LTC_4 synthase a candidate gene for asthma, with regard to both disease severity and disease management. LTC_4 synthase, FLAP, and a recently recognized type II microsomal GSH S-transferase appear to be members of a novel gene family. These molecules are each 18 kDa integral membrane proteins involved in cysteinyl leukotriene biosynthesis with significant homology at the nucleotide and amino acid levels. Their evolutionary divergence is evident, however, in the differences in intron sizes and 5′ regulatory elements of LTC_4 synthase and FLAP and the separate chromosomal localization of each.

References

1. Kellaway CH, Trethewie WR. The liberation of a slow reacting smooth muscle-stimulating substance in anaphylaxis. Q J Exp Physiol 1940; 30:121–145.
2. Brocklehurst WE. Occurrence of an unidentified substance during anaphylactic shock in cavy lung. J Physiol 1953; 120:16–17.
3. Brocklehurst WE. The release of histamine and formation of slow-reacting substance (SRS-A) during anaphylactic shock. J Physiol 1960; 151:416–435.
4. Lewis RA, Wasserman SI, Goetzl EJ, Austen KF. Formation of slow-reacting substance of anaphylaxis in human lung tissue and cells before release. J Exp Med 1974; 140:113–1146.
5. Murphy RC, Hammarstrom S, Samuelsson B. Leukotriene C: a slow reacting substance from murine mastocytoma cells. Proc Natl Acad Aci USA 1979; 76:4275–4279.
6. Lewis RA, Drazen JM, Austen KF, Clark DA, Corey EJ. Identification of the c(6)-S-conjugate of leukotriene A with cysteine as naturally occurring slow reacting sub-

stance of anaphylaxis (SRS-A). Importance of the 11-cis-geometry for biological activity. Biochem Biophys Res Commun 1980; 96:271–277.

7. Lewis RA, Austen KF, Drazen JM, Clark DA, Marfat A, Corey EJ. Slow reacting substances of anaphylaxis: Identification of leukotrienes C-1 and D from human and rat sources. Proc Natl Acad Sci USA 1980; 73:3710–3714.
8. Dahlen S-E, Bjork J, Hedqvist P, Arfors KE, Hammarstrom S, Lindgren JA, Samuelsson B. Leukotriene promotes plasma leakage and leukocyte adherence in post capillary venules: in vivo effects with relevance to the acute inflammatory response. Proc Natl Acad Sci USA 1981; 78:3887–3891.
9. Soter NA, Lewis RA, Corey EJ, Austen KF. Local effects of synthetic leukotrienes (LTC_4, LTD_4, and LTB_4) in human skin. J. Invest Derm 1983; 80:115–119.
10. Dahlen S-E, Hedqvist P, Hammarstrom S, Samuelsson B. Leukotrienes are potent constrictors of human bronchi. Nature 1981; 268:484–486.
11. Marom Z, Shelhamer JH, Bach MR, Morton DR, Kaliner M. Slow-reacting substances, leukotrienes C_4 and D_4, increase the release of mucus from human airways in vitro. Am Rev Respir Dis 1982; 126:449–451.
12. Weller PF, Lee CW, Foster DW, Corey EF, Austen KF, Lewis RA. Generation and metabolism of 5-lipoxygenase pathway leukotrienes by human eosinophils: predominant production of leukotriene C_4. Proc Natl Acad Sci USA 1983; 80:7626–7630.
13. MacGlashan DW Jr, Schleimer RP, Peters SP, Schulman ES, Adams GK III, Newball NH, Lichtenstein LM. Generation of leukotrienes by purified human lung mast cells. J Clin Invest 1982; 70:747–751.
14. Taylor GW, Taylor I, Black P, Maltby NH, Turner N, Fuller RW, Dollery CT. Urinary leukotriene E_4 after antigen challenge and in acute asthma and allergic rhinitis. Lancet 1989; 1:584–588.
15. Smith CM, Christie PE, Hawksworth RJ, Thien F, Lee TH. Urinary leukotriene E_4 levels after allergen and exercise challenge in bronchial asthma. Am Rev Respir Dis 1991; 144:1411–1412.
16. Israel E, Rubin P, Kemp JP, Grossman J, Pierson W, Siegel SC, Tinkelman D, Murray JJ, Busse W, Segal AT, Fish J, Kaiser HB, Ledford D, Wenzel S, Rosenthal R, Cohn J, Lanni C, Pearlman H, Karahalios P, Drazen JM. The effect of inhibition of 5-lipoxygenase by zileuton in mild-to-moderate asthma. Ann Intern Med 1993; 119: 1059–1066.
17. Gaddy J, Margolskee D, Bush RK, Williams VC, Busse W. Bronchodilatation with a potent and selective leukotriene D_4 (LTD_4) receptor antagonist (MK-571) in patients with asthma. Am Rev Respir Dis 1992; 46:358–363.
18. Manning PJ, Watson RM, Margolskee DJ, Williams VC, Schwartz JI, O'Byrne PM. Inhibition of exercise-induced bronchoconstriction by MK-571, a potent leukotriene D_4 antagonist. N Engl J Med 1990; 232:1736–1739.
19. Christie PE, Smith CM, Lee TH. The potent and selective sulfidopeptide leukotriene antagonist SK&F 104353 inhibits aspirin-induced asthma. Am Rev Respir Dis 1991; 144:957–958.
20. Clark JD, Lin LL, Kriz RW, Ramesha CS, Sultzman LA, Lin AY, Milona N, Knopf JL. A novel arachidonic acid-selective cytosolic phospholipase A_2 contains a Ca^{2+}-dependent translocation domain with homology to PKC and GAP. Cell 1991; 65: 1043–1051.

21. Rouzer CA, Kargman S. Translocation of 5-lipoxygenase to the membrane in human leukocytes challenged with ionophore A23187. J Biol Chem 1988; 263:10980–10988.
22. Abramovitz M, Wong E, Cox ME, Richardson CD, Li C, Vickers PJ. 5-Lipoxygenase-activating protein stimulates the utilization of arachidonic acid by 5-lipoxygenase. Eur J Biochem 1993; 215:105–111.
23. Brock TG, Paine R III, Peters-Golden M. Localization of 5-lipoxygenase to the nucleus of unstimulated rat basophilic leukemic cells. J Biol Chem 1994; 269:22059–22066.
24. Rouzer CA, Matsumoto T, Samuelsson B. Single protein from human leukocytes possesses 5-lipoxygenase and leukotriene A_4 synthase activities. Proc Natl Acad Sci USA 1986; 83:857–861.
25. Bach MK, Brashler JR, Morton DR. Solubilization and characterization of the leukotriene C_4 synthetase of rat basophil leukemia cells: a novel, particulate glutathione S-transferase. Arch Biochem Biophys 1984; 230:455–465.
26. Lam BK, Owen WF Jr, Austen KF, Soberman RJ. The identification of a distinct export step following the biosynthesis of leukotriene C_4 by human eosinophils. J Biol Chem 1989; 264:12885–12889.
27. Lam BK, Owen WF Jr, Austen KF, Soberman RJ. Leukotriene C_4 uses a probenecid-sensitive export carrier that does not recognize leukotriene B_4. Proc Natl Acad Sci USA 1989; 89:11598–11602.
28. Anderson ME, Allison RD, Meister A. Interconversion of leukotrienes catalyzed by purified gamma-glutamyl transpeptidase: concomitant formation of leukotriene D_4 gamma-glutamyl amino acid. Proc Natl Acad Sci USA 1982; 79:1088–1091.
29. Lee CW, Lewis RA, Corey EJ, Austen KF. Conversion of leukotriene D_4 to leukotriene E_4 by a dipeptidase released from the specific granules of human polymorphonuclear leukocytes. Immunology 1983; 48:27–35.
30. Tsuchida S, Izumi T, Shimizu T, Ishikawa T, Hatayama I, Sato K. Purification of a new acidic glutathione S-transferase, GST Yn1-Yn1, with high leukotriene C_4 synthase activity from rat brain. Eur J Biochem 1987; 170:159–164.
31. Jakobsson P-J, Mancini JA, Ford-Hutchinson AW. Identification and characterization of a novel human microsomal glutathione S-transferase with leukotriene C_4 synthase activity and significant sequence identity to 5-lipoxygenase-activating protein and leukotriene C_4 synthase. J Biol Chem 1996; 271:22203–22210.
32. Yoshimoto T, Soberman RJ, Spur B, Austen KF. Properties of highly purified leukotriene C_4 synthase of guinea pig lung. J Clin Invest 1988; 81:866–871.
33. Murakami M, Austen KF, Bingham CO III, Friend DS, Penrose JF, Arm JP. Interleukin-3 regulates development of the 5-lipoxygenase/leukotriene C_4 synthase pathway in mouse mast cells. J Biol Chem 1995; 270:22653–22656.
34. Soderstrom M, Mannervik B, Garkov V, Hammarstrom S. On the nature of LTC_4 synthase in human platelets. Arch Biochim Biophys 1992; 294:70–74.
35. Williams JD, Czop JK, Austen KF. Release of leukotrienes by human monocytes on stimulation of their phagocytic receptor for particulate activators. J Immunol 1984; 132:3034–3040.
36. Yoshimoto T, Soberman RJ, Lewis RA, Austen KF. Isolation and characterization

of leukotriene C_4 synthase of rat basophilic leukemia cells. Proc Natl Acad Sci USA 1985; 82:8399–8403.
37. Penrose JF, Gagnon L, Goppelt-Struebe M, Meyer P, Lam B, Jack R, Austen KF, Soberman RJ. Purification of human leukotriene C_4 synthase. Proc Natl Acad Sci USA 1992; 89:11603–11606.
38. Soderstrom M, Bolling A, Hammarstrom S. Induction of leukotriene C_4 synthase activity in differentiating human erythroleukemia cells. Biochem Biophys Res Commun 1992; 189:1043–1049.
39. Nicholson DW, Klemba MW, Rasper DM, Metters KM, Zamboni RJ, Ford-Hutchinson AW. Purification of human leukotriene C_4 synthase from dimethylsulfoxide-differentiated U937 cells. Eur J Biochem 1992; 209:725–734.
40. Nicholson DW, Ali A, Vaillancourt JP, Calycay JR, Mumford RA, Zamboni RJ, Ford-Hutchinson AW. Purification to homogeneity and the N-terminal sequence of human leukotriene C_4 synthase: a homodimeric glutathione S-transferase composed of 18-kDa subunits. Proc Natl Acad Sci USA 1993; 90:2015–2019.
41. Ali A, Ford-Hutchinson AW, Nicholson DW. Activation of protein kinase C down-regulates leukotriene C_4 synthase activity and attenuates cysteinyl leukotriene production in an eosinophilic substrain of HL-60 cells. J Immunol 1994; 153:776–788.
42. Izumi T, Honda Z, Ohishi N, Kitamura S, Tsuchida S, Sato K, Shimizu T, Seyama Y. Solubilization and partial purification of leukotriene C_4 synthase from guinea-pig lung: a microsomal enzyme with high specificity towards 5,6-epoxide leukotriene A_4. Biochim Biophys Acta 1988; 959:305–315.
43. Penrose JF, Spector J, Lam BK, Friend DS, Xu K, Jack RM, Austen KF. Purification of human lung leukotriene C_4 synthase and preparation of a polyclonal antibody. Am J Respir Crit Care Med 1995; 152:283–289.
44. Petric R, Hutchinson DW, Ford-Hutchinson DW. Renal leukotriene C_4 synthase: characterization, partial purification and alterations in experimental glomerulonephritis. Biochim Biophys Acta 1995; 1254:207–215.
45. Feinmark SJ, Cannon PJ. Endothelial cell leukotriene C_4 synthesis results from transfer of leukotriene A_4 synthesized by polymorphonuclear leukocytes. J Biol Chem 1986; 261:16466–16472.
46. Feinmark SJ, Cannon PJ. Vascular smooth muscle leukotriene C_4 synthesis: requirement for transcellular leukotriene A_4 metabolism. Biochim Biophys Acta 1987; 92: 125–135.
47. Wittenberg RH, Willburger RE, Kleemeyer KS, Peskar BA. In vitro release of prostaglandins and leukotrienes from synovial tissue, cartilage, and bone in degenerative joint diseases. Arthritis Rheum 1993; 10:1444–1450.
48. Boyce JA, Lam BK, Penrose JF, Friend DS, Parsons S, Owen WF, Austen KF. Expression of LTC_4 synthase during the development of eosinophils in vitro from cord blood progenitors. Blood 1996; 88:4338–4347.
49. Scoggan DA, Nicholson DW, Ford-Hutchinson AW. Regulation of leukotriene-biosynthetic enzymes during differentiation of myelocytic HL-60 cells to eosinophilic or neutrophilic cells. Eur J Biochem 1996; 239:572–578.
50. Lam BK, Penrose JF, Freeman GJ, Austen KF. Expression cloning of a cDNA for human leukotriene C_4 synthase, an integral membrane protein conjugating reduced glutathione to leukotriene A_4. Proc Natl Acad Sci USA 1994; 91:7663–7667.

51. Vickers PJ, Adam M, Charleson S, Coppolino MG, Evans JF, Mancini JA. Indentification of amino acid residues of 5-lipoxygenase-activating protein essential for the binding of leukotriene biosynthesis inhibitors. Mol Pharmacol 1992; 42:94–102.
52. Welsch DJ, Creely DP, Hauser SD, Mathis KJ, Krivi GG, Isakson PC. Molecular cloning and expression of human leukotriene C_4 synthase. Proc Natl Acad Sci USA 1994; 91:9745–9749.
53. Lam BK, Penrose JF, Rokach J, Xu K, Baldasaro MH, Austen KF. Molecular cloning, expression and characterization of mouse leukotriene C_4 synthase. Eur J Biochem 1996; 238:606–612.
54. Hamasaki Y, Abe M, Matsumoto S, Ichimaru T, Hara N, Miyazaki S. Specific induction of LTC_4 synthase by retinoic acid in rat basophilic leukemia-1 cells. Int Arch Allergy Immunol 1994; 103:260–265.
55. Tornhamre S, Edenius C, Lindgren JA. Receptor mediated regulation of leukotriene C_4 synthase activity in human platelets. Eur J Biochem 1996; 243:513–520.
56. Nicholson DW, Ali A, Klemba MW, Munday NA, Zamboni RJ, Ford-Hutchinson AW. Human leukotriene C_4 synthase expression in dimethyl sulfoxide-differentiated U-937 cells. J Biol Chem 1992; 267:725–734.
57. Penrose JF, Spector JS, Baldasaro M, Xu K, Boyce J, Arm JP, Austen KF, Lam BK. Molecular cloning of the gene for human leukotriene C_4 synthase: organization, nucleotide sequence, and chromosomal localization to 5q35. J Biol Chem 1996; 271: 11356–11361.
58. Kennedy BP, Diehl RE, Boie Y, Adam M, Dixon RAF. Gene characterization and promotor analysis of the human 5-lipoxygenase-activating protein (FLAP). J Biol Chem 1991; 266:8511–8516.
59. Kersanach R, Brinkmann H, Liaud M-F, Zhang D-X, Martin W, Cerff R. Five identical intron positions in ancient duplicated genes of eubacterial origin. Nature 1994; 367:387–389.
60. Bigby TD, Hodulik CR, Arden KC, Fu L. Molecular cloning of the human leukotriene C_4 synthase gene and assignment to chromosome 5q35. Mol Med 1996; 2: 637–646.
61. Smale S. Core promotor architecture for eukaryocytic protein-coding genes. In: Conaway RC, Conaway JW, eds. Transcription: Mechanism and Regulation. New York: Raven Press, 1994:63–81.
62. Angel P, Imagawa M, Chiu R, Stein B, Imbra RJ, Rahmsdork HJ, Jonat C, Herrlich P, Darin M. Phorbol ester-inducible genes contain a common cis element recognized by a TPA-modulated trans-acting factor. Cell 1987; 49:729–739.
63. Imagawa M, Chie R, Darin M. Transcription factor AP-2 mediates induction by two different signal-transduction pathways: protein kinase C and cAMP. Cell 1987; 51: 251–260.
64. Marsh DG, Neely JD, Breazeale DR, Ghosh B, Freidhoff LR, Ehrlich-Kautzky E, Schou C, Krishnaswamy G, Beaty TH. Linkage analysis of IL4 and other chromosome 5q31.1 markers and total serum immunoglobulin E concentration. Science 1994; 264:1152–1156.
65. van Leeuwen BH, Martinson ME, Wevv GC, Young IG. Molecular organization of the cytokine gene cluster, involving the human IL-3, IL-4, IL-5, and GM-CSF genes, on human chromosome 5. Blood 1989; 73:1142–1148.

66. Kobilka BK, Dixon RAF, Frielle T, Dohlman HHG, Bolanowski MA, Sigal IS, Yang-Feng TL, Francke U, Caron MG, Lefkowitz RJ. cDNA for the human B2-adrenergic receptor: a protein with multiple membrane-spanning domains and encoded by a gene whose chromosomal location is shared with that of the receptor for platelet derived growth factor. Proc Natl Acad Sci USA 1987; 84:46–50.
67. Wasmuth JJ, Bishop DT, Westbrook CA. Report of the committee on the genetic constitution of chromosome 5. Cytogenet Cell Genet 1991; 58:261–194.
68. Rothenberg ME, Petersen J, Stevens RL, Silberstein DS, McKenzie DT, Austen KF, Owen WF. IL-5 dependent conversion of normodense eosinophils to the hypodense phenotype uses 3T3 fibroblasts for enhanced viability, accelerated hypodensity, and sustained antibody dependent cytotoxicity. J Immunol 1989; 143:2311–2316.
69. Rothenberg ME, Owen WF, Silberstein DS, Woods J, Soberman RJ, Austen KF, Stevens RL. Human eosinophils have prolonged survival, enhanced function, and become hypodense when exposed to human interleukin 3. J Clin Invest 1988; 81: 1986–1992.
70. Boyce JA, Friend DS, Gurish MF, Austen KF, Owen WF. Differentiation in vitro of hybrid eosinophil/basophil granulocytes: autocrine function of an eosinophil developmental intermediate. J Exp Med 1995; 182:49–57.
71. Rosenwasser LJ, Klemm DJ, Dresback JK, Inamura H, Mascali JJ, Klinnert M, Borish L. Promotor polymorphisms in the chromosome 5 gene cluster in asthma and atopy. Clin Exp Allergy 1995; 25:74–78.
72. Postma DS, Bleecker ER, Amelung PJ, Holroyd KJ, Xu J, Panhuysen CIM, Meyers DA, Levitt RC. Genetic susceptibility to asthma: coinheritance of bronchial hyperresponsiveness with a major gene for atopy. N Engl J Med 1995; 333:894–900.

4

Leukotriene A_4 Hydrolase

JESPER Z. HAEGGSTRÖM

Karolinska Institutet
Stockholm, Sweden

Leukotrienes are recognized as important chemical mediators in a variety of allergic and inflammatory conditions including those affecting the respiratory system. Considering asthma, most of the scientific interest has been focused on the cysteinyl-containing leukotrienes, which can elicit virtually all signs and symptoms of this disease. However, leukotriene (LT) B_4, one of the most powerful chemotactic agents known to data, also seems to play a role in the pathogenesis of asthma, particularly in the recruitment of inflammatory cells into the lung. This chapter reviews the biochemistry and molecular biology of LTA_4 hydrolase, the enzyme catalyzing the final step in the biosynthesis of LTB_4.

I. LTA_4 Hydrolase as a Distal Enzyme in the 5-Lipoxygenase Pathway

In the biosynthesis of leukotrienes, free arachidonic acid is converted into 5(*S*)-hydroperoxy-8,11,14-*cis*-6-*trans*-eicosatetraenoic acid (5-HPETE), which is further dehydrated into 5(*S*)-*trans*-5,6-oxido-7,9-*trans*-11,14-*cis*-eicosatetraenoic acid (LTA_4), in two consecutive reactions catalyzed by 5-lipoxygenase. LTA_4 is then stereoselectively hydrolyzed, by LTA_4 hydrolase, into 5(*S*),12(*R*)-dihydroxy-6,14-*cis*-8,10-*trans*-eicosatetraenoic acid (LTB_4) (1). Alternatively, LTA_4 may be conjugated with glutathione, by a specific GSH-transferase, to produce 5(*S*)-hydroxy-6(*R*)-S-glutathionyl-7,9-*trans*-11,14-*cis*-eicosatetraenoic acid (LTC_4). Hence, LTA_4 hydrolase catalyzes the most distal step in the biosynthetic pathway leading to the proinflammatory compound LTB_4 (Fig. 1). In the following, the conversion of LTA_4 into LTB_4 will be referred to as the enzyme's epoxide hydrolase activity.

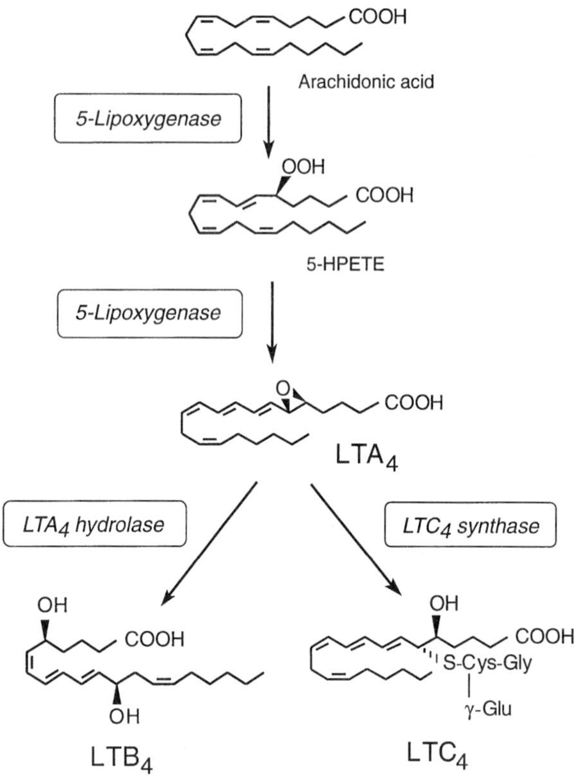

Figure 1 Metabolism of arachidonic acid into leukotrienes. The scheme depicts the key enzymes and intermediates in the biosynthesis of LTB_4 and LTC_4 from arachidonic acid.

II. Purification and Basal Properties of LTA_4 Hydrolase

LTA_4 hydrolase has been purified from a variety of sources as a soluble monomeric protein with a molecular weight of about 70 kDa, and no evidence for posttranslational modification has yet been presented (2–9). It exhibits a narrow substrate specificity and besides LTA_4, the double bond isomers LTA_3 and LTA_5 are the only other accepted substrates known to date (5,10,11). Moreover, all of these leukotriene epoxides inactivate LTA_4 hydrolase during catalysis, a phenomenon referred to as suicide inactivation (4,10). For molecular properties of LTA_4 hydrolase, see Table 1.

Table 1 Molecular Properties of Human Leukotriene A_4 Hydrolase

Subcellular compartment:	Soluble
Protein size (no. of amino acids[a]):	610
Calculated Mw:	69 153 Da[b]
Posttranslational modifications:	No[c]
Isoelectric point:	5.0–5.7
Prosthetic group:	Zinc[d]
Zinc-binding ligands:	His-295, His-299, Glu-318
Putative catalytic residues:	Glu-296, Tyr-383
Gene size:	>35 kbp
Exon no:	19
Putative *cis* elements of promoter region:	XRE, AP2
Chromosomal location:	12q22

[a]Initial methionine excluded.
[b]Computer-assisted calculation.
[c]No known modifications.
[d]1 mol zinc/mol protein.
Source: Refs. 2, 4, 8, 26, 27, 33, 36, 37, 61, 62, 64, 65.

III. Cellular and Subcellular Localization

In all species investigated thus far, LTA_4 hydrolase has been widely spread among organs, tissues, and individual cell types (12). Studies in guinea pig, rat, and human have shown that the enzyme is particularly abundant in the intestine, spleen, lung, and kidney. Also, it was recently reported that *Xenopus laevis* express high levels of LTA_4 hydrolase activity in the reproductive organs (13). In blood, neutrophils, monocytes, lymphocytes, and erythrocytes are rich sources of LTA_4 hydrolase (14–16). In contrast, eosinophils have low levels, and basophils and platelets seem to be virtually devoid of the enzyme (17–19). With respect to the lung, epithelial cells and alveolar macrophages appear to express high levels of LTA_4 hydrolase, whereas mast cells seem to have small amounts of the enzyme (20–23). Considering the fact that leukotriene biosynthesis is generally regarded as a process restricted to the white blood cells and bone marrow, the broad distribution of LTA_4 hydrolase has been difficult to rationalize from a functional point of view. One explanation has been so called transcellular biosynthesis, a phenomenon in which a given intermediate is exported from a donor cell to a recipient cell for further metabolism (see below).

The subcellular localization of LTA_4 hydrolase has never been carefully investigated. It is generally assumed that the activity resides in the cytosol, although in one study, a membrane-bound activity was reported (24). Thus, specific organelles such as nuclei, mitochondria, or peroxisomes have seldom, if ever, been examined as potential sources of a soluble enzyme activity. However, in a recent study by Woods et al., no significant amount of LTA_4 hydrolase immunoreactivity was detected in nuclear fractions of resting human alveolar macrophages, as judged by Western blot analysis (25).

IV. Molecular Cloning, Amino Acid Sequence, and Gene Structure of LTA_4 Hydrolase

A complementary DNA encoding human LTA_4 hydrolase was cloned and sequenced almost a decade ago (26,27). The open reading frame consists of 1833 nucleotides corresponding to 610 amino acids, excluding the first methionine, with a calculated molecular mass of about 69, 153 daltons, in good agreement with early results obtained by SDS-PAGE (Table 1). The deduced amino acid sequence was unique and different from other known epoxide hydrolases. LTA_4 hydrolase has also been cloned from mouse spleen, rat mesangial cells, and guinea pig lung (28–30). The primary structures of the human, mouse, rat, and guinea pig enzymes show a high degree of homology with >90% identity at the amino acid level. For the mouse enzyme, six sites of polymorphism were detected, one of which caused an amino acid change, namely, a conservative shift between an Arg and Lys in position 592. Active recombinant LTA_4 hydrolases have been expressed in *E. coli*, COS-7 cells, and in an insect cell/baculovirus system (28,29,31,32).

The complete gene structure of human LTA_4 hydrolase, including exon/intron organization and approximately 4 kbp of 5′-flanking sequence, was recently reported (33). The gene is >35 kbp, exists in a single copy, and contains 19 exons ranging in size from 24 to 312 bp (Fig. 2). Using fluorescence in situ hybridization, the gene was mapped to chromosome 12q22. The putative promoter region (approx. 4 kbp upstream of the transcription initiation site) contained a phorbol-ester response element (AP2) and two xenobiotic-response elements (XRE) but no definitive TATA box (see Table 1).

V. LTA_4 Hydrolase and the Family of Zinc Metallohydrolases

Cloning and sequencing of rat kidney aminopeptidase M led to the finding that LTA_4 hydrolase exhibits a weak similarity to this enzyme and several other zinc-containing proteases and peptidases (34). The sequence similarity was stronger over a short peptide region encompassing a consensus sequence for a zinc binding site (Fig. 3). Such a motif is characterized by a pentapeptide with the sequence HEXXH in which the histidines are the two zinc-binding ligands. The motif in

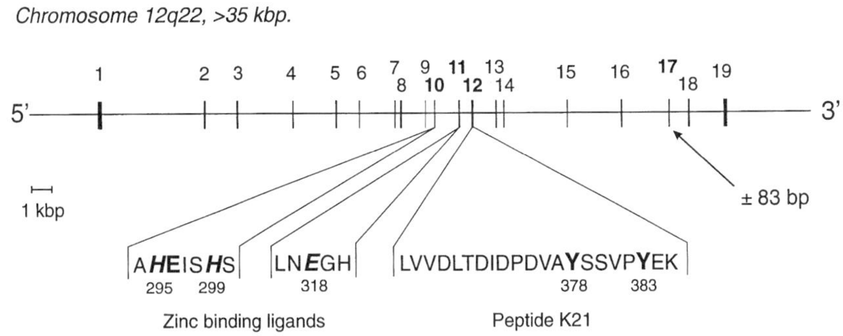

Figure 2 Organization of the human LTA_4 hydrolase gene. The gene is >35 kbp in size, is located at chromosome 12q22 and is composed of 19 exons. All known residues involved in zinc binding, catalyses, or suicide inactivation are located in exons 10, 11, and 12. The gene can be transcribed into two mRNA, one containing all exons and one in which exon 17 (83 bp) has been deleted (see text).

LTA_4 hydrolase conformed to a so-called catalytic zinc site and was very similar to the zinc binding motif in thermolysis (35). A catalytic zinc site is characterized by two primary ligands separated by a short spacer of 1–3 residues, which in turn are separated from a more distant third ligand by a so-called long spacer ranging from 18 to 120 amino acids (35). From sequence alignments of LTA_4 hydrolase and other members of the same group of metallohydrolases, His-295, His-299, and Glu-318 were identified as potential zinc-binding ligands (see below). The discovery of this zinc-binding signature in LTA_4 hydrolase prompted us and others to investigate the possible zinc content of the enzyme (36,37). Thus, treatment of the enzyme with the chelating agents 1,10-phenanthroline and 8-hydroxyquinoline-5-sulfonic acid inhibited the catalytic activity. In contrast, EDTA and 1,7-phenanthroline, a nonchelating analog of 1,10-phenanthroline, were ineffective in this respect. To unequivocally establish the zinc content, we used atomic absorption spectrometry, which revealed the presence of one zinc atom per enzyme molecule, while the amounts of iron, copper, manganese, cobalt, magnesium, nickel, and calcium were negligible (36). Furthermore, enzyme inactivated with 1,10-phenanthroline did not contain any significant amounts of zinc and therefore represented the apoenzyme of LTA_4 hydrolase. However, addition of stoichiometric amounts of zinc to the apoenzyme restored the enzymatic activity, and this effect reached a plateau at a 1:1 molar ratio metal versus protein, i.e., at the same stoichiometry as in the native holoenzyme. Hence, the primary function of the metal seemed to be catalytic rather than structural.

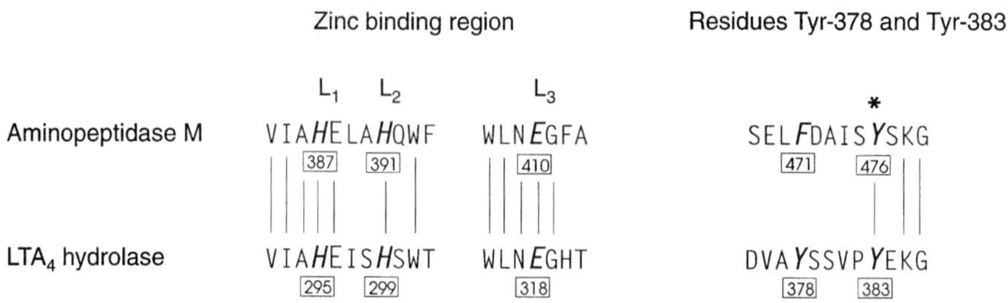

Figure 3 Sequence comparison between human LTA_4 hydrolase and aminopeptidase M. Amino acid sequences corresponding to the zinc-binding motif and a segment centered around the active-site residues Tyr-378 and Tyr-383 of LTA_4 hydrolase are shown. Vertical lines indicate amino acid identities. L, identified or postulated zinc ligands. The putative proton donor residue is indicated with (*).

A. Intrinsic Aminopeptidase Activity of LTA_4 Hydrolase

The identification of LTA_4 hydrolase as a member of a family of zinc metalloproteases suggested that it could possess a peptide-cleaving activity, in addition to its well-characterized epoxide hydrolase activity (the transformation of LTA_4 into LTB_4). This assumption turned out to be true when it was reported that LTA_4 hydrolase could hydrolyze a number of synthetic chromogenic substrates (37,38). Since these compounds were general peptidase substrates, a critical point was to ascertain that the peptide-cleaving activity was an intrinsic property of the enzyme and not the result of contaminating proteases in the enzyme preparations. In our case, we made use of apo-LTA_4 hydrolase and showed that its peptidase activity returned after addition of exogenous metal with the same stoichiometry metal versus protein as for the epoxide hydrolase activity (38). This conclusion was also supported by studies using the competitive inhibitor bestatin, which blocked both the epoxide hydrolase and the peptidase activity of LTA_4 hydrolase (39).

It is also worth mentioning that preparations of aminopeptidases from porcine and hog kidney as well as bovine intestine did not convert LTA_4 into LTB_4 (37,38). Apparently, the presence of a zinc-binding motif in a protein is only indicative of a peptide-cleaving activity. Thus, sequence similarities primarily based on the zinc-binding site have been found between LTA_4 hydrolase and an array of other seemingly unrelated proteases, including the murine phosphorylated cell surface glycoprotein BP-I/6C3 and the lethal factor of *Bacillus anthracis* just to mention two disparate examples (40,41). Of perhaps greater interest was the serendipitous finding of a gene in *Saccharomyces cerevisiae* with >40% sequence identity with LTA_4 hydrolase (42). In this case, the homology was not limited to the zinc signature, as for aminopeptidase M, and it is possible that this yeast enzyme is an ancestor of the mammalian LTA_4 hydrolase (see Fig. 3).

B. Chloride Stimulation of the Peptidase Activity via a Putative Anion-Binding Site

Initial attempts to characterize the peptidase activity in phosphate buffer failed until we realized that the activity was dependent on the presence of certain monovalent anions, in particular chloride ions and thiocyanate ions (43). From kinetic data of the chloride stimulation, we found that the effect obeyed saturation kinetics. An apparent affinity constant for chloride was calculated to approximately 100 mM, which is close to the extracellular concentration of this electrolyte (43). Thus, chloride stimulation of LTA_4 hydrolase appears to be mediated via an anion-binding site. In contrast to the effects on the peptidase activity, no chloride stimulation was observed for the epoxide hydrolase activity. This selective effect on only one catalytic activity may represent a mode of enzyme regulation. Considering the differences in chloride concentration between the intracellular and extracellular compartments, one can speculate that the peptidase activity of LTA_4 hydrolase may only proceed outside the cell, whereas the epoxide hydrolase activity may operate on either side of the cell membrane. Notably, LTA_4 hydrolase activity has been detected in plasma of several mammals and high levels of the enzyme have been found in human bronchoalveolar lavage fluid (44,45). An extracellular role for the peptidase activity is also supported by the finding that albumin, the major protein constituent of plasma, can stimulate the peptidase activity of LTA_4 hydrolase (46).

C. Substrate Specificity of the Peptidase Activity

Apparently, the active site corresponding to the peptidase activity is promiscuous. Thus, an array of different synthetic substrates are cleaved by LTA_4 hydrolase, including nitroanilide and β-naphthylamide derivatives of various amino acids, in particular alanine and arginine (37,38,47). Interestingly, the enzyme was recently shown to cleave the N-terminal arginine from several tripeptides with very high efficiency. For instance, the peptides Arg-Gly-Asp, Arg-Gly-Gly, and Arg-His-Phe were hydrolyzed with specificity constants (k_{cat}/K_m) in the same order of magnitude as for hydrolysis of LTA_4, suggesting that LTA_4 hydrolase is an arginyl tripeptidase (47). Moreover, opioid peptides, substrates of potential physiological importance, have been shown to be hydrolyzed by LTA_4 hydrolase, although with low efficiency (48,49). It may also be worth mentioning that a weak dipeptidase activity toward the cysteinyl-glycyl moiety of LTD_4 has been reported. Notably, the endogenous substrate(s) for the peptidase activity of LTA_4

hydrolase still remains to be identified. Some categories of peptidase substrates are shown in Table 2.

VI. LTA_4 Hydrolase in Transcellular Biosynthesis of LTB_4

Transcellular metabolism means that a certain endogenous compound is exported by a donor cell to a recipient cell for further conversion(s) into metabolites that sometimes none of the participating cell types can generate themselves. This route of biosynthesis has been described for a number of different lipid mediators and in particular for LTA_4 (50). Thus, activated leukocytes can generate LTA_4, which can be metabolized into LTB_4 and LTC_4 as well as lipoxins. As mentioned above, LTA_4 hydrolase has a widespread distribution and is present in many cell types that lack significant 5-lipoxygenase activity and thus the ability to generate the substrate LTA_4, interalia erythrocytes, endothelial cells, and fibroblasts (16,51,52). This uneven distribution of two intimately coupled enzyme activities, i.e., LTA_4 hydrolase and 5-lipoxygenase, has been explained in terms of transcellular biosynthesis, and indeed transfer of LTA_4 from activated leukocytes to a variety of other cell types have been demonstrated in vitro, a phenomenon that is promoted by tight cell-cell interactions (53). With respect to the respiratory system, several studies have indicated that LTB_4 biosynthesis is amplified by transcellular mechanisms involving activated neutrophils as the donor cell and airway epithelial cells or alveolar macrophages as the recipients of LTA_4 (54,55) (Fig. 4). In addition, LTA_4 hydrolase is present in high levels in bronchoalveolar lavage fluid and can convert neutrophil-derived LTA_4 into LTB_4 (45). Inasmuch as LTA_4 hydrolase is a bifunctional enzyme, it is possible that its previously unknown peptide-cleaving activity accounts for the disproportionate distribution of 5-lipoxygenase and LTA_4 hydrolase. Hence, it is possible that the epoxide hydrolase activity is confined to various types of leukocytes, whereas the peptidase activity may predominate in cells not involved in leukotriene biosynthesis or in the extracellular compartment, as discussed above.

VII. Inhibition of LTA_4 Hydrolase by Zinc and Other Divalent Cations

In experiments where apo-LTA_4 hydrolase was reactivated by successive additions of exogenous zinc, we observed that levels of metal exceeding a 1:1 molar ratio caused inhibition of the peptidase activity. Further studies revealed that both enzyme activities were reversibly inhibited by zinc in a dose-dependent manner with IC_{50} values of 10 and 0.1 μM for the epoxide hydrolase and peptidase activity, respectively (56). Divalent cations other than zinc were also found to inhibit LTA_4 hydrolase with different specificity and potency for the two enzyme activi-

Table 2 Substrate Specificity of the Bifunctional Leukotriene A_4 Hydrolase[a]

	Epoxide hydrolase activity				Peptidase activity			
	K_m (μM)	k_{cat} (s^{-1})	k_{cat}/K_m (s^{-1} M^{-1})			K_m (μM)	k_{cat} (s^{-1})	k_{cat}/K_m (s^{-1} M^{-1})
LTA_4	6	0.7	1.3×10^5	Tripeptides	Arg-Ser-Arg	2.2	3.0	1.4×10^6
LTA_5					Arg-His-Phe	30	32	1.1×10^6
LTA_3					Arg-Gly-Gly	210	205	9.8×10^5
				Dipeptides	Arg-Tyr	100	21	2.1×10^5
					Arg-Phe	50	4.9	9.8×10^4
					Arg-Leu	80	3.2	4.0×10^4
				Synthetic amides	Ala-4-NA	500	0.6	1.2×10^3
					Pro-4-NA	100	0.15	1.5×10^3
					Arg-4-NA	200	0.15	7.5×10^2
					Leu-4-NA	300	0.15	5.0×10^2
				Opioid peptides	Leu-enkephalin			
					Met-enkephalin			
					Dynorphin A (1-7)			
					Dynorphin A (1-6)			
				Varia	f-Met-Leu-Phe			
					LTD_4			

[a] Apparent kinetic constants were not determined under identical experimental conditions and therefore values should be regarded as indicative. In particular, values for LTA_4 must be regarded as conservative, considering the instability of this substrate.

Source: Refs. 37, 43, 46, 47, 49.

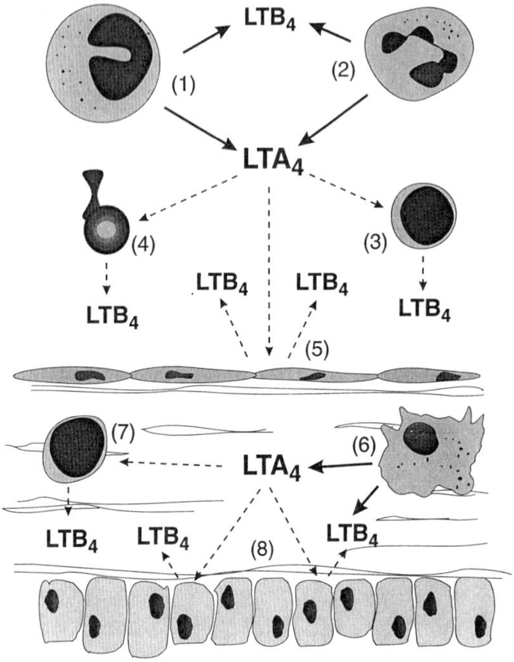

Figure 4 Transcellular biosynthesis of LTB_4. The drawing illustrates potential routes for amplification of LTB_4 biosynthesis by transcellular metabolism of LTA_4. Solid arrows indicate release of LTA_4 (and LTB_4) from activated monocytes (1), neutrophils (2), or tissue macrophages (6). Dashed arrows indicate various routes for metabolism of LTA_4 into LTB_4 via lymphocytes (3), erythrocytes (4), and endothelial cells (5) in the blood vessel, or via lymphocytes (7) and epithelial cells (8) in the tissue.

ties. For instance, Mn^{2+} and Co^{2+}, which inhibited the peptidase activity with IC_{50} values <10 μM, had no effect on the conversion of LTA_4 into LTB_4 at 1 mM concentration (56). Zinc inhibition has previously been reported for thermolysin, presumably via binding of an additional zinc atom to His-231 of the enzyme (57,58). On the other hand, the zinc metalloenzyme carboxypeptidase A is competitively inhibited by zinc via a different mechanism involving a zinc monohydroxide bridge between Glu-270 in the zinc-binding motif and the catalytic zinc atom (59). For LTA_4 hydrolase, the mechanism of zinc inhibition is presently unknown.

VIII. Metal Binding and Catalytic Residues in LTA_4 Hydrolase

The discovery of a zinc-binding motif in LTA_4 hydrolase and its peptide-cleaving activity led to the identification of a series of amino acid residues with a likely role in enzyme function, which could be tested by mutational analysis. It is noteworthy that earlier, virtually nothing was known about which segments or domains of the protein that are catalytically important.

A. Tyrosine and Arginine Residues at the Active Center of LTA_4 Hydrolase

To screen for functionally important amino acids, other than those identified by computer-assisted sequence comparisons, we carried out experiments with chemical modification (60). The tyrosine reagent *N*-acetylimidazole rapidly inactivated both the peptidase and the epoxide hydrolase activity and addition of hydroxylamine restored both catalytic activities, which indicates that the inactivation was due to modification of tyrosines. Furthermore, the competitive inhibitor bestatin could partially protect the enzyme from *N*-acetylimidazole, suggesting that one or several critical tyrosines are located close to, or at, the active site(s). Similar results were obtained with the tyrosine reagent tetranitromethane, and from measurements of nitrated residues by UV, in the presence or absence of bestatin, it was calculated that two out of 22 tyrosines could be protected by the competitive inhibitor.

Two arginine-modifying reagents, namely, 2,3-butanedione and phenylglyoxal, effectively inhibited both enzyme activities. As was the case for *N*-acetylimidazole and tetranitromethane, the enzyme could be protected from inactivation by either bestatin or captopril. From experiments with differential labeling, in which (7-^{14}C)phenylglyoxal was incorporated into unprotected and protected enzyme, we could calculate that three arginines (out of a total of 23), could be protected by captopril. Taken together, the results of chemical modification suggest that two tyrosyl and three arginyl residues are located near or at the active site(s).

B. Identification of the Zinc-Binding Ligands of LTA_4 Hydrolase

From the thermolysin/aminopeptidase M sequence homology, His-295, His-299, and Glu-318 were proposed to be the three ligands involved in zinc coordination (Fig. 3). To investigate the role of these residues in metal-binding and catalytic activities, site-directed mutagenesis was carried out. The codons for His-296, His-299, and Glu-318 were changed to codons for Tyr, Tyr, and Gln, respectively, by PCR mutagenesis (61). The mutated cDNAs were expressed in *E. coli* and the corresponding recombinant enzymes were purified to homogeneity to allow determinations of zinc content and enzyme activities. Thus, insignificant amounts of zinc were detected in all three mutants, as judged by atomic absorption spectrometry. Furthermore, none of the mutated enzymes exhibited significant epoxide hydrolase or peptidase activity. Using this approach, we were able to verify the predictions that His-295, His-299, and Glu-318 are the three zinc-binding ligands of LTA_4 hydrolase (61). Moreover, the properties of the mutated enzymes lent further support to our previous conclusion that the zinc atom is not critical for the maintenance of the tertiary structure of LTA_4 hydrolase, whereas it seems to play a fundamental role in catalyses.

C. Selective Abrogation of the Peptidase Activity by Mutation of Glutamic Acid 296

A conserved glutamic acid, juxtaposed to the first zinc-binding ligand, is a typical feature of the zinc signature of several zinc proteases, e.g., thermolysin, neutral endopeptidase, and aminopeptidase M (Fig. 3). In LTA_4 hydrolase, Glu-296 occupies this position in the zinc binding motif (35). Since earlier data for thermolysin, obtained by X-ray crystallographic analysis, had indicated that the corresponding Glu-143 is involved in the proteolytic reaction catalyzed by this enzyme, we wanted to investigate the role of Glu-296 for the two catalytic activities of LTA_4 hydrolase. To this end, we constructed two mutants in this position, i.e., (E296Q) and (E296A)LTA_4 hydrolase, which were purified to homogeneity to allow metal analysis and enzyme activity determinations (62). Both mutants contained the expected amounts of zinc (~1 eq) and exhibited significant epoxide hydrolase activity (150% and 15% for (E296Q) and (E296A)LTA_4 hydrolase, respectively). In contrast, the two mutated enzymes were virtually inactive with respect to the peptidase activity. Apparently, we had been able to selectively abrogate one of the two catalytic activities of LTA_4 hydrolase. Two important conclusions can be made from these experiments. First, Glu-296 is obviously essential for the peptidase but not for the epoxide hydrolase activity. Second, the selective effect of mutation on only one of the two activities shows that the corresponding active site(s) are not identical but rather overlapping.

D. Tyrosine 383 As a Potential Proton Donor in the Peptidase Reaction

In addition to the zinc-binding motif, computer-assisted sequence comparisons between LTA_4 hydrolase and aminopeptidase M revealed the presence of a conserved nonapeptide centered around a tyrosine residue (63,64) (Fig. 3). This short peptide has been suggested to represent a proton donor motif and in LTA_4 hydrolase, Tyr-383 was proposed to be the proton-donating residue (64). To detail the role of Tyr-383 for the two catalytic activities of LTA_4 hydrolase, we exchanged this residue for a Phe, His, or Gln residue by site-directed mutagenesis

(65). Again, the mutated enzymes were purified to apparent homogeneity to allow enzyme activity determinations. All mutants exhibited significant albeit substantially reduced epoxide hydrolase activities ranging from 11 to 17% of the wild-type enzyme. For the mutant (Y383Q)LTA_4 hydrolase, the reduced activity was mostly due to an increased K_m for LTA_4. Thus, at saturating concentrations of substrate, (Y383Q)LTA_4 hydrolase displayed 60% of the activity expressed by wild-type enzyme. In contrast, none of the mutated enzymes exhibited any significant peptidase activity against alanine-4-nitroanilide (0.3–0.02% of the control) and for (Y383Q)LTA_4 hydrolase, an increased substrate concentration to values 60 times the K_m did not significantly improve the catalytic efficiency. Thus, these results are in agreement with a role of Tyr-383 in the peptidase reaction, perhaps as a proton donor (see below). However, our data do not allow a similar interpretation for the epoxide hydrolase activity.

E. A Possible Reaction Mechanism for the Peptidase Activity

Based on X-ray crystallographic data, two reaction mechanisms have been discussed for the proteolytic activity of thermolysin, which contains a zinc site structurally very similar to that of LTA_4 hydrolase. Thus, the conserved Glu-143 has been suggested to act as a general base or to form an anhydride with the substrate (58,66). In the former and most favored mechanism, water is displaced from the zinc atom by the carbonyl oxygen of the substrate and then polarized by the carboxylate of the glutamic acid to promote an attack on the carbonyl carbon of the scissile peptide bond. Simultaneously, a proton is transferred to the nitrogen of the peptide bond from an adjacent amino acid. Considering the results obtained by mutational analysis (see above), Glu-296 and Tyr-383 would correspond to the base and proton donor in LTA_4 hydrolase, respectively.

IX. Molecular Basis for Suicide Inactivation of LTA_4 Hydrolase

Typically, LTA_4 hydrolase is covalently modified and inactivated by its endogenous lipid substrate LTA_4, a process commonly referred to as suicide inactivation (4,10). This built-in mechanism for enzyme inhibition may be of importance for the overall regulation of LTB_4 biosynthesis in vivo. Using enzyme kinetics, Fitzpatrick and coworkers have shown that suicide inactivation satisfies several criteria which define a mechanism-based process (67,68). For instance, after treatment of LTA_4 hydrolase with LTA_4 or with LTA_4 methyl ester, the epoxide hydrolase and peptidase activities are lost simultaneously and irreversibly in a time-dependent, saturable process that is of pseudo first-order kinetics and dependent upon catalysis. Active-site specificity has been demonstrated by protection with competitive inhibitors, and mass spectrometric analysis has revealed that suicide inactivation occurs predominantly in a 1:1 stoichiometry between lipid and protein, with only little modification of secondary sites.

A. Identification of a Peptide Region Involved in Suicide Inactivation

To study the molecular mechanisms of suicide inactivation, we used differential Lys-specific peptide mapping (69). Thus, samples of untreated and suicide-inactivated (5 × 13 μM LTA_4) enzyme were digested with Lys-C protease, and the resulting peptides were separated by RP-HPLC. Differential analysis showed that one peak was always reduced in peptide maps of suicide-inactivated LTA_4 hydrolase. Material under this peak was subjected to amino acid sequence analysis, which revealed a peptide spanning 21 residues from Leu-365 to Lys-385. Due to the number of amino acids and the fact that it originates from a Lys-C digest, the peptide was denoted K21. Notably, Tyr-383, the previously discussed potential proton donor of the peptidase reaction, was located within peptide K21, lending further support to the conclusion that Tyr-383 is an active-site residue (see Figs. 3 and 5).

To link peptide K21 to suicide inactivation, the loss of enzyme activities upon repetitive additions of LTA_4 was compared with the loss of K21 in corresponding peptide maps. We found a good correlation between these two parame-

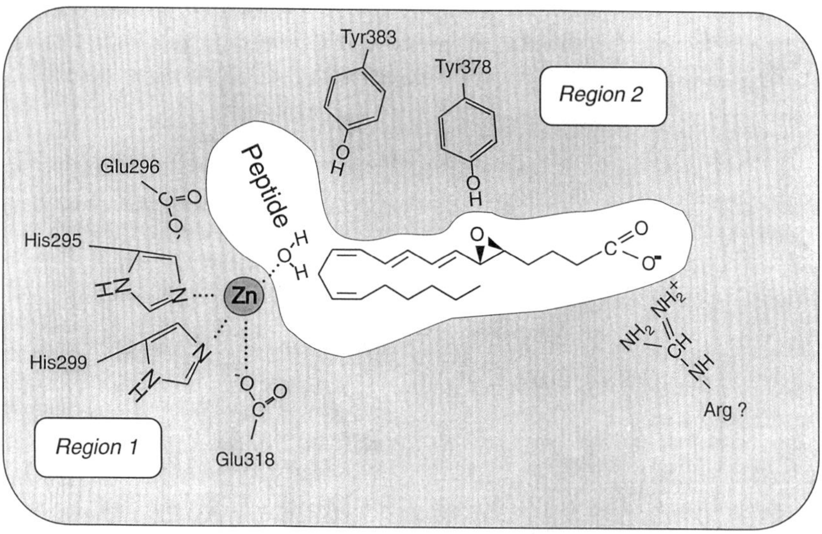

Figure 5 Tentative model for the active site structure of LTA_4 hydrolase. For details see text.

ters, which indicates that the heneicosapeptide is indeed involved in the covalent binding of the substrate LTA_4 to the protein. Further evidence for this conclusion was obtained by the identification of a modified peptide K21, denoted K21-LT (to indicate the content of a leukotriene moiety), which eluted in the more lipophilic part of the HPLC chromatogram. Although the recovery of K21-LT was poor, enough material could be collected to trace the N-terminal amino acid sequence, which was in agreement with the corresponding sequence of K21.

LTA_4 hydrolase can also be suicide inactivated by LTA_4 methyl and ethyl ester. In these cases, the inactivation is more efficient, which may be explained by less depletion of the leukotriene epoxides due to the absence of significant enzymatic conversion and a higher chemical stability of esterified LTA_4 as compared to the free acid. We also tested these LTA_4 analogs in experiments similar to those described above. Again, we found loss of peptide K21 in digests of inactivated enzyme and also observed the simultaneous appearance of modified, more lipophilic peptides. In the case of LTA_4 ethyl ester, the amounts of modified peptide, denoted K21-LTet, was sufficient to allow complete Edman degradation. Thus, the sequence of K21-LTet was identical to the sequence of K21 with the exception of a gap in position 14, corresponding to Tyr-378 of intact LTA_4 hydrolase. Apparently, LTA_4 ethyl ester had bound to Tyr-378 during suicide inactivation of LTA_4 hydrolase (see Figs. 3 and 5).

B. Peptide K21 as Part of a Catalytic Domain

Suicide inactivation and covalent modification (as judged by loss of peptide K21 in peptide maps) by the leukotriene epoxides could be prevented by preincubation of the enzyme with the competitive inhibitor bestatin. Hence, binding of LTA_4 and its esters to peptide K21 is an active-site–directed process and K21 most likely contains active-site residues. In fact, peptide K21 could be considered as a second catalytic domain, in addition to the previously well-characterized zinc-binding site (Fig. 3). Although the borders of K21 are defined by the proteolytic specificity of Lys-C protease, this region would seem to be functionally centered around the two tyrosines in position 378 and 383. In this context it is interesting to note that results obtained with chemical modification had pointed to the presence of two tyrosines located at the active site of LTA_4 hydrolase.

C. Tyrosine 378 as a Major Structural Determinant for Suicide Inactivation

To detail the role of Tyr-378 in suicide inactivation and its potential catalytic function, we carried out a mutational analysis. Thus, we exchanged Tyr for Phe or Gln in two separate mutants (70). In addition, each of two adjacent and potentially reactive residues, Ser-379 and Ser-380, were exchanged for Ala. The mutated enzymes were expressed as $(His)_6$-tagged fusion proteins in *E. coli*, purified to apparent homogeneity, and characterized. Interestingly, enzyme activity determinations and differential peptide mapping, before and after repeated exposure to LTA_4, revealed that wild-type enzyme and the mutants (S379A) and (S380A)LTA_4 hydrolase were equally susceptible to suicide inactivation, whereas the mutants in position 378 were no longer inactivated or covalently modified by LTA_4, as judged by enzyme activity determinations and differential peptide mapping (presence of K21). Furthermore, in (Y378F)LTA_4 hydrolase, the value of k_{cat} for epoxide hydrolysis was increased 2.5-fold over that of the wild-type enzyme. Thus, by a single point mutation in LTA_4 hydrolase, catalysis and covalent modification/inactivation had been dissociated, yielding an enzyme with increased turnover and resistance to mechanism-based inactivation.

D. Formation of a Double-Bond Isomer of LTB_4 by Mutants of Tyrosine 378

A more detailed examination of the catalytic properties of (Y378F), (Y378Q), (S379A), and (S380A)LTA_4 hydrolase revealed that the two mutants in position 378 were able to generate not only LTB_4 but also a second metabolite of LTA_4, in a yield of about 20–30% (71). From data obtained by UV spectrophotometry, GC/MS, UV-induced double-bond isomerization, and comparison with a synthetic standard, the novel metabolite was assigned the tentative structure 5(*S*),12(*R*)-dihydroxy-6,10-*trans*-8,14-*cis*-eicosatetraenoic acid, i.e., Δ^6-*trans*-Δ^8-*cis*-LTB_4. The observation that mutants in position 378 can generate an isomer of LTB_4 further corroborates our previous conclusion that Tyr-378 is an active-site residue (Fig. 5).

E. Possible Role of Tyr-378 in the Hydrolysis of LTA_4 into LTB_4

Leukotriene A_4 is a highly unstable allylic epoxide that is spontaneously hydrolyzed in water with a $t_{1/2} \approx 10$ s at neutral pH. Nonenzymatic hydrolysis of LTA_4 is thought to be initiated via an acid-induced opening of the epoxide moiety, and a carbonium ion with a positive charge delocalized over the triene system would be formed as an intermediate in the reaction. This intermediate will result in a planar sp^2-hybridized configuration at C12, which in turn allows a nucleophilic attack from both sides of the carbon. Accordingly, the two epimers at C12 of 5(*S*),12-dihydroxy-6,8,10-*trans*-14-*cis*-eicosatetraenoic acid, also referred to as Δ^6-*trans*-LTB_4 and Δ^6-*trans*-12-epi-LTB_4, will be formed and are in fact the predominant nonenzymatic hydrolysis products of LTA_4. The structure of LTB_4, formed by enzymatic hydrolysis, differs from the structure of either of the two nonenzymatically formed 5,12-dihydroxy acids in two ways, namely the double-bond geometry and the configuration of the hydroxyl group at C12. Apparently, during enzymatic hydrolysis of LTA_4 into LTB_4, LTA_4 hydrolase ensures a stereoselective introduction of H_2O at C12 as well as the formation of the Δ^6-*cis*-Δ^8-

trans-Δ^{10}-*trans* configuration of the conjugated triene. Interestingly, the mutants at position 378 differ from wild-type enzyme regarding one of these two essential functions of the enzyme, i.e., the positioning of the *cis* double bond in the product. Hence, Tyr-378 appears to be involved in this aspect of catalysis, perhaps by assisting in the proper alignment of LTA_4 in the substrate-binding pocket or by promoting a favorable conformation of a putative carbonium ion intermediate.

X. Active-Site Structure of LTA_4 Hydrolase

If one tries to unify the information that has been generated regarding structural and functional properties of LTA_4 hydrolase into a model of the active site, the result may look as outlined in Figure 5. Since the two enzyme activities are exerted via nonidentical but yet overlapping active sites, one can envisage two immediately adjacent substrate-binding pockets, one containing a peptide substrate and the other, the lipid substrate LTA_4. A water molecule acts on the peptide substrate, activated by the zinc complexed to His-295, His-299, and Glu-318, and the base Glu-296. In addition, Tyr-383 should be positioned in proximity to the peptide bond to make possible a proton transfer. Since both activities are zinc-dependent, the metal should be located at, or at least close to, the junction between the two pockets. Much less is known about amino acid residues involved in the conversion of LTA_4 into LTB_4. It seems likely that a basic residue, perhaps one of the arginines identified by chemical modification, acts as a carboxylate recognition site and contributes to substrate binding. Moreover, Tyr-378 should be positioned in the vicinity of the reactive allylic epoxide and the conjugated triene. However, it must be emphasized that a detailed and correct picture of all structural elements of the active site(s) will only be obtained by X-ray crystallographic analysis of the protein, data which soon may be at hand since crystals of LTA_4 hydrolase are now available (72).

XI. Evidence for the Presence of Isoenzymes of LTA_4 Hydrolase

A number of investigators have shown that there may exist more than one LTA_4 hydrolase protein with slightly different biochemical characteristics. For instance, LTA_4 hydrolase from the human B-lymphocytic cell line *Raji* was reported to contain two pools of the enzyme which differed in kinetic properties and sensitivity to heat (8). Furthermore, purification of LTA_4 hydrolase from guinea pig liver and lung resulted in two enzymatically active protein species with different isoelectric points (6,7). In particular, LTA_4 hydrolase from human airway epithelial cells has been shown to display a number of unusual characteristics. Thus, Bigby and coworkers have reported that these cells contain a hydrolase that exhibits a slower time course for product formation, a reduced susceptibility to suicide inactivation, minute peptidase activity, and reduced sensitivity to inhibition by 1,10-phenanthroline (20,73,74). Clearly, an increasing body of evidence suggests that isoenzymes of LTA_4 hydrolase may exist. Some of these data, such as the lower Mr ≈ 54,000 reported for LTA_4 hydrolase purified from human erythrocytes (4), has been shown not to hold true (67,75), but the possibility of isoenzymes is still open. Interestingly, an explanation that could account for all these somewhat vague and inconclusive observations was recently put forward by Jendraschak and coworkers (76). Using sequential reverse-transcriptase PCR mapping, they were able to identify a novel short transcript of the gene. This mRNA was formed by alternative splicing of an 83 bp exon (no. 17), which in turn leads to an altered reading frame and a preterminal stop after 22 amino acids. As a consequence, the mRNA predicts the expression of an LTA_4 hydrolase isoform with a calculated molecular mass of 59 kDa and a distinct C-terminus. However, whether or not this isoform is enzymatically active or even expressed in vivo remains to be determined.

XII. Inhibitors of LTA_4 Hydrolase

Prior to the identification of LTA_4 hydrolase as a zinc metalloenzyme with peptide-cleaving activity, no reasonably potent or specific enzyme inhibitors were known. An immediate consequence of the homology to zinc proteases was to test the effect of a number of peptidase inhibitors. As a result, bestatin and captopril, classical inhibitors of aminopeptidases and angiotensin-converting enzyme, respectively, were found to be effective inhibitors of LTA_4 hydrolase (39,77). Work in several laboratories has led to the development of more powerful and selective compounds. Thus, based on proposed reaction mechanisms and inhibitor-enzyme interactions for other zinc hydrolases, new compounds were synthesized and tested for their effect on the epoxide hydrolase and peptidase activity of LTA_4 hydrolase. Among more than 30 different structures, we found two compounds, an α-keto-β-amino ester and a thioamine, which were potent tight-binding inhibitors with IC_{50} values in the low μM to nM range (78–81). In addition, a series of β-amino hydroxylamine and amino hydroxamic acids were developed, among which one hydroxamate turned out to be as potent as the above-mentioned substances (82) (see Fig. 6). Moreover, the α-keto-β-amino ester, the thioamine, and the hydroxamate are all potent and selective inhibitors of LTB_4 biosynthesis in intact human leukocytes (81,82). Other investigators have found that the hydroxamic acid containing peptide kelatorphan, a known inhibitor of enkephalin-degrading enzymes, and several related analogs are potent inhibitors of both the epoxide hydrolase and peptidase activity of LTA_4 hydrolase (83). However, these compounds were all relatively poor inhibitors of LTB_4 biosynthesis in whole

	IC_{50} (μM) / K_i (μM)		
	$LTA_4 \rightarrow LTB_4$	Peptidase activity	LTB_4 synthesis intact cells
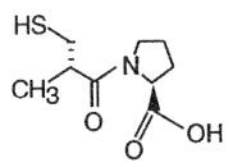 Captopril	14	0.1*	360¶
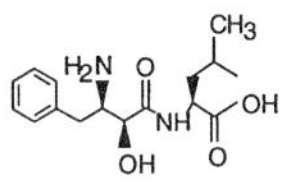 Bestatin	4	0.2*	40¶
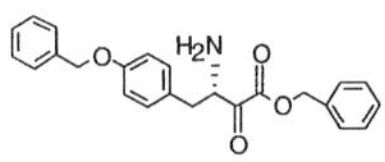 α-Keto-β-amino ester	2	0.02*	0.2
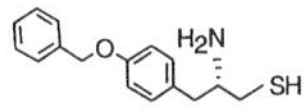 Thioamine	0.2	0.015*	0.1
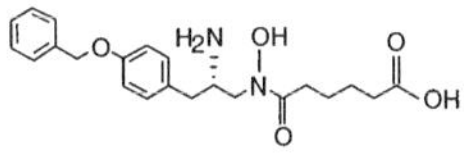 Amino hydroxamic acid	0.15	0.002*	0.3
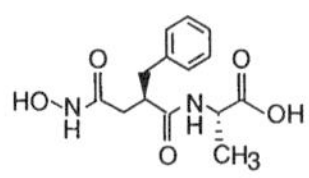 Kelatorphan	0.005	0.007	>8
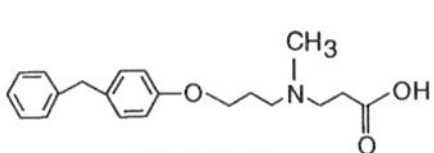 SC-57461	–	–	0.05

Figure 6 Inhibitors of LTA_4 hydrolase. The structures of some of the most potent and selective inhibitors of LTA_4 hydrolase are shown together with IC_{50} or K_i (indicated with *) values toward the epoxide hydrolase and peptidase activity of purified enzyme as well as LTB_4 biosynthesis in intact leukocytes or whole blood. The peptidase activity was measured with Ala-4-NA, Leu-4-NA, or Lys-4-NA. (Values from Refs. 39, 77, 81–83, 86.)

cells. Furthermore, a class of ω-[(ω-arylalkyl)aryl]alkanoic acids, were reported to inhibit LTA_4 hydrolase in the low μM range, one of which was metabolically stable after oral administration to rats (84). Some of these substances were also shown to bind to the LTB_4 receptor (85). Perhaps the most interesting and promising inhibitors of LTA_4 hydrolase were recently presented by Searle. Particularly SC-57461, *N*-methyl-*N*-[3-[4-(phenylmethyl)-phenoxy]propyl]-β-alanine, blocked ionophore-induced LTB_4 production in human whole blood with an IC_{50} of only 49 nM (86). Notably, this compound was orally active and showed very promising results in an animal model of colitis (87). The structures of some of the most potent inhibitors of LTA_4 hydrolase are shown in Figure 6.

Acknowledgments

The author is most grateful to Anders Wetterholm, Juan F. Medina, Martin J. Mueller, Martina Blomster Andberg, Filippa Strömberg, Eva Ohlson, and Bengt Samuelsson for their contributions to the studies described in this chapter. Work in the author's laboratory was financially supported by The Swedish Medical Research Council (O3X-10350), The European Union (BMH4-CT960229), Konung Gustav V:s 80-årsfond, Vårdalstiftelsen, and Petrus och Augusta Hedlunds stiftelse.

References

1. Borgeat P, Samuelsson, B. Arachidonic acid metabolism in polymorphonuclear leukocytes: Unstable intermediate in formation of dihydroxy acids. Proc Natl Acad Sci USA 1979; 76:3213–3217.
2. Rådmark O, Shimizu T, Jörnvall H, Samuelsson B. Leukotriene A_4 hydrolase in human leukocytes: purification and properties. J Biol Chem 1984; 259:12339–12345.
3. Evans JF, Dupuis P, Ford-Hutchinson AW. Purification and characterisation of leukotriene A_4 hydrolase from rat neutrophils. Biochim Biophys Acta 1985; 840:43–50.
4. McGee J, Fitzpatrick F. Enzymatic hydration of leukotriene A_4: purification and characterization of a novel epoxide hydrolase from human erythrocytes. J Biol Chem 1985; 260:12832–12837.
5. Ohishi N, Izumi T, Minami M, Kitamura S, Seyama Y, Ohkawa S, Terao S, Yotsumoto H, Takaku F, Shimizu T. Leukotriene A_4 hydrolase in the human lung: Inactivation of the enzyme with leukotriene A_4 isomers. J Biol Chem 1987; 262:10200–10205.
6. Haeggström J, Bergman T, Jörnvall H, Rådmark O. Guinea-pig liver leukotriene A_4 hydrolase: purification, characterization and structural properties. Eur J Biochem 1988; 174:717–724.

7. Bito H, Ohishi N, Miki I, Minami M, Tanabe T, Shimizu T, Seyama Y. Leukotriene A_4 hydrolase from guinea pig lung: The presence of two catalytically active forms. J Biochem 1989; 105:261–264.
8. Odlander B, Claesson H-E, Bergman T, Rådmark O, Jörnvall H, Haeggström J Z. Leukotriene A_4 hydrolase in the human B-lymphocytic cell line Raji: Indications of catalytically divergent forms of the enzyme. Arch Biochem Biophys 1991; 287:167–174.
9. Iversen L, Kristensen P, Nissen JB, Merrick WC, Kragballe K. Purification and characterization of leukotriene A_4 hydrolase from human epidermis. FEBS Lett 1995; 358:316–322.
10. Evans JF, Nathaniel DJ, Zamboni RJ, Ford-Hutchinson AW. Leukotriene A_3: a poor substrate but a potent inhibitor of rat and human neutrophil leukotriene A_4 hydrolase. J Biol Chem 1985; 260:10966–10970.
11. Nathaniel DJ, Evans JF, Leblanc Y, Leveille C, Fitzsimmons B, Ford-Hutchinson AW. Leukotriene A_5 is a substrate and inhibitor of rat and human neutrophil LTA_4 hydrolase. Biochem Biophys Res Commun 1985; 131:827–835.
12. Samuelsson B, Funk CD. Enzymes involved in the biosynthesis of leukotriene B_4. J Biol Chem 1989; 264:19469–19472.
13. Strömberg F, Hamberg M, Rosenqvist U, Dahlén S-E, Haeggström JZ. Formation of a novel metabolite of leukotriene A_4 in tissues of *Xenopus laevis*. Eur J Biochem 1996; 238:599–605.
14. Williams JD, Czop JK, Austen KF. Release of leukotrienes by human monocytes on stimulation of their phagocytic receptor for particulate activators. J Immunol 1984; 132:3034–3040.
15. Odlander B, Jakobsson P-J, Rosén A, Claesson H-E. Human B and T lymphocytes convert leukotriene A_4 into leukotriene B_4. Biochem Biophys Res Commun 1988; 153:203–208.
16. Fitzpatrick FA, Ligget W, McGee J, Bunting S, Morton D, Samuelsson B. Metabolism of leukotriene A_4 by human erythrocytes. A novel cellular source of leukotriene B_4. J Biol Chem 1984; 259:11403–11407.
17. Weller PF, Lee CW, Foster DW, Corey EJ, Austen KF, Lewis RA. Generation and metabolism of 5-lipoxygenase pathway leukotrienes by human eosinophils: Predominant production of leukotriene C_4. Proc Natl Acad Sci USA 1983; 80:7626–7630.
18. Shaw RJ, Crowell O, Kay AB. Preferential generation of leukotriene C_4 by human eosinophils. Clin Exp Immunol 1984; 56:716–722.
19. Warner JA, Freeland HS, MacGlashan Jr. DW, Lichtenstein LM, Peters SP. Purified human basophils do not generate LTB_4. Biochem Pharmacol 1987; 36:3195–3199.
20. Bigby TD, Lee DM, Meslier N, Gruenert DC. Leukotriene A_4 hydrolase activity of human airway epithelial cells. Biochem Biophys Res Commun 1989; 164:1–7.
21. Brown GP, Monick MM, Hunninghake GW. Human alveolar macrophage arachidonic acid metabolism. Am J Physiol 1988; 254:C809–C815.
22. Peters SP, MacGlashan Jr. DW, Schulman ES, Schleimer RP, Hayes EC, Rokach J, Adkinson Jr NF, Lichtenstein LM. Arachidonic acid metabolism in purified human lung mast cells. J Immunol 1984; 132:1972–1979.
23. Freeland HS, Schleimer RP, Schulman ES, Lichtenstein LM, Peters SP. Generation

of leukotriene B_4 by lung fragments and purified human lung mast cells. Am Rev Respir Dis 1988; 138:389–394.
24. Gut J, Goldman DW, Jamieson GC, Trudell JR. Conversion of leukotriene A_4 to leukotriene B_4: Catalysis by human liver microsomes under anaerobic conditions. Arch Biochem Biophys 1987; 259:497–509.
25. Woods JW, Coffey MJ, Brock TG, Singer II, Petersgolden M. 5-lipoxygenase is located in the euchromatin of the nucleus in resting human alveolar macrophages and translocates to the nuclear envelope upon cell activation. J Clin Invest 1995; 95:2035–2046.
26. Funk, CD, Rådmark O, Fu JY, Matsumoto T, Jörnvall H, Shimizu T, Samuelsson B. Molecular cloning and amino acid sequence of leukotriene A_4 hydrolase. Proc Natl Acad Sci USA 1987; 84:6677–6681.
27. Minami M, Ohno S, Kawasaki H, Rådmark O, Samuelsson B, Jörnvall H, Shimizu T, Seyama Y, Suzuki K. Molecular cloning of a cDNA coding for human leukotriene A_4 hydrolase. J Biol Chem 1987; 262:13873–13876.
28. Medina JF, Rådmark O, Funk CD, Haeggström JZ. Molecular cloning and expression of mouse leukotriene A_4 hydrolase cDNA. Biochem Biophys Res Commun 1991; 176:1516–1524.
29. Makita N, Funk CD, Imai E, Hoover RL, Badr KF. Molecular cloning and functional expression of rat leukotriene A_4 hydrolase using the polymerase chain reaction. FEBS Lett 1992; 299:273–277.
30. Minami M, Mutoh H, Ohishi N, Honda ZI, Bito H, Shimizu T. Amino-acid sequence and tissue distribution of guinea-pig leukotriene A_4 hydrolase. Gene 1995; 161:249–251.
31. Minami M, Minami Y, Emori Y, Kawasaki H, Ohno S, Suzuki K, Ohishi N, Shimizu T, Seyama Y. Expression of human leukotriene A_4 hydrolase cDNA in *Escherichia coli*. FEBS Lett 1988; 229:279–282.
32. Gierse JK, Luckow VA, Askonas LJ, Duffin KL, Aykent S, Bild GS, Rodi CP, Sullivan PM, Bourner MJ, Kimack NM, Krivi GG. High-level expression and purification of human leukotriene A_4 hydrolase from insect cells infected with a baculovirus vector. Protein Express Purif 1993; 4:358–366.
33. Mancini JA, Evans JF. Cloning and characterization of the human leukotriene A_4 hydrolase gene. Eur J Biochem 1995; 231:65–71.
34. Malfroy B, Kado-Fong H, Gros C, Giros B, Schwartz J-C, Hellmiss R. Molecular cloning and amino acid sequence of rat kidney aminopeptidase M: A member of a super family of zinc-metallohydrolases. Biochem Biophys Res Commun 1989; 161: 236–241.
35. Vallee BL, Auld DS. Zinc coordination, function, and structure of zinc enzymes and other proteins. Biochemistry 1990; 29:5647–5659.
36. Haeggström JZ, Wetterholm A, Shapiro R, Vallee BL, Samuelsson B. Leukotriene A_4 hydrolase: A zinc metalloenzyme. Biochem Biophys Res Commun 1990; 172: 965–970.
37. Minami M, Ohishi N, Mutoh H, Izumi T, Bito H, Wada H, Seyama Y, Toh H, Shimizu T. Leukotriene A_4 hydrolase is a zinc-containing aminopeptidase. Biochem Biophys Res Commun 1990; 173:620–626.
38. Haeggström JZ, Wetterholm A, Vallee BL, Samuelsson B. Leukotriene A_4 hydrolase:

an epoxide hydrolase with peptidase activity. Biochem Biophys Res Commun 1990; 173:431–437.

39. Örning L, Krivi G, Fitzpatrick FA. Leukotriene A_4 hydrolase: Inhibition by bestatin and intrinsic aminopeptidase activity establish its functional resemblance to metallohydrolase enzymes. J Biol Chem 1991; 266:1375–1378.
40. Wu Q, Lahti JM, Air GM, Burrows PD, Cooper MD. Molecular cloning of the murine BP-1/6C3 antigen: A member of the zinc-dependent metallopeptidase family. Proc Natl Acad Sci USA 1990; 87:993–997.
41. Ménard A, Mock M, Montecucco C. Similarities between the lethal factor of bacillus anthracis and leukotriene A_4 hydrolase. Mol Microbiol 1995; 18:991–992.
42. Nasr F, Bécam AM, Herbert CJ. The sequence of 12.8 kb from the left arm of chromosome XIV reveals a sigma element, a pro-tRNA and six complete open reading frames, one of which encodes a protein similar to the human leukotriene A_4 hydrolase. Yeast 1996; 12:493–499.
43. Wetterholm A, Haeggström JZ. Leukotriene A_4 hydrolase: an anion activated peptidase. Biochim Biophys Acta 1992; 1123:275–281.
44. Fitzpatrick FA, Haeggström J, Granström E Samuelsson B. Metabolism of leukotriene A_4 by an enzyme in blood plasma: a possible leukotactic mechanism. Proc Natl Acad Sci USA 1983; 80:5425–5429.
45. Munafo DA, Shindo K, Baker JR, Bigby TD. Leukotriene A_4 hydrolase in human bronchoalveolar lavage fluid. J Clin Invest 1994; 93:1042–1050.
46. Örning L, Fitzpatrick FA. Albumins activate peptide hydrolysis by the bifunctional enzyme LTA_4 hydrolase/aminopeptidase. Biochemistry 1992; 31:4218–4223.
47. Orning L, Gierse JK, Fitzpatrick FA. The bifunctional enzyme leukotriene A_4 hydrolase is an arginine aminopeptidase of high efficiency and specificity. J Biol Chem 1994; 269:11269–11273.
48. Griffin KJ, Gierse J, Krivi G, Fitzpatrick FA. Opioid peptides are substrates for the bifunctional enzyme LTA_4 hydrolase/aminopeptidase. Prostaglandins 1992; 44:251–257.
49. Nissen JB, Iversen L, Kragballe K. Characterization of the aminopeptidase activity of epidermal leukotriene A_4 hydrolase against the opioid dynorphin fragment 1–7. Br J Dermatol 1995; 133:742–749.
50. MacLouf J, Fitzpatrick FA, Murphy RC. Transcellular biosynthesis of eicosanoids. Pharmacol Res 1989; 21:1–7.
51. Claesson H-E, Haeggström J. Human endothelial cells stimulate leukotriene synthesis and convert granulocyte released leukotriene A_4 into leukotrienes B_4, C_4, D_4 and E_4. Eur J Biochem 1988; 173:93–100.
52. Medina JF, Barrios C, Funk CD, Larsson O, Haeggström J, Rådmark O. Human fibroblasts show expression of the leukotriene A_4 hydrolase gene, which is increased after SV-40 transformation. Eur J Biochem 1990; 191:27–31.
53. Brady HR, Serhan CN. Adhesion promotes transcellular leukotriene biosynthesis during neutrophil–glomerular endothelial cell interactions–inhibition by antibodies against CD18 and L-selectin. Biochem Biophys Res Commun 1992; 186:1307–1314.
54. Zhou SY, Stark JM, Leikauf GD. Leukotriene B_4 formation–human neutrophil airway epithelial cell interactions. J Appl Physiol 1995; 78:1396–1403.

55. Grimminger F, Sibelius U, Seeger W. Amplification of LTB_4 Generation in AM-PMN cocultures—transcellular 5-lipoxygenase metabolism. Am J Physiol 1991; 261:L195–L203.
56. Wetterholm A, Macchia L, Haeggström JZ. Zinc and other divalent cations inhibit purified leukotriene A_4 hydrolase and leukotriene B_4 biosynthesis in human polymorphonuclear leukocytes. Arch Biochem Biophys 1994; 318:263–271.
57. Holmquist B, Vallee BL. Metal substitutions and inhibition of thermolysin: Spectra of the cobalt enzyme. J Biol Chem 1974; 249:4601–4607.
58. Kester WR, Matthews BW. Crystallographic study of the binding of dipeptide inhibitors to thermolysin: Implications for the mechanism of catalysis. Biochemistry 1977; 16:2506–2516.
59. Larsen KS, Auld DS. Carboxypeptidase A: mechanism of zinc inhibition. Biochemistry 1989; 28:9620–9625.
60. Mueller MJ, Samuelsson B, Haeggström JZ. Chemical modification of leukotriene A_4 hydrolase. Indications for essential tyrosyl and arginyl residues at the active site. Biochemistry 1995; 34:3536–3543.
61. Medina JF, Wetterholm A, Rådmark O, Shapiro R, Haeggström JZ, Vallee BL, Samuelsson, B. Leukotriene A_4 hydrolase: determination of the three zinc-binding ligands by site-directed mutagenesis and zinc analysis. Proc Natl Acad Sci USA 1991; 88: 7620–7624.
62. Wetterholm A, Medina JF, Rådmark O, Shapiro R, Haeggström JZ, Vallee BL, Samuelsson B. Leukotriene A_4 hydrolase: Abrogation of the peptidase activity by mutation of glutamic acid-296. Proc Natl Acad Sci USA 1992; 89:9141–9145.
63. Watt VM, Yip CC. Amino acid sequence deduced from a rat kidney cDNA suggests it encodes the Zn-peptidase aminopeptidase N. J Biol Chem 1989; 264:5480–5487.
64. Minami M, Bito H, Ohishi N, Tsuge H, Miyano M, Mori M, Wada H, Mutoh H, Shimada S, Izumi T, Abe K, Shimizu T. Leukotriene A_4 hydrolase, a bifunctional enzyme. Distinction of leukotriene A_4 hydrolase and aminopeptidase activities by site-directed mutagenesis at Glu-297. FEBS Lett 1992; 309:353–357.
65. Blomster M, Wetterholm A, Mueller MJ, Haeggstrom JZ. Evidence for a catalytic role of tyrosine 383 in the peptidase reaction of leukotriene A_4 hydrolase. Eur J Biochem 1995; 231:528–534.
66. Pangburn MK, Walsh KA. Thermolysin and neutral protease: mechanistic considerations. Biochemistry 1975; 14:4050–4054.
67. Orning L, Jones DA, Fitzpatrick FA. Mechanism-based inactivation of leukotriene A_4 hydrolase during leukotriene B_4 formation by human erythrocytes. J Biol Chem 1990; 265:14911–14916.
68. Orning L, Gierse J, Duffin K, Bild G, Krivi G, Fitzpatrick FA. Mechanism-based inactivation of leukotriene A_4 hydrolase/aminopeptidase by leukotriene A_4. Mass spectrometric and kinetic characterization. J Biol Chem 1992; 267:22733–22739.
69. Mueller MJ, Wetterholm A, Blomster M, Jörnvall H, Samuelsson B, Haeggström JZ. Leukotriene A_4 hydrolase: mapping of a heneicosapeptide involved in mechanism-based inactivation. Proc Natl Acad Sci USA 1995; 92:8383–8387.
70. Mueller MJ, Blomster M, Opperman UCT, Jörnvall H, Samuelsson B, Haeggström JZ. Leukotriene A_4 hydrolase: protection from mechanism-based inactivation by mutation of tyrosine-378. Proc Natl Acad Sci USA 1996; 93:5931–5935.

71. Mueller MJ, Blomster M, Samuelsson B, Haeggström JZ. Leukotriene A_4 hydrolase: mutation of tyrosine-383 allows conversion of leukotriene A_4 into an isomer of leukotriene B_4. J Biol Chem 1996; 271:24345–24348.
72. Tsuge H, Ago H, Aoki M, Furuno M, Noma M, Miyano M, Minami M, Izumi T, Shimizu T. Crystallization and preliminary X-ray crystallographic studies of recombinant human leukotriene A_4 hydrolase complexed with bestatin. J Mol Biol 1994; 238:854–856.
73. Bigby TD, Lee DM, Minami M, Ohishi N, Shimizu T, Baker JR. Characterization of human airway epithelial cell leukotriene A_4 hydrolase. Am J Respir Cell Mol Biol 1994; 11:615–624.
74. Baker JR, Kylstra TA, Bigby TD. Effects of metalloproteinase inhibitors on leukotriene A_4 hydrolase in human airway epithelial cells. Biochem Pharmacol 1995; 50: 905–912.
75. Rådmark O, Haeggström J. Properties of leukotriene A_4 hydrolase. Adv Prostaglandin Leukotriene Thromboxane Res 1990; 20:35–45.
76. Jendraschak E, Kaminiski WE, Kiefl R, von Schacky C. The human leukotriene A_4 hydrolase gene is expressed in two alternatively spliced mRNA forms. Biochem J 1996; 314:733–737.
77. Örning L, Krivi G, Bild G, Gierse J, Aykent S, Fitzpatrick FA. Inhibition of leukotriene A_4 hydrolase/aminopeptidase by captopril. J Biol Chem 1991; 266:16507–16511.
78. Yuan W, Zhong Z, Wong CH, Haeggström JZ, Wetterholm A, Samuelsson B. Probing the inhibition of leukotriene A_4 hydrolase based on its aminopeptidase activity. Bioorg Med Chem Lett 1991;1:551–556.
79. Yuan W, Wong C-H, Haeggström JZ, Wetterholm A, Samuelsson B. Novel tight-binding inhibitors of leukotriene A_4 hydrolase. J Am Chem Soc 1992;114:6552–6553.
80. Yuan W, Munoz B, Wong C-H, Haeggström JZ, Wetterholm A, Samuelsson B. Development of selective tight-binding inhibitors of leukotriene A_4 hydrolase. J Med Chem 1993; 36:211–220.
81. Wetterholm A, Haeggström JZ, Samuelsson B, Yuan W, Munoz B, Wong C-H. Potent and selective inhibitors of leukotriene A_4 hydrolase: effects on purified enzyme and human polymorphonuclear leukocytes. J Pharmacol Exp Ther 1995; 275: 31–37.
82. Hogg JH, Ollmann IR, Haeggström JZ, Wetterholm A, Samuelsson B, Wong C-H. Amino hydroxamic acids as potent inhibitors of LTA_4 hydrolase. Bioorg Med Chem 1995; 3:1405–1415.
83. Penning TD, Askonas LJ, Djuric SW, Haack RA, Yu SS, Michener ML, Krivi GG, Pyla EY. Kelatorphan and related analogs—potent and selective inhibitors of leukotriene A_4 hydrolase. Bioorg Med Chem Lett 1995; 5:2517–2522.
84. Labaudinière R, Hilboll G, Leon-Lomeli A, Lautenschläger H-H, Parnham M, Kuhl P, Dereu N. ω-[(ω-Arylalkyl)aryl]alkanoic acids—a new class of specific LTA_4 hydrolase inhibitors. J Med Chem 1992; 35:3156–3169.
85. Labaudinière R, Hilboll G, Leon-Lomeli A, Terlain B, Cavy F, Parnham M, Kuhl P, Dereu N. ω-[(ω-Arylalkyl)thienyl]alkanoic acids: from specific LTA_4 hydrolase inhibitors to LTB_4 receptor antagonists. J Med Chem 1992; 35:3170–3179.

86. Yuan JH, Birkmeier J, Yang DC, Hribar JD, Liu N, Bible R, Hajdu E, Rock M, Schoenhard G. Isolation and identification of metabolites of leukotriene A_4 hydrolase inhibitor SC-57461 in rats. Drug Metab Dispos 1996; 24:1124–1133.
87. Smith WG, Russell MA, Liang C, Askonas LA, Kachur JF, Kim S, Souresrafil N, Price DV, Clapp NK. Pharmacological characterization of selective inhibitors of leukotriene A_4 hydrolase. Prostaglandins Leukotrienes Essent Fatty Acids 1996; 55:13.

5

Leukotriene Export in Human Leukocytes

BING K. LAM

Harvard Medical School
and Brigham and Women's Hospital
Boston, Massachusetts

I. Introduction

Leukotrienes are lipid mediators with profound biologic effects. Leukotriene B_4 (LTB_4), a dihydroxy leukotriene, is a potent modulator of polymorphonuclear leukocytes (PMN). It induces chemotaxis, chemokinesis, aggregation, and degranulation of PMN (1–3) and causes PMN to adhere to endothelial cells (4). LTB_4 can act synergistically with vasodilators to promote vascular leakage (5). These effects implicate LTB_4 as mediators of certain inflammatory diseases. The cysteinyl leukotrienes, LTC_4, LTD_4, and LTE_4, are cystine-containing leukotrienes that are historically known as slow-reacting substances of anaphylaxis (SRS-A) (6). The cysteinyl leukotrienes are the most potent contractile agonists for human bronchial smooth muscle (7) and thus are implicated in the pathogenesis of asthma.

II. Roles of Cysteinyl Leukotrienes in Asthma

The specific involvement of leukotrienes in asthma is suggested by their potent biological activities, their presence in the airways of individuals with asthma, and the beneficial effects of 5-lipoxygenase inhibitors and LTD_4 receptor antagonists in various types of asthma. Both inhaled LTC_4 and LTD_4 are 1000-fold, and LTE_4 10-fold, more potent than histamine in compromising airway function in normal individuals. In individuals with asthma the cysteinyl leukotrienes are almost equipotent in compromising pulmonary function, and their effects are greater than in normal individuals (8). These lipid mediators stimulate mucus secretion from bronchial epithelial cells and increase pulmonary vascular permeability through endothelial cell contraction at the postcapillary venules (9–11). The cysteinyl leukotrienes have been recovered from the airways of individuals with asthma at rest (12). Cysteinyl leukotrienes are released in the airways after either allergen challenge (13) or isocapnic hyperventilation (14). The newly developed leukotriene antagonists, 5-lipoxygenase inhibitors, and 5-lipoxygenase activating protein inhibitors have permitted a definitive examination of the role of leukotrienes in bronchial asthma. The administration of these pharmacological agents, which are devoid of intrinsic bronchodilatory activity, leads to bronchodilatation in individuals with asthma (15,16), suggesting that leukotrienes contribute to the abnormal resting tone in asthmatic airways. These agents inhibit the acute asthmatic response to exercise (17,18), cold dry air (19), allergen (20), and aspirin (21,22). They also decrease the late asthmatic response to allergen and the accompanying increase in airway hyperresponsiveness (20) and improve the severity of chronic asthma (23).

III. Biosynthesis of Leukotrienes

Leukotriene biosynthesis is initiated by agonist stimulation of human leukocytes such as mast cells and eosinophils (Fig. 1). On cell activation, cytosolic phospholipase A_2 (PLA_2) is translocated to the perinuclear membrane (24) and releases arachidonic acid from membrane phospholipids. The 5-lipoxygenase–activating

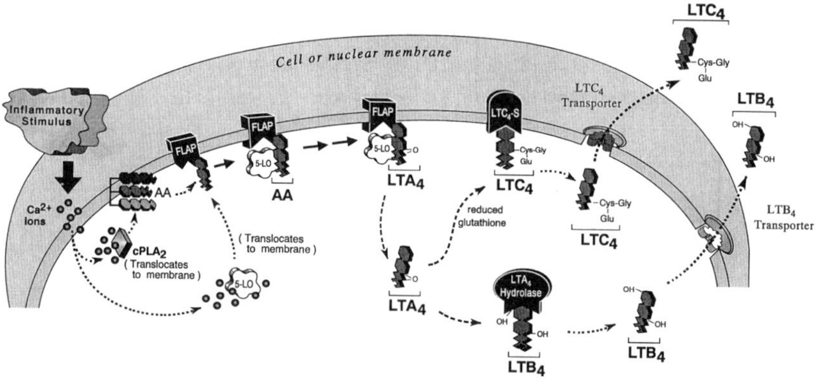

Figure 1 Schematic representation of the biosynthesis and release of LTB_4 and LTC_4. $cPLA_2$, Cytosolic phospholipase A_2; AA, arachidonic acid; 5-LO, 5-lipoxygenase; FLAP, 5-lipoxygenase–activating protein; LTC_4-S, LTC_4 synthase.

protein, a perinuclear membrane protein, binds the released arachidonic acid and presents it to the 5-lipoxygenase. The 5-lipoxygenase that also translocated to the perinuclear membrane on cell activation (25) metabolizes arachidonic acid in two sequential steps to form an epoxide intermediate, LTA_4 (26). In PMN, LTA_4 is metabolized to LTB_4 by LTA_4 hydrolase. In eosinophils and mast cells, LTA_4 is conjugated to reduced glutathione by LTC_4 synthase to form LTC_4 (27,28), the parent compound of the cysteinyl leukotrienes. LTB_4 and LTC_4 are subsequently exported from their cells of origin by specific membrane carriers (Fig. 1) (29–31). Once released, LTC_4 is metabolized extracellularly to form receptor-active LTD_4 and LTE_4.

IV. Transport of Leukotrienes in Human Granulocytes and Leukemic Cell Lines

The determination that the release of leukotrienes from human granulocytes is a carrier-mediated process was based on the criteria that define a carrier-mediated transport process (30). These criteria include exhibition of saturation kinetics, temperature dependence, substrate specificity, and competition by its substrate analogs, and inhibition by available pharmacological transport inhibitors.

A. LTC_4 Export

LTC_4 is exported from human eosinophils in accordance with saturation kinetics. When eosinophils were incubated with increasing concentrations of LTA_4 at 37°C for 10 minutes, there was a concentration-dependent increase in LTC_4 generation and release. At LTA_4 concentrations below 7.5 μM, all the LTC_4 formed appeared in the supernatant. When the concentration of LTA_4 reached 7.5 μM or higher, LTC_4 generation continued to increase, but the amount of LTC_4 released into the supernatant remained constant. This finding suggested that the release of LTC_4 is saturable (30).

When peripheral blood eosinophils isolated from patients with cancer undergoing treatment with interleukin-2 were incubated at 0°C with LTA_4, the cells converted LTA_4 to LTC_4; however, all the LTC_4 was retained in the cell pellet (30). This phenomenon indicates that the release of LTC_4 is a temperature-dependent process. Because LTC_4 synthase can function at 0°C but LTC_4 cannot be released, it was possible to study the release process of preformed LTC_4 in human eosinophils and leukemic cell lines by incubating the cells at 0°C with LTA_4, washing away the unreacted LTA_4, and resuspending the cells at 37°C. When KG-1 cells were preloaded with increasing intracellular amounts of LTC_4 and then resuspended at 37°C buffer, there was a concentration-dependent release of

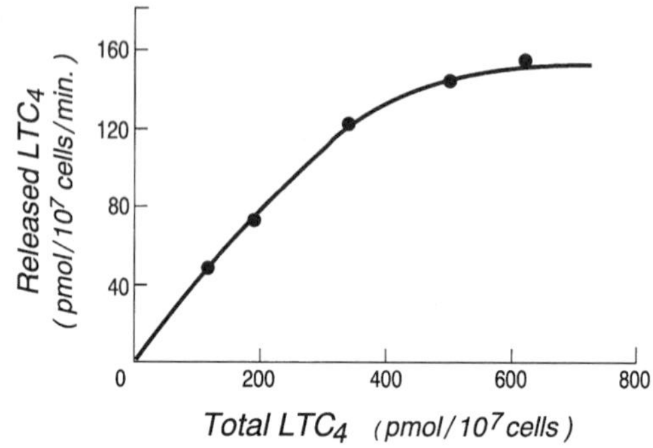

Figure 2 Concentration-dependent release of LTC_4 from KG-1 cells.

LTC_4 that plateaued at 600 pmol/10^7 cells of intracellular LTC_4 (Fig. 2). The K_m and V_{max} were determined to be 80.0 pmol/10^6 cells and 38.5 pmol/10^6 cells/min, respectively, in KG-1 cells (Table 1). This finding suggested that the release of LTC_4 is a saturable process.

The temperature dependency of LTC_4 export was demonstrated in human eosinophils, KG-1 cells, and DMSO-differentiated HL-60 cells. When these cells were preloaded with intracellular LTC_4, resuspended in buffer at various temperatures, and incubated at that temperature for 3 minutes, they released LTC_4 into the supernatant in a temperature-dependent fashion. These data were plotted on an Arrhenius plot, and the Q_{10} (temperature quotation at 10 degrees) value and energy of activation were calculated. Q_{10} values obtained for eosinophils, KG-1 cells, and the DMSO-differentiated HL-60 cells were 3.7, 3.3, and 3.4, respec-

Table 1 Parameters of LTC_4 and LTB_4 Export in Intact Cell Systems

Cell type	Substrate(s)	Q_{10}	Energy of activation (kcal/mol)	K_m (kcal/10^6 cells)	V_{max} (kcal/10^6 cells/min)	Probenecid (IC_{50})
KG-1 cells	LTC_4	3.3	23.0	80.0[a]	38.5[a]	5 mM
Eosinophils	LTC_4	3.7	28.2	N.D.	N.D.	2 mM
DMSO-dHL-60	LTC_4	3.4	27.8	N.D.	N.D.	2 mM
HL-60 cells	LTB_4	N.D.	N.D.	N.D.	N.D.	No effect
PMN	LTB_4	3.0	19.9	79.8	114.9	N.D.

DMSO-dHL-60, DMSO-differentiated HL-60 cells; N.D., not determined.
[a]Values from B. K. Lam et al., unpublished.
Source: Refs. 29, 31.

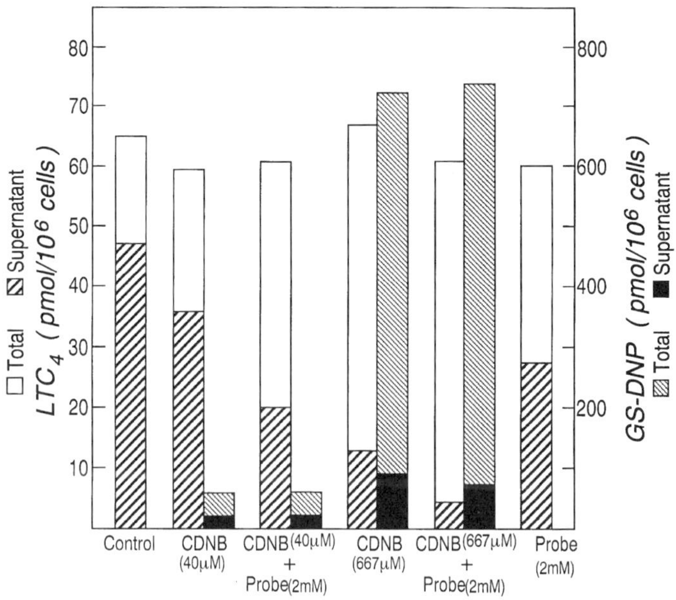

Figure 3 Effect of GS-DNP and probenecid on LTC_4 release from KG-1 cells. CDNB, 1-chloro-2,4-dinitrobenzene. (From Ref. 31.)

tively (Table 1) (31). The energy of activation values for LTC_4 export were determined to be 28.2, 23.0, and 27.8 kcal/mol, respectively, for eosinophils, KG-1 cells, and HL-60 cells (Table 1) (31). These values are too high for simple diffusion.

When eosinophils were preloaded with a fixed amount of intracellular LTC_4 and then incubated with increasing concentrations of LTA_5, the substrate analog of LTA_4, the release of LTC_4 was inhibited in a dose-dependent fashion, with the total amount of LTC (LTC_4 + LTC_5) in the supernatant being constant. This finding again suggested that the release of LTC_4 is saturable. In addition, LTC_4 release was inhibited by the intracellular glutathione conjugates GS-DNP (glutathione conjugate of 1-chloro-2,4-dinitrobenzene) (Fig. 2) (30,31) and S-(*p*-azidophenacyl)-glutathione (B.K. Lam et al., unpublished observation). Furthermore, LTC_4 export is inhibited by the organic acid transport inhibitor probenecid. When added to human eosinophils, KG-1 cells, and DMSO-differentiated HL-60 cells preloaded with intracellular LTC_4 at 37°C, probenecid inhibited the release of LTC_4 from these cells in a dose-dependent fashion (31). The effect of probenecid and the glutathione conjugate GS-DNP together was additive (Fig. 3) (31).

The demonstrations that LTC_4 release is a saturable and temperature-depen-

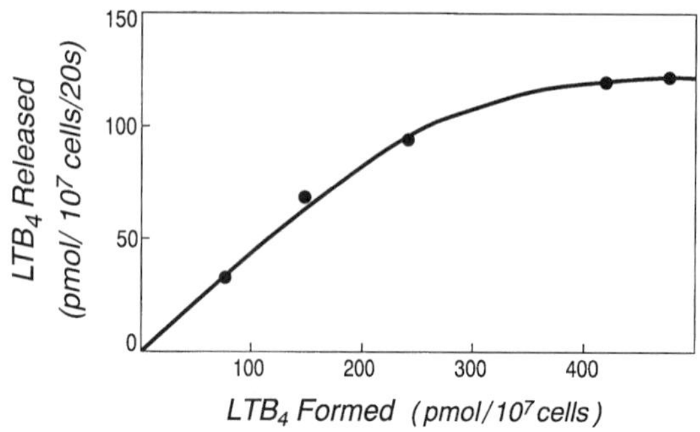

Figure 4 Concentration-dependent release of LTB_4 from human PMN. (Modified from Ref. 29.)

dent process, competition by its substrate analog and can be inhibited by a transport inhibitor fulfill the criteria for a carrier-mediated process.

B. LTB_4 Export

LTB_4 is less polar than LTC_4 and does not contain a glutathione moiety. PMN is the major cell type that generates LTB_4. Under the same criteria as LTC_4 for defining a carrier-mediated process, LTB_4 release in human PMN was determined to be a carrier-mediated export process. LTB_4 export is temperature dependent with a Q_{10} value of 3.0 and energy of activation value of 19.9 kcal/mol (Table 1) (29). The rate of LTB_4 release is about 60-fold faster than its metabolite 20-hydroxy-LTB_4. LTB_4 export in human PMN is a concentration-dependent and saturable process (Fig. 4), with a calculated K_m of 79.8 pmol/10^6 cells and V_{max} of 114.9 pmol/min/10^6 cells (Table 1). Like LTC_4 export, the release of LTB_4 is inhibited by its structural analog LTB_5. In contrast, LTB_4 release in nondifferentiated HL-60 cells is not inhibited by probenecid (Fig. 5), thereby indicating that the carrier that exports LTB_4 is different from that for LTC_4 (31).

V. Multidrug-Resistance Protein and Adenosine Triphosphate-Dependent Transport of LTC_4 in Membrane Vesicles

The finding that LTC_4 export in intact cells is a carrier-mediated process was also observed in an inside-out membrane vesicle system. LTC_4 inhibited the adenosine triphosphate (ATP)–dependent uptake of GS-DNP by inside-out vesicles (32),

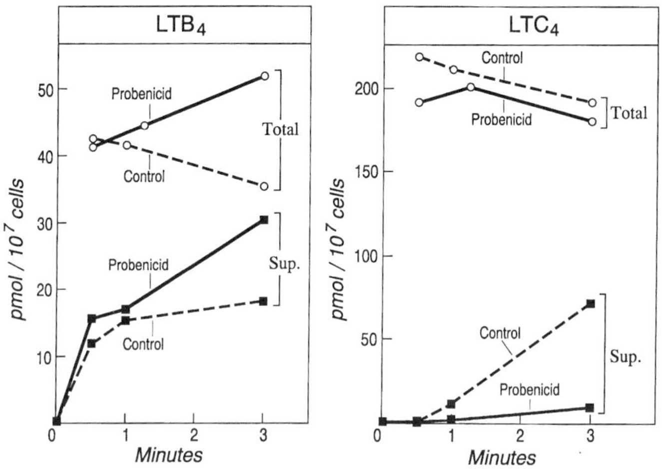

Figure 5 Effect of probenecid on LTB_4 and LTC_4 release from nondifferentiated HL-60 cells. (Modified from Ref. 31.)

thereby confirming the finding in intact cells that LTC_4 and glutathione conjugate utilize the same export carrier. Ishikawa et al. (33) demonstrated that LTC_4 is among the most effective glutathione conjugates in inhibiting the ATP-dependent uptake of GS-DNP by rat heart sarcolemma inside-out vesicles. ATP-dependent uptake of LTC_4 was also observed in rat liver canalicular vesicles, and this carrier was absent in rats with genetic deficiency in bile salt excretion (34). The ATP-dependent uptake of LTC_4 by membrane vesicles of murine mastocytoma cells is inhibited by the LTD_4 receptor antagonist MK-571 and by cyclosporin A (35). The ATP-dependent uptake of GS-DNP and LTC_4, however, was not inhibited by LTB_4 (36), consistent with the findings in intact cells.

Recently, the cDNA for the multidrug-resistance protein (MRP) was cloned from a human small-cell lung cancer line (37). The deduced amino acid sequence of MRP suggested that it is a member of an ATP-binding cassette superfamily of transmembrane transport proteins. When the MRP cDNA was transfected into HeLa cells, the transfected HeLa cell membrane vesicles displayed an increase in the ATP-dependent uptake of LTC_4 (38). The ATP-dependent uptake of LTC_4 by transfected HeLa cell membrane vesicles is inhibited by MK-571 and cyclosporin A with IC_{50} values of 0.6 μM and 5.0 μM, respectively, similar to that of mastocytoma cells (38). Photoaffinity labeling with $[H^3]LTC_4$ revealed a 190 kDa glycoprotein in both transfected HeLa cells and mastocytoma cells. These results suggest that MRP may be the LTC_4 carrier protein (36,38).

References

1. Ford-Hutchinson AW, Bray MA, Doig MV, Shipley ME, Smith MJH. Leukotriene B, a potent chemokinetic and aggregating substance released from polymorphonuclear leukocytes. Nature 1980; 286:264–265.
2. Palmblad J, Malmsten CL, Uden AM, Radmark O, Engstrot L, Samuelsson B. Leukotriene B_4 is a potent stereospecific stimulator of neutrophil chemotaxis and adherence. Blood 1981; 58:658–661.
3. Showell JH, Naccache PH, Borgeat P, Picard S, Vallerand P, Becker EL, Sha'afi RI. Characterization of the secretory activity of leukotriene B_4 toward rabbit neutrophils. J Immunol 1982; 128:811–816.
4. Rollins TE, Zanolari B, Springer MS, Guindon Y, Zamboni R, Lau CK, Rokach J. Synthetic leukotriene B_4 is a potent chemotaxin but a weak secretagogue for human PMN. Prostaglandins 1983; 25:281–289.
5. Wedmore CV, Williams TJ. Control of vascular permeability by polymorphonuclear leukocytes in inflammation. Nature 1981; 289:646–650.
6. Austen KF. SRS-A leukotrienes: from definition to biologic implications. In: PMH Mazumdar, ed. Immunology 1930–1980. Essay on History of Immunology. Toronto: Wall and Thompson, 1989:232–251.
7. Samuelsson B. Leukotrienes: mediators of immediate hypersensitivity reactions and inflammation. Science 1983; 220:568–575.
8. Arm JP, O'Hickey SP, Hawksworth RJ, Fong CY, Crea AEG, Spur B, Lee TH. Asthmatic airways have a disproportionate hyperresponsiveness to LTE_4, as compared with normal airways, but not to LTC_4, LTD_4, methacholine, and histamine. Am Rev Respir Dis 1990; 142:1112–1118.
9. Marom Z, Shelhamer JH, Bach MK, Morton DR, Kaliner M. Slow-reacting substances, leukotriene C_4 and D_4 increase the release of mucus from human airway in vitro. Am Rev Respir Dis 1982; 126:449–451.
10. Drazen JM, Austen KF, Lewis RA, Clark DA, Goto G, Marfat A, Corey EJ. Comparative airways and vascular activities of leukotrienes C-1 and D in vivo and in vitro. Proc Natl Acad Sci USA 1980; 77:4354–4358.
11. Dahlen SE, Djork J, Hedqvist P, Arfors KE, Hammarstrom S, Lindgren JA, Samuelsson B. Leukotrienes promote plasma leakage and leukocyte adhesion in postcapillary venules: in vivo effects with relevance to the acute inflammatory response. Proc Natl Acad Sci USA 1981; 78:3887–3891.
12. Lam S, Chan H, LeRiche JC, Chan-Yeung M, Salari H. Release of leukotrienes in patients with bronchial asthma. J Allergy Clin Immunol 1988; 81:711–717.
13. Wenzel SE, Larsen GL, Johnston K, Voelkel NF, Westcott JY. Elevated levels of leukotriene C_4 in bronchoalveolar lavage fluid from atopic asthmatics after endobronchial allergen challenge. Am Rev Respir Dis 1990; 142:112–119.
14. Pliss LB, Ingenito EP, Ingram RH, Pichurko B. Assessment of broncho-alveolar cell and mediator response to isocapnic hypernea in asthma. Am Rev Respir Dis 1990; 142:73–78.
15. Hui KP, Barnes NC. Lung function improvement in asthma with a cysteinyl-leukotriene antagonist. Lancet 1991; 1:1062–1063.

16. Gaddy J, Margolskee D, Bush RK, Williams VC, Busse W. Bronchodilatation with a potent and selective leukotriene D_4 (LTD_4) receptor antagonist (MK-571) in a patient with asthma. Am Rev Respir Dis 1992; 146:358–363.
17. Manning PJ, Watson RM, Margolskee DJ, Williams VC, Schwartz JI, O'Byrne PM. Inhibition of exercise-induced bronchoconstriction by MK-571, a patent leukotriene D4-receptor agonist. N Engl J Med 1990; 323:1736–1739.
18. Makker HK, Lau LC, Thomson HW, Binks SM, Holgate ST. The protective effect of inhaled leukotriene D(4) receptor antagonist ICI-204,219 against exercise-induced asthma. Am Rev Respir Dis 1993; 147:1413–1418.
19. Israel E, Dermarkarian R, Rosenberg M, Sperling R, Taylor G, Rubin P, Drazen JM. The effects of 5-lipoxygenase inhibitor. N Engl J Med 1990; 323:1740–1744.
20. Taylor IK, O'Shaughnessy KM, Fuller RW, Dollery CT. Effect of cysteinyl-leukotriene receptor antagonist ICI 204,219 on allergen induced bronchoconstriction and airway hyperreactivity in atopic subjects. Lancet 1991; 337:690–694.
21. Christie PE, Smith CM, Lee TH. The potent and selective sulfidopeptide leukotriene antagonist, SK&F 104353, inhibits aspirin-induced asthma. Am Rev Respir Dis 1991; 144:957–958.
22. Israel E, Fischer AR, Rosenberg MA, Lilly CM, Callery JC, Shapiro J, Cohn J, Rubin P, Drazen JM. The pivotal role of 5-lipoxygenase products in the reaction of aspirin-induced asthma. Am Rev Respir Dis 1993; 148:1447–1451.
23. Israel E, Rubin P, Kemp JP, Grossman J, Pierson W, Siegal SC, Tinkleman D, Murray JJ, Busse W, Segal AT. The effect of inhibition of 5-lipoxygenase by zileuton in mild-to-moderate asthma. Ann Intern Med 1993; 119:1059–1066.
24. Clark JD, Lin LL, Kriz RW, Ramesha CS, Sultzman LA, Lin AY, Milona NM, Knopf JL. A novel arachidonic acid-selective cytosolic phospholipase A_2 contains a Ca^{2+}-dependent translocation domain with homology to PKC and GAP. Cell 1991; 65:1043–1051.
25. Abramovitz M, Wong E, Cox ME, Richardson CD, Li C, Vickers PJ. 5-Lipoxygenase-activating protein stimulates the utilization of arachidonic acid by 5-lipoxygenase. Eur J Biochem 1993; 215:105–111.
26. Rouzer CA, Matsumoto T, Samuelsson B. Single protein from human leukocytes possesses 5-lipoxygenase and leukotriene A_4 synthase activities. Proc Natl Acad Sci USA 1986; 83:857–861.
27. Yoshimoto T, Soberman RJ, Spur B, Austen KF. Properties of highly purified leukotriene C_4 synthase of guinea pig lung. J Clin Invest 1988; 81:866–871.
28. Izumi T, Honda Z, Ohishi N, et al. Solubilization and partial purification of leukotriene C_4 synthase from guinea-pig lung: a microsomal enzyme with high specificity toward 5,6-epoxide leukotriene A_4. Biochem Biophys Acta 1988; 959:305–315.
29. Lam BK, Gagnon L, Austen KF, Soberman RJ. The mechanism of leukotriene B_4 export from human polymorphonuclear leukocytes. J Biol Chem 1990; 265:13438–13441.
30. Lam BK, Owen WF Jr, Austen KF, Soberman RJ. The identification of a distinct export step following the biosynthesis of leukotriene C_4 by human eosinophils. J Biol Chem 1989; 264:12885–12889.
31. Lam BK, Xu K, Atkins MB, Austen KF. Leukotriene C_4 uses a probenecid-sensitive

export carrier that does not recognize leukotriene B_4. Proc Natl Acad Sci USA 1992; 89:11598–11602.

32. Ishikawa T. Leukotriene C4 inhibits ATP-dependent transport of glutathione S-conjugate across rat heart sarcolemma: implication for leukotriene C4 translocation mediated by glutathione S-conjugate carrier. FEBS Lett 1989; 246:177–180.
33. Ishikawa T. ATP/Mg^{2+}-dependent cardiac transport system for glutathione S-conjugates: a study using rat heart sarcolemma vesicles. J Biol Chem 1989; 264:17343–17348.
34. Ishikawa T, Muller M, Klunemann C, Schaub T, Keppler D. ATP-dependent primary active transport of cysteinyl leukotrienes across liver canalicular membrane: role of the ATP-dependent transport system for glutathione S-conjugates. J Biol Chem 1990; 265:19279–19286.
35. Leier I, Jedlitschky G, Buchholz U, Keppler D. Characterization of the ATP-dependent leukotriene C_4 export carrier in mastocytoma cells. Eur J Biochem 1994; 220: 599–606.
36. Leier I, Muller M, Jedlitschky G, Keppler D. Leukotriene uptake by hepatocytes and hepatoma cells. Eur J Biochem 1992; 209:281–289.
37. Cole SPC, Bhardwaj G, Gerlach JH, Mackie JE, Grant CE, Almquist KC, Stewart AJ, Kurz EU, Duncan AMV, Deeley RG. Overexpression of a transporter gene in a multidrug-resistant human lung cancer cell line. Science 1992; 258:1650–1654.
38. Leier I, Jedlitschky G, Buchholz U, Coles SPC, Deeley RG, Keppler D. The MRP gene encodes an ATP-dependent export pump for leukotriene C_4 and structurally related conjugates. J Biol Chem 1994; 269:27807–27810.

6

Pathways of Leukotriene Metabolism in Isolated Cell Models and Human Subjects

ROBERT C. MURPHY and PAT WHEELAN

National Jewish Medical and Research Center
Denver, Colorado

I. Introduction

The reaction of molecular oxygen with free arachidonic acid, catalyzed by 5-lipoxygenase, leads to the formation of the progenitor leukotriene, namely, leukotriene A_4 (LTA_4) (1,2). While there is no evidence for any direct LTA_4 biological activity, its rapid conversion either into leukotriene B_4 (LTB_4) or the sulfidopeptide leukotriene [leukotriene C_4 (LTC_4)] has been the subject of numerous investigations (3,4). It is interesting to note a parallelism between the metabolic conversion of LTA_4 into the dihydroxy product LTB_4 catalyzed by LTA_4 hydrolase and conjugation of LTA_4 with glutathione to form LTC_4, with the metabolic events known to occur for electrophilic species produced during normal cellular metabolic processes. The reaction of epoxides with epoxide hydrolase (5) or glutathione-S-transferase (6) has been widely studied for many xenobiotics exposed to mammalian cells and tissues. However, the processing of LTA_4 within the cell is carried out by rather specific and unique enzymes highlighting the important roles these lipid products play in normal physiology and pathophysiology. While LTA_4 hydrolase is widely distributed in most cell types (7), the expression of LTC_4 synthase is largely restricted to cells that have been derived from the bone marrow (8).

The further processing of the primary leukotrienes by metabolic pathways (catabolic) within the cell is now known to play the central role in the regulation of leukotriene biological activity. For these leukotrienes to act as mediators of the inflammatory response, there needs to be a mechanism by which their action can be limited. As a general principle, covalent alteration of the leukotrienes into chemically different compounds is the process that terminates the biological activity of these lipid mediators. Furthermore, metabolic inactivation within cells of close proximity to the site of biosynthesis is likely since lipid mediators act locally and do not circulate with the body.

The metabolism of related lipid mediators, the prostaglandins, has been studied for approximately 20 years, and a general picture of the metabolic events transforming these cyclooxygenase products has emerged (9,10). Many cells contain the enzyme 15-hydroxy prostaglandin dehydrogenase, which oxidizes the 15-hydroxy group present in all prostaglandins, yielding the 15-oxo moiety, thereby terminating biological activity (11). Further processing occurs with the reduction of the double bond at carbon-13; both of these metabolic events often take place within the tissue of biosynthetic origin. Prostaglandins as well as the 15-oxo-prostaglandin metabolites are also metabolized after transport to and uptake into specialized metabolic cells such as hepatocytes. After formation of a coenzyme A (CoA) ester at the carboxy terminus, β-oxidation in mitochondria or peroxisomes takes place along pathways existing for metabolic degradation of fatty acids and polyunsaturated fatty acids (12). In addition, cytochrome P-450 in the endoplasmic reticulum of hepatocytes can oxidize the methyl terminus of the prostaglandin leading to the 20-hydroxy and 20-carboxy metabolites (13). The prostaglandin metabolites eventually eliminated into the urine of human subjects are typically the result of multiple metabolic reactions leading to chain-shortening by β-oxidation from the C-1 terminus, oxidation of the methyl terminus to a carboxyl moiety, and oxidation of the 15-hydroxy group and reduction of the carbon-13 double bond (10). As discussed below, leukotriene metabolism is similar in many respects to these metabolic events taking place for the prostaglandins; however, important differences do exist. For example, little β-oxidation from the C-1 terminus of leukotrienes has been observed. This rather surprising difference in metabolism of the otherwise structurally similar eicosanoids suggests an important role played by the double bond at carbon-5 present in the prostaglandins, but absent in the leukotrienes.

The relatively recent investigations of the in vitro and in vivo metabolism of leukotrienes have been greatly facilitated by advances made in techniques of mass spectrometry. The structure elucidation of many of the prostaglandin metabolites involved gas chromatography to separate chemically derivatized metabolites and gas chromatography/mass spectrometry (GC/MS) to structurally characterize the derivatives through studies of their electron ionization mass spectral behavior (14). Electron ionization leads to a rich population of fragment ions, many of which reveal important clues necessary for structure elucidation of the metabolite. Nevertheless, some prostanoid metabolites formed in vitro and in vivo, such as conjugates with glucuronic acid or taurine, cannot be directly analyzed by electron ionization mass spectrometry. Development of fast atom bombardment ionization and, more recently, electrospray ionization mass spectrometry has made a major contribution to the study of eicosanoid metabolism (15). These techniques do not require that the metabolite become volatile prior to the ionization event, rather ions are formed in the gas phase directly from the condensed phase. Both fast atom bombardment and electrospray ionization typically form protonated molecular ions as positive ions as well as carboxylate anions as abundant negative ions and few, if any, decomposition ions (16). This feature emphasizes the importance of the development of tandem mass spectrometry as a critical tool to provide detailed information of the structurally unknown leukotriene metabolite. Collisional activation of the molecular ion species in the tandem instrument (MS/MS) leads to a population of decomposition ions, which can be analyzed by the terminal mass spectrometer to yield the collisionally activated mass spectrum (17). Detailed analysis of the decomposition processes for polyunsaturated and oxidized fatty acids has revealed a rich ion chemistry, often suitable for structural characterization of the metabolite (18,19). Electrospray ionization also permits direct coupling of the HPLC effluent with the mass spectrometer, enabling on-line LC/MS and LC/MS/MS operation. LC/MS with electrospray ionization obviates the need to form volatile derivatives of the metabolite and thermally unstable, nonvolatile metabolites can be directly analyzed including taurine, glutathione, and glucuronide conjugates. Equally important is that these newer techniques in mass spectrometry are substantially more sensitive, compared to electron ionization mass spectrometric techniques, and structural studies are possible when metabolites are only available in subnanomole or smaller quantities. These newer techniques in mass spectrometry have made possible the rapid progress in understanding many of the pathways of both LTB_4 metabolism as well as the metabolism of the cysteinyl leukotrienes.

II. Cysteinyl Leukotriene Metabolism

Leukotriene C_4 is a glutathione adduct of LTA_4, and as such can be substrate for a number of ubiquitous peptidases found in virtually all cells and present in circulating plasma. The peptidic cleavage of the γ-glutamyl amino acid from LTC_4 by γ-glutamyl transpeptidase (20) converts this leukotriene into leukotriene D_4 (LTD_4) (Scheme 1). Subsequent to this reaction is removal of the glycine residue of LTD_4 catalyzed by several dipeptidases including aminopeptidases (21). In circulating blood, ectopeptidases of the vascular endothelium had been found to metabolize LTC_4 into LTE_4, explaining the short half-life of LTC_4 (0.2–2 min) in the circulation of monkeys (22,23). Whole blood also contains peptidases, which can convert LTC_4 into LTE_4, but plasma contains less γ-glutamyl transpeptidase that can convert LTC_4 into LTD_4 (24). As expected, the liver contains a large quantity of peptidases that efficiently degrade LTC_4 and LTD_4 into LTE_4, including cathepsin H, which can act as a dipeptidase converting LTD_4 into LTE_4

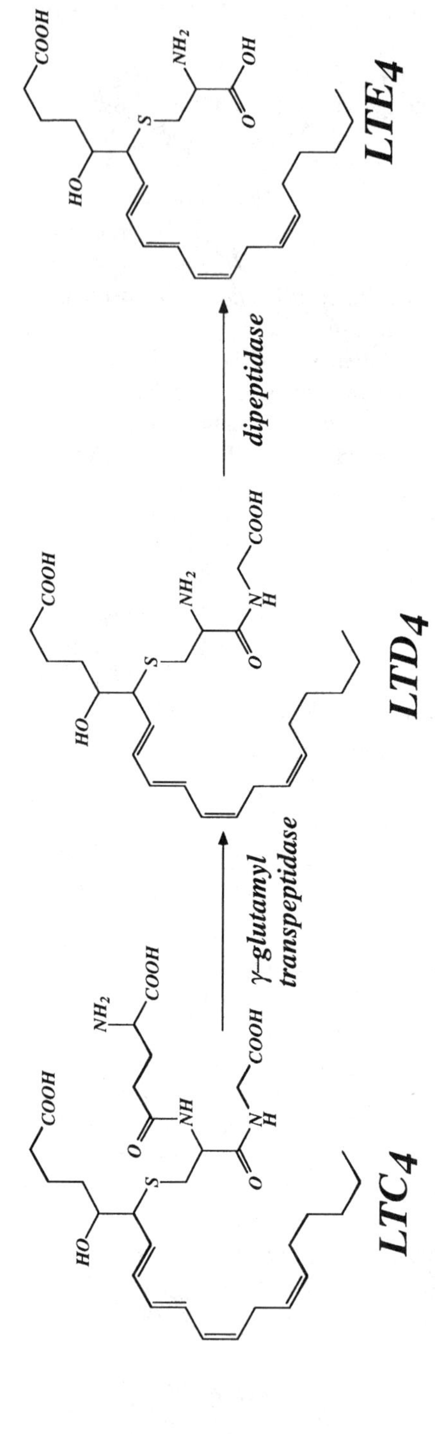

Scheme 1

(25). This metabolic transformation of the initially formed sulfidopeptide leukotriene, LTC_4, alters to some extent the biological activity of the parent LTC_4. However, in many species, including humans, LTD_4 and LTE_4 are sufficiently potent to still be responsible for many of the biological actions of slow-reacting substance of anaphylaxis (26). Further metabolic transformation of LTE_4 is required to terminate its biological action.

Studies with various isolated cells and tissues have revealed a similar story of rapid conversion of LTC_4 into LTE_4, but little further metabolic processing. The exception to this general pattern is the liver hepatocyte, which carries out extensive oxidative degradation of cysteinyl leukotrienes. An understanding of the metabolic processes involved in cysteinyl leukotriene metabolism at the tissue level is incomplete at the present time, but suggests that termination of cysteinyl leukotriene action may involve rapid elimination into blood for transport to the major metabolic site—the hepatocyte. Studies of instillation of LTC_4 into the isolated perfused lung have revealed a rapid appearance of LTE_4 in the perfusate with a half-life of less than one minute (27). This is in contrast to prostaglandin E_2, which is quantitatively metabolized by the isolated perfused lung in a single pass to the 15-oxo metabolite because of the abundant expression of 15-hydroxy prostaglandin dehydrogenase in this organ (28).

In certain animal species such as the rodent, a major pathway of metabolic inactivation is that of *N*-acetylation (29). Formation of *N*-acetyl-LTE_4 is catalyzed by *N*-acetyl-transferase found in many tissues and abundantly in liver, kidney, and lung. Furthermore, *N*-acetyl-LTE_4 has also been found to be excreted in high concentrations in rat bile (30). This metabolite is substantially less active than the parent LTE_4 (29). *N*-acetylation of LTE_4 is not a major metabolic pathway in human subjects, but has been found as a minor metabolite excreted in human urine (31).

A. Human Granulocytes

Incubation of LTC_4 with isolated human polymorphonuclear leukocytes followed by stimulation of the respiratory burst with phorbol ester led to the rapid conversion of LTC_4 into a series of metabolites (32). These metabolites were structurally characterized as two diastereomeric sulfoxides and two diastereomeric sulfones as well as two 6-*trans*-LTB_4 epimers. This metabolic process could be completely inhibited by the addition of catalase and azide, suggesting a requirement of H_2O_2 and myeloperoxidase. The formation of the LTC_4 sulfones and 6-*trans*-LTB_4 isomers likely were a result of the formation of an intermediate *S*-chlorosulfonium ion as an initial product of the reaction of hyperchloric acid generated by the stimulated neutrophil. The rapidity of this reaction led investigators to suggest that the respiratory burst of the neutrophil may be an important facet in controlling local inactivation of the cysteinyl leukotrienes in vivo (32).

Similar reactions were found to be catalyzed by eosinophil peroxidase, hydrogen peroxide, and chloride ions found in the circulating eosinophil (33). Porcine alveolar macrophages and rat peritoneal mononuclear cells were found to convert LTC_4 into LTD_4 and LTE_4 by the above-mentioned peptidase reactions (34). More extensive metabolic transformation of this cysteinyl leukotriene by the human monocyte and monocyte-derived macrophage has been reported when this cell type was stimulated to undergo an oxidative burst by phorbol ester (30). The bacterial enzyme cysteinyl-conjugated β-lyase was found to metabolically inactivate LTE_4 into 5-hydroxy-6-mercapto-7,9,11,14-eicosatetraenoic acid; however, the importance of these reactions in vivo is not clear (36).

B. Hepatic Metabolism of Cysteinyl Leukotrienes

Hepatic metabolism of cysteine-containing leukotriene has been the focus of numerous investigations because of the rapid peripheral conversion of LTC_4 and LTD_4 into LTE_4 and the observed rapid uptake of all three molecules into the hepatocyte (37). Involvement of a leukotriene-binding protein has been suggested to be responsible for the avidity of this uptake (38). Using positron emission tomography, within 1 minute after intravenous injection of [^{11}C]N-acetyl-LTE_4 into normal monkeys, only the liver and kidney were found to contain labeled LTE_4 and metabolites (39). After 8 minutes, only the liver was found to contain detectable quantities of radiolabeled metabolites. The hepatocyte has also been found to have an ATP-dependent export carrier for cysteinyl leukotrienes to remove these eicosanoids from the hepatocyte and excrete them into bile. The uptake of leukotrienes into the hepatocyte was strongly influenced by this ATP-dependent exporter (40).

Rat liver microsomes were found to contain a cytochrome P-450 system that could catalyze the ω-oxidation of LTE_4 with the formation of 20-hydroxy-LTE_4 and 20-carboxy-LTE_4 (41). Molecular oxygen and NADPH were required for this reaction. The oxidation of 20-hydroxy-LTE_4 was also found to be catalyzed by NAD^+-dependent alcohol dehydrogenase found in the cytosol of hepatocytes (41).

The metabolism of LTE_4 in intact rat hepatocytes led to the structural identification of six LTE_4 metabolites separated by reverse-phase HPLC shown in Figure 1 (42). Structural characterization of these metabolites was carried out by fast atom bombardment mass spectrometry and reductive cleavage of the cysteine residue followed by chemical derivatization, since intact cysteinyl leukotrienes were not amenable to electron ionization mass spectrometry, let alone GC/MS analysis.

The metabolic processing of LTE_4 by oxidative pathways in the rat proceed after initial acetylation of the free amino of cysteine of LTE_4. Oxygenation of the terminal methyl group of the arachidonate backbone (ω-oxidation) is likely

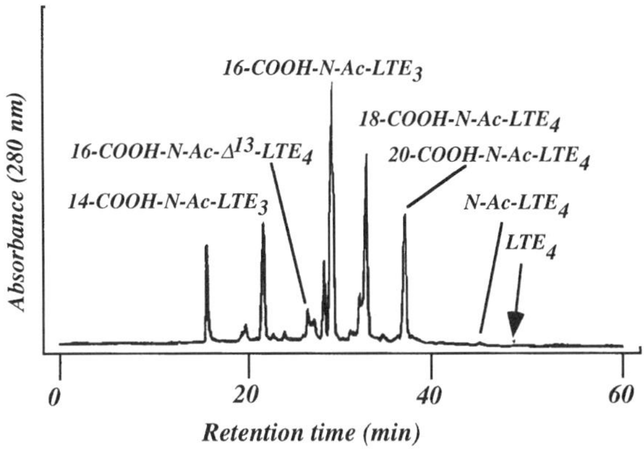

Figure 1 Reverse-phase HPLC separation of the metabolites of LTE_4 following incubation with isolated rat hepatocytes. Identification of the metabolites was carried out by mass spectrometry supporting the metabolic pathway outlined in Scheme 2. (Adapted from Ref. 42.)

mediated by a cytochrome P-450 (41) to yield 20-hydroxy-N-acetyl-LTE_4 as outlined in Scheme 2. This metabolite was also found to be a substrate for cytosolic alcohol dehydrogenase which could participate in the formation of 20-carboxy-LTE_4. Once the new carboxylic acid moiety is formed at carbon-20 of the arachidonate backbone, CoA ester formation takes place prior to uptake into peroxisomes and further metabolic transformation. Several metabolites of LTE_4 have been identified as products of the β-oxidation of CoA intermediates outlined in Scheme 3. The first complete β-oxidation product, *N*-acetyl-18-carboxy-LTE_4 CoA ester, is reduced by an NADPH-dependent 2,4-dienoyl-CoA reductase leading to the unexpected β-oxidation product 16-carboxy-tetranor-*N*-acetyl-LTE_3. A related metabolite, 16-carboxy-tetranor-Δ^{13}-*N*-acetyl-LTE_4 is likely a product of the action of $\Delta^{3,2}$ isomerase that places the initially formed double bond at C-14 (original arachidonate carbon number designation) into conjugation with the conjugated triene. Formation of 14-carboxy-hexanor-N-acetyl-LTE_3 is a result of further β-oxidation of 16-carboxy-tetranor-N-acetyl-LTE_3. These pathways are summarized in Scheme 3.

C. Metabolism of Cysteinyl Leukotrienes in Animal Models

The metabolism of cysteinyl leukotrienes has been studied in several animal models including rat (43,44), monkey (45–48), and human (49–51). Urinary metabolites of LTC_4 in the rat were structurally characterized as *N*-acetyl-LTE_4 and 20-

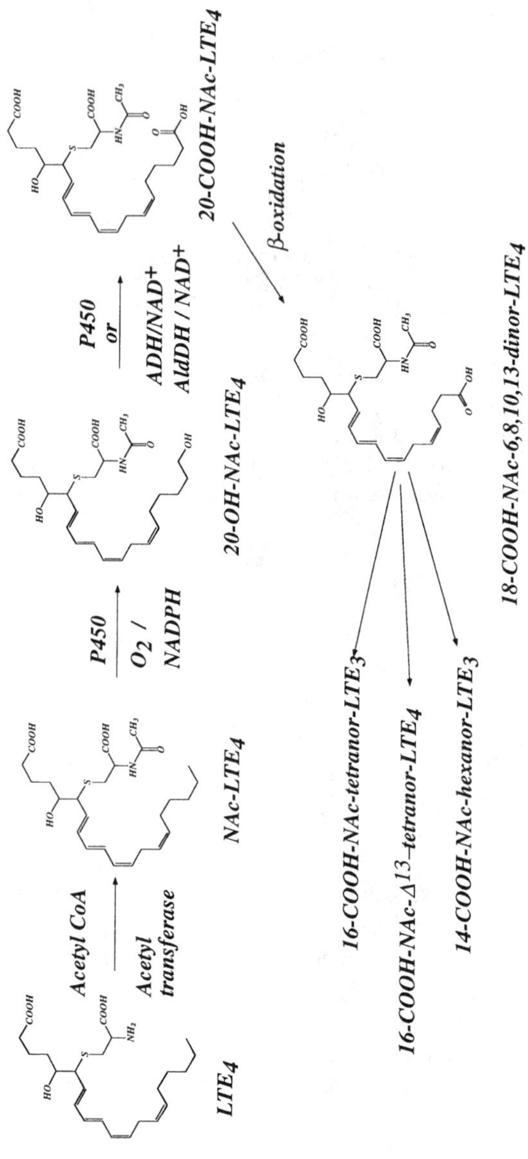
LTE4
Acetyl CoA
Acetyl transferase
NAc-LTE4
P450
O2 / NADPH
20-OH-NAc-LTE4
P450
or
ADH/NAD+
AldDH / NAD+
20-COOH-NAc-LTE4
β-oxidation
18-COOH-NAc-6,8,10,13-dinor-LTE4
16-COOH-NAc-tetranor-LTE3
16-COOH-NAc-Δ13-tetranor-LTE4
14-COOH-NAc-hexanor-LTE3

Scheme 2

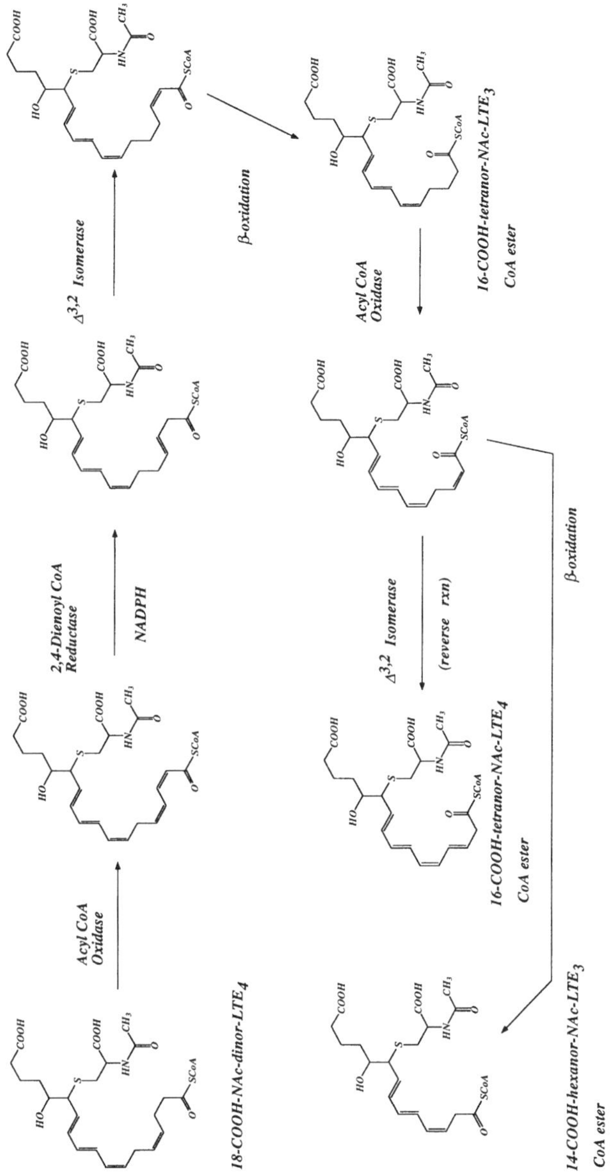
18-COOH-NAc-dinor-LTE4
Acyl CoA Oxidase
2,4-Dienoyl CoA Reductase
NADPH
Δ3,2 Isomerase
β-oxidation
16-COOH-tetranor-NAc-LTE3 CoA ester
Acyl CoA Oxidase
Δ3,2 Isomerase
(reverse rxn)
16-COOH-tetranor-NAc-LTE4 CoA ester
β-oxidation
14-COOH-hexanor-NAc-LTE3 CoA ester

Scheme 3

carboxy-*N*-acetyl-LTE_4 (43). However, numerous other metabolites were also formed, but not structurally identified.

The metabolism of LTE_4 in the cynomolgus monkey has also been reported (46). Only two inactive metabolites were structurally characterized, those being 20-hydroxy-LTE_4 and 20-carboxy-LTE_4, and these identifications were based upon comparison of radiolabeled metabolites with HPLC retention times of available synthetic standards (46). The major simian urinary metabolite of intravenously injected LTC_4 was found to be LTE_4 itself (47). For this primate model there was no acetylation of the free amino group present on the cysteinyl residue of LTE_4 and the ω/β-oxidized metabolites were only observed for LTE_4, suggesting that in vivo oxidative metabolism of cysteinyl leukotrienes occurred subsequent to peptidase degradation of LTC_4 into LTE_4.

The metabolism of LTC_4 in human subjects has been reported by several laboratories to result in excretion of numerous metabolites. HPLC separation of radiolabeled urinary metabolites of ^{35}S-LTC_4 injected into a human subject (51) is shown in Figure 2. Mass spectrometry played the central role in the structural characterization of these urinary metabolites, and the negative ion chemical ionization MS/MS spectrum of reduced and derivatized metabolites led to the structural characterization of the two predominant metabolites excreted 2 hours after infusion as 14-carboxy-hexanor-LTE_3 and a conjugated tetraene, 16-carboxy-Δ^{13}-tetranor-LTE_4 (51,52). These two products were likely the result of combined pathways of metabolism including cytochrome P-450–mediated formation of 20-carboxy-LTE_4 followed by β-oxidation and intermediate reduction of the double bond between carbons 14 and 15 described above. These same metabolites were observed to be formed following intravenous injection of radiolabeled LTC_4 into human subjects (53). The major pathway of LTC_4 metabolism in humans leading to excretion of the metabolic products was one of initial peptide cleavage reactions to form LTE_4, which was excreted intact; however, further ω-oxidation and β-oxidation of LTE_4, leading to 14-carboxy-LTE_3 and 16-carboxy-LTE_4 metabolites were significant pathways that accounted for metabolites that continued to be excreted up to 24 hours following intravenous injection of LTC_4. These human metabolic pathways are summarized in Scheme 4.

D. Urinary LTE_4 Entry Rate

The detailed understanding of the metabolic pathways associated with LTC_4 degradation and the observation that LTE_4 was a major urinary metabolite led to studies of LTE_4 excretion levels to assess the formation rate of sulfidopeptide leukotrienes in human subjects. A relationship between the concentration of LTE_4 observed in urine to the quantity of LTC_4 entering into the vascular system was required to make this correlation. Using LTC_4 at various doses, the absolute quantity of LTE_4 excreted into urine was found to be approximately 5% of the injected

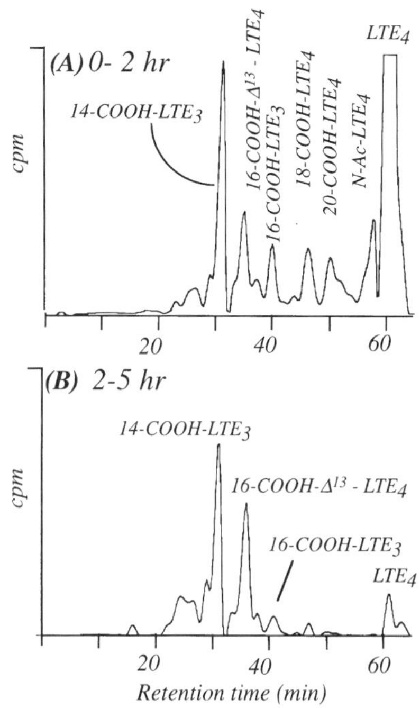

Figure 2 Reverse-phase HPLC separation of the radioactive urinary metabolites of [^{35}S]LTE_4 injected into a human subject. The urine was extracted and partially purified prior to reverse-phase separation. (A) Urinary metabolites during the first 2 hours of urinary collection. (B) Urinary metabolites present in the second collection period between 2 and 5 hours following injection of radiolabeled LTE_4. Metabolites were identified by mass spectrometry and support the suggested metabolic pathway outlined in Scheme 4. (Adapted from Ref. 51.)

LTC_4 dose (53). Furthermore, the quantity of intravenously infused LTC_4 led to a dose-dependent concentration of LTE_4 excreted into the urine. Based upon the linear relationship determined in this experiment (Fig. 3), it was possible to calculate the entry rate of LTC_4 into the normal human subject as 0.063 ± 0.01 pmol/kg/min (53).

Since measurement of the LTE_4 concentration in urine was found to be a good index of the appearance of LTC_4 into the vascular compartment, measurement of urinary LTE_4 concentration has become a valuable index of cysteinyl leukotriene biosynthesis in humans. Elevation in LTE_4 excretion has been observed in asthmatic patients during the early- and late-phase asthmatic response (54). Elevation in LTE_4 concentration was also found in subjects with liver cirrho-

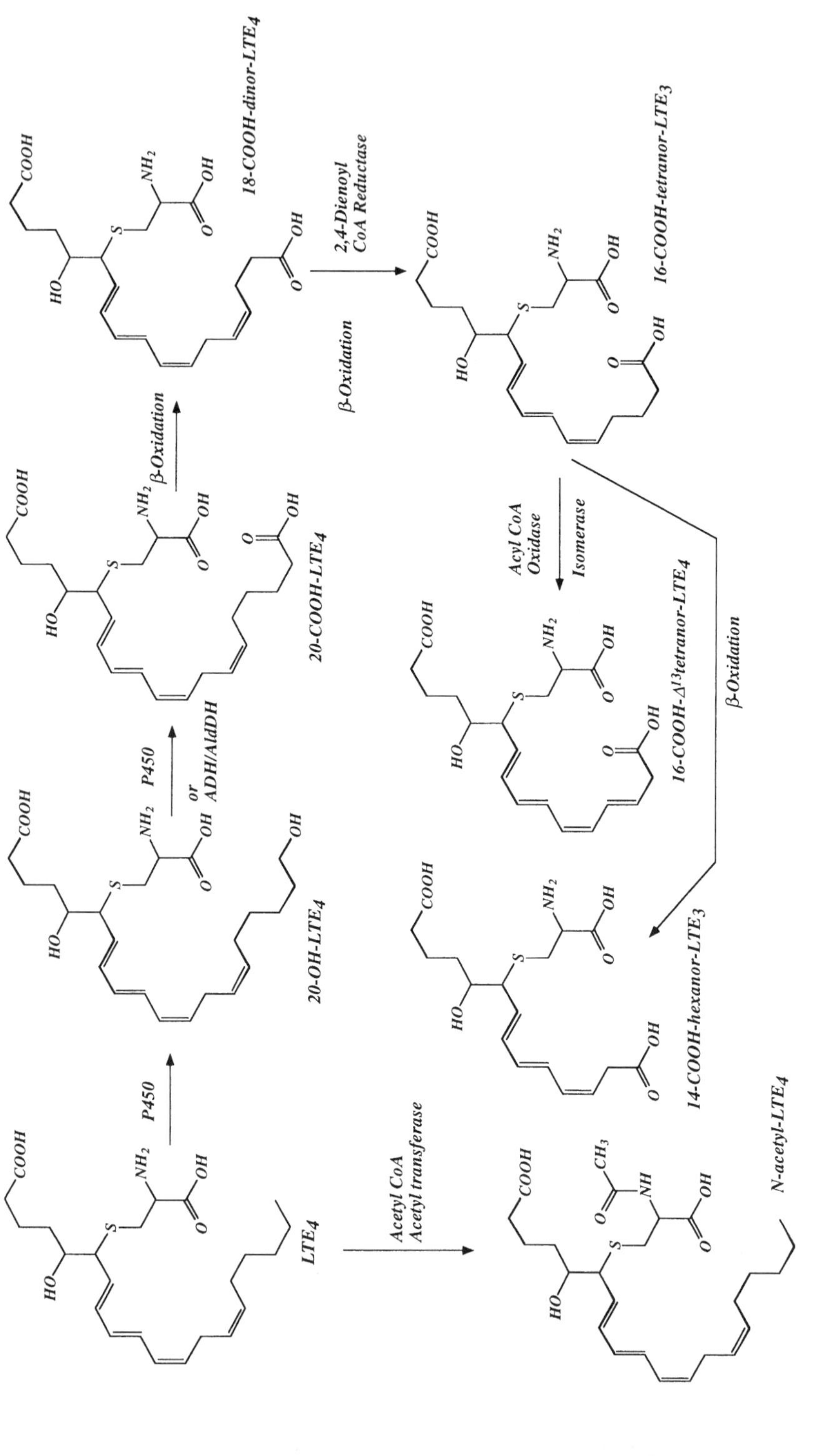
LTE4
P450
20-OH-LTE4
P450
or
ADH/AldDH
20-COOH-LTE4
β-Oxidation
18-COOH-dinor-LTE4
β-Oxidation
2,4-Dienoyl
CoA Reductase
16-COOH-tetranor-LTE3
Acyl CoA
Oxidase
Isomerase
16-COOH-Δ13tetranor-LTE4
β-Oxidation
14-COOH-hexanor-LTE3
Acetyl CoA
Acetyl transferase
N-acetyl-LTE4

Scheme 4

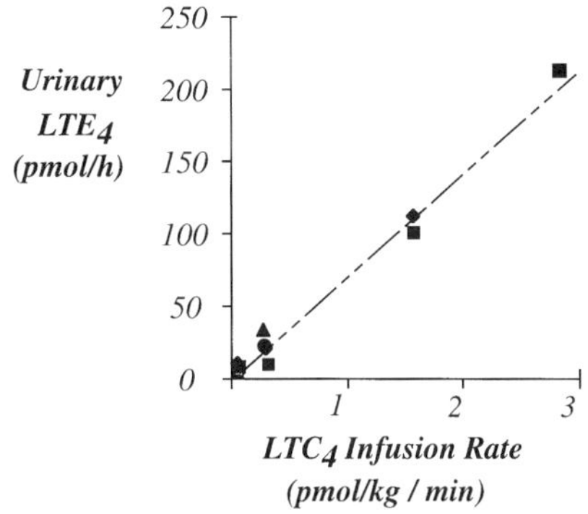

Figure 3 Relationship between an intravenous infused quantity of LTC_4 and resultant urinary concentration of LTE_4 excreted in the immediate first 2 hours. By extrapolation to zero infused LTC_4, it was possible to assess the normal entry rate of LTC_4 into the circulation of normal human subjects as 0.063 ± 0.01 pmol/kg/min. (Adapted from Ref. 53.)

sis (31) and individuals with hepatorenal syndrome (31,55). Excretion of LTE_4 has also been used in studies of airway obstruction in spontaneous acute asthma (56), nocturnal asthma (57), and exercise-induced asthma (58).

III. Metabolism of Leukotriene B_4

Leukotriene B_4 is substantially different in structure from the cysteinyl leukotrienes because of the lack of the peptide conjugate attached to the arachidonic acid backbone as well as the presence of a double bond at carbon-6 in LTB_4. These features significantly alter the metabolism of LTB_4 relative to that of LTC_4. Studies of the metabolism of LTB_4 began as early as the initial investigations into the biosynthesis of LTB_4 since those cells capable of synthesizing LTB_4 were also found to be catabolic as well.

A. Human Polymorphonuclear Leukocytes

Shortly after the discovery of LTB_4, it was found that the human neutrophil could also metabolize LTB_4 into two separable products (59,60). This is illustrated in Figure 4 as the HPLC separation of LTB_4 and its metabolites produced following opsonized zymosan stimulation of neutrophil phagocytosis. In this experiment, electrospray tandem mass spectrometry and multiple reaction monitoring was used to detect the appearance of LTB_4 (*m/z* 335 → 195), 20-hydroxy-LTB_4 (*m/z* 351 → 195), and 20-carboxy-LTB_4 (*m/z* 365 → 195) (61). LTB_4 is a sub-

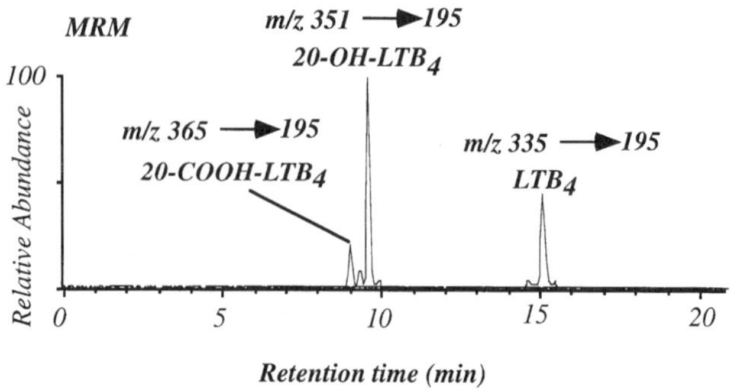

Figure 4 Reverse-phase HPLC and online tandem mass spectrometric analysis of LTB_4 and its ω-oxidized products 20-hydroxy-LTB_4 and 20-carboxy-LTB_4 obtained by stimulation of phagocytosis of human neutrophils with opsonized zymosan. Tandem mass spectrometry was used to specifically detect the emergence of these metabolites from the HPLC column by monitoring specific ion transitions in the multiple reaction monitoring mode (MRM) with the ions indicated. (From Ref. 61.)

strate for a specific NADPH-dependent cytochrome P-450 found in the membrane fraction of the human polymorphonuclear leukocyte (62). This P-450, termed P-$450_{LTB\omega}$, has been cloned and found to be a member of the CYP4 family of P-450 enzymes (63). The initial ω-oxidation product of this reaction, 20-hydroxy-LTB_4 does retain significant biological activity (64), but it can be further oxidized by this cytochrome P-450 to the biologically inactive 20-carboxy-LTB_4. This second step of ω-oxidation was found to involve formation of an intermediate, 20-oxo-LTB_4, which has been isolated and identified (65). The ω-oxidation pathway of LTB_4 metabolism is summarized in Scheme 5.

The human polymorphonuclear leukocyte contains 5-lipoxygenase as well as LTA_4 hydrolase and is thus able to synthesize LTA_4 as well as LTB_4. However, the identification of the metabolic pathways within the human neutrophil has led to speculations as to whether or not LTB_4 is released from neutrophils prior to metabolism (66). Recent studies have suggested that at least 70% of the LTA_4 synthesized by the neutrophil is in fact released intact from the neutrophil (67). The LTB_4 synthesized in the studies of neutrophil stimulation is therefore likely to represent released LTA_4 from the neutrophil followed by reuptake by adjacent neutrophils for metabolic conversion by LTA_4 hydrolase. Only then would LTB_4 be available for subsequent metabolic inactivation by neutrophil cytochrome P-450. It is possible that the stimulation of LTA_4 biosynthesis within the human polymorphonuclear leukocyte in vivo does not involve concomitant transformation into LTB_4 and metabolism within the same neutrophil, rather cellular cooperation and transcellular biosynthesis may play a major role in ultimate LTB_4 bio-

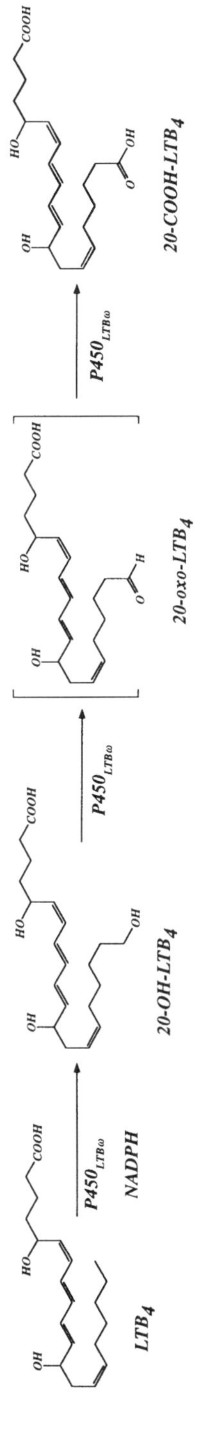
LTB4
P450LTBω
NADPH
20-OH-LTB4
P450LTBω
20-oxo-LTB4
P450LTBω
20-COOH-LTB4

Scheme 5

synthesis (68). Nevertheless, the neutrophil may play an important role in terminating the activity of LTB_4.

Metabolism of 6-*trans*-LTB_4 isomers (6-*trans*-LTB_4 and 6-*trans*-12-epi-LTB_4) by the human polymorphonuclear leukocyte (Fig. 5A) has also been studied (69–71). Two novel reduced metabolites, retaining a conjugated diene rather than a conjugated triene, were observed in these metabolic investigations (69). The structures of these conjugated diene metabolites (from both isomers) were identified as 6,7-dihydro-5-oxo-LTB_4 and 6,7-dihydro-LTB_4 (71). The defining characteristic of the metabolism of these nonenzymatic hydrolysis products of LTA_4 was the reduction of the double bond adjacent to the 5-hydroxy group at carbon-6. However, identification of an oxidized 5-oxo metabolite suggested an important role of this new structural unit in subsequent metabolic steps. This oxidative step was found to be catalyzed by a NAD^+-dependent 5-hydroxy eicosanoid dehydrogenase. Following this oxidation step, the reduction of the 6,7 double bond occurs to form the conjugated diene, a process catalyzed by a Δ^6-reductase (71). The absence of such a metabolic transformation of LTB_4 suggests the geometry of the double bond at carbon-6 is the primary determinant of substrate specificity for this 5-hydroxy dehydrogenase (Scheme 6).

Several additional metabolites of 6-*trans*-LTB_4 were structurally characterized when this eicosanoid was incubated with HepG2 cells (Fig. 5B), including 5-oxo-6,7-dihydro-LTB_4 and 6,7-dihydro-LTB_4 consistent with the operation of the 5-hydroxy dehydrogenase/Δ^6-reductase pathway (71). Subsequent β-oxidation of the 5-oxo-6,7-dihydro-LTB_4 would likely lead to a 3,5-β-diketone, which could be directly cleaved by keto thiolase to yield another metabolite—8-hydroxy-4,6,10-hexadecatrienoic acid. Two more steps of β-oxidation would then yield the most abundant metabolite observed—4-hydroxy-6-dodecanoic acid. It is interesting to note that double bond geometry at carbon-6 in the *trans* position leads to extensive and rapid metabolism of 6-*trans*-LTB_4 into the substantially chain-shortened 12-carbon hydroxy acid, whereas the *cis* double bond at carbon-6, which occurs for LTB_4, substantially reduces the rate of metabolic transformation.

B. Nonhuman Cells In Vitro

Studies of LTB_4 metabolism in circulating polymorphonuclear leukocytes present in animals other than human subjects was found to yield a series of novel reduced metabolites that no longer contained the original conjugated triene present in LTB_4, but a conjugated diene moiety. The rat neutrophil formed these reduced metabolites (72) as did the porcine leukocyte (73). Structural elucidation of this metabolite by mass spectrometry revealed the formation of 10,11-dihydro-LTB_4 and a related compound, 10,11-dihydro-12-oxo-LTB_4. The pathway leading to the formation of this metabolite was found to proceed through a common interme-

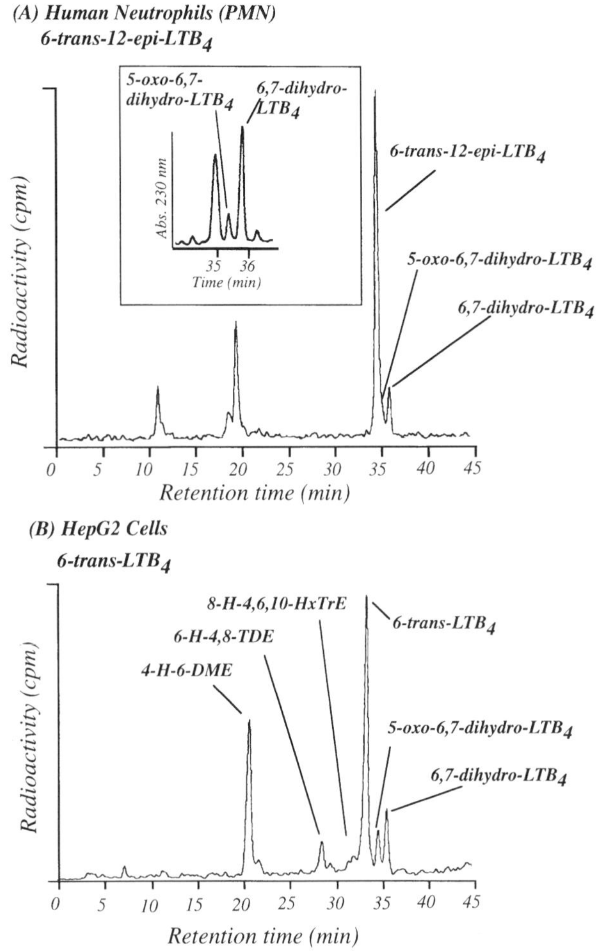

Figure 5 (A) Reverse-phase HPLC separation of the radioactive metabolites of 6-*trans*-12-epi-[^{3}H]LTB$_4$ incubated with human polymorphonuclear leukocytes. (B) Reverse-phase HPLC separation of the radioactive metabolites of 6-trans-[^{3}H]LTB$_4$ incubated with HepG2 cells. Designations used to identify hydroxy fatty acid metabolites follow the suggested rules for abbreviations (96). The metabolic pathway leading to the 6,7-dihydro-LTB$_4$ metabolites is outlined in Scheme 6. (Adapted from Ref. 71.)

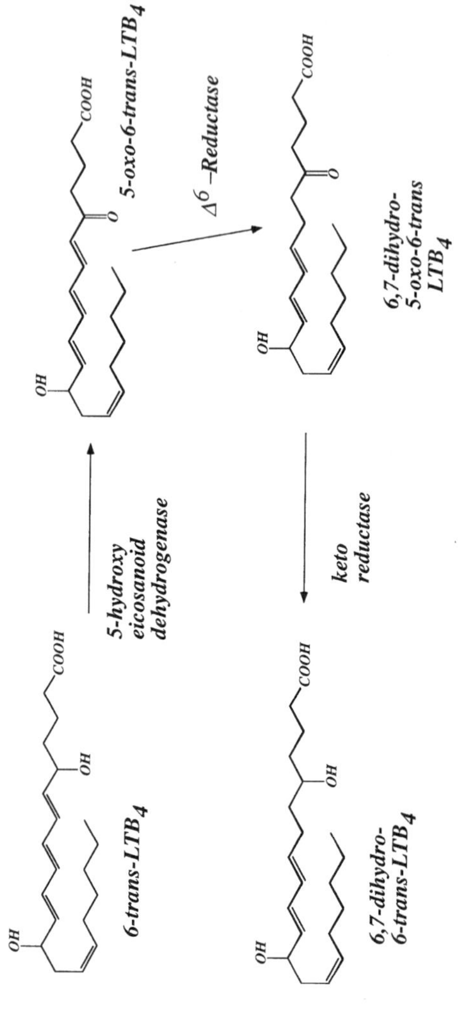
6-trans-LTB4
5-hydroxy eicosanoid dehydrogenase
5-oxo-6-trans-LTB4
Δ6 –Reductase
6,7-dihydro-5-oxo-6-trans LTB4
keto reductase
6,7-dihydro-6-trans-LTB4
OH
COOH
O

Scheme 6

diate, 12-oxo-LTB_4. The enzyme present in the rat neutrophil responsible for this metabolic pathway was found to reside in the endoplasmic reticulum and require NAD^+ as cofactor. The enzyme was termed 12-hydroxyeicosanoid dehydrogenase (74). A further enzyme found in the neutrophil cytosol reduced the double bond at carbon-10 conjugated to the 12-oxo group and part of the conjugated triene. This auxiliary enzyme, termed Δ^{10}-reductase, along with the 12-hydroxyeicosanoid dehydrogenase, accounted for the production of 10,11-dihydro-12-oxo-LTB_4, which was subsequently reduced by keto reductases to the corresponding 10,11-dihydro-LTB_4 metabolites.

This reductase pathway of LTB_4 metabolism has been observed in several other cells including human mesangial cells (75), bone marrow–derived macrophages (76), human monocytes (77), as well as human lung tissue (78). Porcine kidney was found to convert LTB_4 into 12-oxo-LTB_4, 10,11-dihydro-LTB_4, and a further reduced metabolite, 10,11,14,15-tetrahydro-12-oxo-LTB_4 (79). In these latter studies, the initial oxidation of the 12-hydroxy group occurred in the cytosol and required $NADP^+$. The cytosolic 12-hydroxyeicosanoid dehydrogenase has been cloned and its distribution in human tissues studied by Northern blot analysis revealing high expression in kidney, liver, and intestine, but not leukocytes (80) (Scheme 7).

C. Other Human-Derived Cells

The 12-hydroxy-dehydrogenase/Δ^{10}-reductase pathway of LTB_4 metabolism was found to be a major metabolic process for a number of human-derived cells. Human lung macrophages were found to metabolize LTB_4 into a more lipophilic metabolite, tentatively identified as dihydro-LTB_4 (81). Human monocytes also formed 10,11-dihydro- and 10,11-dihydro-12-oxo-LTB_4 (77).

Studies of the metabolism of LTB_4 by human keratinocytes in primary culture (Fig. 6) led to the identification of six previously unidentified metabolites (82). Many of the metabolites were derived from the 12-hydroxyeicosanoid dehydrogenase/Δ^{10}-reductase pathway but included metabolites that were additionally chain-elongated and chain-shortened by β-oxidation. One of the major metabolites was 10-hydroxyoctadecatrienoic acid (10-HOTrE), which contained a conjugated diene and lost the original hydroxy group present at carbon-5.

Perhaps the most interesting keratinocyte metabolites were glutathione adducts of 12-oxo-LTB_4, which likely arose through a 1,8-glutathione conjugation reaction and led to a series of metabolites characterized by a thioether bond linking the sulfur atom of glutathione with the carbon-6 atom of the arachidonic acid backbone of LTB_4. These metabolites were of interest structurally because the carboxy terminus from carbon-1 to carbon-10 was identical to that of LTC_4, whereas the methyl terminus of these metabolites from carbon-20 to carbon-12

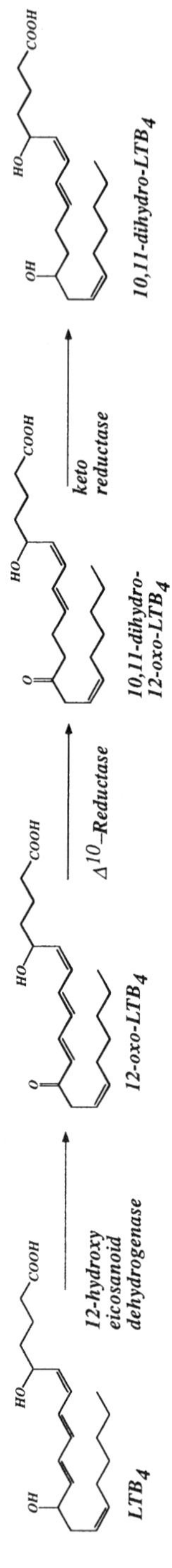
LTB4
12-hydroxy eicosanoid dehydrogenase
12-oxo-LTB4
Δ10-Reductase
10,11-dihydro-12-oxo-LTB4
keto reductase
10,11-dihydro-LTB4
OH
HO
O
COOH

Scheme 7

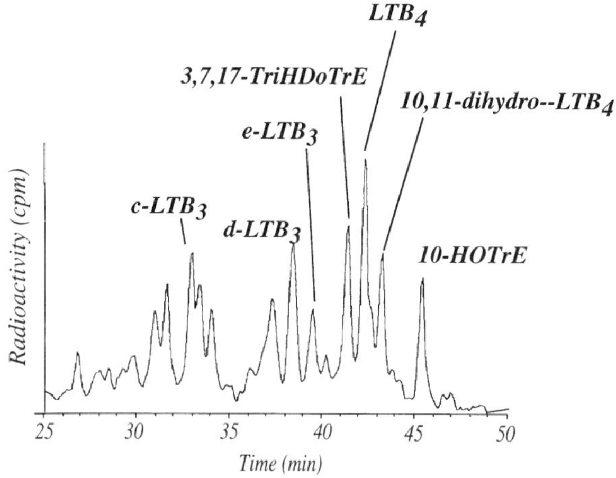

Figure 6 Reverse-phase HPLC separation of radioactive metabolites following incubation of LTB_4 with human keratinocytes in primary culture. All metabolites were derived from the 12-hydroxyeicosanoid dehydrogenase/Δ^{10}-reductase pathway (Scheme 7), including the unique metabolites containing glutathione (c-LTB_3), cysteinyl glycine (d-LTB_3), and cysteine (e-LTB_3) as Michael addition adducts of the intermediate 12-oxo-LTB_4 with glutathione. (Adapted from Ref. 82.)

was identical to that of LTB_4. The glutathione-derived metabolites were structurally characterized using fast atom bombardment ionization and tandem mass spectrometry since volatile metabolites could not be made for gas phase analysis by electron ionization or other GC/MS techniques (83). These techniques had been previously used to characterize LTE_4 (Fig. 7A) present in human urine by collision-induced decomposition of m/z 438 $[M\text{-}H]^-$ to yield an abundant β-elimination ion at m/z 351 and m/z 333 after a further loss of H_2O (83). The tandem mass spectrum of the metabolite corresponding to the cysteinyl adduct of the LTB_4 backbone (e-LTB_3) is shown in Figure 7B with collision-induced decomposition of m/z 456, the carboxylate anion $[M\text{-}H]^-$ of this metabolite. The presence of the cysteine residue could be assigned from abundant ions corresponding β-elimination at m/z 369 and loss of H_2O at m/z 351, as indicated in Figure 7B. These metabolic pathways were quite novel and illustrate additional steps of LTB_4 metabolism not previously appreciated.

D. Hepatocyte Metabolism

The isolated rat hepatocyte was found to rapidly metabolize LTB_4 into several novel metabolites that had not been previously identified (Fig. 8). The structures

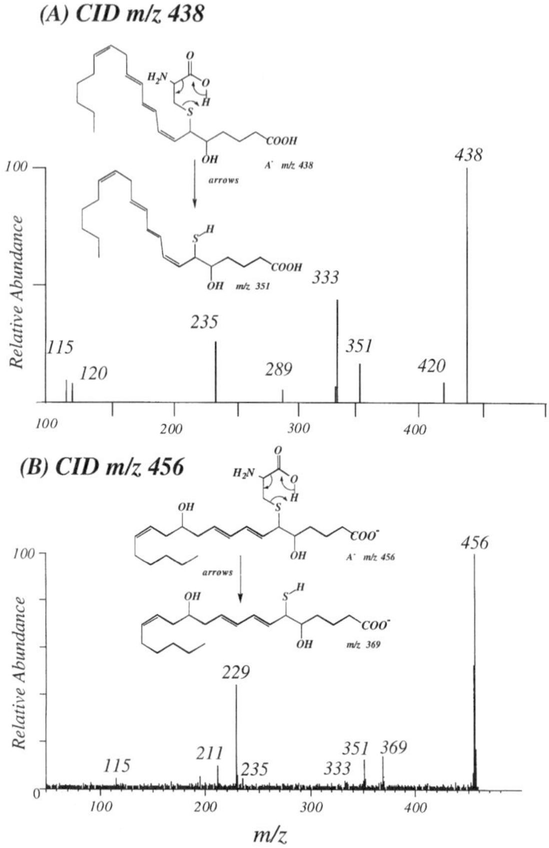

Figure 7 Tandem mass spectrometry of the carboxylate anions obtained from (A) LTE_4 and (B) e-LTB_3, a metabolite of LTB_4 isolated from human keratinocytes. A suggested mechanism leading to the formation of the structurally significant fragment ion at *m/z* 351 for LTE_4 and *m/z* 369 e-LTB_3 are illustrated in the figures corresponding to a β-elimination reaction induced by collisional activation of the carboxylate anions.

of these metabolites were elucidated using mass spectrometry and included 20-hydroxy-LTB_4, 20-carboxy-LTB_4, as well as 18-carboxy-dinor-LTB_4, the taurine conjugate of 18-carboxy-dinor-LTB_4 and 16-carboxy-LTB_3 (84).

Electrospray ionization mass spectrometry and collision-induced decomposition can yield significant structural information, as illustrated in Figure 9A for the collision-induced decomposition of the carboxylate anion from the LTB_4, *m/z* 335. Detailed analysis of the ion chemistry involved and the formation of

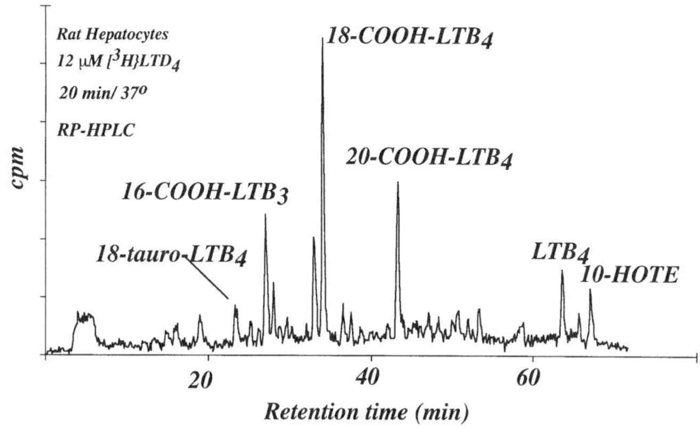

Figure 8 Reverse-phase HPLC separation of radioactive metabolites of [^{3}H]LTB$_4$ following incubation of LTB$_4$ (12 μM) with 2 × 10^6 rat hepatocytes (1 mL) for 20 min at 37°C. Metabolites were structurally characterized using electrospray mass spectrometry and the structures of the metabolites and their pathway of metabolic formation are outlined in Scheme 8.

these ions has been reported (18,19), including a likely mechanism responsible for the appearance of the most abundant decomposition ion at *m/z* 195. This ion would correspond to cleavage of the bond between carbons 11 and 12 driven by a complex series of double bond rearrangements with charge localized on the oxygen atom at carbon-12. Thus, this ion contains many of the structural features inherent in LTB$_4$ and its metabolites. The collision-induced decomposition of the metabolite, which had a carboxylate anion at *m/z* 337, revealed that this metabolite was likely unaltered between carbons 1 and 11 from the LTB$_4$ structure (Fig. 9B). In contrast, the collision induced decomposition of *m/z* 337 from 10,11-dihydro-LTB$_4$ was completely lacking this ion at *m/z* 195 (Fig. 9C). The clue to the exact structural alteration of this LTB$_4$ metabolite (Fig. 9B) comes in part from the abundant ion at *m/z* 113, which would be formed by a charge-remote fragmentation with transfer of the C-12 hydroxy proton to C-15 followed by loss of the neutral aldehyde (C-1 through C-12) with formation of the observed terminal C-18 carboxylate anion (19). The identification of these metabolites was the first indication that LTB$_4$ would participate in β-oxidation of the initially formed 20-carboxy-LTB$_4$.

Keppler and coworkers (85) found that rat liver cytosol contained enzymes that could rapidly oxidize 20-hydroxy-LTB$_4$ into 20-carboxy-LTB$_4$ when exogenous NAD$^+$ was added. This suggested involvement of alcohol dehydrogenase and aldehyde dehydrogenase in this oxidation pathway rather than a membrane-

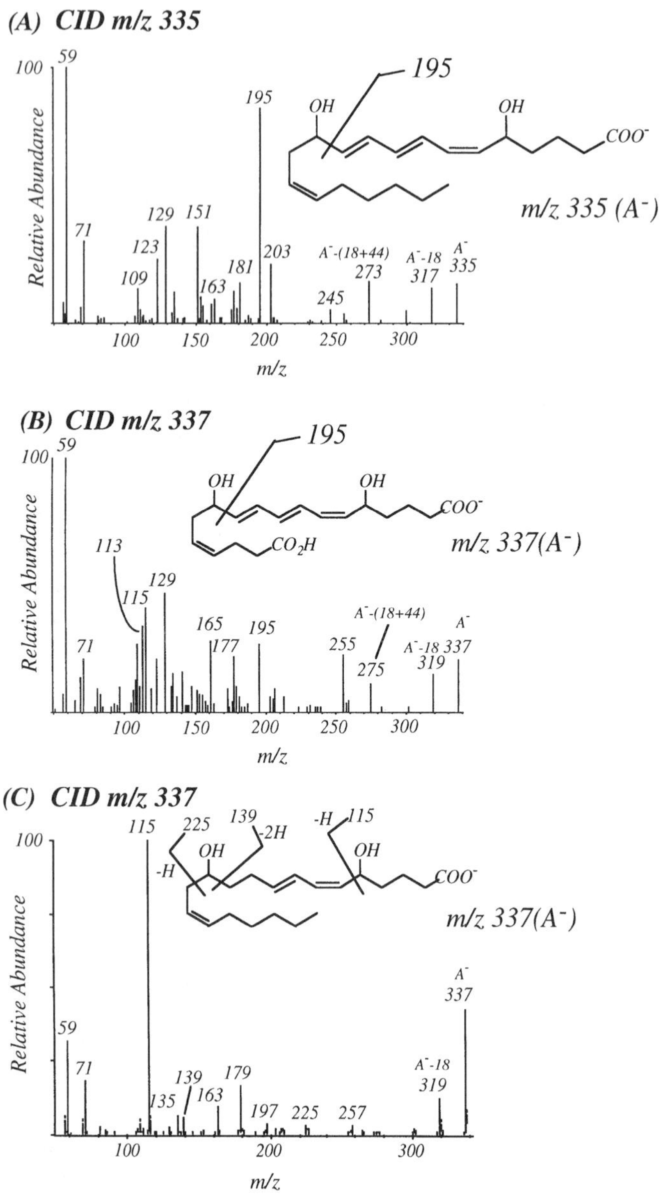

Figure 9 Collision-induced decomposition (CID) of the carboxylate anion of LTB_4 and metabolites in a tandem quadrupole mass spectrometer. The abundant product ions are characteristic of the molecular structure of each of the metabolites (19). The most abundant product ion for LTB_4 (A) as well as 18-carboxy-LTB_4 (B) was *m/z* 195. The product ion spectrum of 10,11-dihydro-LTB_4 (C) does not lead to this abundant ion, rather the most abundant ion observed at *m/z* 115.

associated cytochrome P-450 for the conversion of the primary alcohol at C-20 to a carboxylate moiety. A cytochrome P-450 was found in the hepatocyte that could hydroxylate LTB_4 at the ω-position, but this P-450 was substantially different in its enzymatic characteristics, namely, a substantially higher case of K_m, from that measured for human neutrophil $P\text{-}450_{LTB\omega}$ (86).

The taurine conjugate of 18-carboxy-LTB_4 and 16-carboxy-LTB_3 suggested that further enzymatic processing of the 18-carboxy-LTB_4 CoA ester takes place within the hepatocyte. The conjugation of the amino acid taurine with 18-carboxy-LTB_4 likely targeted export of this metabolite into the bile. The reduction of the double bond at carbon-14 of LTB_4 was a key structural alteration leading to the 16-carboxy-tetranor-LTB_3 metabolite. This reduction process likely involved 2,4-dienoyl-CoA reductase during the β-oxidation of 18-carboxy-dinor-LTB_4 and the intermediate formation of the requisite conjugated diene of the CoA ester. The requirement of NADPH in the formation of this metabolite was established by Keppler and coworkers (87).

β-Oxidation of LTB_4 (Scheme 8) was found to take place in both the peroxisomes and mitochondria in studies of the subcellular localization of hepatocyte LTB_4 metabolism (87). The cysteinyl leukotrienes were found to be metabolized by β-oxidation from the ω-oxidized LTE_4 exclusively within the peroxisome (87).

The involvement of alcohol dehydrogenase in the major hepatic pathway of LTB_4 metabolism, namely conversion of 20-hydroxy-LTB_4 into 20-carboxy-LTB_4, suggested that it may be possible to inhibit LTB_4 metabolism by ethanol at concentrations relevant to human subject ingestion (88). Furthermore, ethanol causes an alteration in the $NADPH/NAD^+$ ratio, and these cofactors are required in intermediate steps of LTB_4 β-oxidation. The reduction of the overall rate of metabolism of LTB_4 was observed when hepatocytes were treated with ethanol as well as an accumulation of 20-hydroxy-LTB_4 (88), the formation of a new metabolite, 3-hydroxy-LTB_4 (89), and cytochrome P-450 metabolites with a 3-hydroxyl substituent. Interestingly, the addition of ethanol reduced the metabolic inactivation of LTB_4 since 20-hydroxy-LTB_4 and 3-hydroxy-LTB_4 were found to be potent chemotactic agents (90). The identification of 3-hydroxy-LTB_4 was the first indication that β-oxidation from the C-1 carboxy terminus of LTB_4 could take place under appropriate circumstances. This metabolite likely accumulated in the β-oxidation pathway because the next step of β-oxidation involves the oxidation of the 3-hydroxy-LTB_4 CoA ester and conversion into 3-oxo-LTB_4 CoA ester, which required NAD^+ as a cofactor. The accumulation of these chemotactic eicosanoids has led to the hypothesis that a new chemotactic gradient may exist in individuals with chronic exposure to ethanol and may be responsible, in part, for the phenomenon referred to as alcoholic hepatitis where the polymorphonuclear leukocyte accumulates in the liver (90).

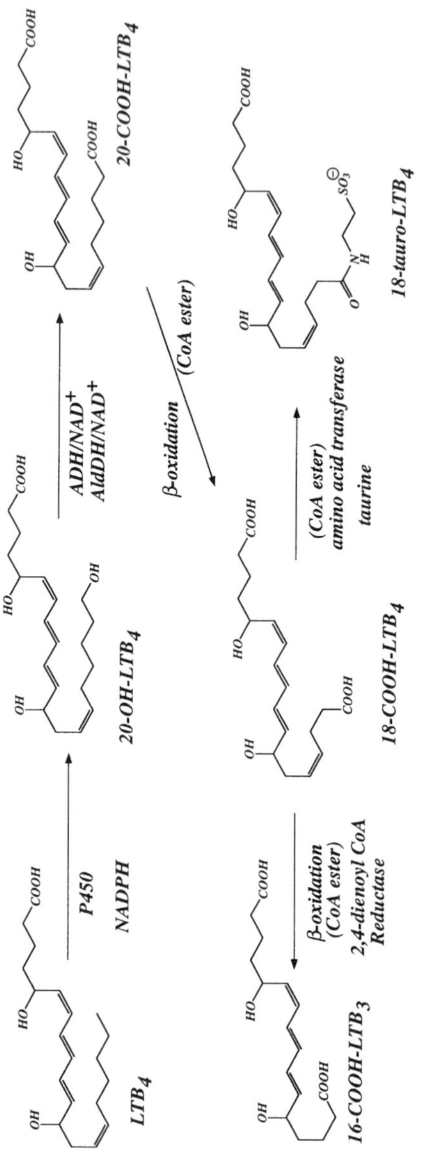
LTB4
P450
NADPH
20-OH-LTB4
ADH/NAD+
AldDH/NAD+
20-COOH-LTB4
β-oxidation
(CoA ester)
18-COOH-LTB4
(CoA ester)
amino acid transferase
taurine
18-tauro-LTB4
β-oxidation
(CoA ester)
2,4-dienoyl CoA
Reductase
16-COOH-LTB3

Scheme 8

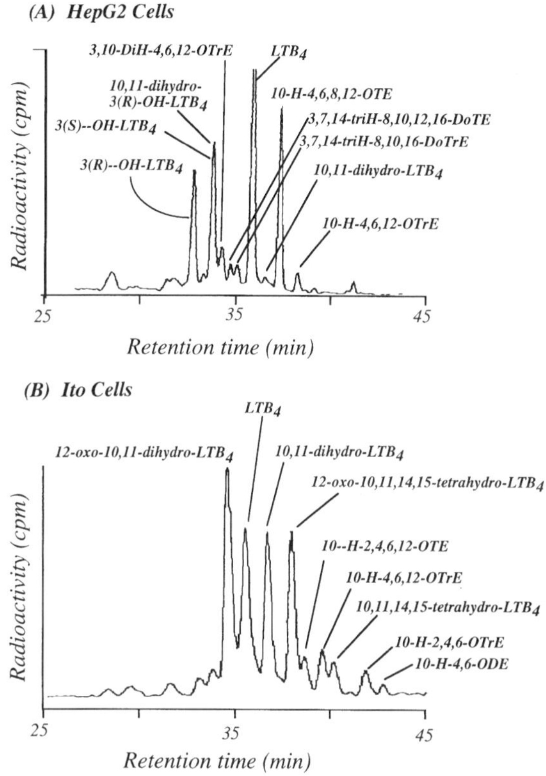

Figure 10 Reverse-phase HPLC separation of radioactive metabolites obtained following incubation of [^{3}H]LTB$_4$ with (A) HepG2 cells and (B) Ito cells. Designations used to identify the hydroxy fatty acid metabolites follow the suggested rules for abbreviation (96). (Adapted from Refs. 91 and 92.)

E. Cultured Cells of Hepatic Origin

Incubation of LTB$_4$ with HepG2 cells, a human-derived hepatoma cell line, yielded several metabolites, as indicated in Figure 10A (91). Structural identification of the major metabolite, which eluted after LTB$_4$ on this HPLC chromatogram, was found to be 10-hydroxy-4,6,8,12-octadecatetraenoic acid (10-HOTE) (91). This metabolite unexpectedly involved chain-shortening from β-oxidation from the carboxy terminus of LTB$_4$, but was missing the hydroxy group at carbon-5 in the parent leukotriene. The mechanism for this unique metabolic transformation is currently unknown; however, it was suggested to involve β-oxidation.

Other metabolites included chain-elongation and β-oxidation leading to 3-

hydroxy-LTB_4 epimers. These metabolites would all involve intermediate formation of the LTB_4 CoA ester. The HepG2 cell also produced metabolites of the 12-hydroxy-dehydrogenase/Δ^{10}-reductase pathway described previously.

Analysis of the metabolites obtained following incubation of LTB_4 with normal rat liver, fat-storing stellate cells, termed Ito cells, was found to lead to extensive metabolism by various pathways (92). In addition to the above-mentioned 12-hydroxyeicosanoid dehydrogenase/Δ^{10}-reductase pathways, a series of major metabolites resulted from the reduction of the double bond at carbon-14 (Fig. 10B). This Δ^{14}-reductase pathway (Scheme 9) accounted for approximately 20% of the metabolized LTB_4 in this cell type. This pathway had also been observed during incubation of LTB_4 with porcine kidney (79).

F. LTB_4 Metabolism In Vivo

Only a few studies have been reported concerning the metabolism of LTB_4 in vivo. The metabolism of high specific activity tritium-labeled LTB_4 in rats was reported where bile and urine was collected for one hour after intravenous injection (93). The bile was found to contain 20–25% of the injected LTB_4, whereas urine contained substantially less than 10% of the injected dose. The structure elucidation of these bile and urinary metabolites was not carried out; however, HPLC analysis of the bile revealed several metabolites with substantially shorter retention time on reverse-phase HPLC, suggesting chain-shortening of the LTB_4 structure consistent with ω/β-oxidation.

Shortly after the structure elucidation of LTB_4, one study was reported of the metabolism of LTB_4 in the intact monkey (94). When urine was collected following injection of fairly low specific activity [^3H]LTB_4, 25% of the infused radioactivity appeared in the urine after 24 hours. In order to reduce the toxicity of LTB_4 in this study since large amounts of LTB_4 were infused (5 mg), a stepwise LTB_4 infusion was carried out to desensitize the circulating neutrophils to the effects of LTB_4. Purification of the radiolabeled metabolites appearing in the urine was carried out, and one metabolite was found to coelute with 20-hydroxy-LTB_4. The structures of the other urinary metabolites was not reported although several metabolites could be separated from each other.

The presence of metabolites of LTB_4 in the urine of human subjects with genetic disorders has been reported. Eight infant subjects with Zellweger syndrome and neonatal adrenal leukodystrophy were found to have measurable levels of LTB_4 in the urine as well as ω-carboxy-LTB_4 (95). Individuals with Zellweger syndrome lack peroxisomes in their hepatocytes, which are likely involved as a major metabolic subcellular organelle for LTB_4 metabolism. Certainly these observations of urinary LTB_4 and 20-carboxy-LTB_4 highlight the importance of peroxisomal metabolism of LTB_4 in normal human subjects.

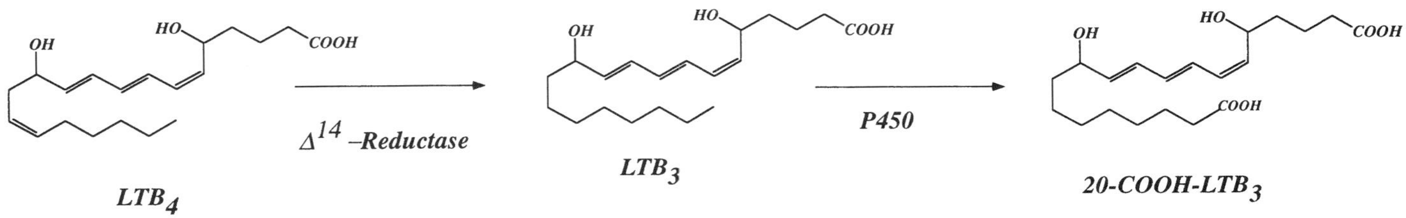

Scheme 9

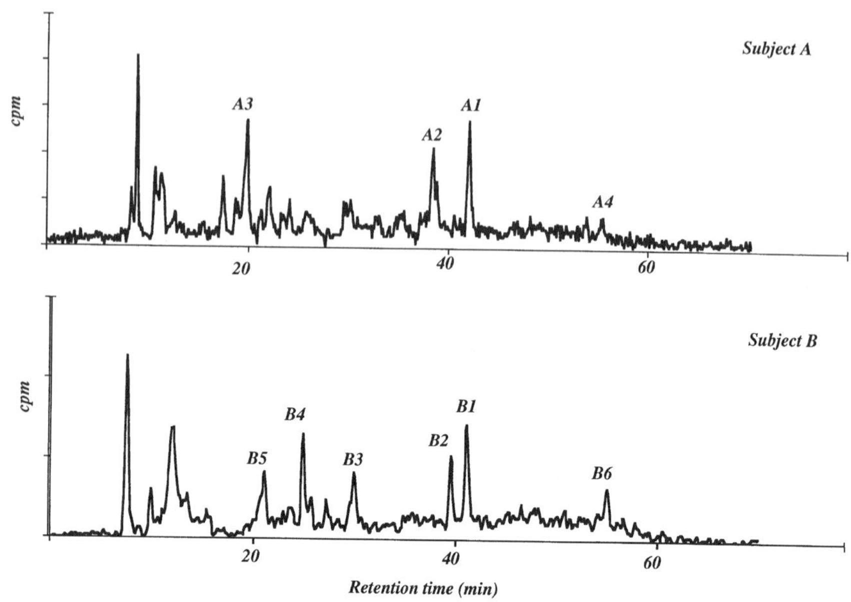

Figure 11 Reverse-phase separation of radioactive, urinary metabolites of [^{3}H]LTB$_4$ infused into two separate human subjects (A and B), excreted within the first 2 hours following infusion. The urine was partially purified by solvent extraction prior to reverse-phase HPLC separation. Unique urinary metabolites in the urine of each subject have been labeled. The metabolite eluting shortly after 40 minutes is likely similar in structure for both subject A (A1) and subject B (B1).

Studies of the metabolism of LTB$_4$ in human subjects have been carried out with high specific activity [^{3}H]LTB$_4$ in order to reduce any potential pharmacological properties of LTB$_4$ in the metabolic studies. Several urinary metabolites have been observed as illustrated for two subjects in Figure 11. For example, a common metabolite appears to elute from reverse-phase HPLC at a retention time similar, but not identical to that of 20-carboxy-LTB$_4$. In fact, none of the metabolites observed as HPLC peaks in this figure coelute with the known metabolites of LTB$_4$ produced by human or animal cells. This suggests the operation of multiple pathways of metabolism in the ultimate disposition of LTB$_4$ before appearance of a metabolite in urine. These results do support the suggestion that a urinary metabolite of LTB$_4$ may serve as a useful index of LTB$_4$ production in vivo and that a quantitative relationship may be able to relate the absolute quantity of

LTB_4 metabolite appearing in urine and the quantity of LTB_4 emerging into the circulation prior to metabolism. The structure characterization of the human LTB_4 urinary metabolites is currently under investigation.

IV. Conclusions

The leukotrienes are a family of novel metabolites of arachidonic acid from the 5-lipoxygenase cascade. The sulfidopeptide leukotrienes and LTB_4 are potent molecules and serve as important lipid mediators in normal physiology as well as pathophysiology. Metabolism of these primary leukotrienes plays a central role in the termination of the biological activity of these molecule in vivo. Partial metabolism is thought to take place very close to the site of biosynthesis of these molecules, likely within these same tissues. Several pathways of metabolism are available for both the cysteinyl leukotrienes as well as the dihydroxy leukotrienes. Cytochrome P-450 metabolism of the methyl terminus of the arachidonate backbone appears to be a general process leading to inactivation of all the leukotrienes. This cytochrome P-450–dependent pathway is the predominant pathway of leukotriene metabolism in the liver, which is probably the metabolic organ responsible for a significant amount of leukotriene metabolism in vivo. Unlike the prostaglandins, β-oxidation and subsequent chain-shortening of the leukotriene from the carboxyl terminus is not a major pathway for hepatic metabolism. The action of hepatic cytochrome P-450 results in a pathway of initial ω-oxidation followed by β-oxidation from the ω-terminus. However, β-oxidation from the carboxy terminus (C-1) does appear to be a metabolic pathway for leukotrienes when the cytochrome P-450 pathway is not predominant. Leukotriene B_4 is metabolized in some cells by a series of unique pathways of hydroxyl oxidation and subsequent reduction of the conjugated ketone structural unit. The 12-hydroxyeicosanoid dehydrogenase/Δ^{10}-reductase pathway appears to be a major pathway of metabolism in many human-derived cells and 12-hydroxyeicosanoid dehydrogenase is expressed in many human tissues including liver.

Measurement of the urinary metabolites of the cysteinyl leukotrienes, as well as LTB_4 metabolites, in the future, will likely play an increasingly important role in assessing in vivo production of these 5-lipoxygenase metabolite. The metabolism of leukotrienes in the human subject is extensive, and significant advances made within the past several years have led to an appreciation of the various pathways that lead to covalent alteration of the leukotriene structure. The understanding of these detailed pathways of metabolism and the individual enzymes involved in the inactivation of leukotrienes may shed additional light on the altered biochemistry in individuals with defects in these enzymatic pathways.

Acknowledgments

This work was supported, in part, by grants from the National Institutes of Health (HL25785).

References

1. Borgeat P, Samuelsson, B. Arachidonic acid metabolism in polymorphonuclear leukocytes: unstable intermediate in formation of dihydroxy acids. Proc Natl Acad Sci 1979; 76:3213–3217.
2. Ford-Hutchinson AW, Gresser M, Young RN. 5-Lipoxygenase. Annu Rev Biochem 1994; 63:383–417.
3. Corey EJ. Chemical studies on slow reacting substances/leukotrienes. Experientia 1982; 38:1259–1381.
4. Hay DW, Torphy TJ, Undem BJ. Cysteinyl leukotrienes in asthma: old mediators up to new tricks. Trends Pharmacol Sci 1995; 16:304–309.
5. Ota K, Hammock BD. Cytosolic and microsomal epoxide hydrolases: differential properties in mammalian liver. Science 1980; 207:1479–1481.
6. Tsuchida S, Sato K. Glutathione transferases and cancer. Crit Rev Biochem Mol Biol 1992; 27:337–384.
7. Ohishi N, Minami M, Kobayashi J, Seyama Y, Hata J, Yotsumoto H, Takaku F, Shimizu T. Immunological quantitation and immunohistochemical localization of leukotriene A_4 hydrolase in guinea pig tissues. J Biol Chem 1990; 265:7520–7525.
8. Penrose JF, Spector J, Lam BK, Friend DS, Xu K, Jack RM, Austen KF. Purification of human lung leukoctriene C_4 synthase and preparation of a polyclonal antibody. Am J Respir Crit Care Med 1995; 152:283–289.
9. Patrono C. Biosynthesis and pharmacological modulation of thromboxane in humans. Circulation 1990; 81:I12–I15.
10. Diczfalusy U. β-Oxidation of eicosanoids. Prog Lipid Res 1994; 33:403–428.
11. Hansen HS. 15-Hydroxy prostaglandin dehydrogenase: a review. Prostaglandins 1976; 12:647–679.
12. Schulz H. Beta oxidation of fatty acids. Biochim Biophys Acta 1991; 1081:109–120.
13. Holm KA, Park SS, Gelboin HV, Kupfer D. Monoclonal antibody-directed characterization of rat hepatic P450 catalyzing the omega-1 and omega-2 hydroxylation of prostaglandins. Arch Biochem Biophys 1989; 269:664–677.
14. Pace-Asciak CR. Advances in Prostaglandin, Thromboxane, and Leukotriene Research. Vol. 18. New York: Raven Press, 1989.
15. Murphy RC. Lipid mediators, leukotrienes, and mass spectrometry. J Mass Spectrom 1995; 30:5–16.
16. Murphy RC. Handbook of Lipid Research: Mass Spectrometry of Lipids. Vol. 7. New York: Plenum Press, 1993.
17. Dettoffmann E. Tandem mass spectrometry: a primer. J Mass Spectrom 1996; 31: 129–137.

18. Wheelan P, Zirrolli JA, Murphy RC. Electrospray ionization and low energy tandem mass spectrometry of polyhydroxy unsaturated fatty acids. J Am Soc Mass Spectrom 1996; 7:140–149.
19. Wheelan P, Zirrolli JA, Murphy RC. Negative ion electrospray tandem mass spectrometric structural characterization of leukotriene B_4 (LTB_4) and LTB_4-derived metabolites. J Am Soc Mass Spectrom 1996; 7:129–139.
20. Orning L, Hammarstrom S, Samuelsson B. Leukotriene D: a slow reacting substance from rat basophilic leukemia cells. Proc Natl Acad Sci USA 1980; 77:2014–2017.
21. Bernstrom K, Hammarstrom S. Metabolism of leukotriene D by porcine kidney. J Biol Chem 1981; 256:9579.
22. Keppler D, Guhlmann A, Huber M. Metabolism and actions of leukotrienes in vivo. Prog Appl Microcirc 1990; 17:129–141.
23. Keppler D, Huber M, Hagmann W, Ball HA, Guhlmann A, Kastner S. Metabolism and analysis of endogenous cysteinyl leukotrienes. Ann NY Acad Sci 1988; 524: 68–74.
24. Keppler D, Huber M, Baumert T, Guhlmann A. Metabolic inactivation of leukotrienes. In: Weber G, ed. Advances in Enzyme Regulation. New York: Pergamon Press, 1989:307–319.
25. Yokota K, Shono F, Yamamoto S, Kominami E, Katunuma N. Transformation of leukotriene D4 catalyzed by lysosomal cathepsin H of rat liver. J Biochem 1983; 94:1173–1178.
26. Joris I, Majno G, Corey EJ, Lewish RA. The mechanism of vascular leakage induced by leukotriene E_4. Am J Pathol 1987; 127:19–24.
27. Harper TW, Westcott JY, Voelkel N, Murphy RC. Metabolism of leukotrienes B_4 and C_4 in the isolated perfused rat lung. J Biol Chem 1984; 259:14437–14440.
28. Hayman AL, Spannhake EW, Kadowitz PJ. Prostaglandins and the lung. Am Rev Respir Dis 1978; 117:111–135.
29. Orning L, Norin E, Gustafsson B, Hammarstrom S. In vivo metabolism of leukotriene C_4 in germ-free and conventional rats: fecal excretion of N-acetyl leukotriene E_4. J Biol Chem 1986; 261:766–771.
30. Hagmann W, Denzlinger C, Rapp S, Weckbecker G, Keppler D. Identification of the major endogenous leukotriene metabolite in the bile of rats as N-acetyl leukotriene E_4. Prostaglandins 1986; 31:239–251.
31. Huber M, Kastner S, Scholmerich J, Gerok W, Keppler D. Analysis of cysteinyl leukotrienes in human urine: Enhanced excretion in patients with liver cirrhosis and hepatorenal syndrome. Eur J Clin Invest 1989; 19:53–60.
32. Lee CW, Lewis RA, Corey EJ, Barton A, Oh H, Tauber AI, Austen KF. Oxidative inactivation of leukotriene C_4 by stimulated human polymorphonuclear leukocytes. Proc Natl Acad Sci USA 1982; 79:4166–4170.
33. Goetzl EJ. The conversion of leukotriene C_4 to isomers of leukotriene B_4 by human eosinophil peroxidase. Biochem Biophys Res Commun 1982; 106:270–275.
34. Paterson NAM. Metabolism of leukotriene D_4 by porcine alveolar macrophages. Am Rev Respir Dis 1984; 129:274–278.
35. Neill MA, Henderson WR, Klebanoff SJ. Oxidative degradation of leukotriene C_4 by human monocytes and monocyte-derived macrophages. J Exp Med 1985; 162: 1634–1644.

36. Bernstrom K, Larsen GL, Hammarstrom S. Metabolism of leukotriene E_4 to 5-hydroxy-6-mercapto-7,9-trans-11,14-cis-eicosatetraenoic acid by microfloral cysteine-conjugate B-lyase and rat cecum contents. Arch Biochem Biophys 1989; 275:531–539.
37. Keppler D. Leukotrienes: biosynthesis, transport, inactivation, and analysis. Rev Physiol Biochem Pharmacol 1992; 121: 1–30.
38. Falk E, Muller M, Huber M, Keppler D, Kurz G. Direct photoaffinity labeling of leukotriene binding sites. Eur J Biochem 1989; 186:741–747.
39. Guhlmann A, Krauss K, Oberdorfer F, Siegel T, Scheuber PH, Muller J, Csuk-Glanzer B, Ziegler S, Ostertag H, Keppler D. Noninvasive assessment of hepatobiliary and renal elimination of cysteinyl leukotrienes by positron emission tomography. Hepatology 1995; 21:1568–1575.
40. Ishikawa T, Muller M, Klunemann C, Schaub T, Keppler D. ATP-dependent primary active transport of cysteinyl leukotrienes across liver canalicular membrane. Role of the ATP-dependent transport system for glutathione S-conjugates. J Biol Chem 1990; 265:19279–19286.
41. Orning L. ω-Oxidation of cysteine-containing leukotrienes by rat-liver microsomes: Isolation and characterization of ω-hydroxy and ω-carboxy metabolites of leukotriene E_4 and N-acetyl leukotriene E_4. Eur J Biochem 1987; 170:77–85.
42. Stene DO, Murphy RC. Metabolism of leukotriene E_4 in isolated rat hepatocytes. Identification of beta-oxidation products of sulfidopeptide leukotrienes. J Biol Chem 1988; 263:2773–2778.
43. Perrin P, Zirrolli J, Stene DO, Lellouche JP, Beaucourt JP, Murphy RC. In vivo formation of β-oxidized metabolites of leukotriene E_4 in the rat. Prostaglandins 1988; 37:53–60.
44. Foster A, Fitzsimmons B, Rokach J, Letts G. Evidence of in vivo ω-oxidation of peptide leukotrienes in the rat: Biliary excretion of 20-CO_2H N-acetyl LTE_4. Biochem Biophys Res Commun 1987; 148:1237–1245.
45. Ball HA, Keppler D. ω-Oxidation products of leukotriene E_4 in bile and urine of the monkey. Biochem Biophys Res Commun 1987; 148:664–670.
46. Tagari P, Foster A, Delorme D, Girard Y, Rokach J. Metabolism and excretion of exogenous $[^3H]LTC_4$ in primates. Prostaglandins 1989; 37:629–640.
47. Denzlinger C, Guhlmann A, Scheuber PH, Wilker D, Hammer DK, Keppler D. Metabolism and analysis of cysteinyl leukotrienes in the monkey. J Biol Chem 1986; 261:15601–15606.
48. Huber M, Muller J, Leier I, Jedlitschky G, Ball HA, Moore KP, Taylor GW, Williams R, Keppler D. Metabolism of cysteinyl leukotrienes in monkey and man. Eur J Biochem 1990; 194:309–315.
49. Orning L, Kaijser L, Hammarstrom S. In vivo metabolism of leukotriene C_4 in man: urinary excretion of leukotriene E_4. Biochem Biophys Res Commun 1985; 130:214–220.
50. Verhagen J, Bel EH, Kijne GM, Sterk PJ, Bruynzeel PLB, Veldink GA, Vliegenthart JFG. The excretion of leukotriene E_4 into urine following inhalation of leukotriene D_4 by human individuals. Biochem Biophys Res Commun 1987; 148:864–868.

51. Sala A, Voelkel N, Maclouf J, Murphy RC. Leukotriene E_4 elimination and metabolism in normal human subjects. J Biol Chem 1990; 265:21771–21778.
52. Murphy RC, Sala A, Voelkel N, Maclouf J. Appearance of urinary metabolites of LTE_4 in human subjects. Ann NY Acad Sci 1991; 629:105–111.
53. Maclouf J, Antoine C, De Caterina R, Sicari R, Murphy RC, Patrignani P, Loizzo S, Patrono C. Entry rate and metabolism of leukotriene C_4 into vascular compartment in healthy subjects. Am J Physiol 1992; 263:H244–H249.
54. Manning PJ, Rokach J, Malo JL, Ethier D, Cartier A, Girard Y, Charleson S, O'Byrne PM. Urinary leukotriene E_4 levels during early and late asthmatic responses. J Allergy Clin Immunol 1990; 86:211–220.
55. Moore KP, Taylor GW, Maltby NH, Siegers D, Fuller RW, Dollery CT, Williams R. Increased production of cysteinyl leukotrienes in hepatorenal syndrome. J Hepatol 1990; 11:263–271.
56. Drazen JM, O'Brien J, Sparrow D, Weiss ST, Martins MA, Israel E, Fanta CH. Recovery of leukotriene E_4 from the urine of patients with airway obstruction. Am Rev Respir Dis 1992; 146:104–108.
57. Wenzel SE, Trudeau JB, Kaminsky DA, Cohn J, Martin RJ, Westcott JY. Effect of 5-lipoxygenase inhibition on bronchoconstriction and airway inflammation in nocturnal asthma. Am J Respir Care Med 1995; 152:897–905.
58. Taylor IK, Wellings R, Taylor GW, Fuller RW. Urinary leukotriene E_4 excretion in exercise-induced asthma. J Appl Physiol 1992; 73:743–748.
59. Hansson G, Lindgren JA, Dahlen SE, Hedqvist P, Samuelsson B. Identification and biological activity of novel omega-oxidized metabolites of leukotriene B_4 from human leukocytes. FEBS Lett 1981; 130:107–112.
60. Lindgren JA, Hansson G, Samuelsson B. Formation of novel hydroxylated eicosatetraenoic acids in preparations of human polymorphonuclear leukocytes. FEBS Lett 1981; 128:329–335.
61. Wheelan P, Murphy RC. Quantitation of 5-lipoxygenase products by electrospray mass spectrometry: effect of ethanol on zymosan-stimulated production of 5-lipoxygenase by human neutrophils. Anal Biochem 1997; 244:110–115.
62. Shak S, Goldstein IM. Leukotriene B_4 ω-hydroxylase in human polymorphonuclear leukocytes: Partial purification and identification as a cytochrome P-450. J Clin Invest 1985; 76:1218–1228.
63. Kikuta Y, Kusunose E, Endo K, Yamamoto S, Sogawa K, Fujii-Kuriyama Y, Kusunose M. A novel form of cytochrome P-450 family in human polymorphonuclear leukocytes: cDNA cloning and expression of leukotriene B_4 omega-hydroxylase. J Biol Chem 1993; 268:9376–9380.
64. Clancy RM, Dahinden CA, Hugli TE. Oxidation of leukotrienes at the ω end: demonstration of a receptor for the 20-hydroxy derivative of leukotriene B_4 on human neutrophils and implications for the analysis of leukotriene receptors. Proc Natl Acad Sci USA 1984; 81:5729–5733.
65. Soberman RJ, Sutyak JP, Okita RT, Wendelborn DF, Roberts LJ, Austen KF. The identification and formation of 20-aldehyde leukotriene B_4. J Biol Chem 1988; 263: 7996–8002.
66. McMillan RM, Foster SJ, Dieppe PA. Leukotriene B4 metabolism in human leukocytes: fact or artefact? Agents Actions 1987; 21:355–357.

67. Sala A, Bolla M, Zarini S, Muller-Peddinghaus R, Folco G. Release of leukotriene A_4 versus leukotriene B_4 from human polymorphonuclear leukocytes. J Biol Chem 1996; 271:17944–17948.
68. Maclouf J, Fitzpatrick FA, Murphy RC. Transcellular biosynthesis of eicosanoids. Pharmacol Res 1989; 21:1–7.
69. Powell WS. Novel pathway for the metabolism of 6-trans-leukotriene B_4 by human polymorphonuclear leykocytes. Biochem Biophys Res Commun 1986; 136:707–712.
70. Powell WS, Gravelle F. Metabolism of 6-trans isomers of leukotriene B_4 to dihydro products by human polymorphonuclear leukocytes. J Biol Chem 1988; 263:2170–2177.
71. Wheelan P, Murphy RC. Metabolism of 6-trans isomers of leukotriene B_4 in cultured hepatoma cells and in human polymorphonuclear leukocytes: Identification of a Δ^6-reductase metabolic pathway. J Biol Chem 1995; 270:19845–19852.
72. Powell WS. Conversion of leukotriene B_4 to dihydro and 19-hydroxy metabolites by rat polymorphonuclear leukocytes. Biochem Biophys Res Commun 1987; 145: 991–998.
73. Powell WS, Gravelle F. Metabolism of leukotriene B_4 to dihydro and dihydro-oxo products by porcine leukocytes. J Biol Chem 1989; 264:5364–5369.
74. Wainwright SL, Powell WS. Mechanism for the formation of dihydro metabolites of 12-hydroxyeicosanoids: conversion of leukotriene B_4 and 12-hydroxy-5,8,10,14-eicosatetraenoic acid to 12-oxo intermediates. J Biol Chem 1991; 266:20899–20906.
75. Kaever V, Bruuns J, Wunder J, Damerau B, Zimmer G, Fauler J. Human glomerular mesangial cells inactivate leukotriene B_4 by reduction into dihydro-leukotriene B_4 metabolites. Life Sci 1990; 46:1465–1470.
76. Kaever V, Martin M, Fauler J, Marx K-H, Resch K. A novel metabolic pathway for leukotriene B_4 in different cell types: primary reduction of a double bond. Biochim Biophys Acta 1987; 922:337–344.
77. Fauler J, Marx K-H, Kaever V, Frolich JC. Human monocytes convert leukotriene B_4 to two dihydro-leukotriene B_4-metabolites. Prostaglandins Leukotrienes Essent Fatty Acids 1989; 37:193–196.
78. Kumlin M, Falck JR, Raud J, Harada Y, Dahlen S-E, Granstrom E. Identification and biological activity of dihydro-leukotriene B_4: a prominent metabolite of leukotriene B_4 in the human lung. Biochem Biophys Res Commun 1990; 170:23–29.
79. Yokomizo T, Izumi T, Takahashi T, Kasama T, Kobayashi Y, Sato F, Taketani Y, Shimizu T. Enzymatic inactivation of leukotriene B_4 by a novel enzyme found in the porcine kidney. Purification and properties of leukotriene B_4 12-hydroxydehydrogenase. J Biol Chem 1993; 268:18128–18135.
80. Yokomizo T, Ogawa Y, Uozumi N, Kume K, Izumi T, Shimizu T. cDNA cloning, expression, and mutagenesis study of leukotriene B_4 12-hydroxydehydrogenase. J Biol Chem 1996; 271:2844–2850.
81. Schonfeld W, Schluter R, Hilger R, Konig. Leukotriene generation and metabolism in isolated human lung macrophages. Immunology 1988; 65:529–536.
82. Wheelan P, Zirrolli JA, Morelli JG, Murphy RC. Metabolism of leukotriene B_4 by cultured human keratinocytes. Formation of glutathione conjugates and dihydro metabolites. J Biol Chem 1993; 268:25439–25448.

83. Sala A, Kayganich K, Zirrolli JA, Murphy RC. Negative ion tandem mass spectrometry of leukotriene E_4 and LTE_4 metabolites: identification of LTE_4 in human urine. J Am Soc Mass Spectrom 1991; 4:314–321.
84. Shirley MA, Murphy RC. Metabolism of leukotriene B_4 in isolated rat hepatocytes. Involvement of 2,4-dienoyl-coenzyme A reductase in leukotriene B_4 metabolism. J Biol Chem 1990; 265:16288–16295.
85. Gotoh Y, Sumimoto H, Takeshige K, Minakami S, Keppler D. NAD^+-dependent oxidation of 20-hydroxyleukotriene B_4 to 20-carboxyleukotriene B_4 by rat liver cytosol. Biochim Biophys Acta 1988; 960:342–350.
86. Romano MC, Eckardt RD, Bender PE, Leonard TB, Straub KM, Newton JF. Biochemical characterization of hepatic microsomal leukotriene B_4 hydroxylases. J Biol Chem 1987; 262:1590–1595.
87. Jedlitschky G, Huber M, Volkl A, Muller M, Leier I, Muller J, Lehmann WD, Fahimi HD, Keppler D. Peroxisomal degradation of leukotrienes by beta-oxidation from the omega-end. J Biol Chem 1991; 266:24763–24772.
88. Baumert T, Huber M, Mayer D, Keppler D. Ethanol-induced inhibition of leukotriene degradation by omega-oxidation. Eur J Biochem 1989; 182:223–229.
89. Shirley MA, Murphy RC. Novel 3-hydroxylated leukotriene B_4 metabolites from ethanol-treated rat hepatocytes. J Am Soc Mass Spectrom 1992; 3:762–768.
90. Shirley MA, Reidhead CT, Murphy RC. Chemotactic LTB_4 metabolites produced by hepatocytes in the presence of ethanol. Biochem Biophys Res Commun 1992; 185:604–610.
91. Wheelan P, Murphy RC. Metabolism of leukotriene B_4 in cultured hepatoma cells. Arch Biochem Biophys 1995; 321:381–389.
92. Wheelan P, Simon FR, Murphy RC. GC/MS analysis of oxo and chain-shortened leukotriene B_4 metabolites: leukotriene B_4 metabolism in Ito cells. J Mass Spectrom 1996; 31:236–246.
93. Hagmann W, Korte M. Hepatic uptake and metabolic disposition of leukotriene B_4 in rats. Biochem J 1990; 267:467–470.
94. Serafin WE, Oates JA, Hubbard WC. Metabolism of leukotriene B_4 in the monkey. Identification of the principal nonvolatile metabolite in the urine. Prostaglandins 1983; 27:899–911.
95. Mayatepek E, Lehmann W-D, Fauler J, Tsikas D, Frolich JC, Schutgens RBH, Wander RJA, Keppler D. Impaired degradation of leukotrienes in patients with peroxisome deficiency disorders. J Clin Invest 1993; 91:881–888.
96. Smith WL, Borgeat P, Hamberg M, Roberts LJI, Willis AL, Yamamoto S, Ramwell PW, Rokach J, Samuelsson B, Corey EJ. Nomenclature. Meth Enzymol 1990; 187: 1–9.

7

Cell Biology of the 5-Lipoxygenase Pathway

Amplification and Generation of Leukotrienes and Lipoxins by Transcellular Biosynthesis

TIMOTHY D. BIGBY

University of California
Department of Veterans Affairs Medical Center
San Diego, California

BRUCE D. LEVY and CHARLES N. SERHAN

Harvard Medical School
and Brigham and Women's Hospital
Boston, Massachusetts

I. Introduction

Leukotrienes are oxygenated products of arachidonic acid produced by the action of 5-lipoxygenase via the epoxide intermediate leukotriene A_4 (LTA_4). The term leukotriene was originally coined because these products were synthesized from arachidonic acid by leukocytes and carried conjugated trienes (1). Since their discovery, leukotrienes have been implicated as key mediators in a wide variety of disorders, including asthma. This chapter reviews the cell biology of the 5-lipoxygenase pathway. The first half of this chapter focuses on the spectrum of cells capable of biosynthesis of 5-lipoxygenase–derived products, their relative ability to generate bioactive products, variations among species, the stimuli for biosynthesis, the regulation of expression of the enzymatic machinery necessary for leukotriene formation, and the unique properties of the 5-lipoxygenase pathway in the lung, especially in asthma. The second half of this chapter focuses on leukotriene and lipoxin transcellular biosynthesis, defined as the cooperative formation of products by two or more cell types, the impact of select cytokines and cell adhesion on 5-lipoxygenase–derived eicosanoid formation, the relationship between leukotriene and lipoxin biosynthesis, lipoxin generation in vivo, and transcellular arachidonate metabolism in respiratory tissues. Except where specifically noted, we will focus on eicosanoid biosynthesis in human cell types and tissues because of significant species differences that exist in features of the 5-lipoxygenase pathway. These species differences will also be specifically reviewed in the hope that this knowledge may provide insights into eicosanoid biochemistry and biology, as well as insights into human diseases, including asthma.

II. Cellular Leukotriene Generation

A. Cellular Distribution of the 5-Lipoxygenase Pathway

Myeloid Cells

Neutrophils

The initial molecular evidence for the existence of a 5-lipoxygenase pathway was reported by Borgeat et al., who demonstrated that rabbit neutrophils were capable of synthesis of 5-(*S*)-hydroxy-6-*trans*-8,11,14-*cis*-eicosatetraenoic acid (5-HETE) when challenged with arachidonic acid (2). The formation of dihydroxy-eicosatetraenoic derivatives of arachidonic acid was first discovered by Borgeat and Samuelsson when glycogen-elicited rabbit neutrophils obtained from the peritoneum were incubated with arachidonic acid (3). They found that neutrophils converted from 0.5 to 2% of the substrate to a dihydroxy acid that was stereochemically pure at C-5 and C-12. Borgeat and Samuelsson further delineated the dihydroxy metabolites of rabbit neutrophils (4) by characterizing their structures and, subsequently, the total chemical synthesis of leukotriene B_4 (LTB_4) by Corey and colleagues allowed definitive assignment of the stereochemistry of this compound as 5(*S*),12(*R*)-dihydroxy-6,14-*cis*-8,10-*trans*-eicosatetraenoic acid (5). We now recognize that virtually all cells of myeloid origin are capable of generating substantial quantities of products from the 5-lipoxygenase pathway. Neutrophils are perhaps the best characterized in this regard. The principal 5-lipoxygenase products of isolated human neutrophils are LTB_4 and 5-HETE (6) (Table 1). Neutrophils, prepared free of platelets and eosinophils, do not generate LTC_4 (7), but these cells, and other leukocytes, release up to 50% of their LTA_4 without further metabolism prior to release (8–10). These data suggest that neutrophils and other inflammatory cells can participate in transcellular biosynthesis of leukotrienes in the presence of cells that carry LTA_4 hydrolase or LTC_4 synthase activity (see Sec. III).

Mononuclear Phagocytes

Mononuclear phagocytes, including peripheral blood monocytes (11–13) and tissue macrophages, are capable of synthesizing 5-lipoxygenase products (13–15). In humans, these products again appear to be principally LTB_4 and 5-HETE (Table 1). Mononuclear phagocytes also release LTA_4, which can be utilized for the synthesis of LTB_4 (16,17) or LTC_4 (18) by other cell types. In addition, mononuclear phagocytes may be able to synthesize cysteinyl leukotrienes, as suggested

Table 1 5-Lipoxygenase Products of Inflammatory Cells

Cell type	5-Lipoxygenase product	Relative-amount (pmol/10^6 cells)	Ref.
Neutrophils	LTB_4	30–60 pmol/10^6 cells	6,7,51,68
	5-HETE	Similar	6,7,51
	LTA_4		10
Macrophages	LTB_4	>180 pmol/10^6 cells	13–15
	5-HETE	>160 pmol/10^6 cells	13
	LTA_4		13
	LTC_4		19,22
Monocytes	LTB_4	>16 pmol/10^6 cells	11–13,18
	5-HETE	>18 pmol/10^6 cells	13,18
	LTC_4		
	LTA_4	5–10 pmol/10^6 cells	18
Eosinophils	LTC_4	150 pmol/10^6 cells	27,69
	5-HETE	Similar	27
Basophils	LTC_4	90 pmol/10^6 cells	32–34
	5-HETE	Similar	
Mast cells	LTC_4	~90 pmol/10^6 cells	30,31
	5-HETE		
	LTB_4	Trace	

by a variety of studies (19–21). Although not examined in detail, macrophages from different tissue sites may have different capacities for 5-lipoxygenation of arachidonic acid and different profiles of 5-lipoxygenase products. Two independent studies indicate that human peritoneal macrophages are capable of synthesis of LTC_4, in addition to LTB_4 and 5-HETE (19,22). Alveolar and interstitial macrophages in the lung may also differ in their profile and capacity for 5-lipoxygenation of arachidonic acid. This is a difficult comparison with human cells, but when examined with mouse cells both quantities and profiles of 5-lipoxygenase products may be different (23). When monocytes and lung macrophages are directly compared, lung macrophages obtained by bronchoalveolar lavage have about 10-fold greater capacity for 5-lipoxygenation of arachidonic acid (13). This is due to an 8- to 10-fold greater quantity of immunoreactive 5-lipoxygenase (24,25) and a 40-fold increase in FLAP (25). Additional work will be required to demonstrate definitively whether mononuclear phagocytes in normals, or in humans with disease, contain appreciable amounts of leukotriene C_4 synthase.

Eosinophils

Eosinophils are a prominent pathological feature of allergic inflammation and are found in large numbers of the airways of most asthmatics (26). Eosinophils were first described by Weller and colleagues to release LTC_4 and very modest amounts of LTB_4 in response to the calcium ionophore, A23187 (27) (Table 1). More recent data suggest that these cells have not only a potent 5-lipoxygenase pathway, but also have a prominent 15-lipoxygenase pathway, as will be discussed subsequently. However, we now recognize that this latter enzyme also can generate LTA_4 via the action of 15-lipoxygenase as an LTA_4 synthase (28).

Mast Cells and Basophils

Mast cells are important resident inflammatory cells of the lungs and airways. They are increased in a variety of lung diseases, most prominently in asthma, where they are found primarily in a subepithelial location within the airway (29). However, modest numbers of mast cells are also present within the airway lumen. More limited information is available on lung mast cell arachidonic acid metabolism because of the difficulty in obtaining adequate human tissue and the problem of isolating these cells in a functional state. However, mast cells do contain a potent lipoxygenase pathway. The principal lipoxygenase product of stimulated mast cells is LTC_4; however, they also release modest amounts of LTB_4 (30,31) (Table 1). Basophils also have a potent 5-lipoxygenase pathway, and LTC_4 is the predominant product (32,33). Basophils do not, however, release measurable amounts of LTB_4 upon cell stimulation (34).

Lymphocytes

Lymphocytes are the principal cell type mediating specific immune responses. However, via the release of a variety of cytokines and a variety of other functions, they may also participate in nonspecific inflammatory responses (35). Until recently, lymphocytes were presumed to not contain a 5-lipoxygenase pathway based on stimulation of intact lymphocytes. To the contrary, B lymphocytes and lymphoblastoid B cells have clearly been shown to contain 5-lipoxygenase activity and to convert arachidonic acid to LTB_4 (17). Additional studies have demonstrated that B cells express 5-lipoxygenase and FLAP, but T cells express only FLAP (36). Stimulated 5-lipoxygenase activity in B cells is relatively modest; however, when these cells are treated with some reducing agents, stimulated 5-lipoxygenase activity is increased, suggesting that this activity varies with the redox status of the cell (36).

Nonmyeloid Cells

A variety of cells other than myeloid cells have been suggested to express 5-lipoxygenase activity. Leukotrienes and other lipoxygenase products have been suggested to play a variety of roles in the brain including in neurotransmission, ischemia-reperfusion injury, brain edema, regulation of permeability of the blood-brain barrier, and brain tumors (for review see Ref. 37). The cells of origin in the brain have been investigated in animal models primarily, and few data exist from studies performed in human tissues. However, in addition to microglial cells and inflammatory cells, specific neurons, including some human brain tumors, may express 5-lipoxygenase and FLAP (38). Interestingly, these cells appear to contain a multitranscript family for 5-lipoxygenase, which has not been reported in inflammatory cells. However, a detailed discussion of this area is beyond the scope of the present review.

Epithelial cell arachidonic acid metabolism has been extensively examined. The overwhelming balance of data indicates that human airway epithelial cells contain a 15-lipoxygenase pathway (39). By contrast, human intestinal epithelial cells express 12-lipoxygenase, at least in the setting of inflammatory bowel disease (40). Primary isolates of normal human epithelial cells have not convincingly been demonstrated to contain 5-lipoxygenase activity (41). A variety of studies in human cell lines have, however, indicated that gastrointestinal epithelial cells may express 5-lipoxygenase activity (39). The gastric cancer cell line AGS has been shown to produce leukotrienes B_4, C_4, and D_4 (42). Likewise, the Caco-2 colonic epithelial cell line also is capable of synthesis of modest amounts of LTB_4 in response to the calcium ionophore A23187 (43). The human intestinal epithelial cell line, 407, releases both 5-HETE and LTB_4 when stimulated with A23187 (44). Only limited studies have been performed examining human epithelial cell lines with antibody or cDNA probes for 5-lipoxygenase or FLAP (45). In these studies, intestinal epithelial cell lines such as HT-29 and Caco-2 were found to have FLAP mRNA by Northern blots, but only HT-29 cells also contained mRNA for 5-lipoxygenase. These findings raise the possibility that LTB_4 synthesis by Caco-2 cells may occur via another pathway for synthesis of this product (45). These studies also raise serious doubts that native epithelial cells contain significant quantities of 5-lipoxygenase and FLAP, and it is doubtful that these cells synthesize significant quantities of leukotrienes. Recent studies have, however, again raised the possibility that 5-lipoxygenase activity may be expressed in epithelial cells under specific circumstances. Lung cancer cells, including a variety of squamous and nonsquamous lung cancer cell lines, express mRNA encoding for both 5-lipoxygenase and FLAP in response to insulinlike growth factor-1 and gastrin-releasing peptide (46,47). Blockade of the 5-lipoxygenase pathway induces apoptosis in these cells. Furthermore, in situ hybridization in both squamous and nonsquamous lung cancers reveals mRNA encoding for 5-lipoxygenase. Thus, the airway epithelium may be able to participate in the development of inflammation via 5-lipoxygenase activity in some circumstances. Because 5-lipoxygenase products may modulate cell growth (47,48), it is reasonable to consider the possibility that they may be involved in oncogenesis.

B. Stimuli for Biosynthesis of 5-Lipoxygenase Products

The biologically relevant stimuli for the 5-lipoxygenase pathway have been relatively difficult to establish (Table 2). However, stimulation of the 5-lipoxygenase

Table 2 Stimuli for the 5-Lipoxygenase Pathway

Cell type	Stimulus	Ref.
Neutrophils	A23187	4,6,7
	Arachidonic acid	3
	Zymosan	56
	FMLP	63
	Plasmin	61,62
	C5a	63
	Urate crystals	58,59
Macrophages	A23187	13–15
	Zymosan	52–54
	IgE	57
Monocytes	A23187	11–13
	Zymosan	13,55
	Aggregated Ig	21
Eosinophils	A23187	27,69
	IgE	27
	FMLP	64
Basophils	A23187	32–34
	IgE	32
	C5a	33
Mast cells	A23187	30
	IgE	30

pathway is associated with a substantial influx of extracellular calcium into the cell. Likewise, stimulation of the 5-lipoxygenase pathway can be prevented by removing calcium from the extracellular medium irrespective of the stimulus (49). Stimulation results in a burst of lipoxygenase activity that is relatively short-lived (<30 min) (13). The explanation for this short duration of activity is unknown, but is probably due to suicide inactivation of 5-lipoxygenase.

Many in vitro studies examining 5-lipoxygenase have utilized nonbiological stimuli, such as the calcium ionophore A23187. This has been an extremely valuable tool in order to determine the maximal capacity for 5-lipoxygenation of arachidonic acid in specific cell types. Essentially all inflammatory cells respond to A23187 or other calcium ionophores by releasing 5-lipoxygenase products (50). Elicited rabbit neutrophils have also been shown to release 5-lipoxygenase products when incubated simply with high concentrations of arachidonic acid (3). However, elicited cells are probably primed by the harvesting process for the generation of lipoxygenase products. Very high concentrations of arachidonic acid can also mimic detergent-like actions on cells. In contrast, under most experimental conditions, inflammatory cells do not release significant quantities of 5-lipoxygenase products in response to exogenous arachidonic acid alone (13,51).

Particulate stimuli have been shown to stimulate 5-lipoxygenase in cells that are capable of phagocytosis. Zymosan, a component of yeast cell walls that can fix complement, has been utilized in both unopsonized (52) and opsonized forms (53,54) to stimulate 5-lipoxygenase activity. Zymosan stimulates monocytes (55) and neutrophils (56) via the beta glucan receptor. Aggregated IgE also stimulates macrophage 5-lipoxygenase activity (57), and aggregated immunoglobulins G, A, and E stimulate leukotriene release from human monocytes (21). The potency of these stimuli for 5-lipoxygenase activity is about one-fourth that of ionophore, based on the results of these studies. IgE that is aggregated or bound to antigen is also a potent stimulus for both mast cell (30) and basophil (32) 5-lipoxygenase activity. Eosinophils are also stimulated by IgE (27). Another class of particulate triggers for leukotriene formation includes crystals, such as monosodium urate, which can lead to gouty arthritis and can activate suspensions of mixed leukocytes in vitro to generate leukotrienes with potency equivalent to opsonized microbes (58,59). These results suggest that products of the 5-lipoxygenase pathway may play a role in the pathobiology of crystal-induced inflammatory diseases, such as asbestosis.

A number of soluble stimuli for 5-lipoxygenase activity other than immunoglobulin have also been examined. Although phorbol myristate acetate is known to stimulate arachidonic acid release it does not stimulate 5-lipoxygenase activity in macrophages by itself (60). In the presence of the calcium ionophore A23187, however, there is a 50-fold increase in 5-lipoxygenase product release from macrophages when compared to macrophages treated with A23187 alone. Contact-activated plasma is known to stimulate 5-lipoxygenase activity in peripheral blood monocytes (61), and this is due to selective stimulation of 5-lipoxygenase by plasmin (62). Of note, the cyclooxygenase pathway is not stimulated by plasmin in this system. The bacterial peptide, f-met-leu-phe, has been studied by a variety of investigators, though there are conflicting reports regarding its ability to stimulate 5-lipoxygenase activity in inflammatory cells obtained from humans (63,64). This is also the case for the complement components C5a and C3a (23,63,65). A general consensus would be that, by themselves, fMLP, C5a, and C3a induce little, if any, 5-lipoxygenase product release from neutrophils isolated from healthy individuals, but more recent results indicate that these stimuli can be important triggers for leukotriene production in the presence of a co-stimulus or a priming agent (66,67).

C. Relative Quantitative Synthesis of 5-Lipoxygenase Products by Inflammatory Cells

In addition to the specific products released by inflammatory cells, the relative quantities of these products synthesized by these cells is important in determining their role in inflammatory diseases. Resident human lung macrophages have a very potent 5-lipoxygenase pathway. They release more than 180 pmol of LTB_4 and more than 160 pmol of 5-HETE per million cells when maximally stimulated (13,15) (Table 1). By contrast, peripheral blood monocytes, the precursors to mature tissue macrophages, release only 16 pmol of LTB_4 and 18 pmol of 5-HETE per million cells with an identical stimulus (13). Neutrophils release 30–60 pmol of LTB_4 and similar amounts of 5-HETE in response to maximal stimulation (6,7,68). Although these three inflammatory cells—macrophages, monocytes, and neutrophils—are represented in the largest numbers in both the resident state and in inflammatory diseases, neutrophils are the overwhelmingly predominant cell present at sites of acute inflammation. Therefore, the 3- or more-fold potency of the 5-lipoxygenase in macrophages is perhaps irrelevant at sites of acute inflammation, and, therefore, the neutrophil is the most likely source of the vast majority of LTB_4 at these sites.

Eosinophils are also a powerful source of products of the 5-lipoxygenase pathway. When maximally stimulated, these cells release large quantities (up to 150 pmol per million cells) of cysteinyl leukotrienes but produce no significant quantities of LTB_4 (27,69). Substantially fewer data are available regarding quantitative leukotriene synthesis in basophils and mast cells. Basophils, when maximally stimulated, have the capacity to release about 90 pmol of LTC_4 per million cells (32). Mast cells release similar quantities of LTC_4 with stimulation (30,31), although accurate quantitative data are more difficult to obtain because of the difficulty of obtaining pure mast cells in an intact state from human tissues.

D. The 5-Lipoxygenase Pathway in Other Mammals

The 5-lipoxygenase pathway was first discovered and characterized in neutrophils obtained from rabbits (3). In subsequent studies performed in humans and a variety of other mammals, substantial species differences have become evident. Some of these differences are dramatic and instructive. For example, macrophages obtained from animals, such as mice (23,52) or rats (54), contain a potent 5-lipoxygenase pathway but synthesize large quantities of LTC_4 when stimulated, instead of LTB_4, as seen with human macrophages (13–15).

Likewise, in some animals the distribution of 5-lipoxygenase does not appear to be limited to inflammatory cells. For example, the canine airway epithelium has been demonstrated to release significant quantities of LTB_4 and 5-HETE in response to exogenous arachidonic acid and the calcium ionophore, A23187 (70,71). The release of LTC_4 has also been reported from these canine cells (71). Some investigators have found that bovine airway epithelial cells release LTB_4 when stimulated (72); however, the predominance of evidence suggests that these cells contain principally 12-lipoxygenase activity (73).

Table 3 Priming of 5-Lipoxygenase Activity

Cell type	Priming agent	Ref.
Neutrophils	GM-CSF	63,75–78
	TNF-α	76,79
	LPS	81
	LTB_4	51,83,84
Macrophages	IFN-γ	54
Monocytes	LPS	82
Eosinophils	GM-CSF	64,69,74
	TNF-α	79
	IL-3	124
Basophils	NGF	80

E. Priming of the 5-Lipoxygenase Pathway

Priming is a term frequently used by inflammatory cell biologists to suggest that an agent augments a cell activity, but does not actually stimulate it. The molecular events for priming the 5-lipoxygenase pathway have not been examined in detail, but are unlikely to be the same for all known stimuli of pathway activity. Thus, a variety of cytokines have been found to have short-term effects on 5-lipoxygenase activity (Table 3). Granulocyte-macrophage colony-stimulating factor (GM-CSF) primes eosinophils for leukotriene synthesis (69,74). GM-CSF has also been shown to have similar effects on neutrophils (63,75,76). This priming effect of GM-CSF is no longer seen if exogenous arachidonic acid is provided, suggesting that the principal effect of the priming agent is to induce arachidonic acid release (77). Although the mechanism of action of GM-CSF in this setting has not been extensively explored, pertussis toxin can inhibit the priming effect of GM-CSF, suggesting a G-protein–mediated effect (78).

Tumor necrosis factor-α (TNF-α) primes neutrophils and eosinophils (79), and interferon-γ (IFN-γ) can prime lung macrophages for leukotriene release (54). Likewise, nerve growth factor (NGF) primes basophils for LTC_4 synthesis and release in response to the complement fragment C5a (80). This effect is apparently mediated via the trk receptor on the basophil surface.

Perhaps one of the most important priming agents for the 5-lipoxygenase pathway is lipopolysaccharide. Priming of the 5-lipoxygenase pathway by this agent was first demonstrated in neutrophils (81). Conditioning of human neutrophils with relatively large quantities of lipopolysaccharide (10 μg/ml) for 30 minutes induced a 10-fold enhancement in 5-lipoxygenase product release when they were subsequently stimulated with f-met-leu-phe. Lower concentrations of lipopolysaccharide (1–10 ng/ml) were also demonstrated to exert a significant effect. Likewise, similar effects are observed when cells are stimulated with C5a (81). The effect of lipopolysaccharide on 5-lipoxygenase activity in neutrophils is dependent on the presence of plasma and is apparently mediated via the CD14 cell surface receptor. Lipopolysaccharide has virtually identical effects on peripheral blood monocytes, and these also are mediated via the CD14 receptor (82).

The role of LTB_4 in priming the 5-lipoxygenase pathway has also been examined. Some of these studies indicate that LTB_4 can itself stimulate LTB_4 formation by augmenting arachidonic acid release from cellular stores (83). LTB_4 may also enhance 5-lipoxygenase activity directly as measured using the surrogate substrate, 15-hydroperoxyeicosatetraenoic acid (84). Additional studies have further demonstrated that LTB_4 plays a pivotal role in priming neutrophils for 5-lipoxygenase activity. Thus, exogenous LTB_4 enhances 5-lipoxygenase in vigorously stimulated neutrophils by a factor of approximately two (51). Furthermore, inhibitors of the enzyme LTA_4 hydrolase, which have no direct effect on 5-lipoxygenase, significantly inhibit 5-lipoxygenase activity in intact neutrophils stimulated with the calcium ionophore, A23187 (7). More importantly, potent LTB_4 receptor antagonists almost completely inhibit 5-lipoxygenase activity in intact neutrophils, but have no effect on this enzyme directly (51). These data strongly indicate that LTB_4 plays a pivotal role in priming the neutrophil for 5-lipoxygenase activity in vivo, and that it does so by binding to its extracellular receptor. Although this effect may be at the level of arachidonic acid release (83,84), translocation of 5-lipoxygenase is also enhanced by exogenous LTB_4 and is inhibited by a potent LTB_4 receptor antagonist (51). The importance of 5-lipoxygenase translocation from cytosol to membranes upon cellular activation was first recognized in studies with colchicine, a microtubule inhibitor which disrupts the topological relationship between enzyme and substrate (58,59). This concept, namely translocation of 5-lipoxygenase from cytosol to membrane with cellular activation, has resulted in the development of a line of inhibitors which interfere with 5-LO-FLAP interaction (e.g., MK-886) (reviewed in Ref. 143). Although the mechanism of priming by LTB_4 remains unclear, evidence does indicate that LTB_4 may augment the translocation of 5-lipoxygenase to the nuclear membrane.

F. Regulation of Expression of the 5-Lipoxygenase Pathway

A number of features of the 5-lipoxygenase pathway have limited in-depth investigations examining the mechanism of cell-specific expression. These include the fact that many cells that express enzymes of this pathway are short-lived (e.g., neutrophils), difficult to isolate, and difficult to maintain in culture. Another factor is that, even when circumstances are ideal, inflammatory cells rapidly lose 5-lipoxygenase activity in culture (85). Moreover, adequate models using cell lines have proven difficult to develop. However, from these difficulties have come

Table 4 Regulators of 5-Lipoxygenase Pathway Expression

Enzyme	Agent	Cell type	Ref.
5-Lipoxygenase	GM-CSF	Monocytes, THP-1	86,95
		Neutrophils	87,89
	IL-3	Monocytes, THP-1	86,95
	Melatonin	Lymphocytes	90
	Retinoic acid, vitamin D	HL-60 cells	91
	DMSO	HL-60 cells	92,94
	TGF-β	HL-60 cells	92–94
	Glucocorticoids	Monocytes, THP-1	95
FLAP	GM-CSF	Monocytes, THP-1	86,95
		Neutrophils	88
	IL-3	Monocytes, THP-1	86,95
	DMSO	HL-60	94
	Glucocorticoids	Monocytes, THP-1	95
	Oxidized LDL	U937,HL-60	106
LTC_4 synthase	GM-CSF	Eosinophils	69,74
	IL-3	Eosinophils	124
	PMA, Vitamin D, DMSO	Mouse mast cells	125
		HEL cells	126

some clues as to the regulation of expression of enzymes in the 5-lipoxygenase pathway (Table 4).

Studies in Primary Isolates of Inflammatory Cells

Some evidence suggests that maturation of inflammatory cells, thus terminal differentiation, is in some manner linked to the expression of the 5-lipoxygenase pathway. When human peripheral blood monocytes and lung macrophages are compared, lung macrophages have 10-fold greater stimulated 5-lipoxygenase activity than their circulating counterparts (13). Lung macrophages also contain greater quantities of 5-lipoxygenase (24) and FLAP (25) than monocytes. Mononuclear phagocytes are more long-lived in vitro than other inflammatory cells, and, therefore, these cells have proven useful in efforts to characterize cell-specific expression of the 5-lipoxygenase pathway in vitro. When human peripheral blood monocytes are isolated in a highly pure form and are placed in culture, they lose all 5-lipoxygenase activity, as measured after A23187 stimulation, within 7 days (85). This loss in activity is associated with a corresponding loss in protein and mRNAs encoding for 5-lipoxygenase and FLAP. This loss in activity occurs in the face of these cells assuming the morphological characteristics of mature macrophages (so-called ''monocyte-derived macrophages''), suggesting that expression of 5-lipoxygenase and FLAP is not simply associated with maturation of monocytes into macrophages. However, when these same cells are co-cultured with lymphocytes under identical conditions, they increase their stimulated 5-lipoxygenase activity (86). Under these conditions, activated lymphocytes release soluble factors that increase 5-lipoxygenase activity by stimulating increases in mRNA encoding for 5-lipoxygenase and FLAP, resulting in increases in both 5-lipoxygenase and FLAP proteins. Both GM-CSF and interleukin-3 (IL-3) contribute to this effect (86).

Studies in human neutrophils have also demonstrated that GM-CSF increases immunoreactive 5-lipoxygenase (87) and FLAP (88). One group has found that in the case of 5-lipoxygenase, mRNA encoding for 5-lipoxygenase and the stability of this message are unchanged, suggesting that the effect of GM-CSF might be at a translational level in the neutrophil (87). Another group has found, in contrast, that GM-CSF does increase mRNA encoding for 5-lipoxygenase and that this change is at a transcriptional level as demonstrated by nuclear run-on assays (89). By contrast, studies in human B lymphocytes suggest that 5-lipoxygenase gene expression may be under negative regulation via melatonin binding to a subtype of the retinoid Z receptor (RZRα) (90). In general, more details are needed, based on experimental studies in primary cells, regarding the regulation of 5-lipoxygenase expression by GM-CSF.

Regulation in Inflammatory Cell Lines

A variety of cell lines have been utilized in studies examining the cellular expression of 5-lipoxygenase and FLAP. HL-60 cells can be differentiated into granulocytic, monocytic, and macrophage-like cells by a number of agents including DMSO, retinoic acid, dibutyryl cAMP, and 1,25-dihydroxyvitamin D_3 (91). This differentiation is associated with changes in expression of both 5-lipoxygenase and FLAP. DMSO has been utilized to differentiate HL-60 cells along the granulocyte lineage, and such cells have been shown to respond to serum with increased 5-lipoxygenase activity (92). The active factor in this response appears to be heat stable (93). Transforming growth factor-β, activated by heat treatment of serum, appears to be the principal constituent in serum responsible for changes in 5-lipoxygenase and FLAP expression in the HL-60 cell line when they are preconditioned with DMSO (94). Although prior studies have failed to demonstrate that the THP-1 cell line was a good monocyte-like cell model to study 5-lipoxygenase pathway expression, recent studies demonstrate that THP-1 cells respond to activated lymphocyte supernatants in a manner similar to primary monocytes. Thus, these cells demonstrate increased 5-lipoxygenase activity due to increased expression of 5-lipoxygenase and FLAP at both a protein and mRNA level (95). Again, these changes appear to be mediated via GM-CSF and IL-3. Of interest, GM-CSF and IL-3 do indeed appear to play a role in inflammatory cell survival, maturation, and activation (96,97).

Glucocorticoids are widely accepted to inhibit 5-lipoxygenase activity based on rational knowledge of glucocorticoid function (98) and limited experimental data (99–101). However, data exist to the contrary, indicating that glucocorticoids have stimulatory effects on 5-lipoxygenase activity (102–105). Based on the recognition that the 5′-flanking region of the FLAP gene contains a putative glucocorticoid response element, neutrophils, conditioned with glucocorticoid, have been analyzed for FLAP protein and steady-state mRNA (88). In these studies FLAP mRNA and protein were increased in neutrophils by conditioning with glucocorticoid. Additional studies have shown that glucocorticoids increase 5-lipoxygenase activity, immunoreactive 5-lipoxygenase and FLAP, and steady mRNA for 5-lipoxygenase and FLAP in both monocytes and in the monocyte-like cell line, THP-1 (95). Thus, in contrast to the prevailing belief, glucocorticoids have potent, direct effects in stimulating the expression of mRNA encoding for 5-lipoxygenase and FLAP. In turn, these proteins, and, finally, these cells have increased capacity for lipoxygenation of arachidonic acid. Other regulatory mechanisms appear to exist for 5-lipoxygenase and FLAP expression in inflammatory cells. In the mononuclear cell line, U937, and in HL-60 cells, oxidized low-density lipoproteins increase 5-lipoxygenase activity by increasing expression of FLAP (106).

LTA_4 hydrolase, the downstream enzyme in the 5-lipoxygenase pathway responsible for metabolizing LTA_4 to the potent chemotactic agent LTB_4 (107), has been found in virtually all tissues in the guinea pig (108), and this also appears to be the case in humans (109). LTA_4 hydrolase is 69 kDa protein and is a metalloproteinase (110) with aminopeptidase activity (111). Attempts to examine cell-specific expression and to determine if the expression of this enzyme can be modulated have been relatively unproductive. However, this issue may need to be reconsidered based on currently available information. For example, cells capable of synthesizing large quantities of cysteinyl leukotrienes such as eosinophils (27,69), basophils (32,33), and mast cells (30,31) make significantly less or no LTB_4. However, quantitative differences in LTA_4 hydrolase expression between these cells and other cell types have not been examined using antibody or cDNA probes and, therefore, the question remains unresolved. Additional data also suggest that not all cells express LTA_4 hydrolase equally or express the same isoform. For example, human erythrocytes contain LTA_4 hydrolase with some unique characteristics, one of which is a smaller estimated molecular size (112). Human airway epithelial cells contain substantial quantities of LTA_4 hydrolase activity, but this enzyme demonstrates unique characteristics, such as a slower time course of product generation (16), nonlinear kinetics (113), lack of significant aminopeptidase activity (113), and a different inhibitor profile (114) when compared to LTA_4 hydrolase in neutrophils. Recent work has demonstrated that human LTA_4 hydrolase can be expressed in two alternatively spliced mRNA forms (115). The short mRNA represents a deletion of an 83 bp exon in the 3′-

coding region and predicts an isoform with a predicted molecular mass of 59 kDa and a distinct C-terminus. However, this isoform of the protein has not been isolated or expressed to date to allow characterization of its functional properties.

LTC_4 synthase, the enzyme responsible for the first committed step in cysteinyl leukotriene synthesis (116), has a more restricted distribution, which includes some inflammatory cells but does not correspond well to the distribution of 5-lipoxygenase and FLAP. Thus, LTC_4 synthase activity is found in eosinophils (27), basophils (32), mast cells (30), endothelial cells (117), and platelets (18,118,119). Only eosinophils, basophils, and mast cells are known to synthesize cysteinyl leukotrienes without an extracellular source of intermediate substrate, namely LTA_4. Although LTC_4 synthase has now been purified to homogeneity (116), its cDNA cloned (120,121), and its gene cloned (122,123), little is known about the expression of its biosynthetic capacity in these cells. Only a few studies have examined the issue of expression of LTC_4 synthase in cells directly. Thus, human eosinophils incubated in the presence of 3T3 fibroblasts and GM-CSF (69,74) or IL-3 (124) show a 2- to 3-fold increase in capacity for LTC_4 synthase. Mouse mast cell LTC_4 synthase activity expression has also been examined and can be induced by interleukin-3 (125). However, the mechanism of this increase has not been fully explored. Studies in human erythroleukemia (HEL) cells demonstrate that when these cells are differentiated with phorbol myristate acetate, 1,25-dihydroxyvitamin D, or DMSO, cellular LTC_4 synthase enzymatic activity is increased (126), suggesting that a greater mass of this enzyme may be induced by these agents. DMSO has also been used to induce a 10-fold increase in expression of LTC_4 synthase in U937 cells (127). However, in contrast to findings in HEL cells, phorbol myristate acetate has been found to attenuate LTC_4 synthase activity in HL-60 cells (128). Further investigations suggest that LTC_4 synthase may be a phosphoregulated protein (129). Phorbol myristate acetate also decreases LTC_4 synthase activity in mixed human granulocytes (130). However, these latter studies did not directly assess the effect of the phorbol ester on LTC_4 synthase mass.

In summary, the regulation of expression of the components of the 5-lipoxygenase pathway can only be commented on definitively at this time with respect to 5-lipoxygenase and FLAP. These two proteins both appear to be upregulated by conditioning cells with agents such as DMSO, retinoic acid, dibutyryl cAMP, and 1,25 dihydroxyvitamin D_3. Cytokines and growth factors, including GM-CSF, IL-3, and TGF-β, also appear to modulate these two proteins. Surprisingly, glucocorticoids also induce expression of 5-lipoxygenase and FLAP. However, for all positive modulators of expression discussed, the molecular mechanism of action has not been definitively determined, nor is it clear at what level they influence expression (e.g., transcriptional, posttranscriptional, translational, or posttranslational). Finally, melatonin has been identified as a negative regulator of 5-lipoxygenase expression and this agent appears to act at the level of transcription.

G. The 5-Lipoxygenase Pathway in Inflammatory Cells of Asthmatics

The lung is a rich source of metabolites of arachidonic acid, especially those of the 5-lipoxygenase pathway (131). A number of studies have demonstrated that leukotrienes are released in asthmatics. For example, leukotrienes have been found in bronchoalveolar lavage fluid in asthmatics after antigen challenge (132), and leukotriene levels also correlate with development of the late asthmatic response (133). Urinary LTE_4, used as a marker of cysteinyl leukotriene release into plasma, is also elevated in asthmatics (134) and, in aspirin-sensitive asthmatics, is increased after antigen challenge (135). Cysteinyl leukotrienes are also released into nasal fluid after aspirin challenge in aspirin-sensitive asthmatics (136,137). These and other data provide a convincing case that leukotrienes, especially the cysteinyl leukotrienes, are released in the lungs and, in some circumstances, the upper airways of asthmatics. Urinary leukotriene measurements further suggest ongoing production of leukotrienes in asthmatics and that leukotriene release is still further increased after airway challenge.

These data are consistent with increased recruitment of inflammatory cells to the lung, greater stimulation of these cells in the lung, and increased expression of enzymes of the 5-lipoxygenase pathway within the lung. All of these mechanisms are likely to be operative. It is well documented that eosinophils, mast cells, macrophages, monocytes, basophils, and lymphocytes are present in increased numbers in the airways of asthmatics (26). Although mechanisms for stimulation of these cells in asthma have not been broadly examined, at least in the case of antigen, enhanced stimulation is likely to be the case both in the sense that there are greater numbers of target ligands and antibodies, but also that receptors for a variety of stimuli appear to be increased by cytokines (26). Further, the possibility that enzyme expression is modulated in asthma is supported by data indicating that cytokines and growth factors modulate the expression of these enzymes in inflammatory cells (86,125,138). At least some of these cytokines are known to be increased in asthma (139,140).

Expression of enzymes of the 5-lipoxygenase pathway in the inflammatory cells of asthmatics has not been examined adequately to date. Furthermore, little information is available on novel locations for expression of enzymes of the 5-lipoxygenase pathway in asthma. LTA_4 hydrolase in known to be present in large quantities in lung lining fluid of normals, and the amount of this enzyme increased about fourfold in smokers (141). No information is available in asthmatics, but an increase in this enzyme might provide a mechanism to amplify inflammation in the lungs of asthmatics. Recent preliminary work in this area suggests that expression of the 5-lipoxygenase pathway may, in fact, be enhanced in the inflammatory cells of asthmatics and that the enzymatic activity may be tonically active (142). In these studies, circulating neutrophils were found to spontaneously release large quantities of LTB_4, whereas neutrophils from normals did not. Furthermore, asthmatic neutrophils were found to contain increased immunoreactive 5-lipoxygenase. Although additional work is needed in this area, these data suggest that stimulation of 5-lipoxygenase activity in asthma may be a systemic process.

III. Transcellular Eicosanoid Biosynthesis

As exemplified by asthma, 5-lipoxygenase–derived eicosanoids play critical roles in multicellular events such as host defense, inflammation, and reperfusion injury (143). Elicitation of these important mediators is of interest because they are present in vivo during human illness and influence leukocyte adherence, migration, and activation, as well as tissue responses, such as smooth muscle contraction, vascular permeability, airway mucus secretion, and fibroblast chemotaxis (144,145). While some cell types are capable of generating leukotrienes and lipoxins directly from endogenous arachidonic acid, most require donation or transcellular transfer of eicosanoid biosynthetic intermediates. This requirement is largely explained (1) for leukotriene generation, by the discrepant cellular distributions of 5-lipoxygenase and the leukotriene-forming enzymes, LTA_4 hydrolase (146) and LTC_4 synthase (147), and (2) for lipoxin formation, by the general segregation of each of the three major mammalian lipoxygenase (5-, 12-, or 15-LO) activities into individual cell types (148). Circulating leukocytes and resident cells of the vasculature and tissues come in close proximity at sites of inflammation or injury, and upon activation by cellular or bacterial products in the local milieu, these cells release arachidonate and can exchange labile eicosanoid intermediates. These interactions between cells with distinct enzymatic capacities enable the transcellular biosynthesis of both leukotrienes, lipoxins, and the recently identified aspirin-triggered 15-epimer lipoxins.

Initial examination of cell types in isolation led to the determination of the basic profile of arachidonic acid–derived products for a triad of cell types known to interact in vivo, namely neutrophils, platelets, and endothelial cells, so it was possible to investigate the impact of one cell type on arachidonic acid metabolism in a second cell population. The development of specific thromboxane synthetase inhibitors for potential antithrombotic therapy revealed that during platelet–vessel wall interactions, accumulated endoperoxide intermediates formed in platelets could be released and converted to prostacyclin by endothelial cells (the "steal hypothesis") (149–151). However, the study of isolated platelets and leukocytes during coincubations in vitro provided the first direct evidence for the impact of cell-cell interactions in the biosynthesis of lipoxygenase-derived products (118). By labeling arachidonic acid stores of an isolated cell population before coincubation with a second cell type, it was possible to determine the identities of lipoxygenase-derived products catalyzed by the second cell type that carried radiolabel from the cell population of origin. This line of investigation demonstrated that novel eicosanoids could be generated via cellular interactions during coincubations of two cell types that were not products of either isolated cell population. The second half of this chapter on the cell biology of the 5-lipoxygenase pathway focuses on the critical role of this enzyme in transcellular eicosanoid biosynthesis.

A. Transcellular Leukotriene Formation

As discussed above, leukotriene biosynthesis is initiated by 5-lipoxygenase, which catalyzes the dioxygenation of arachidonic acid to 5-H(p)ETE and, in a second step, the conversion of 5-H(p)ETE to the pivotal epoxide intermediate, LTA_4 (50). Not just an intracellular intermediate, over 45% of LTA_4 generated by leukocytes is released from cells (8–10). Although extremely labile in aqueous environments (typically hydrolyzing to inactive products within seconds), it can be stabilized (minutes to hours) in vitro by interacting with phospholipid bilayers (9) or albumin (152). In addition, pulmonary surfactant, which lines alveoli and is composed of phospholipids and hydrophobic proteins, can also delay the non-enzymatic hydrolysis of LTA_4 in vitro, and in this form, LTA_4 remains available for further enzymatic conversion via transcellular biosynthesis to either leukotrienes or lipoxins (153). By transferring eicosanoid intermediates (e.g., LTA_4), cells expressing LTA_4 hydrolase and/or LTC_4 synthase can generate LTB_4 and cysteinyl leukotrienes, respectively, even when these cells lack endogenous 5-lipoxygenase activity. This paradigm was originally described during platelet-neutrophil coincubations (Fig. 1), but it has been extended to other cell types and, in vivo, other settings.

Dihydroxy LTs

LTA_4 hydrolase is present in a wide variety of cells, such as human erythrocytes (154), leukocytes (155), endothelial cells (146), airway epithelial cells (145), and lung fibroblasts (156), and several tissues including human lung, liver and kidney (109). Of all these human cell types and tissues, only neutrophils, monocytes/macrophages, and transformed lymphocytes are known to also possess high levels of 5-lipoxygenase activity (157). Because the other cell types lack substantial 5-lipoxygenase activity and thus the ability to generate the substrate for LTA_4 hydrolase, they require donation of LTA_4 to generate LTB_4. In support of this transcellular biosynthetic route, activated neutrophils generate increased amounts of LTB_4 in the presence of increasing numbers of erythrocytes, presumably via

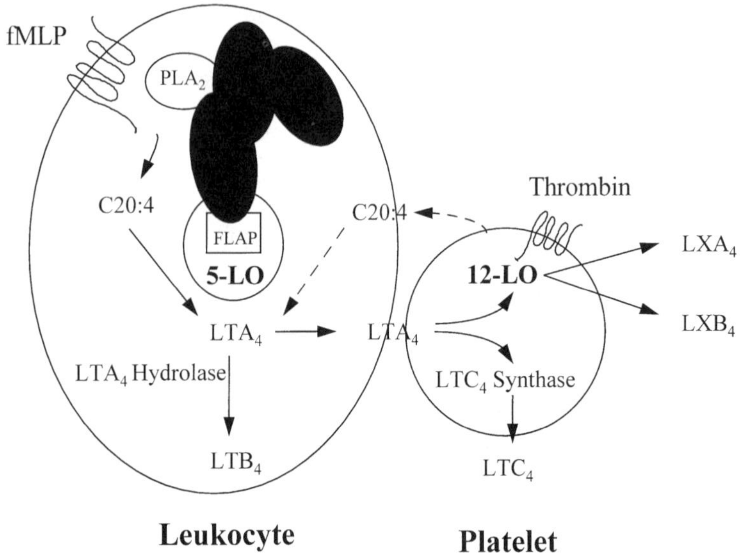

Figure 1 Platelet-leukocyte interactions: a model of transcellular biosynthesis of leukotrienes and lipoxins.

the conversion of neutrophil-derived LTA_4 by erythrocyte LTA_4 hydrolase (158,159). This conversion of donated LTA_4 to LTB_4 by recipient cells has also been reported with human endothelial cells (160) (Fig. 2), airway epithelial cells (16) (Fig. 3), T lymphocytes (161), and epidermal cells (162). LTB_4 levels are elevated in asthmatic lung and contribute to leukocyte recruitment and activation in the airways (50,131,163,164). Because there are several distinct mechanisms and cellular routes for the transcellular biosynthesis of dihydroxyleukotrienes, they are likely to be important during multicellular responses, such as inflammation or host defense.

Cysteinyl LTs

Three cysteinyl leukotrienes, LTC_4, LTD_4, and LTE_4, comprise the slow-reacting substance of anaphylaxis, a life-threatening systemic inflammatory response, and have been demonstrated in vivo during several human diseases of inflammation (50). LTC_4 synthase converts the 5-lipoxygenase-derived intermediate LTA_4 into the parent compound, LTC_4 (122,123,165). Sequential elimination of glutamic acid and glycine from LTC_4 results in the formation of LTD_4 and LTE_4, respectively (166,167). Unlike 5-lipoxygenase, which is present within myeloid cells, LTC_4 synthase activity is more widely distributed (147). Although identified in

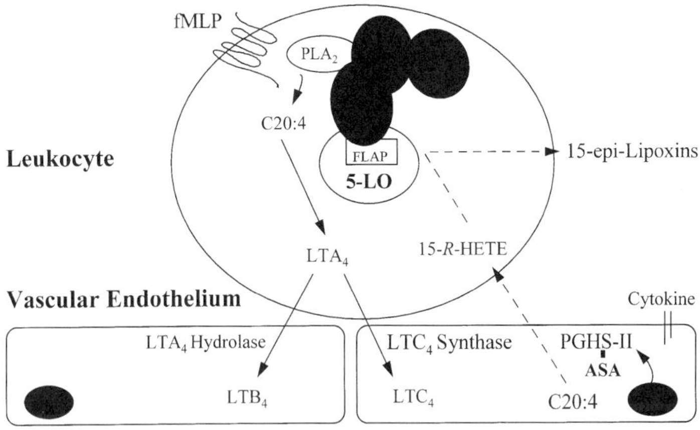

Figure 2 Transcellular eicosanoid biosynthesis: leukocyte-endothelial cell.

eosinophils, monocytes/macrophages, and mast cells that possess additional 5-lipoxygenase activity, cells without the ability to generate LTA_4, such as endothelial cells (168,169), platelets (67,170), smooth muscle (171), and mesangial cells (172), also demonstrate LTC_4 synthase activity. Early studies investigating transcellular biosynthesis of LTC_4 by leukocytes utilized mixed-cell suspensions that

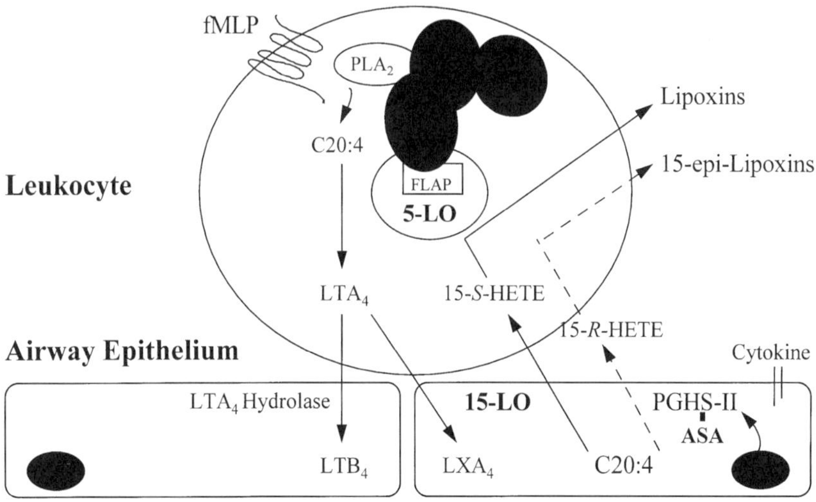

Figure 3 Transcellular eicosanoid biosynthesis: leukocyte-epithelial cell.

were activated by monosodium urate crystals (59). Similarly, activated leukocyte suspensions from hypereosinophilic donors also generated LTC_4 (173).

Platelets and leukocytes interact at sites of vascular inflammation and damage and, because of the ease of their isolation in sufficient number from peripheral blood, have been studied in vitro as a more convenient model to examine eicosanoid transcellular biosynthesis (66,118,174,175). Platelets lack 5-lipoxygenase mRNA and 5-lipoxygenase catalytic activity, but possess LTC_4 synthase activity and convert exogenous LTA_4 to LTC_4, LTD_4 and LTE_4 (170) (Fig. 1). In addition, platelets can generate LTC_4 from neutrophil-derived LTA_4 (119). Furthermore, coincubation of autologous human platelets and granulocytes results in two- to threefold increase in Ca^{2+} ionophore–induced LTC_4 formation, which peaks at 5 minutes with subsequent catabolism to LTD_4 and LTE_4, which predominates by 30 minutes (176,177). A similar increase in platelet LTC_4 formation has been observed from monocyte-derived LTA_4 (18). Transcellular LTC_4 formation is augmented dramatically by neutrophil priming with granulocyte/monocyte colony-stimulating factor (GM-CSF), a cytokine produced by activated T_H2-lymphocytes during specific inflammatory diseases, such as asthma (178). GM-CSF increases 5-lipoxygenase expression in leukocytes (87), thereby enhancing the generation of LTA_4, and subsequently LTC_4, during coincubations of neutrophils and platelets in the presence of the receptor-mediated stimuli, fMLP, and thrombin (67).

Compared to cell activation with stimuli, such as Ca^{2+} ionophore, which bypass cell receptors, physiologically relevant stimuli often lead to a quantitatively different profile of lipoxygenase-derived products. Table 5 reviews the stimuli used to activate cells during coincubations performed to investigate LO-derived eicosanoid formation. During platelet-neutrophil interactions, maximal leukotriene formation occurs in the presence of both cell types and both agonists, and increasing the number of platelets relative to neutrophils also results in increasing amounts of cysteinyl leukotrienes. Initial labeling of only platelet arachidonate stores leads to the production of radiolabeled cysteinyl leukotrienes during coincubations with neutrophils, indicating bidirectional transfer of eicosanoid intermediates (Fig. 1). Upon activation, platelet arachidonate is released and converted by neutrophil 5-lipoxygenase to LTA_4, which is subsequently returned to the platelet for further metabolism to LTC_4 (67). Here, cell–cell interactions result in the formation of novel lipoxygenase-derived products beyond the enzymatic capacity of the individual cell types in isolation.

The interaction of activated leukocytes with vascular endothelium is critical to the coordinated extravasation of these circulating leukocytes during host defense or inflammatory responses (179). The development of appropriate cell culture techniques has permitted the evaluation of essentially pure populations of endothelial cells in vitro. Endothelial cells express LTC_4 synthase but not lipoxygenase mRNA or catalytic activity (180). In contrast to incubations of either cell

Table 5 Diverse Agonists Stimulate Formation of LO-Derived Eicosanoids from Endogenous Arachidonate During Cell–Cell Interactions

A. Cell-cell interactions	Receptor bypass	Product	Ref.
Neutrophil-Platelet	Ca^{2+} ionophore	LT	118
Neutrophil-Platelet	Urate crystals	LT	58,59
Neutrophil-RBC	Ca^{2+} ionophore	LT	158
Granulocyte-Eos	Ca^{2+} ionophore	LT & LX	173
Granulocyte-Platelet	Ca^{2+} ionophore	LT & LX	170,175
Neutrophil-Endothelial cell	Ca^{2+} ionophore	LT	160
Monocyte-Platelete	Ca^{2+} ionophore	LT	18
Monocyte-Endothelial cell	Ca^{2+} ionophore	LT	168
Granulocyte-Lung tissue	Ca^{2+} ionophore	LT &LX	224
Monocyte-Raji cell	Ca^{2+} ionophore	LT	146
Alveolar macrophage-Epithelial cell	Ca^{2+} ionophore	LT & LX	232
Neutrophil-Epidermal cell	Ca^{2+} ionophore	LT	162
B. Cell-cell interactions	**Receptor-Mediated**	**Product**	**Ref.**
Neutrophil-Platelet	FMLP, thrombin	LT & LX	66
Neutrophil-Platelet	GM-CSF & FMLP, thrombin	LT & LX	67
Monocyte-Astroglial cell	IL-1β and TNF-α	LT & LX	233
Neutrophil-Platelet	GM-CSF & FMLP, thrombin or PDGF-AB	LX	230
Neutrophil-Endothelial cell	IL-1β, TNFα, or LPS & FMLP or PMA, thrombin (+ASA)	15-epi-LX	208
Neutrophil-Epithelial cell	IL-1β (+ASA)	15-epi-LX	46

type alone, coincubations of neutrophils and endothelial cells generate significant quantities of LTC_4 in the presence of Ca^{2+} ionophore (117). These results indicate the conversion of neutrophil-derived LTA_4 by endothelial cell LTC_4 synthase (Fig. 2). By increasing neutrophil 5-lipoxygenase activity, GM-CSF also enhances LTC_4 formation during coincubations with endothelial cells (180). These results indicate that cell-cell interactions, at sites of inflammation, can amplify the formation of leukotrienes, which can mediate, in part, the bioactions relevant to the asthmatic diathesis, such as vasoconstriction, bronchoconstriction, plasma exudation, and leukocyte migration.

B. Lipoxin Generation

In humans, LX biosynthesis is an example of lipoxygenase interactions via transcellular routes (144). Lipoxins can be generated by one of three routes that can be operative either independently or in concert, since these biosynthetic pathways are assembled during cell-cell interaction and/or when cells are primed by cytokines (see below).

15-LO–Initiated Pathway

Recognition of the carbon 15 position of arachidonic acid as the site for insertion of molecular oxygen was an integral step in the first described biosynthetic route for the generation of lipoxins (181). With oxygen inserted predominantly in the *S* configuration, the involvement of 15-lipoxygenase in the generation of bioactive molecules was inferred. An important role for human 15-LO in lipoxin formation is now clear and of interest, because 15-lipoxygenase (reviewed in Ref. 182), present in eosinophils (183), alveolar macrophages (184), monocytes (185), and epithelial cells (186), is under cytokine control and regulated primarily by IL-4 and IL-13 (184,185,187), two cytokines that are implicated as negative regulators of the inflammatory response or ''anti-inflammatory'' cytokines (178). Recent studies on the actions of LX implicate both LXA_4 and B_4 as potential anti-inflammatory mediators (144), suggesting that lipoxins may serve as effectors of the local actions of these cytokines.

15-Lipoxygenase inserts oxygen at the C15 postion of arachidonic acid, resulting in the generation of 15-H(p)ETE and/or 15S-HETE. Each of these biosynthetic intermediates can serve as a substrate for further metabolism by 5-lipoxygenase, transformations that occur within the cell type of origin or, more commonly, via transcellular routes (Fig. 3). 5-Lipoxygenase is abundant in human neutrophils and monocytes and, like 15-LO, is regulated by cytokines (e.g., GM-CSF and IL-3) (86,87). 5-Lipoxygenase converts 15-H(p)ETE into 5*S*-hydroperoxy,15*S*-hydro(peroxy)-DiH(p)ETE, which, after transformation to a 5(6)epoxytetraene, can be nonenzymatically converted to lipoxin A_4, 5*S*,6*R*, 15*S*-trihydroxy-7,9,13-*trans*-11-*cis*-eicosatetraenoic acid, or, via lipoxin B_4 hydrolase, to lipoxin B_4, 5*S*,14*R*,15*S*-trihydroxy-6,10,12-*trans*-8-*cis*-eicosatetraenoic acid. Both LXA_4 and B_4 have proven to be vasoactive and primarily vasodilatory in most isolated organs and in vivo models tested (188), and they both regulate leukocyte functions, perhaps serving as down regulatory molecules.

Although initial reports of 15-HETE as a substrate for lipoxins implicated 15-lipoxygenase products as ''anti-inflammatory'' (189,190), a series of in vitro experiments suggested that 15-lipoxygenase, via the oxidation of low-density lipoprotein (LDL), had pro-atherogenic properties and contributed to the chronic inflammation characteristic of atherosclerosis (191). To this end, macrophage-rich areas of atherosclerotic plaques co-localized by immunohistochemistry with 15-LO mRNA, protein, and activity (192–195). Purified 15-LO oxidized LDL in a cell-free system (196), and when overexpressed in fibroblasts, 15-LO, in the presence of LDL, generated increased amounts of lipoperoxides (197), a process inhibitable by LO inhibitors (196). In addition, gene transfer of 15-LO resulted in enhanced LDL oxidation in rabbit iliac arteries (198), and 15-LO–specific LDL oxidation products increased in rabbits on a high-cholesterol diet (194). Together, these results suggest that if 15-LO could directly access LDL, it possesses the capacity to oxidize LDL in vitro, however, the quantitative impact of this reaction on atherosclerosis had not been demonstrated in vivo. More recently and in contrast to these in vitro findings, 15-LO transgenic rabbits fed a high-fat and high-cholesterol diet were determined to have a reduction in aortic atherosclerosis when compared with nontransgenic littermates (199). These results, a surprise to the investigators in this line of inquiry, once again found evidence for an antiatherogenic action of 15-LO, and therefore, provide further evidence for an ''anti-inflammatory'' role for 15-LO activation and the eicosanoids it generates in protection against vascular inflammation and atherosclerosis (see Ref. 144).

In addition to the agonist-induced transcellular metabolism of donated 15-HETE by recipient cell 5-lipoxygenase to lipoxins, recent evidence indicates that primed leukocytes from individuals with inflammatory disorders, such as asthma, can generate lipoxins entirely from endogenous sources of arachidonic acid from a single cell type. The ability of primed cells (67) and cells from the peripheral blood of individuals with various diseases, including asthma (200,201), to generate lipoxins from endogenous sources of arachidonic acid indicates the importance of determining the temporal relationship in eicosanoid generation. A better understanding of this relationship will help elucidate the roles of leukotrienes and lipoxins in the regulation of pathobiological responses.

5-LO–Initiated Lipoxin Biosynthesis

Interactions between leukocytes and platelets exemplify the second recognized pathway for lipoxin biosynthesis. In this biosynthetic scheme, 5-LO within human neutrophils and the 12-lipoxygenase, abundant in human platelets (66,67,147,175), transform arachidonate into lipoxins A_4 and B_4. Neutrophils from healthy individuals do not generate lipoxins on their own in appreciable quantities, and much of their LTA_4, formed from 5-lipoxygenase, is released into the extracellular milieu (9). Platelets adherent to neutrophils convert the LTA_4, via 12-LO to lipoxins in a reaction mechanism similar to the 15-LO (66,202–204). Platelet 12-lipoxygenase abstracts hydrogen at carbon 13 and inserts molecular oxygen into the C15 position of LTA_4 and, unlike 15-LO, converts it to a carbonium cation intermediate that opens either to lipoxin B_4, when attacked by water at the C14 position, or LXA_4, when attacked by water at the C6 position (205–207) (Fig. 1). The formation of both LXB_4 and LXA_4 is unique to 12-LO; 15-LO converts LTA_4 to the 5(6)-epoxytetraene and then nonenzymatically opens to LXA_4 and its isomers without a high yield generation of LXB_4 (202) (Fig. 2). This activity of 12-lipoxygenase in platelets, confirmed with recombinant 12-lipoxygenase (207), indicates a functional role for the enzyme as a lipoxin synthase in the conversion of LTA_4 to both LXA_4 and LXB_4. It is of interest that 12-lipoxygenase undergoes suicide inactivation with LTA_4 as substrate for LXB_4 but continues to generate LXA_4. This distinctive regulatory mechanism suggests unique bioactions for lipoxin A_4 and B_4 when generated at sites of vascular inflammation or injury (148).

Aspirin-Triggered 15-epi-Lipoxin Biosynthesis

In this third major pathway for lipoxin biosynthesis, aspirin acetylates cyclooxygenase-2 (PGHS-II), when induced in either endothelial cells (Fig. 2) or epithelial cells (Fig. 3) via pro-inflammatory cytokines such as IL-1β, LPS, or TNFα, and switches its catalytic activity to convert arachidonic acid to 15-*R*-HETE in lieu of prostaglandin endoperoxide (46,208). Prostaglandin biosynthesis by both PGHS-I and PGHS-II are inhibited by aspirin (209). When acetylated at serine 530, PGHS-II converts endogenous stores of arachidonate to 15-*R*-HETE. This biosynthetic intermediate is released and can be transformed by 5-lipoxygenase in adherent leukocytes, via transcellular routes, to form 15-epi-lipoxins. Oxygenation of 15-*R*-HETE by 5-LO leads to a 5(6) epoxytetraene and both 15-epi-lipoxin A_4 and 15-epi-lipoxin B_4. As evident from their names, the *R* configuration from the precursor 15-*R*-HETE is preserved in the epimeric lipoxins at the C15 position. These 15-epimer lipoxins interact with native lipoxin receptors (210), previously characterized on human leukocytes (211–214), but differ from native lipoxins in the potency of their resultant bioactions. 15-epi-LXA_4 is more potent than LXA_4 in inhibiting neutrophil adhesion to endothelial cells (208), and 15-epi-LXB_4 inhibits cell proliferation more potently than either LXA_4 or LXB_4 (46). PGHS-II is abundant in endothelial and epithelial cells during inflammatory reactions and in disease states (39,209,215) and, therefore, likely to be present when individuals take aspirin, suggesting that 15-*R*-HETE and 15-epi-lipoxin formation in vivo may contribute to aspirin's beneficial actions.

These emerging findings indicate that aspirin not only inhibits prostaglandin biosynthesis, but also triggers formation of novel eicosanoids, namely, the 15-epi-lipoxins (46,208). These lipid-derived mediators display bioactions of potential endogenous anti-inflammatory signals and may be responsible for some of aspirin's therapeutic benefits, including the prevention of myocardial infarction and certain human malignancies (216–220).

Summary of Transcellular LX Biosynthetic Circuits

Operating independently or in concert, at least three major transcellular routes can lead to the formation of lipoxins (148). For example, GM-CSF–primed neutrophils can interact with platelets at sites of vascular inflammation. Upon activation, platelets adhere to neutrophils (221,222) and can convert LTA_4 released by neutrophils to lipoxins via platelet 12-LO (66,223) (Fig. 1). Because aspirin or other NSAIDs do not inhibit transcellular leukotriene or lipoxin biosynthesis, aspirin-triggered lipoxins could be generated simultaneously within the vasculature. In this setting, 15-epi lipoxin formation can occur when endothelial cell COX-2, upregulated by pro-inflammatory cytokines, is acetylated by aspirin and 5-lipoxygenase is present in activated, adherent leukocytes (Fig. 2). Bidirectional transcellular lipoxin biosynthesis also occurs when leukocytes interact with epithelial surfaces during respiratory, renal, or GI inflammation. In one biosynthetic circuit, epithelial cell 15-HETE is released and converted to LX by neutrophil 5-lipoxygenase. Alternatively, neutrophil-released LTA_4 can be converted by epithelial cell 15-LO, particularly abundant in tracheal epithelial cells, to generate lipoxins (224) (Fig. 3). Thus, LTA_4 is a substrate for the 15-LO, in addition to 12-LO, and can be converted to LX (184,224). 5,6-Dihydroxyeicosanoids are also substrates for LX in the presence of either 15-LO or 12-LO activity (225).

Of particular interest in pulmonary tissues, LX biosynthesis during inflammation can occur via a new form of priming with the esterification of 15-HETE into inositol-containing phospholipids in the membranes of human neutrophils (226). These leukocytes rapidly esterify 15-HETE into their inositol-containing lipids, which, following agonist stimulation, can release 15-HETE from this membrane source. Thus, cell membranes can be primed with their plasma and/or subcellular membranes carrying esterified mono-HETEs, which can then be released following receptor activation and transformed, in this case, to LX, or perhaps to other eicosanoids that have yet to be discovered that may also carry biological actions. This acylation and deacylation pathway also suggests that precursors of LX biosynthesis can be stored within membranes of inflammatory cells and then released by stimuli activating PLA_2 (226). Membranes primed with 15-HETE also utilize unique second messengers, such as 15-hydroxy-PIP_2 and diglyceride, which contain esterified 15-HETE that may alter intracellular signaling properties. In addition to 15-*S*-HETE, 15-*R*-HETE is also esterified into membrane phospholipids and can serve as a substrate for 15-epi lipoxin formation (46). 15-*R*-HETE can also be generated through the P450 oxygenation of native arachidonic acid (227). Therefore, 15-epi-lipoxin formation can also occur in the absence of aspirin in tissues with abundant P450 to produce the precursor, 15-*R*-HETE. Diverse biosynthetic routes are available for LX formation, likely reflecting an essential role for these mediators in homeostasis and human disease.

C. Impact of Cytokines on Transcellular Eicosanoid Biosynthesis

The profile of cytokines in a given microenvironment is closely related to LT and LX formation and action at that site. The expression of cycloxygenases and lipoxygenases is regulated by individual cytokines, which primes cells for LT and LX transcellular biosynthesis (Table 5). Cell–cell interactions, for example, neutrophil and platelet microaggregates, have been demonstrated in vivo (221,222). Therefore, the regulation of eicosanoid biosynthetic enzymes by specific cytokines (187,228) can have a direct impact on the formation (169) and actions of LT and LX (144). Cytokines and growth factors, in general, exert important regulatory roles within the eicosanoid signaling cascade and can specifically regulate the induction of key enzymes and the profile of products generated by cells after stimulation (143). In HL-60 cells, 5-LO activity is upregulated by transforming growth factor β, whose action is enhanced in the presence of TNF-α and GM-CSF (138). Priming of neutrophils by exposure to pM concentrations of GM-CSF leads to enhanced release of arachidonic acid and its conversion to lipoxygenase products (88). GM-CSF enhances LT and LX generation by priming neutrophils during receptor-mediated neutrophil and platelet interactions (67). Similarly, human peripheral blood monocyte 5-lipoxygenase activity is also increased in the presence of activated lymphocytes expressing GM-CSF and interleukin-3 (86), and rat macrophage 5-lipoxygenase activity is increased twofold by interferon-γ (54). Platelet-derived growth factor is a cytokine believed to act on both neutrophils and platelets (229). When added to coincubations of GM-CSF primed neutrophils and platelets, PDGF stimulates a concentration- and time-dependent formation of LXA_4 from endogenous sources of arachidonate (230). In addition, T_H2 lymphocytes produce IL-4 and IL-13, which (1) result in the appearance of 15-lipoxygenase mRNA and activity in monocytes (185,187,228), human alveolar macrophages (184), and airway epithelial cells (231) and (2) enable these cell types to participate in transcellular LX formation (184,232). HIV-infected mononuclear cells cultured in the presence of astroglial cells generate substantial amounts of LXA_4, in addition to LTB_4 and LTD_4 (233). Because formation of these LO-derived products was associated with increased levels of

IL-1β and TNF-α, LT and LX may mediate the local effects of these cytokines in the brain during infection and play a role in resultant neuronotoxicity. LX generation in this setting presumably occurs via conversion of monocyte-derived LTA_4 by astroglial cells, which possess 12-LO activity (234). Thus, an in vivo microenvironment, particularly in a certain disease state, is highly likely to contain specific cytokines that can regulate elaboration of lipoxins and other novel bioactive mediators.

D. Adhesion in Transcellular Eicosanoid Biosynthesis

Adhesion between cell types engaged in transcellular metabolism appears to facilitate the exchange or transfer of intermediates involved in the formation of both leukotrienes and lipoxins. Initial adhesive events between neutrophils and endothelial cells are mediated by selectins, followed by integrin adhesion molecules (CD11/CD18) of the neutrophil (179). Exposure to anti-CD18 and anti-Sel adhesion blocking antibodies inhibits agonist-induced LTC_4 formation via transcellular metabolism (169). Although cell–cell contact enhances eicosanoid formation, it is not absolutely required for transcellular eicosanoid biosynthesis, because it is well established that exogenous substrates can be added to cells and transformed without activation or involvement of adhesion molecules (reviewed in Ref. 144). Lipoxygenase-derived products of these cellular interactions carry interesting regulatory bioactions in vivo. For example, LTD_4 stimulates expression of P-selectin on endothelial cells that is temporally regulated by lipoxin A_4 (235). At nanomolar levels and for short duration (<15 min), both lipoxin A_4 and lipoxin B_4 inhibit leukotriene-induced expression of P-selectin and neutrophil adherence (235), whereas longer endothelial cell exposure to LXA_4 induces hyperadhesiveness of endothelial cells that appears to involve platelet-activating factor generation (236). These results suggest that neutrophil-endothelial cell interactions promote the formation of LT and LX and that the balance of proinflammatory and anti-inflammatory LO-derived products regulates selectin-mediated cellular adhesion.

Similarly, human platelets adhere to neutrophils upon activation during coincubations via interactions that involve P-selectin (237). Disruption of neutrophil-platelet contact inhibits agonist-induced LX generation (230). In an animal model of glomerular nephritis, platelet-leukocyte interactions in vivo result in the generation of LX (223). Inhibition of this interaction with monoclonal antibodies against P-selectin attenuates transcellular LX biosynthesis both in vitro and during ConA-F glomerulonephritis in vivo (238). Similarly, P-selectin "knockout" mice develop more marked neutrophil infiltration during acute nephrotoxic serum nephritis and have a reduced efficiency of transcellular LX generation (223). Infusion of wild-type platelets into null animals restores renal LXA_4 levels in this model and negates the difference in neutrophil infiltration. The process of adhesion appears to promote or facilitate transcellular eicosanoid metabolism by enhancing the duration and contact of the cells involved. Together these reports indicate that platelet-neutrophil adherence itself may be an important inflammatory event in the regulation of leukocyte recruitment via the formation of endogenous lipid mediators that ultimately suppress the proinflammatory response. Thus, the generation of LX by platelets may have an important role in regulating the entry of infiltrating neutrophils.

E. Relationship Between Leukotriene and Lipoxin Biosynthesis

Exemplified by the model of platelet-neutrophil interactions, transcellular biosynthetic routes can yield both leukotrienes and lipoxins. During the biosynthesis of lipoxins, leukotriene biosynthesis is blocked at the 5-lipoxygenase level (189). To this end, an inverse relationship has been observed between leukotriene and lipoxin biosynthesis from LTA_4 as a precursor. Because lipoxins block the actions of both LTB_4 and cysteinyl leukotrienes (reviewed in Ref. 189), this change in the profile of lipoxygenase products is likely to have functional consequences. If lipoxins act as a braking signal or as an endogenous stop signal for the recruitment of leukocytes, it is likely that molecular switches are thrown that direct eicosanoid product profiles from a pro-inflammatory to an anti-inflammatory phenotype. In this regard, cytokines as well as the redox potential of the inflammatory environment play important roles in the generation of LX, particularly in platelets. In this respect, agents that reduce the intracellular platelet level of glutathione, such as nitroprusside or DNCB, enhance the conversion of LTA_4 by platelets to LX and block the conversion of LTA_4 to cysteinyl-containing LT (67).

F. Amounts of Lipoxins Generated In Vivo

Experiments performed in vitro have determined lipoxin formation by both isolated cell types and coincubations of cells that undergo transcellular metabolism (reviewed in Ref. 148). In these settings, cell activation results in lipoxin generation from endogenous sources of arachidonate in the nanogram range (66,175,200,201,239). To more accurately represent in vivo production, LXA_4 formation by activated whole blood was examined using physical methods of detection and found to be in the nanomolar range (240). After coronary angioplasty (241) in patients with coronary artery disease and in an animal model of immune complex glomerulonephritis (238), LXA_4 is rapidly produced in vivo in nanogram amounts. Picogram to nanogram levels of immunoreactive LXA_4 are evident in nasal lavage fluids from aspirin-challenged aspirin-sensitive asthmatics (230), and nanogram amounts of lipoxins were generated by activated cells from rheumatoid arthritis (201) and asthma patients (200). The profile of LO-derived eicosanoids in the presence of receptor-mediated stimuli differs from that observed with stimuli, such as calcium ionophore, which bypasses cell receptors.

Cells activated by receptor-mediated stimuli generate lipoxins in amounts on the same order of magnitude as leukotrienes (67,184), whereas LT formation predominates with calcium ionophore.

Lipoxins have demonstrated bioactions, such as the inhibition of leukocyte migration or cell proliferation (242,243), in the nanomolar range; amounts which are achieved in both in vitro and in vivo settings (reviewed in Ref. 144). It is also theoretically possible that even higher concentrations of lipoxins may be generated at intracellular or sequestered sites in vivo. The recent design and development of stable lipoxin analogs will permit more detailed study of the paracrine or autacoid actions of LX and evaluation of their efficacy in vivo in modulating disease (242).

G. Respiratory Tissues: Transcellular Arachidonate Metabolism

Since the original description of the slow-reacting substance of anaphylaxis generated during antigenic challenge of sensitized lung, leukotriene formation in respiratory tissues has been implicated in human pulmonary disease (50,131, 157,244). During allergic conditions, fluids lavaged from both upper and lower respiratory tracts are rich in cysteinyl leukotrienes. These compounds have potent pharmacological effects on human central and peripheral airways resulting in bronchoconstriction that is more than 1000-fold greater than the reference agonist, histamine (50). Cysteinyl leukotriene receptors have been described in human lung and can be blocked by receptor antagonists (245). As mentioned above, the cellular distribution of LTC_4 synthase differs from 5-lipoxygenase, necessitating an exchange of eicosanoid intermediates during cell–cell interactions for cysteinyl leukotriene production.

During pulmonary inflammation, leukocytes migrate into respiratory tissues and airways. Once activated in the local microenvironment and in close proximity to resident cells of the lung, arachidonate is released for further metabolism to lipoxygenase-derived eicosanoids. The 5-lipoxygenase product LTA_4 can be released from activated leukocytes (8) and transformed to LTB_4 by LTA_4 hydrolase, present in airway epithelial cells, alveolar macrophages, and extracellularly in alveolar spaces (16,141,246). Of interest is the markedly enhanced ability of pulmonary macrophages to generate LTB_4 compared with peripheral blood monocytes (13), indicating the important role of leukotrienes in the alveolar macrophages' contribution to host defense. Several cell types present in respiratory tissues, including endothelial and mast cells, can also convert released LTA_4 to LTC_4 (reviewed in Ref. 244). During specific pulmonary diseases, other cells with LTC_4 synthase activity, such as eosinophils and platelets, may be present in the lung and can amplify cysteinyl LT production by resident cells. Thus, diverse pathways exist in respiratory tissues for transcellular LT formation.

Because human lung is rich in lipoxygenase activities, particularly 5- and

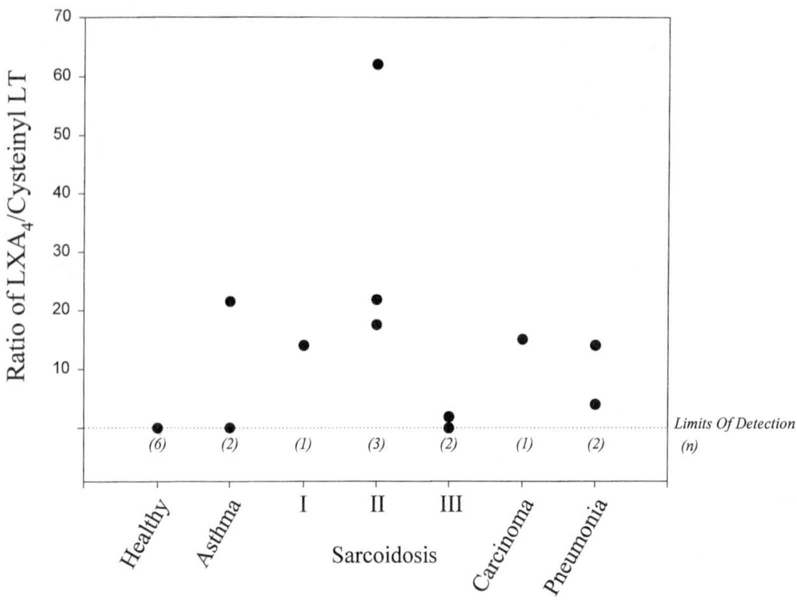

Figure 4 Relationship between lipoxin A_4 and cysteinyl leukotrienes in bronchoalveolar lavage fluid from patients with respiratory diseases.

15-lipoxygenase, it might also be expected to generate lipoxins. In addition to the 5-lipoxygenase–derived leukotrienes, 15-HETE, a substrate for lipoxin formation, has been detected in elevated amounts in bronchoalveolar lavage fluid from asthmatic patients at rest and at increased levels after antigen challenge (247). GC/MS analysis of blinded samples of bronchoalveolar lavage fluid from patients with respiratory illnesses, such as asthma, sarcoid, carcinoma, and slowly resolving pneumonia, demonstrated LXA_4 in amounts ranging from 0.4 to 3.1 ng/ml (248). In contrast, LXA_4 could not be detected in bronchoalveolar lavage fluid from any of six healthy volunteer subjects. For those with detectable levels of LXA_4, the ratio of lipoxin to cysteinyl leukotriene formation varied between 1.9 and 62 (mean = 19) (Fig. 4). The highest LX/LT ratios were seen in fluid from patients with asthma and radiographic stage II sarcoidosis.

Lipoxins can also be recovered from the upper respiratory tract after challenge of aspirin-sensitive asthmatics (230). In a double-blind, cross-over design, five aspirin-sensitive asthmatics underwent nasal lavage 2–3 hours after receiving a predetermined threshold dose of aspirin or placebo for ingestion. In contrast with placebo, all subjects receiving aspirin had detectable increases in lavage fluid LXA_4 (maximal levels: 41.7–318.9 pg $iLXA_4$/ml) after the development

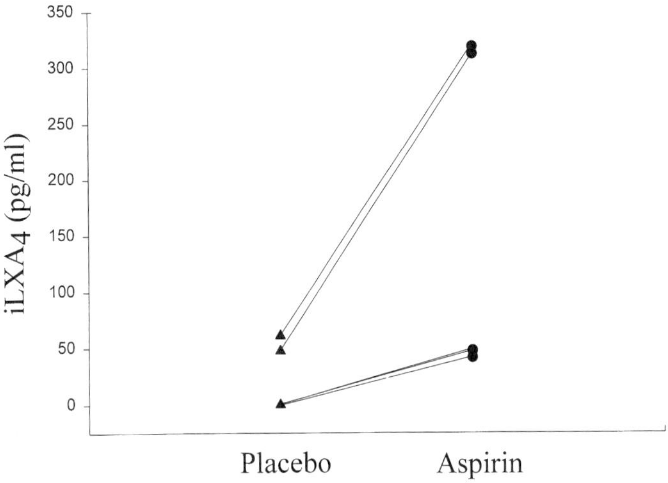

Figure 5 Formation of lipoxin A_4 by aspirin-sensitive asthmatics in vivo after aspirin challenge.

of oculo-nasal symptoms and bronchospasm (Fig. 5). These results demonstrate agonist-induced formation of LXA_4 in vivo by human asthmatics.

Although lipoxins have been identified in the respiratory tract of patients with pulmonary disorders, the cellular origin of these eicosanoids has not been determined. LXA_4 is generated from endogenous arachidonate in leukocyte suspensions enriched with eosinophils, obtained from hypereosinophilic donors, when challenged with Ca^{2+} ionophore (173). Eosinophils are rich in 15-lipoxygenase activity (183) and are present in lung tissue during diseases such as asthma (249). Thus, eosinophils can also contribute to lipoxin formation by serving as a source of 15-HETE or in the transformation of LTA_4, by 15-lipoxygenation, to the 5(6)-epoxytetraene lipoxin intermediate. LTA_4 is a substrate for 15-lipoxygenase in vitro with isolated enzyme (202) and in bronchial tissues (224). Also, coincubations of nasal polyps with leukocytes result in lipoxin formation, presumably via the donation of LTA_4 by activated leukocytes to airway epithelial cells or eosinophils for transformation by 15-lipoxygenase to lipoxins (224). In addition, 15-HETE generation by these cell types can result in lipoxin generation by the 5-lipoxygenase activity of leukocytes.

Alveolar macrophages are a predominant cell type in bronchoalveolar lavage fluids and can participate in 15-HETE formation and lipoxin production (184). Alveolar macrophages obtained by lavage of healthy volunteer donors generate lipoxins from endogenous sources when exposed to stimuli in vitro (184).

These cells transformed LTA_4 to lipoxins that could be modulated by the presence of a pulmonary surfactant (153). The half-life of this labile, epoxide-containing intermediate was dramatically increased by pulmonary surfactant, suggesting that surfactant could play a regulatory role by altering the half-life or further metabolism of lipid mediators. LTB_4 is the major product, from endogenous stores of arachidonic acid, when alveolar macrophages are exposed to Ca^{2+} ionophore (250), however, receptor-mediated stimuli, such as fMLP, result in LX formation on the same order of magnitude as LT (184).

Human alveolar macrophages also generate leukotrienes and lipoxins during cell-cell interactions. In the presence of LTA_4, these cells further metabolize this pivotal, 5-lipoxygenase–derived intermediate to both LTB_4 and lipoxins (184). When exposed to 15-HETE, alveolar macrophages can also convert it to lipoxins (232). In addition, coincubations of alveolar macrophages and epithelial cells generate lipoxins, presumably via 15-HETE produced by the epithelial cells as substrate for 5-lipoxygenation by the macrophages (232). The generation of lipoxins by these and undoubtedly several other biosynthetic circuits in the lung is relevant to human respiratory disease as LXA_4 has effects on human airway responses, including the modulation of LTC_4-induced airway obstruction in asthmatics (251).

IV. Summary

Products of 5-lipoxygenase and subsequent reactions leading to bioactive compounds, such as leukotrienes and lipoxins, are formed by asthmatics in vivo (131,230) and play critical roles during inflammation and other multicellular responses (148). Although select cell types can generate these products solely from endogenous stores of arachidonate, the distribution of 5-lipoxygenase differs, in general, from that of the leukotriene-forming enzymes as well as the other lipoxygenases which in human cell types are required for lipoxin production. Complex cell–cell interactions occur as leukocytes are recruited into multicellular inflammatory environments, and transcellular eicosanoid biosynthesis amplifies the array and amounts of lipoxygenase-derived products at sites of inflammation. While leukotrienes stimulate experimental inflammation in animal and human models, lipoxins inhibit neutrophil functions critical to host defense and stimulate monocyte recruitment that ultimately inactivates both LXA_4 and LXB_4 (252). Aspirin-triggered 15-epimeric lipoxins also inhibit neutrophil adhesion to endothelium (208) and block cell proliferation of airway epithelium from adenocarcinoma (46). The novel downregulatory actions of lipoxins on leukocyte trafficking suggest that the intensity of an inflammatory response at any given time point during host defense or disease reflects a tightly regulated balance between proinflammatory and anti-inflammatory factors. This interaction was recently demonstrated in vivo with 16-phenoxy-LXA_4, an LXA_4 analog, which by topical application inhibits LTB_4-induced neutrophil infiltration into mouse ear skin with a potency of inhibition equivalent to dexamethasone (253). Because the inflammatory response is normally a self-limited event, lipoxins may represent natural stop signals or ''chalones'' for inflammatory cells. Both leukotrienes and lipoxins, 5-lipoxygenase-derived eicosanoids, have been identified in human asthma. Elucidation of the temporal relationship between leukotriene and lipoxin formation may lead to a better understanding of their respective roles in the pathobiology of airway inflammation. Pharmacological manipulations of lipoxins may result in the development of novel anti-inflammatory agents and contribute to the efficacy of established anti-inflammatory drugs such as glucocorticoids.

Acknowledgments

Experiments in the CNS laboratory were supported in part by National Institutes of Health grants GM38765 and P01-DK50305. TDB is funded in part by a Merit Review Grant from the Department of Veterans Affairs, a Career Investigator Award from the American Lung Association, and the National Institutes of Health (DK 47756).

References

1. Samuelsson B, Hammarström S. Nomenclature for leukotrienes. Prostaglandins 1980; 19:645–648.
2. Borgeat P, Hamberg M, Samuelsson B. Transformation of arachidonic acid and homo-gamma-linolenic acid by rabbit polymorphonuclear leukocytes. Monohydroxy acids from novel lipoxygenases. J Biol Chem 1976; 251:7816–7820.
3. Borgeat P, Samuelsson B. Transformation of arachidonic acid by rabbit polymorphonuclear leukocytes. J Biol Chem 1979; 254:2643–2646.
4. Borgeat P, Samuelsson B. Metabolism of arachidonic acid in polymorphonuclear leukocytes. Structural analysis of novel hydroxylated compounds. J Biol Chem 1979; 254:7865–7869.
5. Corey EJ, Marfat A, Goto G, Brion F. Leukotriene B. Total synthesis and assignment of stereochemistry. J Am Chem Soc 1980; 102:7984–7985.
6. Borgeat P, Samuelsson B. Arachidonic acid metabolism in polymorphonuclear leukocytes: effects of ionophore A23187. Proc Natl Acad Sci USA 1979; 76:2148–2152.
7. Shindo K, Baker JR, Munafo DA, Bigby TD. Captopril inhibits neutrophil synthesis of leukotriene B_4 in vitro and in vivo. J Immunol 1994; 153:5750–5759.
8. Dahinden CA, Clancy RM, Gross M, Chiller JM, Hugli TE. Leukotriene C_4 production by murine mast cells: evidence of a role for extracellular leukotriene A_4. Proc Natl Acad Sci USA 1985; 82:6632–6636.

9. Fiore S, Serhan CN. Phospholipid bilayers enhance the stability of leukotriene A_4 and epoxytetraenes: stabilization of eicosanoids by liposomes. Biochem Biophys Res Commun 1989; 159:477–481.
10. Sala A, Bolla M, Zarini S, Muller-Peddinghaus R, Folco G. Release of leukotriene A_4 versus leukotriene B_4 from human polymorphonuclear leukocytes. J Biol Chem 1996; 271:17944–17948.
11. Goldyne ME, Burrish GF, Poubelle P, Borgeat P. Arachidonic acid metabolism among human mononuclear leukocytes. Lipoxygenase-related pathways. J Biol Chem 1984; 259:8815–8819.
12. Pawlowski NA, Kaplan G, Hamill AL, Cohn ZA, Scott WA. Arachidonic acid metabolism by human monocytes. Studies with platelet-depleted cultures. J Exp Med 1983; 158:393–412.
13. Bigby TD, Holtzman MJ. Enhanced 5-lipoxygenase activity in lung macrophages compared to monocytes from normal subjects. J Immunol 1987; 138:1546–1550.
14. Fels AO, Pawlowski NA, Cramer EB, King TKC, Cohn ZA, Scott WA. Human alveolar macrophages produce leukotriene B_4. Proc Natl Acad Sci USA 1982; 79: 7866–7870.
15. Martin TR, Altman LC, Albert RK, Henderson WR. Leukotriene B_4 production by the human alveolar macrophage: a potential mechanism for amplifying inflammation in the lung. Am Rev Respir Dis 1984; 129:106–111.
16. Bigby TD, Lee DM, Meslier N, Gruenert DC. Leukotriene A_4 hydrolase activity of human airway epithelial cells. Biochem Biophys Res Commun 1989; 164:1–7.
17. Jakobsson P-J, Odlander B, Steinhilber D, Rosen A, Claesson H-E. Human B lymphocytes possess 5-lipoxygenase activity and convert arachidonic acid to leukotriene B_4. Biochem Biophys Res Commun 1991; 178:302–308.
18. Bigby TD, Meslier N. Transcellular lipoxygenase metabolism between monocytes and platelets. J Immunol 1989; 143:1948–1954.
19. Du LT, Foegh M, Maddox Y, Ramwell PW. Human peritoneal macrophages synthesize leukotriene B_4 and C_4. Biochim Biophys Acta 1983; 753:159–163.
20. Damon M, Chavis C, Godard P, Michel FB, Crastes de Paulet A. Purification and mass spectrometry identification of leukotriene D_4 synthesized by human alveolar macrophages. Biochem Biophys Res Commun 1983; 111:518–524.
21. Ferreri NR, Howland WC, Spiegelberg HL. Release of leukotriene C_4 and B_4 and prostaglandin E_2 from human monocytes stimulated with aggregated IgG, IgA, and IgE. J Immunol 1986; 136:4188–4193.
22. Laviolette M, Carreau M, Coulombe R, Cloutier D, Dupont P, Rioux J, Braquet P, Borgeat P. Metabolism of arachidonic acid through the 5-lipoxygenase pathway in normal human peritoneal macrophages. J Immunol 1988; 141:2104–2109.
23. Rouzer CA, Scott WA, Hamill AL, Cohn ZA. Synthesis of leukotriene C and other arachidonic acid metabolites by mouse pulmonary macrophages. J Exp Med 1982; 155:720–733.
24. Pueringer RJ, Bahns CC, Hunninghake GW. Alveolar macrophages have greater amounts of the enzyme 5-lipoxygenase than do monocytes. J Appl Physiol 1992; 73:781–786.
25. Coffey MJ, Wilcoxen SE, Peters-Golden M. Increases in 5-lipoxygenase activating

protein expression account for enhanced capacity for 5-lipoxygenase metabolism that accompanies differentiation of peripheral blood monocytes into alveolar macrophages. Am J Respir Cell Mol Biol 1994; 11:153–158.
26. Bigby TD, Nadel JA. Chapter 44: Asthma. In: Gallin JI, Goldstein IM, Snyderman R, eds. Inflammation: Basic Principles and Clinical Correlates. New York: Raven Press, 1992:889–906.
27. Weller PF, Lee CW, Foster DW, Corey EJ, Austen KF, Lewis RA. Generation and metabolism of 5-lipoxygenase pathway leukotrienes by human eosinophils: predominant production of leukotriene C_4. Proc Natl Acad Sci USA 1983; 80:7626–7630.
28. MacMillan DK, Hill E, Sala A, Sigal E, Shuman T, Henson PM, Murphy RC. Eosinophil 15-lipoxygenase is a leukotriene A_4 synthase. J Biol Chem 1994; 269: 26663–26668.
29. Peters SP, Schleimer RP, Naclerio RM, MacGlashan DW Jr, Togias AG, Proud D, Freeland HS, Fox C, Adkinson NF Jr, Lichtenstein LM. The pathophysiology of human mast cells. In vitro and in vivo function. Am Rev Respir Dis 1987; 135: 1196–1200.
30. MacGlashan DW, Schleimer RP, Peters SP. Generation of leukotrienes by purified human lung mast cells. J Clin Invest 1982; 70:747–751.
31. Levi-Schaffer F, Austen KF, Caulfield JP, Hein A, Gravallese PM, Stevens RL. Co-culture of human lung-derived mast cells with mouse 3T3 fibroblasts: morphology and IgE-mediated release of histamine, prostaglandin D_2, and leukotrienes. J Immunol 1987; 139:494–500.
32. MacGlashan DW, Peters SP, Warner J, Lichenstein LM. Characteristics of human basophil sulfidopeptide leukotriene release: releasability defined as the ability of the basophil to respond to dimeric cross-links. J Immunol 1986; 136:2231–2239.
33. Kurimoto Y, de Weck AL, Dahinden CA. Interleukin 3-dependent mediator release in basophils triggered by C5a. J Exp Med 1989; 170:467–479.
34. Warner JA, Freeland HS, MacGlashan DWJ, Lichtenstein LM, Peters SP. Purified human basophils do not generate LTB_4. Biochem Pharmacol 1987; 36:3195–3199.
35. Paul WE. Development and function of lymphocytes. In: Gallin JI, Goldstein IM, Snyderman R, eds. Inflammation: Basic Principles and Clinical Correlates. New York: Raven Press, 1992:775–790.
36. Jakobsson P-J, Steinhilber D, Odlander B, Radmark O, Claesson H-E, Samuelsson B. On the expression and regulation of 5-lipoxygenase in human lymphocytes. Proc Natl Acad Sci USA 1992; 89:3521–3525.
37. Simmet T, Peskar BA. Lipoxygenase products of polyunsaturated fatty acid metabolism in the central nervous system: biosynthesis and putative functions. Pharmacol Res 1990; 22:667–682.
38. Boado RJ, Pardridge WM, Vinters HV, Black KL. Differential expression of arachidonate 5-lipoxygenase transcripts in human brain tumors: evidence for the expression of a multitranscript family. Proc Natl Acad Sci USA 1992; 89:9044–9048.
39. Holtzman MJ, Zhang V, Hussain H, Roswit WT, Wilson JD. Prostaglandin H synthase and lipoxygenase gene families in the epithelial cell barrier. Ann NY Acad Sci 1994; 744:58–77.

40. Shannon VR, Stenson WF, Holtzman MJ. Induction of epithelial arachidonate 12-lipoxygenase at active sites of inflammatory bowel disease. Am J Physiol 1993; 264:G104–111.
41. Barrett KE, Bigby TD. New roles for eicosanoids as regulators of epithelial function and growth. News Physiol Sci 1995; 10:153–159.
42. Shimakura S, Boland CR. Eicosanoid production by the human gastric caner cell line AGS and its relation to cell growth. Cancer Res 1992; 52:1744–1749.
43. Dias VC, Wallace JL, Parsons HG. Modulation of cellular phospholipid fatty acids and leukotriene B_4 synthesis in the human intestinal epithelial cell (CaCo-2). Gut 1992; 33:622–627.
44. Sjolander A, Schippert A, Hammarstrom S. A human epithelial cell line, intestine 407, can produce 5-hydroxyeicosatetraenoic acid and leukotriene B_4. Prostaglandins 1993; 45:85–96.
45. Cortese JF, Spannhake EW, Eisinger W, Potter JJ, Yang VW. The 5-lipoxygenase pathway in cultured human intestinal epithelial cells. Prostaglandins 1995; 49:155–166.
46. Claria JE, Lee MH, Serhan CN. Aspirin-triggered lipoxins (15-epi-LX) are generated by the human lung adenocarcinoma line (A549)-neutrophil interactions and are potent inhibitors of cell proliferation. Mol Med 1996; 2:583–596.
47. Avis IM, Jett M, Boyle T, Vos MD, Moody T, Treston AM, Martinez A, Mulshine JL. Growth control of lung cancer by interruption of 5-lipoxygenase-mediated growth factor signaling. J Clin Invest 1996; 97:806–813.
48. Maxion H, Chorné N, Bigby TD, Barrett KE. Effect of leukotriene B_4 on intestinal epithelial cell proliferation and function. J Invest Med 1995; 43(suppl):109A.
49. Krump E, Pouliot M, Naccache PH, Borgeat P. Leukotriene synthesis in calcium-depleted human neutrophils: arachidonic acid release correlates with calcium influx. Biochem J 1995; 310:681–688.
50. Samuelsson B. Leukotrienes: mediators of immediate hypersensitivity reactions and inflammation. Science 1983; 220:568–575.
51. Serio KJ, Baker JR, Ring WL, Riddick CA, Bigby TD. Leukotriene B_4 co-stimulates 5-lipoxygenase activity in neutrophils via increased 5-lipoxygenase translocation. Am J Physiol 1997; 272(4 pt 1):C1329–C1334.
52. Rouzer CA, Scott WA, Cohn ZA, Blackburn P, Manning JM. Mouse peritoneal macrophages release leukotriene C in response to a phagocytic stimulus. Proc Natl Acad Sci USA 1980; 77:4928–4932.
53. MacDermot J, Kelsey CR, Waddell KA, Richmond R, Knight RK, Cole PJ, Dollery CT, Landon DN, Blair IA. Synthesis of leukotriene B_4 and prostaglandins by alveolar macrophages: analysis by gas chromatography/mass spectrometry. Prostaglandins 1984; 27:163–179.
54. Meslier N, Aldrich AJ, Bigby TD. Effect of interferon-gamma on the 5-lipoxygenase pathway of rat lung macrophages. Am J Respir Cell Mol Biol 1992; 6:93–99.
55. Czop JK, Austen KF. Generation of leukotrienes by human monocytes upon stimulation of their beta-glucan receptor during phagocytosis. Proc Natl Acad Sci USA 1985; 82:2751–2755.
56. Czop JK, Puglisi AV, Miorandi DZ, Austen KF. Perturbation of beta-glucan recep-

tors on human neutrophils initiates phagocytosis and leukotriene B_4 production. J Immunol 1988; 141:3170–3176.
57. Rouzer CA, Scott WA, Hamill AL, Liu F-T, Katz DH, Cohn ZA. Secretion of leukotriene C and other arachidonic acid metabolites by macrophages challenged with immunoglobulin E immune complexes. J Exp Med 1982; 156:1077–1086.
58. Serhan CN, Lundberg U, Weissmann G, Samuelsson B. Formation of leukotrienes and hydroxy acids by human neutrophils and platelets exposed to monosodium urate. Prostaglandins 1984; 27:563–581.
59. Serhan CN, Lundberg U, Lindgren JA, Weissmann G, Samuelsson B. Formation of leukotriene C_4 by human leukocytes exposed to monosodium urate crystals. FEBS Lett 1984; 167:109–112.
60. Tripp CS, Mahoney M, Needleman P. Calcium ionophore enables soluble agonists to stimulate macrophage 5-lipoxygenase. J Biol Chem 1985; 260:5895–5898.
61. Weide I, Simmet T. Leukotriene formation by peripheral monocytes in contact-activated human blood. Thromb Res 1993; 71:185–192.
62. Weide I, Römisch J, Simmet T. Contact activation triggers stimulation of the monocyte 5-lipoxygenase pathway via plasmin. Blood 1994; 83:1941–1951.
63. Dahinden CA, Zingg J, Maly FE, de Weck AL. Leukotriene production in human neutrophils primed by recombinant human granulocyte/macrophage colony-stimulating factor and stimulated with complement component C5a and FMLP as second signals. J Exp Med 1988; 167:1281–1295.
64. Owen W, Peterson J, Austen KF. Eosinophils altered phenotypically and primed by culture with granulocyte/macrophage colony-stimulating factor and 3T3 fibroblasts generate leukotriene C_4 in response to FMLP. J Clin Invest 1991; 87:1958–1963.
65. Haines KA, Giedd KN, Rich AM, Korchak HM, Weissmann G. The leukotriene B_4 paradox: neutrophils can, but will not, respond to ligand-receptor interactions by forming leukotriene B_4 or its omega-metabolites. Biochem J 1987; 241:55–62.
66. Serhan CN, Sheppard KA. Lipoxin formation during human neutrophil-platelet interactions. Evidence for the transformation of leukotriene A_4 by platelet 12-lipoxygenase in vitro. J Clin Invest 1990; 85:772–780.
67. Fiore S, Serhan CN. Formation of lipoxins and leukotrienes during receptor-mediated interactions of human platelets and recombinant human granulocyte/macrophage colony-stimulating factor-primed neutrophils. J Exp Med 1990; 172:1451–1457.
68. Sun FF, McGuire JC. Metabolism of arachidonic acid by human neutrophils. Characterization of the enzymatic reactions that lead to the synthesis of leukotriene B_4 Biochim Biophys Acta 1984; 794:56–64.
69. Owen WF Jr, Soberman RJ, Yoshimoto T, Sheffer AL, Lewis RA, Austen KF. Synthesis and release of leukotriene C_4 by human eosinophils. J Immunol 1987; 138:532–538.
70. Holtzman MJ, Aizawa H, Nadel JA, Goetzl EJ. Selective generation of leukotriene B_4 by tracheal epithelial cells from dogs. Biochem Biophys Res Commun 1983; 114:1071–1076.
71. Eling TE, Danilowicz RM, Henke DC, Sivarajah K, Yankaskas JR, Boucher RC. Arachidonic acid metabolism by canine tracheal epithelial cells. Product formation and relationship to chloride secretion. J Biol Chem 1986; 261:12841–12849.

72. Leikauf GD, Driscoll KE, Wey HE. Ozone-induced augmentation of eicosanoid metabolism in epithelial cells from bovine trachea. Am Rev Respir Dis 1988; 137: 435–442.
73. Hansbrough JR, Atlas AB, Turk J, Holtzman MJ. Arachidonate 12-lipoxygenase and cyclooxygenase: PGE isomerase are predominant pathways for oxygenation in bovine tracheal epithelial cells. Am J Respir Cell Mol Biol 1989; 1:237–244.
74. Silberstein DS, Owen WF, Gasson JC, DiPersio JF, Golde DW, Bina JC, Soberman R, Austen KF, David JR. Enhancement of human eosinophil cytotoxicity and leukotriene synthesis by biosynthetic (recombinant) granulocyte-macrophage colony-stimulating factor. J Immunol 1986; 137:3290–3294.
75. Krump E, Borgeat P. Kinetics of 5-lipoxygenase activation, arachidonic acid release, and leukotriene synthesis in human neutrophils: effects of granulocyte-macrophage colony-stimulating factor. Biochem Biophys Acta 1994; 1213:135–139.
76. Palmantier R, Surette ME, Sanchez A, Braquet P, Borgeat P. Priming for the synthesis of 5-lipoxygenase products in human blood ex vivo by human granulocyte-macrophage colony-stimulating factor and tumor necrosis factor-α. Lab Invest 1994; 70:696–704.
77. DiPersio JF, Naccache PH, Borgeat P, Gasson JC, Nguyen MH, McColl SR. Characterization of the priming effects of human granulocyte-macrophage colony-stimulating factor on human neutrophil leukotriene synthesis. Prostaglandins 1988; 36: 673–691.
78. McColl SR, Kreis C, DiPersio JF, Borgeat P, Nacchache PH. Involvement of guanine nucleotide binding proteins in neutrophil activation and priming by GM-CSF. Blood 1989; 73:588–591.
79. Roubin R, Elsas PP, Fiers W, Dessein AJ. Recombinant tumor necrosis factor (rTNF) enhances leukotriene biosynthesis in neutrophils and eosinophils stimulated with the Ca^{2+} ionophore A23187. Clin Exp Immunol 1987; 70:484–490.
80. Burgi B, Otten UH, Ochensberger B, Rihs S, Heese K, Ehrhard PB. Basophil priming by neurotrophic factors. Activation through the trk receptor. J Immunol 1996; 157:5582–5588.
81. Surette ME, Palmantier R, Gosselin J, Borgeat P. Lipopolysaccharides prime whole human blood and isolated neutrophils for the increased synthesis of 5-lipoxygenase products by enhancing arachidonic acid availability: involvement of the CD14 antigen. J Exp Med 1993; 178:1347–1355.
82. Surette ME, Nadeau M, Borgeat P, Gosselin J. Priming of human peripheral blood mononuclear cells with lipopolysaccharides for enhanced arachidonic acid release and leukotriene synthesis. J Leuk Biol 1996; 59:709–715.
83. McDonald PP, McColl SR, Braquet P, Borgeat P. Autocrine enhancement of leukotriene synthesis by endogenous leukotriene B_4 and platelet-activating factor in human neutrophils. Br J Pharmacol 1994; 111:852–860.
84. McDonald PP, McColl SR, Naccache PH, Borgeat P. Activation of human neutrophil 5-lipoxygenase by leukotriene B_4. Br J Pharmacol 1992; 107:226–232.
85. Ring WL, Riddick CA, Baker JR, Munafo DA, Bigby TD. Human monocytes lose 5-lipoxygenase and FLAP as they mature into monocyte-derived macrophages in vitro. Am J Physiol (Cell Physiol) 1996; 271:C372–C377.

86. Ring WL, Riddick CA, Baker JR, Munafo DA, Bigby TD. Lymphocytes stimulate expression of 5-lipoxygenase and its activating protein in monocytes in vitro via granulocyte macrophage colony-stimulating factor and interleukin 3. J Clin Invest 1996; 97:1293–1301.
87. Pouliot M, Khamzina L, Borgeat P, McColl SR. Granulocyte-macrophage colony-stimulating factor enhances 5-lipoxygenase levels in human polymorphonuclear leukocytes. J Immunol 1994; 152:851–858.
88. Pouliot M, McDonald PP, Borgeat P, McColl SR. Granulocyte/macrophage colony-stimulating factor stimulates the expression of the 5-lipoxygenase-activating protein (FLAP) in human neutrophils. J Exp Med 1994; 179:1225–1232.
89. Stankova J, Rola-Pleszczynski, M, Dubois CM. Granulocyte-macrophage colony-stimulating factor increases 5-lipoxygenase gene transcription and protein expression in human neutrophils. Blood 1995; 85:3719–3726.
90. Steinhilber D, Brungs M, Werz O, Wisenberg I, Danielsson C, Kahlen JP, Nayeri S, Schrader M, Carlberg C. The nuclear receptor for melatonin represses 5-lipoxygenase gene expression in human B lymphocytes. J Biol Chem 1995; 270:7037–7040.
91. Bennett CF, Chiang MY, Monia BP, Crooke ST. Regulation of 5-lipoxygenase and 5-lipoxygenase activating protein expression in HL-60 cells. Biochem J 1993; 289: 33–39.
92. Steinhilber D, Hoshiko S, Grunewald J, Rådmark O, Samuelsson B. Serum factors regulate 5-lipoxygenase activity in maturing HL-60 cells. Biochim Biophys Acta 1993; 1178:1–8.
93. Steinhilber D, Rådmark O, Samuelsson B. A heat stable serum factor upregulates 5-lipoxygenase activity in HL-60 cells, modulation by TNF-α or GM-CSF. Biochem Biophys Res Commun 1993; 193:1083–1090.
94. Steinhilber D, Rådmark O, Samuelsson B. Transforming growth factor β upregulates 5-lipoxygenase activity during myeloid cell maturation. Proc Natl Acad Sci USA 1993; 90:5984–5988.
95. Riddick CA, Ring WL, Baker JR, Hodulik CR, Bigby TD. Dexamethasone increases expression of 5-lipoxygenase and its activating protein in human monocytes and THP-1 cells. Eur J Biochem 1997; 246(1):112–118.
96. Robin G, Markovich S, Athamna A, Keisari Y. Human recombinant granulocyte-macrophage colony-stimulating factor augments viability and cytotoxic activities of human monocyte-derived macrophage in long-term cultures. Lymphokine Cytokine Res 1991; 10:257–263.
97. Nissimov RDL, Keisari Y. Effect of human recombinant granulocyte-macrophage colony-stimulating factor and IL-3 on the expression of surface markers of human monocyte-derived macrophages in long-term cultures. Lymphokine Cytokine Res 1994; 13:239–245.
98. Schleimer RP. Effects of glucocorticosteroids on inflammatory cells relevant to their therapeutic applications in asthma. Am Rev Respir Dis 1990; 141:S59–S69.
99. Peters-Golden M, Thebert P. Inhibition by methylprednisolone of zymosan-induced leukotriene synthesis in alveolar macrophages. Am Rev Respir Dis 1987; 135: 1020–1026.
100. Fuller RW, Kelsey CR, Cole PJ, Dollery CT, MacDermont J. Dexamethasone inhib-

its the production of thromboxane B_2 and leukotriene B_4 by human alveolar and peritoneal macrophages in culture. Clin Sci 1984; 67:653–656.

101. Sebaldt RJ, Sheller JR, Oates JA, Roberts II LJ, Fitzgerald GA. Inhibition of eicosanoid synthesis by glucocorticoids in humans. Proc Natl Acad Sci USA 1990; 87: 6974–6978.
102. Manso G, Baker AJ, Taylor IK, Fuller RW. In vivo and in vitro effects of glucocorticosteroids on arachidonic acid metabolism and monocyte function in non-asthmatic humans. Eur Respir J 1992; 5:712–716.
103. O'Shaughnessy KM, Wellings R, Gillies B, Fuller RW. Differential effects of Fluticasone propionate on allergen-evoked bronchoconstriction and increased leukotriene E_4 excretion. Am Rev Respir Dis 1993; 147:1472–1476.
104. Naray-Fejes-Toth A, Rosenkranz B, Frolich JC, Fejes-Toth G. Glucocorticoid effect on arachidonic acid metabolism in vivo. J Steroid Biochem 1988; 30:155–159.
105. Thomas E, Leroux JL, Blotman F, Descomps B, Chavis C. Enhancement of leukotriene A_4 biosynthesis in neutrophils from patients with rheumatoid arthritis after a single glucocorticoid dose. Biochem Pharmacol 1995; 49:243–248.
106. Fair A, Pritchard KA. Oxidized low density lipoprotein increases U937 cell 5-lipoxygenase activity: induction of 5-lipoxygenase activating protein. Biochem Biophys Res Commun 1994; 201:1014–1020.
107. Rådmark O, Shimizu T, Jornvall H, Samuelsson B. Leukotriene A_4 hydrolase in human leukocytes. Purification and properties. J Biol Chem 1984; 259:12339–12345.
108. Ohishi N, Minami M, Kobayashi J, et al. Immunological quantitation and immunohistochemical localization of leukotriene A_4 hydrolase in guinea pig tissues. J Biol Chem 1990; 265:7520–7525.
109. Fu JY, Haeggstrom J, Collins P, Meijer J, Radmark O. Leukotriene A_4 hydrolase: analysis of some human tissues by radioimmunoassay. Biochim Biophys Acta 1989; 1006:121–126.
110. Toh H, Minami M, Shimizu T. Molecular evolution and zinc ion binding motif of leukotriene A_4 hydrolase. Biochem Biophys Res Commun 1990; 171:216–221.
111. Haeggström JZ. Leukotriene A_4 hydrolase: an epoxide hydrolase with peptidase activity. Biochem Biophys Res Commun 1990; 173:431–437.
112. McGee J, Fitzpatrick F. Enzymatic hydration of leukotriene A_4. Purification and characterization of a novel epoxide hydrolase from human erythrocytes. J Biol Chem 1985; 260:12832–12837.
113. Bigby TD, Lee DM, Minami M, Ohishi N, Shimizu T, Baker JR. Characterization of human airway epithelial cell leukotriene A_4 hydrolase. Am J Respir Cell Mol Biol 1994; 11:615–624.
114. Baker JR, Kylstra TA, Bigby TD. Effects of metalloproteinase inhibitors on leukotriene A_4 hydrolase in human airway epithelial cells. Biochem Pharmacol 1995; 50:905–912.
115. Jendraschak E, Kaminski WE, Kiefl R, von Schacky C. The human leukotriene A_4 hydrolase gene is expressed in two alternatively spliced mRNA forms. Biochem J 1996; 314:733–737.
116. Nicholson DW, Ali A, Vaillancourt JP, Calaycay JR, Mumford RA, ZambonI RJ, Ford-Hutchinson AW. Purification to homogeneity and the N-terminal sequence of

human leukotriene C_4 synthase: a homodimeric glutathione *S*-transferase composed of 18-kDa subunits. Proc Natl Acad Sci USA 1993; 90:2015–2019.
117. Feinmark SJ, Cannon PJ. Endothelial cell leukotriene C_4 synthesis results from intercellular transfer of leukotriene A_4 synthesized by polymorphonuclear leukocytes. J Biol Chem 1986; 261:16466–16472.
118. Marcus AJ, Broekman MJ, Safier LB, Ullman HL, Islam N, Serhan CN, Rutherford LE, Korchak HM, Weissmann G. Formation of leukotrienes and other hydroxy acids during platelet-neutrophil interactions in vitro. Biochem Biophys Res Commun 1982; 109:130–137.
119. Maclouf JA, Murphy RC. Transcellular metabolism of neutrophil-derived leukotriene A_4 by human platelets. A potential cellular source of leukotriene C_4. J Biol Chem 1988; 263:174–181.
120. Lam BK, Penrose JF, Freeman GJ, Austen KF. Expression cloning of a cDNA for human leukotriene C_4 synthase, an integral membrane protein conjugating reduced glutathione to leukotriene A_4. Proc Natl Acad Sci USA 1994; 91:7663–7667.
121. Welsch DJ, Creely DP, Hauser SD, Mathis KJ, Krivi GG, Isakson PC. Molecular cloning and expression of human leukotriene C_4 synthase. Proc Natl Acad Sci USA 1994; 91:9745–9749.
122. Bigby TD HC, Arden KC, Fu L. Molecular cloning of the human LTC_4 synthase gene and assignment to chromosome 5q35. Mol Med 1996; 2:637–646.
123. Penrose JF, Spector J, Baldasaro M, Xu K, Boyce J, Arm JP, Austen KF, Lam BK. Molecular cloning of the gene for human leukotriene C_4 synthase. Organization, nucleotide sequence, and chromosomal localization to 5q35. J Biol Chem 1996; 271:11356–11361.
124. Rothenberg ME, Owen WF, Silberstein DS, Woods J, Soberman RJ, Austen KF, Stevens RL. Human eosinophils have prolonged survival, enhanced functional properties, and become hypodense when exposed to human interleukin 3. J Clin Invest 1988; 81:1986–1992.
125. Murakami M, Austen KF, Bingham CO, Friend DS, Penrose JF, Arm JP. Interleukin-3 regulates development of the 5-lipoxygenase/leukotriene C_4 synthase pathway in mouse mast cells. J Biol Chem 1995; 270:22653–22656.
126. Söderström M, Bolling A Hammarström S. Induction of leukotriene C_4 synthase activity in differentiating human erythroleukemia cells. Biochem Biophys Res Commun 1992; 189:1043–1049.
127. Nicholson DW, Ali A, Klemba MW, Munday NA, Zamboni RJ, Ford-Hutchinson AW. Human leukotriene C_4 synthase expression in dimethyl sulfoxide-differentiated U937 cells. J Biol Chem 1992; 267:17849–17857.
128. Ali A, Ford-Hutchinson AW, Nicholson DW. Activation of protein kinase C down-regulates leukotriene C_4 synthase activity and attenuates cysteinyl leukotriene production in an eosinophil substrain of HL-60 cells. J Immunol 1994; 153:776–788.
129. Kargman S, Ali A, Vaillancourt JP, Evans JF, Nicholson DW. Protein kinase C-dependent regulation of sulfidopeptide leukotriene biosynthesis and leukotriene C_4 synthase in neutrophilic HL-60 cells. Mol Pharmacol 1994; 45:1043–1049.
130. Sjölinder M, Tornhamre S, Werga P, Edenius C, Lindgren JA. Phorpbol ester-induced suppression of leukotriene C_4 synthase activity in human granulocytes. FEBS Lett 1995; 377:87–91.

131. Drazen JM, Austen KF. State of art. Leukotrienes and airway responses. Am Rev Respir Dis 1987; 136:985–998.
132. Wenzel SE, Larsen GL, Johnston K, Voelkel N, Westcott JY. Elevated levels of leukotriene C_4 in bronchoalveolar lavage fluid from atopic asthmatics after endobronchial allergen challenge. AM Rev Respir Dis 1990; 142:112–119.
133. Wenzel SE, Westcott JY, Larsen GL. Bronchoalveolar lavage fluid mediator levels 5 minutes after allergen challenge in atopic subjects with asthma: relationship to the development of late asthmatic responses. J Allergy Clin Immunol 1991; 87: 540–548.
134. Drazen JM, O'Brien J, Sparrow D, Weiss ST, Martins MA, Israel E, Fanta CH. Recovery of leukotriene E_4 from the urine of patients with airway obstruction. Am Rev Respir Dis 1992; 146:104–108.
135. Christie PE, Tagari P, Ford-Hutchinson AW, Charlesson S, Chee P, Arm JP, Lee TH. Urinary leukotriene E_4 concentrations increase after aspirin challenge in aspirin-sensitive asthmatic subjects. Am Rev Respir Dis 1991; 143:1025–1029.
136. Ferreri NR, Howland WC, Stevenson DD,Spiegelberg HL. Release of leukotrienes, prostaglandins, and histamine into nasal secretions of aspirin-sensitive asthmatics during reaction to aspirin. Am Rev Respir Dis 1988; 137:847–854.
137. Picado C, Ramis I, Rosello J, Prat J, Bulbena O, Plaza V, Montserrat JM, Gelpi E. Release of peptide leukotriene into nasal secretions after local instillation of aspirin in aspirin-sensitive asthmatic patients. Am Rev Respir Dis 1992; 145:65–69.
138. Steinhilber D, Radmark O, Samuelsson B. Transforming growth factor beta upregulates 5-lipoxygenase activity during myeloid cell maturation. Proc Natl Acad Sci USA 1993; 90:5984–5988.
139. Broide DH, Lotz M, Cuomo AJ, Coburn DA, Federman EC, Wasserman SI. Cytokines in symptomatic asthma airways. J Allergy Clin Immunol 1992; 89:958–967.
140. Broide DH, Paine MM, Firestein GS. Eosinophils express interleukin 5 and granulocyte macrophage-colony-stimulating factor mRNA at sites of allergic inflammation in asthmatics. J Clin Invest 1992; 90:1414–1424.
141. Munafo DA, Shindo K, Baker JR, Bigby TD. Leukotriene A_4 hydrolase in human bronchoalveolar lavage fluid. J Clin Invest 1994; 93:1042–1050.
142. Munafo DA, Fu L, Ring WL, Riddick CA, Bigby TD. Increased immunoreactive 5-lipoxygenase in neutrophils of asthmatic patients. Am J Respir Crit Care Med 1996; 153:A416.
143. Serhan CN, Haeggstrom JZ, Leslie CC. Lipid mediator networks in cell signaling: update and impact of cytokines. FASEB J 1996; 10:1147–1158.
144. Serhan CN. Lipoxin biosynthesis and its impact in inflammatory and vascular events. Biochim Biophys Acta 1994; 1212:1–25.
145. Bigby TD. Transcellular metabolism of leukotrienes in the lung. Adv Exp Med Biol 1991; 314:235–250.
146. Claesson HE, Haeggstrom JZ, Odlander B, Medina JF, Wetterholm A, Jakobsson PJ, Radmark O. The role of leukotriene A_4 hydrolase in cells and tissues lacking 5-lipoxygenase. Adv Exp Med Biol 1991; 314:307–315.
147. Lindgren JA, Edenius C. Transcellular biosynthesis of leukotrienes and lipoxins via leukotriene A_4 transfer. Trends Pharmacol Sci 1993; 14:351–354.

148. Serhan CN. Lipoxins and novel aspirin-triggered 15-epi-lipoxins: a jungle of cell-cell interactions or a therapeutic opportunity? Prostaglandins 1997; 53:107–137.
149. Samuelsson B. From studies of biochemical mechanisms to novel biological mediators: prostaglandin endoperoxides, thromboxanes, and leukotrienes. Les prix Nobel. Nobel Prizes, Presentations, Biographies and Lectures. Stockholm: Alqvist & Wiksell, 1982:153–174.
150. Marcus AJ, Weksler BB, Jaffe EA, Broekman MJ. Synthesis of prostacyclin from platelet-derived endoperoxides by cultured human endothelial cells. J Clin Invest 1980; 66:979–986.
151. Marcus AJ. Transcellular metabolism of eicosanoids. Prog Hemost Thromb 1986; 8:127–142.
152. Fitzpatrick FA, Morton DR, Wynalda MA. Albumin stabilizes leukotriene A_4. J Biol Chem 1982; 257:4680–4683.
153. Levy BD, Reilly JJ, Drazen JM, Serhan CN. Pulmonary surfactant (Survanta) stabilizes leukotriene A_4 and alters the profile of both lipoxins and leukotrienes generated by human alveolar macrophages. International Spring Symposium on Prostaglandins, Leukotrienes, Lipoxins and Platelet Activating Factor, Washington, DC, 1991. Vol. XI.
154. Fitzpatrick F, Liggett W, McGee J, Bunting S, Morton D, Samuelsson B. Metabolism of leukotriene A_4 by human erythrocytes. A novel cellular source of leukotriene B_4. J Biol Chem 1984; 259:11403–11407.
155. Radmark O, Shimizu T, Jornvall H, Samuelsson B. Leukotriene A_4 hydrolase in human leukocytes. Purification and properties. J Biol Chem 1984; 259:12339–12345.
156. Medina JF, Barrios C, Funk CD, Larsson O, Haeggstrom J, Radmark O. Human fibroblasts show expression of the leukotriene-A_4-hydrolase gene, which is increased after simian-virus-40 transformation. Eur J Biochem 1990; 191:27–31.
157. Samuelsson B, Dahlen SE, Lindgren JA, Rouzer CA, Serhan CN. Leukotrienes and lipoxins: structures, biosynthesis, and biological effects. Science 1987; 237:1171–1176.
158. McGee JE, Fitzpatrick FA. Erythrocyte-neutrophil interactions: formation of leukotriene B_4 by transcellular biosynthesis. Proc Natl Acad Sci USA 1986; 83:1349–1353.
159. Stern A, Serhan CN. Human red cells enhance the formation of 5-lipoxygenase-derived products by neutrophils. Free Rad Res Commun 1989; 7:335–339.
160. Claesson HE, Haeggstrom J. Human endothelial cells stimulate leukotriene synthesis and convert granulocyte released leukotriene A_4 into leukotrienes B_4, C_4, D_4 and E_4. Eur J Biochem 1988; 173:93–100.
161. Jakobsson PJ, Odlander B, Claesson HE. Effects of monocyte-lymphocyte interaction on the synthesis of leukotriene B_4. Eur J Biochem 1991; 196:395–400.
162. Sola J, Godessart N, Vila L, Puig L, de Moragas JM. Epidermal cell-polymorphonuclear leukocyte cooperation in the formation of leukotriene B_4 by transcellular biosynthesis. J Invest Dermatol 1992; 98:333–339.
163. Driscoll BR, Cromwell O, Kay AB. Sputum leukotrienes in obstructive airways diseases. Clin Exp Immunol 1984; 55:397–404.
164. Wardlaw AJ, Hay H, Cromwell O, Collins JV, Kay AB. Leukotrienes, LTC_4 and

LTB_4, in bronchoalveolar lavage in bronchial asthma and other respiratory diseases. J Allergy Clin Immunol 1989; 84:19–26.
165. Yoshimoto T, Soberman RJ, Lewis RA, Austen KF. Isolation and characterization of leukotriene C_4 synthetase of rat basophilic leukemia cells. Proc Natl Acad Sci USA 1985; 82:8399–8403.
166. Tate SS, Meister A. Gamma-glutamyl transpeptidase: catalytic, structural and functional aspects. Mol Cell Biochem 1981; 39:357–368.
167. Lee CW, Lewis RA, Corey EJ, Austen KF. Conversion of leukotriene D_4 to leukotriene E_4 by a dipeptidase released from the specific granule of human polymorphonuclear leucocytes. Immunology 1983; 48:27–35.
168. Claesson HE, Haeggstrom J. Metabolism of leukotriene A_4 by human endothelial cells: evidence for leukotriene C_4 and D_4 formation by leukocyte-endothelial cell interaction. Adv PG, TX, LT Res 1987; 17A:115–119.
169. Brady HR, Serhan CN. Adhesion promotes transcellular leukotriene biosynthesis during neutrophil-glomerular endothelial cell interactions: inhibition by antibodies against CD18 and L-selection. Biochem Biophys Res Commun 1992; 186:1307–1314.
170. Edenius C, Heidvall K, Lindgren JA. Novel transcellular interaction: conversion of granulocyte-derived leukotriene A_4 to cysteinyl-containing leukotrienes by human platelets. Eur J Biochem 1988; 178:81–86.
171. Feinmark SJ, Cannon PJ. Vascular smooth muscle cell leukotriene C_4 synthesis: requirement for transcellular leukotriene A_4 metabolism. Biochim Biophys Acta 1987; 922:125–135.
172. Badr KF. Cell-cell interactions in the regulation of glomerular inflammation by arachidonate lipoxygenase products. Adv Exp Med Biol 1991; 314:335–346.
173. Serhan CN, Hirsch U, Palmblad J, Samuelsson B. Formation of lipoxin A by granulocytes from eosinophilic donors. FEBS Lett 1987; 217:242–246.
174. Marcus AJ, Safier LB, Broekman MJ, Ullman HL, Islam N, Sorrell TC, Serhan CN, Weissmann G, Oglesby TD, Gorman RR. Production of metabolic products of arachidonic acid during cell-cell interactions. J Allergy Clin Immunol 1984; 74:338–342.
175. Edenius C, Haeggstrom J, Lindgren JA. Transcellular conversion of endogenous arachidonic acid to lipoxins in mixed human platelet-granulocyte suspensions. Biochem Biophys Res Commun 1988; 157:801–807.
176. Edenius C, Stenke L, Lindgren JA. On the mechanism of transcellular lipoxin formation in human platelets and granulocytes. Eur J Biochem 1991; 199:401–409.
177. Fiore S, Brezinski ME, Sheppard KA, Serhan CN. The lipoxin biosynthetic circuit and their actions with human neutrophils. Adv Exp Med Biol 1991; 314:109–132.
178. Anderson GP, Coyle AJ. TH2 and 'TH2-like' cells in allergy and asthma: pharmacological perspectives. Trends Pharmacol Sci 1994; 15:324–332.
179. Carlos TM, Harlan JM. Leukocyte-endothelial adhesion molecules. Blood 1994; 84:2068–2101.
180. Brady HR, Papayianni A, Serhan CN. Leukocyte adhesion promotes biosynthesis of lipoxygenase products by transcellular routes. Kidney Int Suppl 1994; 45:S90–97.
181. Serhan CN, Hamberg M, Samuelsson B. Lipoxins: novel series of biologically ac-

tive compounds formed from arachidonic acid in human leukocytes. Proc Natl Acad Sci USA 1984; 81:5335–5339.

182. Ford-Hutchinson AW. Arachidonate 15-lipoxygenase; characteristics and potential biological significance. Eicosanoids 1991; 4:65–74.
183. Turk J, Maas RL, Brash AR, Roberts LJd, Oates JA. Arachidonic acid 15-lipoxygenase products from human eosinophils. J Biol Chem 1982; 257:7068–7076.
184. Levy BD, Romano M, Chapman HA, Reilly JJ, Drazen J, Serhan CN. Human alveolar macrophages have 15-lipoxygenase and generate 15(S)-hydroxy-5,8,11-cis-13-trans-eicosatetraenoic acid and lipoxins. J Clin Invest 1993; 92:1572–1579.
185. Conrad DJ, Kuhn H, Mulkins M, Highland E, Sigal E. Specific inflammatory cytokines regulate the expression of human monocyte 15-lipoxygenase. Proc Natl Acad Sci USA 1992; 89:217–221.
186. Hunter JA, Finkbeiner WE, Nadel JA, Goetzl EJ, Holtzman MJ. Predominant generation of 15-lipoxygenase metabolites of arachidonic acid by epithelial cells from human trachea. Proc Natl Acad Sci USA 1985; 82:4633–4637.
187. Nassar GM, Morrow JD, Roberts LJ, Lakkis FG, Badr KF. Induction of 15-lipoxygenase by interleukin-13 in human blood monocytes. J Biol Chem 1994; 269: 27631–27634.
188. Dahlen SE, Franzen L, Raud J, Serhan CN, Westlund P, Wikstrom E, Bjorck T, Matsuda H, Webber SE, Veale CA, Puustinen T, Haeggström J, Nicolau KC, Samuelsson B. Actions of lipoxin A_4 and related compounds in smooth muscle preparations and on the microcirculation in vivo. Adv Exp Med Biol 1988; 229:107–130.
189. Serhan CN. On the relationship between leukotriene and lipoxin production by human neutrophils: evidence for differential metabolism of 15-HETE and 5-HETE. Biochim Biophys Acta 1989; 1004:1581–68.
190. Serhan CN. Lipoxins: eicosanoids carrying intra- and intercellular messages. J Bioenerg Biomemb 1991; 23:105–122.
191. Belkner J, Wiesner R, Rathman J, Barnett J, Sigal E, Kuhn H. Oxygenation of lipoproteins by mammalian lipoxygenases. Eur J Biochem 1993; 213:251–261.
192. Yla-Herttuala S, Rosenfeld ME, Parthasarathy S, Glass CK, Sigal E, Witztum JL, Steinberg D. Colocalization of 15-lipoxygenase mRNA and protein with epitopes of oxidized low density lipoprotein in macrophage-rich areas of atherosclerotic lesions. Proc Natl Acad Sci USA 1990; 87:6959–6963.
193. Yla-Herttuala S, Rosenfeld ME, Parthasarathy S, Sigal E, Sarkioja T, Witztum JL, Steinberg D. Gene expression in macrophage-rich human atherosclerotic lesions. 15-Lipoxygenase and acetyl low density lipoprotein receptor messenger RNA colocalize with oxidation specific lipid-protein adducts. J Clin Invest 1991; 87:1146–1152.
194. Kuhn H, Belkner J, Zaiss S, Fahrenklemper T, Wohlfeil S. Involvement of 15-lipoxygenase in early stages of atherogenesis. J Exp Med 1994; 179:1903–1911.
195. Hiltunen T, Luoma J, Nikkari T, Yla-Herttuala S. Induction of 15-lipoxygenase mRNA and protein in early atherosclerotic lesions. Circulation 1995; 92:3297–3303.
196. Sparrow CP, Parthasarathy, S., Steinberg, D. Enzymatic modification of low density lipoprotein by purified lipoxygenase plus phopholipase A_2 mimic cell-mediated oxidative modifications. J Lipid Res 1988; 29:745–753.

197. Benz DJ, Mol M, Ezaki M, Mori-Ito N, Zelan I, Miyanohara A, Friedmann T, Parthasarathy S, Steinberg D, Witztum JL. Enhanced levels of lipoperoxides in low density lipoprotein incubated with murine fibroblast expressing high levels of human 15-lipoxygenase. J Biol Chem 1995; 270:5191–5197.
198. Yla-Herttuala S, Luoma J, Viita H, Hiltunen T, Sisto T, Nikkari T. Transfer of 15-lipoxygenase gene into rabbit iliac arteries results in the appearance of oxidation-specific lipid-protein adducts characteristic of oxidized low density lipoprotein. J Clin Invest 1995; 95:2692–2698.
199. Shen J, Herderick, E., Cornhill JF, Zsigmond E, Kim H-S, Kuhn H, Guervara NV, Chan L. Macrophage-mediated 15-lipoxygenase expression protects against atherosclerosis development. J Clin Invest 1996; 98:2201–2208.
200. Chavis C, Chanez P, Vachier I, Bousquet J, Michel FB, Godard P. 5-15-diHETE and lipoxins generated by neutrophils from endogenous arachidonic acid as asthma biomarkers. Biochem Biophys Res Commun 1995; 207:273–279.
201. Thomas E, Leroux JL, Blotman F, Chavis C. Conversion of endogenous arachidonic acid to 5,15-diHETE and lipoxins by polymorphonuclear cells from patients with rheumatoid arthritis. Inflamm Res 1995; 44:121–124.
202. Serhan CN, Sheppard KA, Fiore S. Lipoxin formation: evaluation of the role and actions of leukotriene A_4. Adv PG, TX LT Res 1990; 20:54–62.
203. Stenke L, Edenius C, Samuelsson J, Lindgren JA. Deficient lipoxin synthesis: a novel platelet dysfunction in myeloproliferative disorders with special reference to blastic crisis of chronic myelogenous leukemia. Blood 1991; 78:2989–2995.
204. Stenke L, Mansour M, Edenius C, Reizenstein P, Lindgren JA. Formation and proliferative effects of lipoxins in human bone marrow. Biochem Biophys Res Commun 1991; 180:255–261.
205. Sheppard KA, Greenberg SM, Funk CD, Romano M, Serhan CN. Lipoxin generation by human megakaryocyte-induced 12-lipoxygenase. Biochim Biophys Acta 1992; 1133:223–234.
206. Romano M, Serhan CN. Lipoxin generation by permeabilized human platelets. Biochemistry 1992; 31:8269–8277.
207. Romano M, Chen XS, Takahashi Y, Yamamoto S, Funk CD, Serhan CN. Lipoxin synthase activity of human platelet 12-lipoxygenase. Biochem J 1993; 296:127–133.
208. Claria J, Serhan CN. Aspirin triggers previously undescribed bioactive eicosanoids by human endothelial cell-leukocyte interactions. Proc Natl Acad Sci USA 1995; 92:9475–9479.
209. Herschman HR. Prostaglandin synthase 2. Biochim Biophys Acta 1996; 1299:125–140.
210. Maddox JF HM, Takano T, Petasis NA, Fokin VV, Serhan CN. Lipoxin A_4 stable analogs are potent mimetics that stimulate human monocytes and THP-1 cells via a G-protein linked lipoxin A_4 receptor. J Biol Chem 1997; 272:6972–6978.
211. Fiore S, Ryeom SW, Weller PF, Serhan CN. Lipoxin recognition sites. Specific binding of labeled lipoxin A_4 with human neutrophils. J Biol Chem 1992; 267: 16168–16176.
212. Fiore S, Romano M, Reardon EM, Serhan CN. Induction of functional lipoxin A_4 receptors in HL-60 cells. Blood 1993; 81:3395–3403.

213. Fiore S, Maddox JF, Perez HD, Serhan CN. Identification of a human cDNA encoding a functional high affinity lipoxin A_4 receptor. J Exp Med 1994; 180:253–260.
214. Fiore S, Serhan CN. Lipoxin A_4 receptor activation is distinct from that of the formyl peptide receptor in myeloid cells: inhibition of CD11/18 expression by lipoxin A_4-lipoxin A_4 receptor interaction. Biochemistry 1995; 34:16678–16686.
215. Hla T, Neilson K. Human cyclooxygenase-2 cDNA. Proc Natl Acad Sci USA 1992; 89:7384–7388.
216. Manson JE, Tosteson H, Ridker PM, Satterfield S, Hebert P, O. Connor GT, Buring JE, Hennekens CH. The primary prevention of myocardial infarction. NEJM 1992; 326:1406–1416.
217. Buring JE, Hennekens CH. Prevention of cardiovascular disease: risks and benefits of aspirin. J Gen Intern Med 1990; 5:S54–57.
218. Giovannucci E, Rimm EB, Stampfer MJ, Colditz GA, Ascherio A, Willett WC. Aspirin use and the risk for colorectal cancer and adenoma in male health professionals. Ann Intern Med 1994; 121:241–246.
219. Giovannucci E, Egan KM, Hunter DJ, Stampfer MJ, Colditz GA, Willett WC, Speizer FE. Aspirin and the risk of colorectal cancer in women. NEJM 1995; 333: 609–614.
220. Egan KM, Stampfer MJ, Giovannucci E, Rosner BA, Colditz GA. Prospective study of regular aspirin use and the risk of breast cancer. J Natl Cancer Inst 1996; 88: 988–993.
221. Lehr HA, Olofsson AM, Carew TE, Vajkoczy P, von Andrian UH, Hubner C, Berndt MC, Steinberg D, Messmer K, Arfors KE. P-selectin mediates the interaction of circulating leukocytes with platelets and microvascular endothelium in response to oxidized lipoprotein in vivo. Lab Invest 1994; 71:380–386.
222. Lehr HA, Frei B, Arfors KE. Vitamin C prevents cigarette smoke-induced leukocyte aggregation and adhesion to endothelium in vivo. Proc Natl Acad Sci USA 1994; 91:7688–7692.
223. Mayadas TN, Mendrick DL, Brady HR, et al. Acute passive anti-glomerular basement membrane nephritis in P-selectin-deficient mice. Kidney Intl 1996; 49:1342–1349.
224. Edenius C, Kumlin M, Bjork T, Anggard A, Lindgren JA. Lipoxin formation in human nasal polyps and bronchial tissue. FEBS Lett 1990; 272:25–28.
225. Tornhamre S, Gigou A, Edenius C, Lellouche JP, Lindgren JA. Conversion of 5,6-dihydroxyeicosatetraenoic acids. A novel pathway for lipoxin formation by human platelets. FEBS Lett 1992; 304:78–82.
226. Brezinski ME, Serhan CN. Selective incorporation of (15S)-hydroxyeicosatetraenoic acid in phosphatidylinositol of human neutrophils: agonist-induced deacylation and transformation of stored hydroxyeicosanoids. Proc Natl Acad Sci USA 1990; 87:6248–6252.
227. Capdevila JH, Falck JR, Estabrook RW. Cytochrome P450 and the arachidonate cascade. FASEB 1992; 6:73173–6.
228. Sigal E, Conrad DJ. Human 15-lipoxygenase: a potential effector molecule for interleukin-4. Adv PG, TX, LT Res 1994; 22:309–316.
229. Tzeng DY, Deuel TF, Huang JS, Senior RM, Boxer LA, Baehner RL. Platelet-

derived growth factor promotes polymorphonuclear leukocyte activation. Blood 1984; 64:1123–1128.

230. Levy BD, Bertram S, Tai HH, Israel E, Fischer A, Drazen JM, Serhan CN. Agonist-induced lipoxin A_4 generation: detection by a novel lipoxin A_4-ELISA. Lipids 1993; 28:1047–1053.
231. Brinckmann R, Topp MS, Zalan I, Heydeck D, Ludwig P, Kuhn H, Berdel WE, Habenicht JR. Regulation of 15-lipoxygenase expression in lung epithelial cells by interleukin-4. Biochem J 1996; 318:305–312.
232. Chavis C, Godard P, Crastes de Paulet A, Damon M. Formation of lipoxins and leukotrienes by human alveolar macrophages incubated with 15(S)-HETE: a model for cellular cooperation between macrophages and airway epithelial cells. Eicosanoids 1992; 5:203–211.
233. Genis P, Jett M, Bernton EW, Boyle T, Gelbard HA, Dzenko K, Keane RW, Resnick L, Mizrachi Y, Volsky DJ. Cytokines and arachidonic metabolites produced during human immunodeficiency virus (HIV)-infected macrophage-astroglia interactions: implications for the neuropathogenesis of HIV disease. J Exp Med 1992; 176:1703–1718.
234. Ishizaki Y, Morita I, Murota S. Arachidonic acid metabolism in cultured astrocytes from rat embryo and in C6 glioma cells. Brain Res 1989; 494:138–142.
235. Papayianni A, Serhan CN, Brady HR. Lipoxin A_4 and B_4 inhibit leukotriene-stimulated interactions of human neutrophils and endothelial cells. J Immunol 1996; 156: 2264–2272.
236. Lerner R, Heimburger M, Palmblad J. Lipoxin A_4 induces hyperadhesiveness in human endothelial cells for neutrophils. Blood 1993; 82:948–953.
237. Nagata K, Tsuji T, Todoroki N, KatagirI Y, Tanoue K, Yamazaki H, Hanai N, Irimura T. Activated platelets induce superoxide anion release by monocytes and neutrophils through P-selectin (CD62). J Immunol 1993; 151:3267–3273.
238. Papayianni A, Serhan CN, Phillips ML, Rennke HG, Brady HR. Transcellular biosynthesis of lipoxin A_4 during adhesion of platelets and neutrophils in experimental immune complex glomerulonephritis. Kidney Int 1995; 47:1295–1302.
239. Chavis C, Vachier I, Chanez P, Bousquet J, Godard P. 5(S),15(S)-dihydroxyeicosatetraenoic acid and lipoxin generation in human polymorphonuclear cells: dual specificity of 5-lipoxygenase towards endogenous and exogenous precursors. J Exp Med 1996; 183:1633–1643.
240. Brezinski DA, Serhan CN. Characterization of lipoxins by combined gas chromatography and electron-capture negative ion chemical ionization mass spectrometry: formation of lipoxin A_4 by stimulated human whole blood. Biol Mass Spectrom 1991; 20:45–52.
241. Brezinski DA, Nesto RW, Serhan CN. Angioplasty triggers intracoronary leukotrienes and lipoxin A_4. Impact of aspirin therapy. Circulation 1992; 86:56–63.
242. Serhan CN, Maddox JF, Petasis NA, Akritopoulou-Zanze I, Papayianni A, Brady HR, Colgan SP, Madara JL. Design of lipoxin A stable analogs that block transmigration and adhesion of human neutrophils. Biochemistry 1995; 34:14609–14615.
243. Stenke L, Reizenstein P, Lindgren JA. Leukotrienes and lipoxins-new potential performers in the regulation of human myelopoiesis. Leuk Res 1994; 18:727–732.
244. Lewis RA, Austen KF, Soberman RJ. Leukotrienes and other products of the 5-

lipoxygenase pathway. Biochemistry and relation to pathobiology in human diseases. NEJM 1990; 323:645–655.
245. Spector SL, Smith LJ, Glass M. Effects of 6 weeks of therapy with oral doses of ICI 204,219, a leukotriene D_4 receptor antagonist, in subjects with bronchial asthma. ACCOLATE Asthma Trialists Group. Am J Respir Crit Care Med 1994; 150:618–623.
246. Laviolette M, Coulombe R, Picard S, Braquet P, Borgeat P. Decreased leukotriene B_4 synthesis in smokers' alveolar macrophages in vitro. J Clin Invest 1986; 77:54–60.
247. Kumlin M, Hamberg M, Granstrom E, Bjorck T, Dahlen B, Matsuda H, Zetterstrom O, Dahlen SE. 15(S)-Hydroxyeicosatetraenoic acid is the major arachidonic acid metabolite in human bronchi: association with airway epithelium. Arch Biochem Biophys 1990; 282:254–262.
248. Lee TH, Crea AE, Gant V, Spur BW, Nicolaou KC, Reardon E, BrezinskI M, Serhan CN. Identification of lipoxin A_4 and its relationship to the sulfidopeptide leukotrienes C_4, D_4, and E_4 in the bronchoalveolar lavage fluids obtained from patients with selected pulmonary diseases. Am Rev Respir Dis 1990; 141:1453–1458.
249. McFadden ER, Jr., Gilbert IA. Asthma. NEJM 1992; 327:1928–1937.
250. Damon M, Chavis C, Crastes de Paulet A, Michel FB, Godard P. Arachidonic acid metabolism in alveolar macrophages. A comparison of cells from healthy subjects, allergic asthmatics, and chronic bronchitis patients. Prostaglandins 1987; 34:291–309.
251. Christie PE, Spur BW, Lee TH. The effects of lipoxin A_4 on airway responses in asthmatic subjects. Am Rev Respir Dis 1992; 145:1281–1284.
252. Maddox JF, Serhan CN. Lipoxin A_4 and B_4 are potent stimuli for human monocyte migration and adhesion: selective inactivation by dehydrogenation and reduction. J Exp Med 1996; 183:137–146.
253. Takano T, Fiore S, Maddox JF, Brady HR, Petasis NA, Serhan CN. Aspirin-triggered 15-epi-lipoxin A_4 and LXA_4 stable analogs are potent inhibitors of acute inflammation: evidence for anti-inflammatory receptors. J Exp Med 1997; 185: 1693–1704.

8

Leukotriene Receptors: Incompletely Defined Targets for Treatment of Asthma and Inflammation

SVEN-ERIK DAHLÉN

Institute of Environmental Medicine
Karolinska Institutet
Stockholm, Sweden

I. Introduction

Drugs that selectively inhibit the formation or action of leukotrienes (LT) are currently being introduced as new therapy in asthma. The primary structure of the enzymes in the 5-lipoxygenase (5-LO) pathway has been defined and great progress has been made with respect to the understanding of their cellular localization and genomic regulation (reviewed in Ref. 1). In the process of developing drugs for inhibition of leukotrienes, FLAP (5-lipoxygenase activation protein) was discovered as an important cofactor and rational target for interference with biosynthesis (2,3). In contrast, despite the development of several potent antagonists of cysteinyl-leukotrienes, the corresponding molecular information about the receptors for leukotrienes is very limited. The available leukotriene receptor antagonists have been developed by conventional screening of new chemical entities in functional or ligand-binding assays. The knowledge about leukotriene receptors is mainly derived from studies of functional responses. This chapter will present the framework that defines our current understanding of leukotriene receptors and raise some of the issues that future research will need to address.

II. Leukotriene B_4

A. Profile of Biological Activity

Leukotriene B_4 was the first leukotriene discovered (4) when the 5-lipoxygenase pathway in human leukocytes was explored (5). With the exception of a contrac-

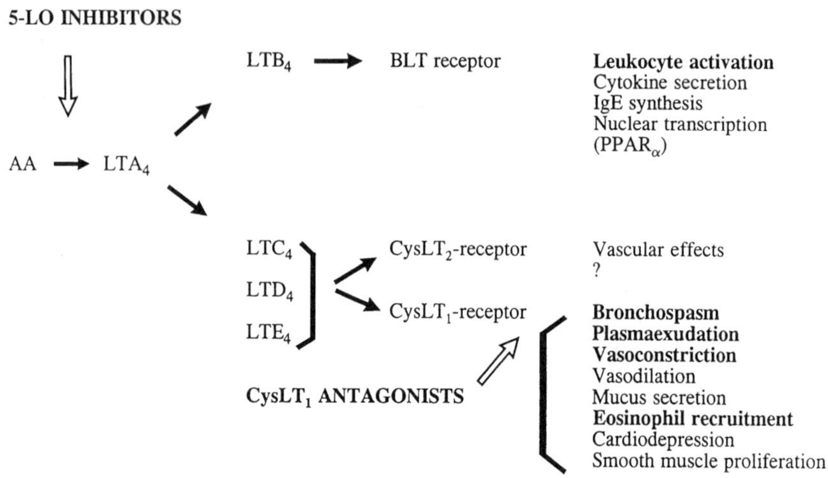

Figure 1 Schematic drawing summarizing the biological actions of leukotrienes, with indications of the receptors which mediate different effects and the points of attack for drugs which inhibit leukotriene formation or action. For effects denoted in bold type, the receptor mediating the response has been established. For other effects, the scheme represents a proposal of the author, but it remains to define the receptor characteristics, in particular for human tissues.

tile effect in the guinea pig lung parenchyma (6–8), LTB_4 has been found to have primarily inflammatory cells as targets for its biological activity (Fig. 1). It is a potent stimulus for activation of leukocytes, eliciting chemokinetic and chemotactic responses in vitro (9). In vivo, LTB_4 increases leukocyte rolling and adhesion to the venular endothelium (10). This initial chemotactic response is followed by emigration of leukocytes into the extravascular space (10). During a short-lasting exposure to LTB_4, polymorphonuclear leukocytes are mainly recruited (11,12). With prolonged exposure to LTB_4, as presumably occurs when LTB_4 is formed in vivo, other granulocytes, including eosinophils, are found in tissues or exudates after challenge with LTB_4 (13). Accordingly, LTB_4 has been shown to be a chemoattractant in interleukin-5–primed eosinophils (14) and to stimulate production of interleukin-5 in T lymphocytes (15).

In addition to effects on leukocyte recruitment, LTB_4 stimulates secretion of superoxide anion and release of different granulae constituents from leukocytes (16,17). Among the effects of LTB_4 on inflammatory cells, it has been observed that LTB_4 may affect expression of low-affinity receptors for IgE on B-lymphocyte cell lines (18) and IgE synthesis induced by interleukin-4 (19). More recently, the observation that LTB_4 is an agonist for the nuclear transcription factor $PPAR_\alpha$ (peroxisome proliferator-activated receptor α) has aroused considerable interest (20). The finding may implicate a role for LTB_4 in the control of central events in lipid metabolism and inflammation (21). The structure-activity relationship for this effect of LTB_4 and the influence of antagonists of LTB_4 on the response remain to be determined, but observations nevertheless suggest the possibility that LTB_4 also has intracellular and nuclear targets, which may participate in long-term control of gene expression.

The ω-oxidized metabolites of LTB_4 generally display effects similar to those of LTB_4, although sometimes with less potency (6,22,23). There was complete cross-tachyphylaxis between LTB_4 and its ω-oxidized metabolites in the guinea pig lung parenchyma (6). The 5*S*,12*R* position of the hydroxyls in LTB_4 appears critical to its biological activity (22,23). For example, 5*S*-HETE and 5*S*,12*S*-DHETE are both less potent than LTB_4 in the guinea pig lung parenchyma (6,23), and the responses elicited by these compounds are also different with respect to time-course and mode of action (6,23). In contrast, a 5*S*,12*R*-DHETE with 6-*trans* and 8-*cis* double bonds (LTB_4 is 6-*cis* and 8-*trans*, otherwise the structure is identical) formed by the LTA_4 hydrolase in *Xenopus laevis* shared the mode of action of LTB_4 in the guinea pig lung strip (24).

B. Receptors for LTB_4

The different profiles of biological activities for LTB_4 and cysteinyl-leukotrienes (Fig. 1) suggested that the two main classes of leukotrienes possessed distinct receptors. The experimental data have indeed established that LTB_4 acts at a specific receptor, which now is designated the BLT receptor (25). Radioligand-binding experiments have been useful in the exploration of the properties of BLT receptors. Thus, specific $[^3H]$-LTB_4 binding has been demonstrated in many tissues including human polymorphonuclear leukocytes (PMNs) (26,27). The binding sites in PMNs were selectively inhibited by guanine nucleotides (28,29), and structurally related metabolites displaced LTB_4 with a potency that correlated with their activities in chemotactic assays (30).

Using different strategies, including structural modifications of partial agonists at the tentative receptor for LTB_4, a number of selective and relatively potent antagonists of LTB_4 have been developed (31). A few compounds have entered into early clinical testing in humans, with LY-293,111 (VML 295) probably being studied the most. This particular compound was recently found to inhibit LTB_4-induced neutrophil responses in vivo and allergen-induced PMN activation, but it had no effect on allergen-induced early or late-phase airway obstruction in asthmatics (32). The results with LY-293,111 in asthmatics argue against an important role for LTB_4 as mediator in asthma but do not exclude that LTB_4 may be involved in other pulmonary reactions.

Pharmacological evidence has accumulated to suggest that BLT receptors are G-protein coupled (28,29), but it was only very recently possible to isolate the cDNA for a BLT receptor in retinoic acid–differentiated HL-60 cells (33). The cDNA encoded a 352-amino-acid cell-surface protein that was G-protein coupled and mediated chemotaxis. Incidentally, this cDNA had previously been described as an orphan receptor possibly mediating chemoattractant responses (34). Northern blotting experiments of human tissues displayed a preferential expression of mRNA for the BLT receptor in PMNs (33). There was also some expression in the spleen and thymus, whereas most other examined tissues, including the lung, showed no or insignificant expression of message for the BLT receptor (33).

It has been observed that especially chemotaxis is mediated at lower agonist concentrations of LTB_4 than are required for degranulation and superoxide generation (17,22,35). Ligand-binding experiments have also demonstrated the presence of low- and high-affinity binding sites (22,36). These observations have been taken as evidence for two subclasses of receptors for LTB_4. However, when tested against competitive antagonists, similar dose ratios are produced for all effects of LTB_4 (29). Likewise, naturally occurring metabolites or synthetic analogs show similar displacement potencies for the low- and high-affinity binding sites (29). Therefore, the apparent high- and low-affinity states may reflect G-protein coupled and uncoupled states of the BLT receptor. The observations suggest that the structural requirements for interaction with the receptor in the two states are quite similar. There is consequently currently no basis for definition of subclasses of receptors for LTB_4, and the developed antagonists appear to block the effects of LTB_4 and its immediate metabolites at a common BLT receptor. However, the recent cloning of the BLT receptor (33) has created an opportunity for new developments in this area.

III. The Cysteinyl-Leukotrienes

A. Profile of Biological Activity

The identification of LTC_4 as a slow-reacting substance in a mouse mastocytoma cell line (37) sparked the recognition that slow-reacting substance of anaphylaxis (SRS-A) was made up of LTC_4 and its two immediate metabolites LTD_4 and LTE_4 (38–45). This in turn led to research on the biological properties of the cysteinyl-leukotrienes along the pathways outlined by the original observations on the properties of biologically generated SRS-A (46). Thus, it was soon documented that, in particular, LTC_4 and LTD_4 were potent inducers of bronchoconstriction in guinea pig airways in vitro and in vivo (47,48) and caused contractions of isolated human bronchi (49–51). When tested in assays that had been used to distinguish SRS-A from other mediators, it was confirmed that LTC_4 and LTD_4

were inactive in systems that had been unresponsive to SRS-A, for example, rabbit bronchus and rat uterus (48).

When injected intravenously into guinea pigs, LTC_4 and LTD_4 caused biphasic changes in blood pressure (47,48). These two cysteinyl-leukotrienes also increased Evans blue accumulation in the skin (47,48), suggesting an increase in microvascular permeability. In the hamster cheek pouch, it was established that LTC_4 and LTD_4 indeed caused exudation of plasma proteins in postcapillary venules (10). In addition, LTC_4 and LTD_4 induced arteriolar constriction, but the plasma exudation was not a consequence of the vasoconstriction (10). In the guinea pig, it was shown that each of LTC_4, LTD_4, and LTE_4 was capable of inducing Evans blue accumulation in the airways (52). Their effects were observed in all airway segments, ranging from the most peripheral small bronchi to trachea, and there was evidence of Evans blue accumulation in superficial as well as deep layers of the airway mucosa.

The biological effects of LTE_4 have generally been studied much less, perhaps because this leukotriene was found to be an incomplete and less potent agonist than LTC_4 and LTD_4 in the guinea pig ileum (53). However, LTE_4 has been documented to possess a bronchoconstrictor activity in vitro and in vivo which is closely similar to that of LTC_4 and LTD_4 (54). It has also been observed that prolonged exposure to LTE_4 may produce enhancement of the responsiveness of smooth muscle to histamine (55,56). Moreover, LTE_4 is a full agonist for contraction of human bronchi in vitro (45,57), and it was not significantly less potent than LTC_4 and LTD_4 (57,58). Apart from a superfusion study that found LTE_4 to be much less potent than LTD_4 on human bronchi (59), investigations using large numbers of tissue specimens and comparable nonflow tissue bath conditions have consistently found LTE_4 to be either equipotent (57,58) or only slightly less potent than LTD_4 or LTC_4 in human bronchi (60). Although the kinetics and transduction mechanisms for the individual cysteinyl-leukotrienes on human airway smooth muscle need to be characterized more extensively, the contention that LTE_4 as a rule is less bioactive than LTC_4 or LTD_4 should be dismissed.

In addition to the bronchospastic and vasoactive properties of the cysteinyl-leukotrienes (Fig. 1), it has been observed that LTC_4 and LTD_4 may stimulate mucus secretion in isolated animal and human airways (61–63). Experiments in isolated perfused hearts also disclosed a depressive effect on cardiac contractility (64,65). The effect correlated with coronary vasoconstriction (65,66), but a direct negative inotropic effect on the myocardium may also be involved (67). More recently, additional effects with potential relevance to the role of cysteinyl-leukotrienes in asthma and pulmonary inflammation have been reported. Thus, increased infiltration of eosinophils into the airway mucosa of asthmatics was observed following inhalation of LTE_4 (68), and inhalation of LTD_4 increased the number of eosinophils in induced sputum samples from asthmatics (69). The capacity of cysteinyl-leukotrienes to promote eosinophil recruitment has recently been confirmed in experimental models (70,71), although the mechanisms involved remain to be defined. There is also experimental data in vitro (72) and in vivo (73) supporting the hypothesis that cysteinyl-leukotrienes may be involved in airway smooth muscle proliferation and remodeling.

Considered together, the spasmogenic and vasoactive properties of cysteinyl-leukotrienes, as well as the effects of LTB_4 on leukocytes and in the microcirculation, have been characterized relatively well, whereas the effects of leukotrienes on many other systems have so far received comparatively little attention. There would seem to be many areas where the effects of leukotrienes need to be explored to obtain more information about possible physiological functions and pathogenetic mechanisms. The large variations in responsiveness to leukotrienes between different animal species may provide important clues in further investigations of leukotriene receptors.

B. Receptors for Cysteinyl-Leukotrienes

When the SRS-A antagonist FPL 55712 (74) was tested against LTC_4 and LTD_4 in guinea pig airway preparations, it was evident that FPL 55712 was a competitive antagonist of LTD_4 but not LTC_4 (47,75,76). When the metabolic conversion of LTC_4 into LTD_4 was inhibited, LTC_4 was as potent an agonist as LTD_4 in the guinea pig trachea, but the effect of LTC_4 was not antagonized by FPL 55712 (76) or subsequently developed antagonist of LTD_4 (77,78). These observations supported the hypothesis of two different receptors for cysteinyl-leukotrienes, tentatively called the LTC_4 and the LTD_4 receptor. The findings with metabolic inhibitors also argued against the hypothesis that LTC_4 only was bioactive after having been transformed into LTD_4 (79).

However, when the influence of FPL 55712 on LTC_4 and LTD_4 was examined in human bronchi in the presence of the conversion inhibitor serine-borate, it was discovered that FPL 55712 antagonized the effect of LTC_4 and LTD_4 in this tissue to the same extent (58). The human airways were thus different from the guinea pig trachea or ileum where LTC_4 and LTD_4 appeared to cause contractions by activation of different receptors. Subsequent studies with more potent antagonists have indeed confirmed that LTC_4 and LTD_4 act at the same receptor in human airways (57,80). Moreover, LTE_4 is also a full and potent agonist at the receptor for cysteinyl-leukotrienes in human bronchi (57,58), and a selective antagonist such as ICI-204,219 (zafirlukast) produces an identical shift in the concentration-response curve for each of LTC_4, LTD_4, and LTE_4 (57).

It has been observed that LTC_4 and LTD_4 contracted human pulmonary vessels (50). When Labat and coworkers examined the effects of antagonists on contractions evoked by cysteinyl-leukotrienes in human pulmonary veins (60), they discovered that the responses were resistant to several potent compounds

(ICI-198,615, MK-571, and SKF 104,353) belonging to the current class of antagonists. The agonist sensitivity was also different from the bronchial preparations, with LTE_4 being a comparatively weak agonist producing only a transient submaximal contraction of the human pulmonary vein. Responses to both LTC_4 and LTD_4 which were resistant to the current class of antagonists had previously been reported in animal tissues such as ferret trachea (81), but did not receive as much attention as the antagonist-resistant effects of LTC_4 in guinea pig ileum (53) and trachea (75–78). The findings in human tissues contributed to the recognition that there seemed to exist at least two different atypical receptors for cysteinyl-leukotrienes, one being preferentially sensitive to LTC_4 (guinea pig ileum and trachea) and the other mediating contractions to both LTC_4 and LTD_4 (human pulmonary vein and ferret trachea).

The effects of LTC_4 and LTD_4 on the human pulmonary vein were antagonized in an apparently competitive manner by the leukotriene analog BAY u9773 (5(*S*)-hydroxy-6(*R*)-(4′-carboxyphenylthio)-7,9-*trans*-11,14-*cis*-eicosatetraenoic acid) (60). This compound has the same C20 backbone as all the natural occurring cysteinyl-leukotrienes but contains a carboxyphenyl group at C6 rather than cysteine or a cysteinyl-containing peptide. The compound BAY u9773 has subsequently been found to be a competitive antagonist of atypical responses to LTC_4 or LTD_4 in guinea pig ileum (82) and trachea (83), sheep bronchus (83) and trachea (84), and ferret trachea (83). However, the compound also antagonizes the effects of cysteinyl-leukotrienes in preparations where the responses are sensitive to the current class of antagonists (83). Therefore, BAY u9773 is not a selective antagonist of atypical responses to cysteinyl-leukotrienes, but it has broader antagonist activities than most other antagonists. It is of interest that there have been suggestions that two other compounds synthesized as leukotriene analogs (SKF 104,353 and MDL 28,753) also display profiles of activity, which in some assays may include broader antagonism than other antagonists of cysteinyl-leukotrienes (85,86).

On the basis of the evidence thus discussed, the IUPHAR (International Union of Pharmacologic Sciences) Nomenclature committee for leukotriene receptors introduced the names $CysLT_1$ and $CysLT_2$ to describe responses that are sensitive and resistant, respectively, to the class of drugs currently being introduced in the clinic (25). The framework shown in Figure 2 introduces a classification on the basis of sensitivity to antagonist drugs rather than agonist properties. As in other fields of pharmacology, the same agonist may activate different receptors. For example, LTC_4 may activate the $CysLT_1$ receptor in human airways, the $CysLT_2$ receptor in human pulmonary veins, and the $CysLT_2$ receptor in guinea pig ileum. An antagonist-based classification is generally considered more appropriate since it is focused on the function of the receptor. (The names $CysLT_1$ and $CysLT_2$ should, according to the nomenclature, be written in italics until their molecular structures have been defined.)

	Receptors for cysteinyl-leukotrienes (LTC_4, LTD_4 and LTE_4)	
	$CysLT_1$	*$CysLT_2$*
Tissue:	Human Bronchus G.P. Trachea & Ileum G.P. Gall Bladder Rat Lung Strip	Human Pulmonary Vein G.P. Trachea & Ileum Sheep Trachea & Bronchus Ferret Trachea
Antagonist:	FPL 55712, LY 171,883 ICI 198,615/ICI 204,219, MK-571/MK-679/MK-476, SKF 104,353/SKF 106,203, ONO 1078/SB 205,312, RG 12,525, CGP 45715, BAY x7195, BAY u9773.	(BAY u9773)

Figure 2 Overview of the *CysLT* receptors and their antagonists. The parentheses around BAY u9773 as $CysLT_2$ antagonist indicates that it is an unselective antagonist with properties as combined $CysLT_1/CysLT_2$ antagonist. As discussed in the text, it is likely that there exist further subclasses of both $CysLT_1$ and $CysLT_2$ receptors.

IV. Controversies and Research Requirements

As indicated in Figure 2, there are tissues such as guinea pig ileum and trachea where both types of receptors coexist, and there are tissues that seem to have homogeneous populations of receptors. For example, $CysLT_1$ receptors predominate in human bronchi (57,58) and rat lung (83), whereas $CysLT_2$ receptors appear to dominate in sheep trachea (84). However, the situation may be more complicated when effects of cysteinyl-leukotrienes are characterized in greater detail. Recently, Ortiz and coworkers revisited human pulmonary vessels and examined the influence of the endothelium on leukotriene responses (87). In addition to the confirmation of $CysLT_2$-mediated contractions of pulmonary veins, they discovered an endothelium-dependent contractile effect that was sensitive to $CysLT_1$ antagonists and a partly endothelium-dependent relaxation, which pharmacologically was classified as $CysLT_2$. Therefore, the presence of opposing and interdependent responses to cysteinyl-leukotrienes highlights the need to obtain more selective antagonists and agonists.

The current classification introducing two main classes of receptors for cysteinyl-leukotrienes is a first step supported by the available evidence but is nevertheless likely to represent an oversimplification. There is, for example, a significant difference in the potency of ICI-198,615 between rat lung and guinea pig trachea (83), which could reflect species differences. However, in the guinea pig, it was found already in an early study using the prototype FPL 55712 (75) that the response to LTD_4 in the ileum was most susceptible to blockade, whereas the trachea and in particular the lung parenchyma required considerably higher concentrations of antagonist. Such differences within the same species have been observed in other studies and may indicate the presence of subclasses of the receptors. The observation that the contraction response to LTD_4 in guinea pig lung parenchyma is poorly inhibited by both potent $CysLT_1$ antagonists such as ICI-198,615 as well as by the combined $CysLT_1/CysLT_2$ antagonist BAY u9773 (83) raises the possibility of a third main subclass ($CysLT_3$).

Likewise, although differences in metabolism between tissues may contribute to differences observed with respect to agonist potency and efficacy for the individual cysteinyl-leukotrienes, it appears likely that the presence of additional receptor subclasses also could explain several apparently disparate observations. For example, the $CysLT_2$ responses in guinea pig ileum or trachea are evoked by LTC_4 alone (53,75–77,82), whereas LTC_4 and LTD_4, and occasionally also LTE_4, may cause their effects through activation of tentative $CysLT_2$ receptors in sheep trachea (84) and human pulmonary vein (60). Conversely, LTC_4 appears inactive at the $CysLT_1$ receptor in guinea pig trachea and ileum, as well as in U-937 cells (88).

As discussed, LTE_4 remains the least studied individual cysteinyl-leukotriene. In addition to striking differences in reported activity of LTE_4 between tissues, there are observations suggesting a separate subclass of $CysLT_1$ receptor for LTE_4 in the guinea pig trachea (89,90). However, differences in the intrinsic agonist activity of LTE_4 compared with LTD_4 and LTE_4 could explain these observations as well. There are additional mechanisms that may contribute to the current set of data, for example, differences between tissues with respect to the number of receptors and the presence of varying numbers of spare receptors.

Another factor that may deserve attention is the localization of receptors to subcellular structures. The recent indications that leukotriene biosynthesis occurs at the perinuclear membrane (91) raises the possibility that certain receptors may be localized in or close to the nucleus, whereas others may be membrane associated. The observation that drugs that affect leukotriene synthesis and receptors may interfere with the cellular transport of LTC_4 (92) is also suggestive of rather complicated interrelations between receptors, biosynthetic enzymes, and transport mechanisms. It is tempting to speculate that there are as yet unknown relationships between, on the one hand, receptors and, on the other hand, transport mechanisms, biosynthetic enzymes, and other proteins, which may compete for the endogenous ligands.

The current classification is mainly derived from results of functional studies. There is supporting evidence from ligand-binding studies, in particular, for the BLT receptor. However, binding studies designed to study cysteinyl-leukotrienes have been more difficult to interpret. Although specific binding sites for LTD_4 have been identified in many tissues (93,94), including the human lung (95), radioligand-binding studies with LTC_4 in lung and other tissues have often shown less evident correlations between binding and functional responses (93,96–98). It has been shown that LTC_4 also binds effectively to a liver glutathione S-transferase (99). In view of the family of related enzymes with capacity to synthesize LTC_4 (100), it appears as if many enzymes and transport mechanisms (92) also display high affinity to LTC_4 and the other cysteinyl-leukotrienes. Increased knowledge about the cell biology of leukotriene synthesis and transport may be required to resolve some of these problems, such as the definition of the molecular structure and anchorage of leukotriene receptors to subcellular constituents. Regrettably, the strategy of using radiolabeled antagonists has been used in only a few studies (101).

The signaling events following activation of leukotriene receptors have not been reviewed. The literature is not extensive, and few studies have a bearing on the characteristic ''slow-reacting'' responses to cysteinyl-leukotrienes in smooth muscle cells. Experimentation with cysteinyl-leukotrienes is associated with certain peculiarities. For example, there is often tachyphylaxis to repeated administration, which means that sequential or cumulative dose-response relations may yield different results (102). The selection of organ bath technique (nonflow vs. superfusion) may also greatly affect the results (102). Some seemingly conflicting data (7,102) have in fact been explained to relate to different methodologies, and the results have fostered the hypothesis that for certain biological effects there may be a unique requirement for a long period of interaction between cysteinyl-leukotrienes and the target tissue (102).

V. Conclusions

The $CysLT_1$ antagonists as a class are currently being introduced as therapy for asthma and may in the future also be used to treat other inflammatory disorders. These achievements have been made by the application of classical strategies such as organic synthesis of new chemical entities, pharmacology screening in smooth muscle bioassays, and subsequent clinical testing in healthy subjects and patients with asthma.

The further exploration of leukotriene effects and the application of currently available antagonist has established that certain effects of cysteinyl-leukotrienes are resistant to inhibition by the present class of antagonists. The effects include both contraction and relaxation of human pulmonary arteries and veins. This has led to the classification of such receptors as $CysLT_2$. There is no selective $CysLT_2$ antagonist available, but the structural analog of cysteinyl-leukotrienes BAY u9773 has been shown to competitively antagonize cysteinyl-leukotrienes at both the $CysLT_1$ and the $CysLT_2$ receptor. Further subclasses of the *CysLT* receptors are, however, to be expected on the basis of, for example, quite remarkable differences in sensitivity to agonists and antagonists between tissues, even in the same species. Although most effects of cysteinyl-leukotrienes that may be involved in the pathogenesis of asthma are believed to be susceptible to $CysLT_1$ antagonism, in humans only the bronchoconstrictive effect of LTD_4 has been unequivocally demonstrated to be inhibited by $CysLT_1$ antagonists. A complete understanding of the role of cysteinyl-leukotrienes in asthma will necessitate not only the molecular characterization of the receptors but also the development of selective agonists and antagonists at different receptor subclasses. This would also help the definition of the role of cysteinyl-leukotrienes in other pulmonary and extrapulmonary diseases. For example, the potent cardiovascular effects of cysteinyl-leukotrienes (64–67,103,104) suggest that it will be of great importance to assess which receptors are involved. In the further evaluation of antileukotrienes as a new strategy for treatment of asthma and other inflammatory disorders, it appears important to focus considerable research efforts on the exploration of the molecular and functional characteristics of the different leukotriene receptors. Presumably more selective antagonists will be required in the future to provide more precise and effective manipulation of leukotrienes. This cannot be achieved without intensified basic research efforts.

Acknowledgments

The author is supported by Karolinska Institutet and the following Swedish foundations: Medical Research Council (project 14X-9071), Heart Lung Foundation, the Foundation for Health Care Sciences and Allergy Research (Vårdal), and the Association Against Asthma and Allergy.

References

1. Funk CD. Molecular biology in the eicosanoid field (review). Progr Nucl Acid Res Mol Biol 1993; 45:67–98.
2. Miller DK, Gillard JW, Vickers PJ, et al. Identification and isolation of a membrane protein necessary for leukotriene production. Nature 1990; 343:278–281.
3. Dixon RAF, Diehl RE, Opas E, et al. Requirement of a 5-lipoxygenase-activating protein for leukotriene synthesis. Nature 1990; 343:282–284.
4. Borgeat P, Samuelsson B. Transformation of arachidonic acid by rabbit polymorphonuclear leukocytes. Formation of a novel dihydroxy eicosanoic acid. J Biol Chem 1979; 254:2643–2646.
5. Borgeat P, Hamberg M, Samuelsson B. Transformation of arachidonic acid and homo-τ-linolenic acid by rabbit polymorphonuclear leukocytes. Monohydroxyacids from novel lipoxygenases. J Biol Chem 1976; 251:7816–7820 (Correction 1977; 252:8772).
6. Hansson G, Lindgren JÅ, Dahlén S-E, Hedqvist P, Samuelsson B. Identification and

biological activity of novel ω-oxidized metabolites of leukotriene B_4 from human leukocytes. FEBS Lett 1981; 130:107–112.
7. Piper PJ, Samhoun MN. Stimulation of arachidonic acid metabolism and generation of thromboxane A_2 by leukotrienes B_4, C_4 and D_4 in guinea-pig lung in vitro. Br J Pharmacol 1982; 77:267–275.
8. Sirois P, Roy S, Borgeat P, Picard S, Vallerand P. Evidence for a mediator role of thromboxane A_2 in the myotropic action of leukotriene B_4 (LTB_4) on the guinea-pig lung. Prostagl Leuko Med 1982; 8:157–170.
9. Ford-Hutchinson AW, Bray MA, Doig MV, Shipley ME, Smith MJH. Leukotriene B_4, a potent chemokinetic and aggregating substance released from polymorphonuclear leukocytes. Nature 1980; 286:264–265.
10. Dahlén S-E, Björk J, Hedqvist P, Arfors K-E, Hammarström S, Lindgren JÅ, Samuelsson B. Leukotrienes promote plasma leakage and leukocyte adhesion in post-capillary venules: in vivo effects with relevance to the acute inflammatory response. Proc Natl Acad Sci USA 1981; 78:3887–3891.
11. Bray MA, Ford-Hutchinson AW, Smith MJH. Leukotriene B_4: an inflammatory mediator *in vivo*. Prostaglandins 1981; 22:213–222.
12. Lindbom L, Hedqvist P, Dahlén S-E, Lindgren JÅ, Arfors KE. Leukotriene B_4 induces extravasation and migration of polymorphonuclear leukocytes in vivo. Acta Physiol Scand 1982; 116:105–108.
13. Smith MJH, Ford-Hutchinson AW, Bray MA. Leukotriene B: a potential mediator of inflammation. J Pharm Pharmacol 1980; 32:517–518.
14. Sehmi R, Wardlaw AJ, Cromwell O, Kurihawa K, Waltman P, Kay AB. Interleukin-5 selectively enhances the chemotactic response of eosinophils obtained from normal but not eosinophilic subjects. Blood 1992; 79:2952–2959.
15. Yamaoka KA, Kolb JP. Leukotriene B_4 induces interleukin-5 generation from human T lymphocytes. Eur J Immunol 1993; 23:2392–2398.
16. Hafström I, Palmblad J, Malmsten C, Rådmark O, Samuelsson B. Leukotriene B_4—a stereospecific stimulator for release of lysosomal enzymes from neutrophils. FEBS Lett 1981; 130:14–17.
17. Rae SA, Smith MJH. The stimulation of lysosomal enzyme secretion from human polymorphonuclear leukocytes by leukotriene B_4. J Pharm Pharmacol 1981; 33: 616–618.
18. Odlander B, Jakobsson PJ, Rosén A, Claesson HE. Human B and T lymphocytes convert leukotriene A_4 into leukotriene B_4. Biochem Biophys Res Commun 1988; 153:203–208.
19. Yamaoka KA, Dugas B, Paul-Eugense N, Mencia-Huerta JM, Braquet P, Kolb JP. Leukotriene B_4 enhances IL-4-induced IgE production from normal human lymphocytes. Cell Immunol 1994; 156:124–134.
20. Devchand PR, Keller H, Peters JM, Vazques M, Gonzalez FJ, Wahli W. The $PPAR_\alpha$-leukotriene B_4 pathway to inflammation control. Nature 1996; 384:39–43.
21. Serhan CN. Signalling the fat controller. Nature 1996; 384:23–24.
22. Goldman DW, Goetzl EJ. Heterogeneity of human polymorphonuclear leukocyte receptors for leukotriene B_4. J Exp Med 1984; 159:1027–1038.

23. Lewis RA, Goetzl EJ, Drazen JM, Soter NA, Austen KF. Functional characterization of synthetic leukotriene B_4 and its stereochemical isomers. J Exp Med 1981; 1243–1248.
24. Strömberg F, Hamberg M, Rosenqvist U, Dahlén S-E, Haeggström JZ. Formation of a novel enzymatic metabolite of leukotriene A_4 in tissues of *Xenopus laevis*. Eur J Biochem 1996; 238:599–605.
25. Coleman RA, Eglen RM, Jones RL, Narumiya S, Shimizu T, Smith WL, Dahlén S-E, Drazen JM, Gardiner PJ, Jackson WT, Jones TR, Krell RD, Nicosia S. Prostanoid and leukotriene receptors: a progress report from the IUPHAR Working Parties on Classification and Nomenclature. In: Samuelsson B, Ramwell PW, Paoletti R, Folco G, Granström E, Nicosia S, eds. Advances in Prostaglandin, Thromboxane and Leukotriene Research, Vol. 23. New York: Raven Press, 1994:283–285.
26. Kreisle RA, Parker CW. Specific binding of leukotriene B_4 to a receptor on human polymorphonuclear leukocytes. J Exp Med 1983; 157:628–632.
27. Lin AH, Ruggsed PL, Gorman RR. Leukotriene B_4 binding to human neutrophils. Prostaglandins 1984; 28:837–845.
28. Goldman DW, Chang FH, Gifford LA, Goetzl EJ, Bourne HR. Pertussis toxin inhibition of chemotactic factor induced calcium mobilization and function in human polymorphonuclear leukocytes. J Exp Med 1985; 162:145–156.
29. Votta B, Mong S. Transition of affinity states for leukotriene B_4 receptor in sheep lung membranes. J Pharm Exp Ther 1990; 265:841–847.
30. Evans JF, Leblanc Y, Fitzsimmons BJ, Chorlesm S, Nathaniel D, Leveille C. Activation of leukocyte movements and displacement of ^{3}H-leukotriene B_4 from leukocyte membrane preparations by (12R)- and (12S)-hydroxyeicosatetraenoic acid. Biochem Biophys Acta 1987; 917:406–410.
31. Morris J, Wishka DG. Synthesis of novel antagonists of leukotriene B_4. Tetrahedron Lett 1988; 29:143–146.
32. Evans DJ, Barnes PJ, Spaethe SM, van Alstyne EL, Mitchell MI, O'Connor BJ. Effects of a leukotriene B_4 receptor antagonist, LY293111, on allergen-induced responses in asthma. Thorax 1996; 51:1178–1184.
33. Yokomizo T, Izumi T, Chang K, Takuwa Y, Shimizu T. A G-protein-coupled receptor for leukotriene B4 that mediates chemotaxis. Nature 1997; 387:620–624.
34. Owman C, Nilsson C, Lolait, SJ. Cloning of cDNA encoding a putative chemoattractant receptor. Genomics 1996; 37:187–194.
35. Feinmark SJ, Lindgren JA, Claesson HE, Malmsten C, Samuelsson B. Stimulation of human leukocyte degranulation by leukotriene B_4 and its ω-oxidized metabolites. FEBS Lett 1981; 136:141–148.
36. Saad M, Wong K. Specific binding of leukotriene B_4 to guinea pig lung membranes. Biochem Biophys Res Commun 1985; 143:364–371.
37. Murphy RC, Hammarström S, Samuelsson B. Leukotriene C: a slow reacting substance from murine mastocytoma cells. Proc Natl Acad Sci USA 1979; 76:4275–4279.
38. Morris HR, Taylor GW, Piper PJ, Tippins JR. Structure of slow-reacting substance of anaphylaxis from guinea-pig lung. Nature 1980; 285:104–106.
39. Parker CW, Falkenhein SF, Huber MM. Sequential conversion of the glutathionyl

side chain of slow reacting substance (SRS) to cysteinyl-glycine and cysteine in rat basophilic leukemia cells stimulated with A 23187. Prostaglandins 1980; 20: 863–886.

40. Örning L, Hammarström S, Samuelsson B. Leukotriene D: a slow reacting substance from rat basophilic leukemia cells. Proc Natl Acad Sci USA 1980; 77:2014–2017.
41. Bach MK, Brashler JR, Brooks CD, Neerken AJ. Slow reacting substances: comparison of some properties of human lung SRS-A and two distinct fractions from ionophore-induced rat mononuclear cells SRS. J Immunol 1980; 122:160–165.
42. Lewis RA, Austen KF, Drazen JM, Clark DA, Marfat A, Corey EJ. Slow reacting substance of anaphylaxis: identification of leukotrienes C-1 and D from human and rat sources. Proc Natl Acad Sci USA 1980; 77:3710–3714.
43. Sok DE, Pai JK, Atrache V, Sih CJ. Characterization of slow reacting substances (SRSs) of rat basophilic leukemia (RBL-1) cells. Effects of cysteine on SRS profile. Proc Natl Acad Sci USA 1980; 77:6481–6485.
44. Bernström K, Hammarström S. Metabolism of leukotriene D by porcine kidney. J Biol Chem 1981; 256:9579–9582.
45. Dahlén S-E, Hansson G, Hedqvist P, Björck T, Granström E, Dahlén B. Allergen challenge of lung tissue from asthmatics elicits bronchial contraction that correlates with the release of leukotrienes C_4, D_4 and E_4. Proc Natl Acad Sci USA 1983; 80: 1712–1716.
46. Orange RP, Austen KF. Slow reacting substance of anaphylaxis. Adv Immunol 1969; 10:105–144.
47. Drazen JM, Austen KF, Lewis RA, Clark DA, Goto G, Corey EJ. Comparative airway and vascular activities of leukotrienes C-1 and D in vivo and in vitro. Proc Natl Acad Sci USA 1980; 77:4354–4358.
48. Hedqvist P, Dahlén S-E, Gustafsson LE, Hammarström S, Samuelsson B. Biological profile of leukotrienes C_4 and D_4. Acta Physiol Scand 1980; 110:331–333.
49. Dahlén S-E, Hedqvist P, Hammarström S, Samuelsson B. Leukotrienes are potent constrictors of human bronchi. Nature 1980; 288:484–486.
50. Hanna CJ, Bach MK, Pare PD, Schellenberg RR. Slow reacting substances (leukotrienes) contract human airway and pulmonary vascular smooth muscle. Nature 1981; 290:343–344.
51. Jones TR, Davies C, Daniel EE. Pharmacological study of the contractile activity of leukotriene C_4 and D_4 on isolated human airway smooth muscle. Can J Physiol Pharmacol 1982; 60:638–643.
52. Hua X-Y, Dahlén S-E, Lundberg JM, Hammarström S, Hedqvist P. Leukotrienes C_4, D_4 and E_4 cause extensive and widespread plasma extravasation in the guinea pig. Naunyn-Schmiedebergk's Arch Pharmacol 1985; 330:136–141.
53. Gardiner PJ, Abram TS, Cuthbert NJ. Evidence for two leukotriene receptor types in the guinea-pig isolated ileum. Eur J Pharmacol 1990; 182:291–299.
54. Weichman BM, Muccitelli RM, Osborn RR, Holden DA, Gleason JG, Wasserman MA. In vitro and in vivo mechanisms of leukotriene-mediated bronchoconstriction in the guinea pig. J Pharm Exp Ther 1982; 222:202–208.
55. Lee TH, Austen KF, Corey EJ, Drazen JM. LTE_4-induced airway hyperresponsiveness of guinea pig tracheal smooth muscle to histamine and evidence for

three separate sulfidopeptide receptors. Proc Natl Acad Sci USA 1984; 81:4922–4925.

56. Jaques CAJ, Spur BW, Johnson M, Lee TH. The mechanism of LTE_4-induced histamine hyperresponsiveness in guinea-pig tracheal and human bronchial smooth muscle in vitro. Br J Pharmacol 1991; 104:859–866.
57. Buckner CK, Fedyna JS, Robertson JL, Will JA, England DM, Krell RD, Saban R. Examination of the influence of the epithelium on contractile responses to peptidoleukotrienes and blockade by ICI 204,219 in isolated guinea-pig trachea and human intralobar airways. J Pharm Exp Ther 1990; 252:77–85.
58. Buckner CK, Krell RD, Laravuso RB, Coursin DB, Bernstein PR, Will JA. Pharmacologic evidence that human intralobar airways do not contain different receptors that mediate contractions to leukotriene C_4 and D_4. J Pharm Exp Ther 1986; 237:558–562.
59. Samhoun MN, Conroy DM, Piper PJ. Pharmacological profile of leukotrienes E_4, N-acetyl-leukotriene E_4 and four of their novel omega- and beta-oxidative metabolites in airways of guinea-pig and man *in vitro*. Br J Pharmacol 1989; 98:1406–1412.
60. Labat C, Ortiz JL, Norel X, Gorenne I, Verkey J, Abram TS, Cuthbert NJ, Tudhope SR, Normann P, Gardiner PJ, Brink C. A second cysteinyl leukotriene receptor in human lung. J Pharm Exp Ther 1992; 263:800–805.
61. Coles SJ, Neill KH, Reid LM, Austen KF, Nii Y, Corey EJ, Lewis RA. Effects of leukotrienes C_4 and D_4 on glycoprotein and lysozyme secretion by human bronchial mucosa. Prostaglandins 1982; 25:155–170.
62. Marom Z, Shelhamer JH, Bach MK, Morton DR, Kaliner M. Slow reacting substances, leukotrienes C_4 and D_4, increase the release of mucus from human airways in vitro. Am Rev Respir Dis 1982; 126:449–451.
63. Peatfield AC, Piper PJ, Richardson PS. The effects of leukotriene C_4 on mucin release into the cat trachea in vivo and in vitro. Br J Pharmacol 1982; 77:391–393.
64. Terashita ZI, Fuki H, Hirata M, Terao S, Ohkawa S, Nishikawa K, Kichuchi S. Coronary vasoconstriction and PGI_2 release by leukotrienes in isolated guinea pig hearts. Eur J Pharmacol 1981; 73:357–361.
65. Letts LG, Piper PJ. The actions of leukotrienes C_4 and D_4 on guinea-pig isolated hearts. Br J Pharmacol 1982; 76:169–176.
66. Michelassi F, Landa L, Hill RD, Lowenstein E, Watkins WD, Petkau AJ, Zapol WM. Leukotriene D_4: a potent coronary artery vasoconstrictor associated with impaired ventricular contraction. Science 1982; 217:841–843.
67. Burke JA, Levi R, Guo Z-g, Corey EJ. Leukotrienes C_4, D_4 and E_4: effects on human and guinea-pig cardiac preparations in vitro. J Pharm Exp Ther 1982; 221:235–241.
68. Laitinen L, Laitinen A, Haahtela T, Vilkka V, Spur B, Lee TH. Leukotriene E_4 causes granulocyte infiltration into asthmatic airways. Lancet 1993; 341:989–990.
69. Diamant Z, Hiltermann JT, van Rensen EL, Callenbach PM, Veselic-Charvat M, van der Veen H, Sont JK, Sterk PJ. The effect of inhaled leukotriene D_4 and methacholine on sputum cell differentials in asthma. Am J Respir Crit Care Med 1977; 155:1247–1253.
70. Underwood DC, Osborn RR, Newsholme SJ, Torphy TJ, Hay DWP. Persistent

airway eosinophilia after leukotriene (LT) D_4 administration in the guinea-pig: Modulation by the LTD_4 receptor antagonist pranlukast or an interleukin-5 monoclonal antibody. Am J Repir Crit Care Med 1996; 154:850–857.
71. Munoz NM, Douglas I, Mayer I, Herrnreiter A, Zhu X, Leff AR. Eosinophil chemotaxis inhibited by 5-lipoxygenase blockade and leukotriene receptor antagonism. Am J Respir Crit Care Med 1997; 155:1398–1403.
72. Peppelenbosch MP, Teretoolen LGJ, Hage WJ, de Laat SW. Epidermal growth factor-induced actin remodeling is regulated by 5-lipoxygenase and cyclooxygenase products. Cell 1993; 74:565–575.
73. Wang CG, Du T, Xu LJ, Martin JG. Role of leukotriene D_4 in allergen-induced increases in airway smooth muscle in the rat. Am Rev Respir Dis 1993; 148:413–417.
74. Augstein J, Farmer JB, Lee TB, Sheard P, Tattersall ML. Selective inhibitor of slow reacting substance of anaphylaxis. Nature N Biol 1973; 245:215–217.
75. Fleisch JH, Rinkema LE, Baker SR. Evidence for multiple leukotriene D_4 receptors in smooth muscle. Life Sci 1982; 31:577–581.
76. Krell RD, Tsai BS, Berdoulay A, Barone M, Giles RE. Heterogeneity of leukotriene receptors in the guinea-pig trachea. Prostaglandins 1983; 25:171–178.
77. Snyder DW, Krell RD. Pharmacologic evidence for a distinct leukotriene C_4 receptor in guinea-pig trachea. J Pharm Exp Ther 1984; 231:616–622.
78. Charette L, Jones TR. Effects of L-Serine borate on antagonism of leukotriene C_4-induced contractions of guinea-pig trachea. Br J Pharmacol 1987; 91:179–188.
79. Morris HR, Taylor GW, Jones CM, Piper PJ, Samhoun MN, Tippins JR. Slow-reacting substances (leukotrienes): enzymes involved in their biosynthesis. Proc Natl Acad Sci USA 1982; 79:4838–4842.
80. Yamaguchi T, Kohrogi H, Honda I, Kawano O, Sugimoto M, Araki S, Ando M. A novel leukotriene antagonist, ONO-1078, inhibits and reverses human bronchial contraction induced by leukotrienes C_4 and D_4, and antigen in vitro. Am Rev Respir Dis 1992; 146:923–929.
81. Snyder DW, Krell RD. Pharmacology of peptide leukotrienes on ferret isolated airway smooth muscle. Prostaglandins 1986; 32:189–200.
82. Bäck M, Wikström-Jonsson E, Dahlén S-E. The cysteinyl-leukotriene antagonist BAY u9773 is a competitive antagonist of leukotriene C_4 in the guinea-pig ileum. Eur J Pharmacol 1996; 317:107–113.
83. Tudhope SR, Cuthbert NJ, Abram TS, Jennings MA, Maxey RJ, Thompson AM, Norman P, Gardiner PJ. BAY u9773, a novel antagonist of cysteinyl-leukotrienes with activity against two receptor subtypes. Eur J Pharmacol 1994; 264:317–323.
84. Wikström-Jonsson E. Functional characterisation of receptors for cysteinyl-leukotrienes in sheep trachealis muscle. Pulm Pharm Ther 1997; 10:29–36.
85. Gieske TH, Sabol JS, Raddatz R. MDL 28,753, an agonist of LTD_4 but an antagonist of LTC_4 in longitudinal muscle of guinea pig ileum. J Pharm Exp Ther 1990; 254:192–197.
86. Mong S, Miller J, Wu HL, Hoffman K, Hall RF, Gleason JG, Crooke ST. SK&F 104,353, a high-affinity antagonist for human and guinea pig lung leukotriene D_4 receptor blocked phosphatidylinositol metabolism and thromboxane synthesis induced by LTD_4. Mol Pharm 1987; 32:223–229.

87. Ortiz JL, Gorenne I, Cortijo J, Seller A, Labat C, Sarria B, Abram TS, Gardiner PJ, Morcillo E, Brink C. Leukotriene receptors on human pulmonary vascular endothelium. Br J Pharmacol 1995; 115:1382–1386.
88. Wetmore LA, Gerard NP, Herron DK, Bollinger NG, Baker SR, Feldman HA, Drazen JM. Leukotriene receptors on U-937 cells: discriminatory responses to leukotrienes C_4 and D_4. Am J Physiol 1991; 261:L164–L171.
89. Aharony D, Catanese CA, Falcone RC. Kinetic and pharmacologic analysis of [^{3}H] leukotriene E_4 binding to receptors on guinea pig lung membranes: evidence for selective binding to a subset of leukotriene D_4 receptors. J Pharm Exp Ther 1989; 248:581–588.
90. Hay DWP, Muccitelli RM, Wilson KA, Wasserman MA, Torphy TJ. Functional antagonism by salbutamol suggests differences in the relative efficacies and dissociation constants of the peptidoleukotrienes in guinea-pig trachea. J Pharmacol Exp Ther 1987; 244:71–78.
91. Woods JW, Evans JF, Ethier D. 5-Lipoxygenase and 5-lipoxygenase activating protein are localized in the nuclear envelope of activated human leukocytes. J Exp Med 1993; 178:1935–1946.
92. Leier I, Jedlitschsky G, Buchholz U, Cole SPC, Deeley RG, Keppler D. The MRP gene encodes an ATP-dependent export pump for leukotriene C_4 and structurally related conjugates. J Biol Chem 1994; 269:27807–27810.
93. Bruns RF, Thomsen WJ, Pugsley TA. Binding of leukotrienes C_4 and D_4 to membranes from guinea-pig lung: regulation by ions and guanine nucleotides. Lif Sci 1983; 33:645–653.
94. Pong SS, DeHaven R. Characterisation of a leukotriene D_4 receptor in guinea pig lung. Proc Natl Acad Sci USA 1983; 80:7415–7420.
95. Lewis MA, Mong S, Veseella RL, Crooke ST. Characterization of leukotriene D_4 receptors in adult and fetal human lung. Biochem Pharmacol 1985; 34:4311–4317.
96. Nicosia S, Crowley HJ, Olivia D, Welton AF. Binding sites for ^{3}H-LTC$_4$ in membranes from guinea pig ileal longitudinal muscle. Prostaglandins 1984; 27:483–494.
97. Rovati GE, Olivia D, Sautebin L, Folco GC, Welton AF, Nicosia S. Identification of specific binding sites for leukotriene C_4 in membranes from human lung. Biochem Pharmacol 1985; 34:2831–2837.
98. Civelli M, Olivia D, Mezzetti M, Nicosia S. Characteristics and distribution of specific binding sites for leukotriene C_4 in human bronchi. J Pharmacol Exp Ther 1987; 242:189–198.
99. Sun FF, Chau L-Y, Spur B, Corey EJ, Lewis RA, Austen KF. Identification of a high affinity leukotriene C_4-binding protein in rat liver cytosol as glutathione S-transferase. J Biol Chem 1986; 261:8540–8546.
100. Jakobsson PJ, Mancini JA, Ford-Hutchinson AW. Identification and characterisation of a novel human microsomal gluthathione S-transferase with leukotriene C_4 synthase activity and significant sequence identity to 5-lipoxygenase activating protein and leukotriene C_4 synthase. J Biol Chem 1996; 271:22203–22210.
101. Aharony D, Falcone RC, Krell RD. Inhibition of ^{3}H-leukotriene D_4 binding to guinea-pig lung receptors by the novel leukotriene antagonist ICI-198,615. J Pharm Exper Ther 1987; 243:921–926.

102. Dahlén S-E, Hedqvist P, Westlund P, Granström E, Hammarström S, Lindgren JÅ, Rådmark O. Mechanisms for leukotriene-induced contractions of guinea pig airways: Leukotriene C_4 has a potent direct action whereas leukotriene B_4 acts indirectly. Acta Physiol Scand 1983; 118:393–403.
103. Smedegård G, Hedqvist P, Dahlén S-E, Revenäs B, Hammarström S, Samuelsson B. Leukotriene C_4 affects pulmonary and cardiovascular dynamics in the monkey. Nature 1982; 295:327–329.
104. Sala A, Rossoni G, Buccellati C, Berti F, Folco G, Maclouf J. Formation of sulphidopeptide-leukotrienes by cell-cell interaction causes coronary vasoconstriction in isolated, cell-perfused heart of rabbit. Br J Pharmacol 1993; 110:1206–1212.

9

Physiological Effects of the Leukotrienes in Humans

NEIL C. BARNES

London Chest Hospital
London, England

LEWIS J. SMITH

Northwestern University Medical School
Chicago, Illinois

I. Introduction

Investigations into the effect of slow-reacting substance of anaphylaxis (SRS-A) in animal models indicate that it is an important allergic mediator with potent activity as a contractor of bronchial smooth muscle (1). Following the elucidation of the structure of SRS-A as leukotrienes (LTs) in 1979 (2), the total chemical synthesis of leukotrienes (3) was described, enabling pharmacologists to study the effect of pure LTs in animal models in vitro and in vivo (4,5). When sufficient quantities of pure LTs became available, studies of the effects of LTs in humans were performed. The majority of these studies have been performed using inhaled cysteinyl leukotrienes, and a more limited number of studies have been performed with systemically administered leukotrienes and LTB_4. Studies of the biological properties of leukotrienes in humans have added significantly to our understanding of the pathophysiological role of leukotrienes in disease and have helped in the evaluation of LTD_4 receptor antagonists.

II. Cysteinyl Leukotrienes in Normal Subjects

The first study of inhaled leukotrienes in humans was performed by Holroyde et al. (6), who studied two normal subjects. They showed that both inhaled leukotrienes, C_4 and D_4, could cause a dose-related bronchoconstriction and that this could be attenuated by the SRS-A antagonist FPL-55712. With the availability of larger quantities of leukotrienes, studies of inhaled LTC_4 and LTD_4 were performed in larger numbers of subjects. These studies showed that leukotrienes C_4 and D_4 were 1000–10,000 times more active than histamine or metacholine on a molar basis (7–10). Both LTC_4 and LTD_4 produced dose-dependent bronchoconstriction. The studies also indicated that LTC_4 and LTD_4 were approximately equipotent as bronchoconstrictors. The onset of action of leukotriene-induced bronchoconstriction was slower than that of histamine, and the LTs had a more prolonged duration of action. One study showed that leukotriene C_4 had a slightly slower onset of action than LTD_4 (9). The probable explanation for this is that LTC_4 is metabolized to LTD_4 before binding to the receptor and causing bronchoconstriction. This explanation is consistent with the finding that inhaled radioactive LTC_4 is metabolized and partially excreted in the urine as LTE_4 (11).

With the initial studies there was considerable concern that leukotrienes would have cardiovascular effects, as they were known to be potent contractors of vascular smooth muscle. However, changes in pulse or blood pressure beyond what would be anticipated with the degree of bronchoconstriction induced were not observed. Inhaled leukotrienes do not cause any significant cough, in contrast to inhaled histamine and inhaled prostaglandins. Although in various experimental models leukotrienes can induce mucus hypersecretion, the production of mucus is not a noticeable symptom following inhalation of leukotrienes in humans.

One controversial aspect of the action of inhaled leukotrienes in normal subjects is their site of action. Guinea pig peripheral airways are more sensitive to leukotrienes than central airways. This is due to the secondary generation of thromboxane A_2 in the peripheral airways, which amplifies the effect of leukotrienes (12). It was therefore suggested that in humans leukotrienes would have a predominantly peripheral action. Bisgaard and Groth (13) found greater effects of inhaled leukotrienes on pulmonary function tests, which are considered measures of small airways function, than on the forced expiratory volume in one second (FEV_1). However, it is difficult to interpret these results, as the nebulizer system used included a settling bag to remove large particles and the size of the particles produced would have caused a more peripheral distribution of the aerosol. Weiss et al. (8) have argued that because the effect of inhaled leukotrienes on flow at low lung volumes is greater than the effect on FEV_1, they have a predominantly peripheral action. However, flow at low lung volumes is a more sensitive measure than FEV_1 and will usually produce greater percentage falls following inhalation of any bronchoconstrictor. Using measures of comparable sensitivity, Barnes et al. (9) have shown similar percentage falls in specific airways conductance (sGaw) and flow at 30% of vital capacity above residual volume ($\dot{V}_{max}30$) for both histamine and inhaled LTD_4. They argue that this is consistent with leukotrienes having the same ratio of central versus peripheral action as histamine. This analysis has been confirmed by Wood-Baker et al. (14). More recently, investigations of drugs acting against the leukotriene pathway have shown improvements in peak expiratory flow rate and FEV_1, and in general the percentage improvement in each is similar (15,16). This again argues against a predominantly peripheral action of the leukotrienes.

A number of studies investigated the reproducibility of leukotriene D_4–induced bronchoconstriction (14,17) and showed the test to be as reproducible as histamine challenge. Reproducibility in normal subjects is usually within one doubling dilution. This excellent reproducibility has enabled leukotriene D_4 challenge testing to be used as a method of evaluating the potency of leukotriene receptor antagonists (18–21).

Leukotriene E_4 has been the subject of fewer studies than have leukotriene C_4 and D_4. In animal models LTE_4 tends to be less potent than LTC_4 or LTD_4, although it may have a longer duration of action (22). Inhaled LTE_4 in humans is one-tenth as potent as LTC_4 or LTD_4, although it still is approximately 100 times more active than histamine or methacholine (23). In one study LTE_4 was shown to have a longer duration of action than LTD_4 (24). It is not clear whether this is due to the slower metabolism of LTE_4 or to the fact that it is inhaled at 10 times the dose to produce an equivalent degree of bronchoconstriction.

III. Studies in Asthmatic Patients

A more limited number of studies of the effect of inhaled leukotrienes has been performed in asthmatic patients. These studies have shown that leukotrienes cause dose-dependent bronchoconstriction in asthmatic patients and that they are more potent than either histamine or methacholine (25–29). However, the potency ratio in asthmatic patients is lower than in normal subjects (Table 1). Whereas in normal subjects leukotrienes are approximately 1000 times more ac-

Table 1 Relative Potency of Leukotrienes Compared with Histamine or Methacholine in Normal and Asthmatic Subjects

	Normals			Asthmatic		
Study	LTC_4	LTD_4	LTE_4	LTC_4	LTD_4	LTE_4
Weiss et al. (7)	3810					
Weiss et al. (8)		6000				
Barnes et al. (9)	800	1000				
Smith et al. (27)		284			404	
Bisgaard and Groth (13)		1608			478	
Roberts et al. (34)		19,400				
Adelroth et al. (26)	1878	3660		603	803	
Davidson et al. (23)			39			13.8
Griffin et al. (25)					14.2	

tive than histamine, in asthmatic patients they are approximately 250 times more active. Expressed another way, if the provocation concentration to histamine is plotted against the provocation concentration to LTD_4, a slope of 0.4 is generated (24,26). The reasons for this difference in relative sensitivity between normal subjects and asthmatic patients is not clear. One suggestion is that the airways of asthmatics are chronically exposed to leukotrienes. As a result, the leukotriene receptors are subject to downregulation and become relatively less sensitive to exogenous leukotrienes (30). Alternatively, the lack of a one-to-one relationship between inhaled leukotrienes and histamine may have no biological significance. Although a one-to-one relation of sensitivity was observed with histamine and methacholine, this relationship is far from perfect. Furthermore, a one-to-one relationship does not hold when comparing responsiveness to other agonist mediators such as histamine versus prostaglandins or adenosine (31,32). As in normal subjects, leukotrienes have a longer duration of action than histamine (29) in asthmatic subjects and leukotriene E_4 is one-tenth as potent as LTC_4 or LTD_4.

IV. Effect of Drugs on Leukotriene-Induced Bronchoconstrictions

The action of a number of different drugs on leukotriene-induced bronchoconstriction has been studied. Leukotriene D_4-induced bronchoconstriction is effectively antagonized by inhaled β_2 agonists, which rapidly reversed the bronchoconstriction (10). As would be anticipated, histamine receptor antagonists do not inhibit LTD_4-induced bronchoconstriction (33), and neither does disodium cromoglycate (34). A large number of studies have demonstrated that leukotriene receptor antagonists, given either orally, intravenously, or by inhalation, can block LTD_4-induced bronchoconstriction. This has become an important technique for evaluating the potency of leukotriene receptor antagonists (18–21). The most potent drugs can shift the dose-response curve to the right by more than 100-fold. Inhaled verapamil protects against LTD_4-induced bronchoconstriction in normal subjects (35), but not against LTD_4 challenge in asthmatic patients (34), and has no effect on methacholine challenge in normal subjects (35). Smith and colleagues found that aerosolized atropine partially protected against LTD_4-induced bronchoconstriction (36), an effect they considered nonspecific and due to the initial bronchodilatation produced.

V. Leukotriene B_4

There are a limited number of studies of inhaled leukotriene B_4 in humans. Black et al. (37) found no change in pulmonary function or in responsiveness to inhaled histamine in normal subjects. Other studies have failed to show any effect of inhaled LTB_4 on pulmonary function (38).

VI. Effects of Leukotrienes on Airway Reactivity in Normal Subjects

The effect of inhaled LTD_4 on airway reactivity in normal subjects has been explored in several studies (Table 2). In one study by Kern and colleagues (10), six subjects inhaled a single dose of LTD_4 or methacholine on separate occasions. The dose inhaled reduced by about 50% both specific airway conductance (sGaw) and the flow rate at 30% of vital capacity measured after a partial forced expiratory maneuver (V30P). When lung function had returned to at least 90% of baseline (about 60 minutes), bronchoprovocation testing was performed with methacholine. In this setting LTD_4 increased airway reactivity to methacholine. It reduced the amount of methacholine required to achieve a 35% decrease in sGaw and a 30% decrease in V30P by 35% and 55%, respectively.

In a second study (39), eight normal subjects received single doses of saline, histamine, LTD_4, or platelet-activating factor (PAF) on separate occasions. The doses administered were designed to reduce sGaw 50%, although this was only achieved for LTD_4. The mean reduction in sGaw was 19% for histamine and 25% for PAF. Methacholine challenges were performed 6 hours and 1, 3, 7, and 14 days later. Using the 95% confidence limits determined for each subject from the saline inhalation followed by the multiple methacholine challenges, six of the eight subjects demonstrated increased airway responsiveness after inhaling LTD_4. No subject had increased airway reactivity after inhaling histamine. Since six of the eight subjects also developed an increase in airway reactivity after inhaling PAF, it is unlikely the LTD_4-induced increase in airway reactivity was due to its preceding bronchoconstriction. The maximal increase in airway responsiveness to methacholine was 46% and occurred between 1 and 7 days after inhaling the LTD_4. In only one subject did airway reactivity increase at 6 hours. Earlier times were not evaluated.

Bel and colleagues (40) also explored the ability of LTD_4 to alter airway reactivity to methacholine in a group of eight nonasthmatic subjects. However, they used a different experimental design. Each individual underwent bronchoprovocation testing with methacholine on the first day, LTD_4 on the second day, and methacholine again 1 and 3 days after the LTD_4 challenge. The maximal bronchoconstrictor response to methacholine measured as PC_{10} FEV_1 and PC_{40} $V40_p$ was increased 24 and 72 hours after the LTD_4 challenge.

These studies suggest that inhalation of a single dose or multiple consecutive doses of LTD_4 can increase airway responsiveness to methacholine in normal subjects, and this increase can persist for an extended period of time.

Table 2 Effects of Cysteinyl Leukotrienes on Airway Reactivity

Study	Subjects	Leukotriene	Challenge	Airway reactivity/response	Time measured
Smith et al. (27)	Normal	LTD_4	Methacholine (PC_{35} sGaw, PC_{30} $V_{30}p$)	Increase	1 hour
Kaye and Smith (39)	Normal	LTD_4	Methacholine (PC_{35} sGaw)	Increase	6 hours–7 days
Bel et al. (40)	Normal	LTD_4	Methacholine (PC_{35} sGaw)	Maximum bronchoconstriction	1 and 3 days
Arm et al. (41)	Normal	LTC_4, D_4, E_4	Histamine (PC_{35} sGaw)	No change	1, 4, 7 hours
Bisgaard and Groth (13)	Normal	LTD_4	Exercise	No effect	2, 6, 10 hours
O'Hickey et al. (42)	Asthma	LTC_4, D_4, E_4	Histamine (PC_{35} sGaw)	Increase	1 hour–2 days
Wood-Baker et al. (14)	Asthma	LTD_4	Histamine	Decrease	2 days
Bianco et al. (43)	Asthma	LTC_4	Distilled water	No effect	7 minutes

Whether LTE_4, the stable metabolite of LTD_4, has a similar effect was first explored by Arm and colleagues (41). Five normal subjects inhaled diluent and LTE_4 on separate occasions. The LTE_4 reduced sGaw nearly 40%. Histamine bronchoprovocation testing was performed 1 hour after the LTE_4 (by which time the sGaw had returned to baseline) as well as at 4 and 7 hours in three of the five individuals. Airway reactivity to histamine, measured as PC_{35}sGaw, did not increase in any of these normal subjects.

The same laboratory studied another group of normal subjects. This time changes in airway reactivity were examined for each of the cysteinyl leukotrienes (42). On separate occasions, six normal subjects inhaled saline, methacholine LTC_4, LTD_4, or LTE_4. Airway responsiveness to histamine (PC_{35}sGaw), measured 1, 4, and 7 hours later, was unchanged after inhaling a bronchoconstricting dose of each leukotriene. In this study and the previous one, patients with asthma developed an increase in airway reactivity to histamine (see below).

There is limited information on the ability of the leukotrienes to increase airway reactivity to other bronchoconstrictor stimuli in normal subjects. In one study, Bisgaard and Groth examined whether LTD_4 leads to exercise-induced bronchoconstriction in normal individuals (13). Fourteen subjects inhaled a single dose of LTD_4 (40 nmol), which resulted in a 40% decrease in V30P. Treadmill exercise testing, designed to increase the pulse rate to 150 beats per minute, was performed before and 2, 6, and 10 hours after inhaling the LTD_4. Exercise-induced bronchoconstriction did not develop in any subject.

VII. Effect on Airway Hyperresponsiveness in Patients with Asthma

A series of studies have been undertaken to determine if the leukotrienes can further increase airway reactivity in patients with asthma, individuals in whom heightened airway responsiveness to multiple stimuli already exists. In the study by Arm and colleagues (41), eight patients with mild asthma inhaled either diluent, methacholine, or LTE_4 on separate occasions. Airway reactivity to histamine (PC_{35}sGaw) was determined one hour later in all subjects and 1, 4, 7, and 24 hours and 4 and 7 days later in four of them. LTE_4 produced a twofold increase in the airway response to histamine at 1 hour. No changes were seen after inhaling methacholine. In the patients who were studied for up to 7 days, the increase in histamine airway reactivity was maximal at 7 hours (3.5-fold increase) and persisted for up to 4 days.

In their other study (42), seven patients with mild-to-moderate asthma inhaled LTC_4, LTD_4, or LTE_4 on separate occasions. All of the patients were atopic, and two of them were using low doses of inhaled corticosteroids. The leukotriene dose administered produced a mean 50% fall in sGaw. All three cysteinyl leukotrienes increased airway reactivity to histamine. The maximal increase, which was three- to fourfold, occurred 4 hours after inhaling the leukotriene.

Wood-Baker and colleagues examined the effect of LTD_4 on the airway response to histamine (14). A majority of the subjects, who had mild-to-moderate asthma, were taking inhaled corticosteroids. Histamine bronchoprovocation testing was performed immediately before and 2 and 7 days after the LTD_4 inhalation challenge. Airway reactivity to histamine decreased 2 days after inhaling LTD_4 and then returned to the pre-LTD_4 value at 7 days. The basis for the reduced airway reactivity, especially in light of the earlier studies demonstrating either no effect or an increase in airway reactivity after inhaling LTD_4, was not apparent or explained. It is possible the rapid reversal of the LTD_4-induced bronchoconstriction with inhaled β-agonist, a unique feature of this study which contrasts with the spontaneous reversal in all previous studies, was responsible.

Bianco and colleagues examined the effect of LTC_4 on airway reactivity to inhaled distilled water in patients with asthma (43). Bronchoconstricting doses of either LTC_4 or methacholine were administered, followed 7–8 minutes later by inhalation of distilled water. Leukotriene C_4 did not increase the airway response to this stimulus. However, the protocol did not permit sufficient time for reversal of the LTC_4- and methacholine-induced bronchoconstriction.

VIII. Interaction of Leukotrienes and Other Bioactive Mediators with Bronchoconstrictor Properties

Barnes and colleagues explored the effects of a subthreshold concentration of LTD_4 (a concentration that had no effect on pulmonary function) on PGF_{2a}-induced bronchoconstriction in six normal subjects (44). The PGF_{2a} was inhaled 10 minutes after the LTD_4. LTD_4 produced a sevenfold shift to the left of the dose-response curve to PGF_{2a}.

Phillips and Holgate investigated the interaction between LTC_4 and either histamine or PGD_2 in patients with asthma (45). Of the nine patients studied, three were taking inhaled corticosteroids. After determining the bronchoconstrictor response to the three mediators individually, patients inhaled the dose of LTC_4, which reduced the FEV_1 12.5%, followed by the dose of either histamine or PGD_2, which decreased the FEV_1 from 12.5 to 25%. The decreases in both FEV_1 and V30P, measured after inhaling LTC_4 followed by either histamine or PGD_2, were greater than predicted based on the responses to the individual mediators alone.

Less data are available on the ability of LTB_4 to increase airway reactivity in normal subjects and patients with asthma. In addition, the protocols used differ from the ones described for the cysteinyl leukotrienes. As noted earlier, Fuller and colleagues (21) examined six nonasthmatic subjects, three of whom were atopic. The first two subjects studied failed to develop increased airway responses to histamine after LTB_4 inhalation; as a result the protocol was modified such that subjects inhaled single doses of PGD_2 or PGD_2 combined with LTB_4. Histamine challenges were performed 30 minutes and 3 and 6 hours later. The primary measure of lung function was sGaw. Neither PGD_2 alone nor PGD_2 plus LTB_4 increased airway reactivity to histamine during this time interval. This is despite the observation that LTB_4 can increase airway reactivity to acetylcholine in dogs (46) and is able to recruit neutrophils into human lungs (47).

Taken together, the current data favor a role for the cysteinyl leukotrienes but not LTB_4 in the airway hyperresponsiveness found in patients with asthma. Possible reasons why some studies failed to demonstrate increased airway reactivity after inhaling the cysteinyl leukotrienes include the use of different patient groups (e.g., normal subjects versus patients with asthma, patients with asthma of different severity receiving different therapies) and dissimilar experimental protocols (e.g., single versus multiple doses of the leukotriene, bronchconstricting versus nonbronchoconstricting doses, the particular leukotriene, the time when airway reactivity is measured, and the test used to assess nonspecific airway reactivity).

IX. Effect of Leukotrienes on Lung Cell Composition and Function

If, as suggested by the above data, the cysteinyl leukotrienes increase airway responsiveness to a variety of stimuli, it should be possible to identify mechanisms by which this may occur. Since the increased airway reactivity has only been demonstrated in short-term studies (hours to days after inhaling the leukotrienes), it is unlikely to be due to effects on cell proliferation or airway remodeling. In contrast, it could be due to the capacity of the leukotrienes to recruit inflammatory cells, activate the recruited cells as well as resident lung cells, enhance mediator release from these cells, and possibly reduce mediator inactivation (see Table 3).

One of the first studies exploring the activation of resident lung cells by the cysteinyl leukotrienes was performed by Chavis and colleagues (48). They obtained alveolar macrophages by bronchoalveolar lavage (BAL) from four patients with asthma. When the cells were incubated in the presence of LTC_4, production of the inflammatory mediators LTB_4 and 5-HETE was enhanced. LTE_4 had a similar effect. In contrast, alveolar macrophages obtained from normal subjects did not demonstrate LTC_4-enhanced synthesis of either LTB_4 or 5-HETE.

Smith and colleagues examined the effect of LTD_4 on BAL fluid and cells in nine normal subjects (49). Increasing concentrations of LTD_4 or methacholine

Table 3 Effect of Cysteinyl Leukotrienes on Lung Cells

Study	Subjects	Leukotriene	Exposure	Effect	Time measured
Chavis et al. (48)	Asthma	LTC_4	In vitro airway macrophages	Increased LTB_4, 5-HETE	2–2.5 hours
Smith et al. (49)	Normal	LTD_4	In vivo BAL cells	Decreased LTB_4 Increased thromboxane	24 hours
Smith et al. (50)	Normal/Asthma	LTD_4	In vitro airway macrophages	Increased LTB_4 in asthma vs. Normals	30 minutes
Laitinen et al. (53)	Asthma	LTE_4	In vivo	Increased eosinophils in lamina propria	4 hours

were inhaled on separate occasions until the sGaw decreased at least 50%. Bronchoscopy with BAL was performed 24 hours later. LTD_4 did not influence the amount of BAL fluid recovered, total and differential cell counts, and BAL fluid protein and histamine concentrations. Alveolar macrophages isolated from the BAL fluid were stimulated in vitro for 30 minutes with either the calcium ionophore A23187 or zymosan; following this LTB4 and thromboxane B_2 were measured in the culture media, while platelet activating factor (PAF) synthesis was measured in the cells. After inhaling LTD_4, calcium ionophore–stimulated LTB_4 synthesis decreased and thromboxane synthesis increased, but PAF synthesis did not change. Although a relationship was not found between the alterations in alveolar macrophage function and airway reactivity to methacholine, this study showed that LTD_4 can influence the alveolar milieu in normal subjects.

In a separate study performed by the same investigators (50), alveolar macrophages were obtained by BAL from normal subjects and patients with mild asthma. The cells were plated on plastic dishes, washed to remove nonadherent cells, incubated with either LTD_4 or its vehicle for 30 minutes, and then stimulated with A23187. Although alveolar macrophages from both the normal subjects and the patients with asthma responded vigorously to the calcium ionophore with a large increase in LTB_4 synthesis, the increase was greater in the patients with asthma.

On the other hand, Balter and colleagues (51) failed to identify increased LTB_4 synthesis by alveolar macrophages recovered from patients with asthma. In their study the cells were incubated overnight before undergoing stimulation with the calcium ionophore. A more recent study reported a reduction in stimulated LTB_4 synthesis by BAL cells from patients with asthma (52). The protocol differed from the other two in that a mixed population of BAL cells, consisting of about 80% alveolar macrophages, was used.

Laitinen and colleagues made a key observation when they examined the effect of inhaled LTE_4 in patients with mild asthma (53). All subjects underwent bronchoscopy with biopsies obtained from the bronchial mucosa. Four subjects then inhaled LTE_4, while the other four inhaled methacholine until sGaw decreased at least 35%. Four hours later the bronchial biopsies were repeated. The subjects who inhaled the LTE_4 had a 10-fold increase in eosinophils in the lamina propria, along with smaller increases in neutrophils and alveolar macrophages. Although only a small number of individuals were studied, this report provided the first direct evidence that the cysteinyl leukotrienes contribute to the airway inflammation characteristic of asthma.

LTB_4 can also recruit inflammatory cells into the lung. Martin and colleagues (55) showed that when LTB_4 was directly instilled into the airways of 11 normal subjects 4 hours later, there was a large increase in the total number of cells recovered by BAL. Most of the cells were neutrophils; there was no increase in eosinophils. A small increase in lavage protein was also found, suggesting an increase in permeability.

Although LTB_4 is a potent neutrophil chemoattractant (55), it appears to have little effect on airway reactivity. In contrast, the cysteinyl leukotrienes, which can recruit eosinophils to the airways (53), increase airway reactivity. Initial clinical studies with leukotriene receptor antagonists and synthesis inhibitors have failed to demonstrate a clear advantage of the synthesis inhibitors (56,57,58,15) over the receptor antagonists. This suggests a more important role for the cysteinyl leukotrienes than LTB_4 in asthma.

X. Mechanism of Cysteinyl Leukotriene–Mediated Effects on Airway Constriction and Hyperreactivity

As described in an earlier chapter, cysteinyl leukotriene receptors are present in human lung. Those felt to be responsible for the bronchoconstrictor effects are almost certainly of the cysLT-1 type. Several studies have shown that potent cysteinyl leukotriene receptor antagonists, such as zafirlukast and MK-571, can shift the dose-response curve to LTD_4 up to and exceeding 100-fold in normal subjects (20) and patients with asthma (59,60). Such findings indicate that the cysteinyl leukotrienes produce bronchoconstriction by a direct action on airway smooth muscle. Whether their effect on airway reactivity is also the result of a direct action on airway smooth muscle is less clear. The studies by Laitinen (53), Chavis (48), and Smith (49,50) indicate that the cysteinyl leukotrienes can recruit inflammatory cells to the lung and activate resident lung cells. All have the capacity to produce mediators, which may contribute to the pathophysiology of asthma. Additional studies have shown that the cysteinyl leukotrienes also have a potent chemotactic effect on eosinophils isolated from nonasthmatic subjects (60). Further, the cysteinyl leukotrienes increase endothelial cell permeability by widening intercellular gaps (61) and enhance the excitability of sensory nerve fibers (at least in guinea pigs) (62). Thus, multiple events appear to contribute to the influence of the cysteinyl leukotrienes on airway reactivity (Table 4).

Table 4 Possible Mechanisms of Cysteinyl Leukotriene–Mediated Increased Airway Reactivity

Direct effect on airway smooth muscle (bronchoconstriction, airway edema, mucus secretion)
Recruit and activate eosinophils and other inflammatory cells with generation of inflammatory mediators, cytokines, or reactive oxygen species
Increased endothelial cell permeability
Enhance excitability of sensory nerve fibers

XI. Summary

Based on studies using human subjects and materials and a much larger body of data from animal and in vitro experiments, one can conclude that the leukotrienes are potent bronchoconstrictors in normal and asthmatic subjects. They exert a major part of their action by a direct effect via the cysLT_1 receptor on airway smooth muscle. There is also evidence for an effect on airway hyperresponsiveness, probably via eosinophil recruitment and activation, airways edema, and airway nerves. Taken together these studies suggest on important role for LTs in asthma, but further detailed study of airway inflammatory responses is needed.

References

1. Brocklehurst WE. Slow-reacting substance and related compounds. Prog Allergy 1962; 6:539–558.
2. Murphy RC, Hammarstrom S, Samuelsson B. Leukotriene C: a slow-reacting substance from murine mastocytoma cells. Proc Natl Acad Sci USA 1979; 76:4275–4279.
3. Corey EJ, Clark DA, Goto G, Marfat A, Mioskowski C, Samuelsson B, Hammarstrom S. Stereospecific total synthesis of a ''slow-reacting substance''of anaphylaxis leukotriene C-1. J Am Chem Soc 1980; 102:1436–1439.
4. Samhoun MN, Conroy DM, Piper PJ. Pharmacological profile of leukotrienes E_4, N-acetyl E_4 and of four of their novel omega- and beta-oxidative metabolites in airways of guinea-pig and man *in vitro*. Br J Pharmacol 1989; 98:1406–1412.
5. Peatfield AC, Piper PJ, Richardson PS. The effect of leukotriene C_4 on mucin release into the cat trachea *in vivo* and *in vitro*. Br J Pharmacol 1982; 77:391–393.
6. Holroyde MC, Altounyan RE, Cole M, Dixon M, Elliott EV. Bronchoconstriction produced in man by leukotrienes C and D. Lancet 1981; ii:17–18.
7. Weiss JW, Drazen JM, Coles N, McFadden ER, Weller PF, Corey EJ, Lewis RA, Austen KF. Bronchoconstrictor effects of leukotriene C in humans. Science 1982; 216:196–198.
8. Weiss JW, Drazen JM, McFadden ER, Weller P, Corey EJ, Lewis RA, Austen KF. Airway constriction in normal humans produced by inhalation of leukotriene D. Potency, time course and effect of aspirin therapy. J Am Med Assoc 1983; 249:2814–2817.
9. Barnes NC, Piper PJ, Costello JF. Comparative effects of inhaled leukotriene C_4, leukotriene D_4, and histamine in normal human subjects. Thorax 1984; 39:500–504.
10. Kern R, Smith LT, Patterson R, Krell RD, Bernstein PR. Characterization of the airway response to inhaled leukotriene D_4 in normal subjects. Am Rev Respir Dis 1986; 133:1127–1132.
11. Kumlin M, Dahlen B, Bjorck T, Zetterstrom O, Granstrom E, Dahlén S-E. Urinary excretion of leukotriene E_4 and 11-dehydro-thromboxone B_2 in response to bronchial

provocations with allergen, aspirin, leukotriene D_4 and histamine in asthmatics. Am Rev Respir Dis 1992; 145:1087–1091.
12. Piper PJ, Samboun MN. Stimulation of arachidonic acid metabolism and generation of thromboxone A_2 by leukotrienes B_4, C_4 and D_4 in guinea pig lung in vitro. Br J Pharm 1982; 77:267–275.
13. Bisgaard H, Groth S. Bronchial effects of leukotriene D_4 inhalation in normal human lung. Clin Sci 1987; 72:585–592.
14. Wood-Baker R, Town IG, Benning B, Holgate ST. The reproducibility and effect on non-specific airway responsiveness of inhaled prostaglandin D_2 and leukotriene D_4 in asthmatic subjects. Br J Clin Pharmacol 1995; 39:119–123.
15. Spector SL, Smith LJ, Glass M. Effects of six weeks of therapy with oral doses of ICI204,219 on leukotriene D_4 receptor antagonists in subjects with bronchial asthma. Am J Respir Crit Care Med 1994; 150:618–623.
16. Barnes NC, Pujet J-C. Pranlukast, a novel leukotriene receptor antagonist: the first European, placebo-controlled, multi centre clinical study in asthma. Thorax 1997; 52:523–527.
17. Barnes NC, Zakrzewski JT, Piper PJ, Costello JF. Reproducibility of histamine and leukotriene D_4 inhalation challenge in normal humans. Br J Clin Pharm 1985; 20: 554P (abstract).
18. Barnes N, Piper PH, Costello JF. The effect of an oral leukotriene antagonist L-649,923 on histamine and leukotriene D_4-induced bronchoconstriction in normal man. J Allergy Clin Immunol 1987; 79:816–821.
19. Evans JM, Barnes NC, Zakrzewski JT, Scibberas D, Stahl E, Piper PH, et al. L648,051 a novel cysteinyl leukotriene antagonist is active by the inhaled route in man. Br J Clin Pharmacol 1989; 28:125–135.
20. Smith LT, Geller J, Elbright L, Glass M, Thyrum PT. Inhibition of leukotriene D_4-induced bronchoconstriction in normal subjects by the oral LTD4 receptor antagonist ICI 204,219. Am Rev Respir Dis 1990; 141:988–992.
21. Fuller RW, Black PN, Dollery CT. Effect of the oral LY171,883 antagonist on inhaled and intradermal challenge with antigen and LTD_4 in atopic subjects. J Allergy Clin Immunol 1989; 83:939–944.
22. Piper PJ, Samboun MN. Comparison of the actions of leukotriene E_4 with those of leukotrienes B_4, C_4 and D_4 guinea pig lung and ideal smooth muscle in vitro. In: Samuelsson B, Paoletti R, Ramwell P, eds. Advances in Prostaglandin, Thromboxane and Leukotriene Research, Vol 12. New York: Raven Press, 1985:127–131.
23. Davidson AB, Lee TH, Scanlon PD, Solway J, McFadden ER. Bronchoconstrictor effects of leukotriene E_4 in normal and asthmatic subjects. Am Rev Respir Dis 1987; 135:333–337.
24. Barnes NC, Piper PJ. The actions of leukotrienes in human lung in vitro oral in vivo. In: Piper PJ, ed. The Leukotrienes: Their Biological Significance. New York: Raven Press, 1986:199–212.
25. Griffin M, Weiss JW, Leitch AG, McFadden ER, Corey EJ, Austen KF, Drazen JM. Effects of leukotriene D, on the airways in asthma. N Engl J Med 1983; 308:436–439.
26. Adelroth E, Morris MM, Hargreave FE, O'Byrne PM. Airway responsiveness to

leukotrienes C_4 and D_4 and the methacholine in patients with asthma and normal contrasts. N Engl J Med 1986; 315:480–484.
27. Smith LJ, Greenberger PA, Patterson R, Krell RD, Bernstein PR. The effect of inhaled leukotriene D_4 in humans. Am Rev Respir Dis 1985; 131:368–372.
28. Bisgaard H, Groth S, Madsen F. Bronchial hyperreactivity to leukotriene D_4 in escugenous asthma. Br Med J 1985; 290:1468–1471.
29. Barnes NC, Piper PJ, Costello JF. Hyperresponsiveness of asthmatics to inhaled leukotriene D_4. Am Rev Respir Dis 1985; 131(4 suppl):A24 (abstract).
30. Drazen JM, Austen KF. Leukotrienes and airway responses. Am Rev Respir Dis 1987; 136:985–998.
31. Hardy CC, Robinson C, Tattersfield AE, Holgate ST. The bronchoconstrictor effect of inhaled prostaglandin D_2 in normal and asthmatic men. N Engl J Med 1984; 311: 209–213.
32. Mann JS, Holgate ST, Renwick ACT, Cushley MJ. Airway effects of purine nucleosides and nucleotides and release with bronchial provocation in asthma. J Appl Physiol 1986; 61:1667–1676.
33. Albazzaz MK, Patel KR. Effect of azelastine on bronchoconstriction induced by histamine and leukotriene C_4 in patients with extrinsic asthma. Thorax 1988; 43: 306–311.
34. Roberts JA, Rodger IW, Thomson NC. Effect of verapamil and sodium cromoglycate on leukotriene D_4-induced bronchoconstriction in patients with asthma. Thorax 1986; 41:753–758.
35. Roberts JA, Giembycz MA, Raeburn D, Rodger IW, Thomson NC. In vitro and in vivo effect of verapamil on human airway responsiveness to leukotriene D_4. Thorax 1986; 41:12–16.
36. Smith LJ, Kern R, Patterson R, Krell RD, Bernstein PR. Mechanism of leukotriene D_4-induced bronchoconstriction in normal subjects. J Allergy Clin Immunol 1987; 80:340–347.
37. Black PN, Fuller RW, Taylor GW, Barnes PJ, Dollery CT. Effect of inhaled leukotriene B_4 alone and in combination with prostaglandin D_2 on bronchial responsiveness to histamine in normal subjects. Thorax 1989; 44:491–495.
38. Sampson SE, Costello JF, Sampson AP. The effect of inhaled leukotriene B_4 in normal and in asthmatic subjects. Am J Respir Crit Care Med 1997; 55:1789–1792.
39. Kaye MG, Smith LJ. Effects of inhaled leukotriene D_4 and platelet-activating factor on airway reactivity in normal subjects. Am Rev Respir Dis 1990; 131:993–997.
40. Bel EH, van der Veen H, Kramps JA, Dijkman JH, Sterk PJ. Maximal airway narrowing to inhaled leukotriene D_4 in normal subjects. Am Rev Respir Dis 1987; 136: 979–984.
41. Arm JP, Spur BW, Lee TH. The effects of inhaled leukotriene E_4 on the airway hyperresponsiveness to histamine in subjects with asthma and normal subjects. J Allergy Clin Immunol 1988; 82:654–660.
42. O'Hickey SP, Hawksworth RJ, Fong CY, Arm JP, Spur BW, Lee TH. Leukotrienes C_4, D_4 and E_4 enhance histamine responsiveness in asthmatic airways. Am Rev Respir Dis 1991; 144:1053–1057.
43. Bianco S, Robushci M, Vaghi A, Simone P, Folco G, Berti F, Pasargiklian M. Effects

of leukotriene C_4 on the bronchial response to an ultrasonic mist of water. In: Herzog H, Perruchoud AP, eds. Progress in Respiratory Research, Vol 19. Asthma and Bronchial Hyperreactivity. Basel: S Karger, 1985:82–86.
44. Barnes NC, Piper PJ, Costello JF. Action of inhaled leukotrienes and their interactions with other allergic mediators. Prostaglandins 1984; 28:629–631.
45. Phillips GD, Holgate ST. Interaction of inhaled LTC_4 with histamine and PGD_2 on airway caliber in asthma. J Appl Physiol 1989; 66:304–312.
46. O'Byrne PM, Leikauf GD, Aizawa H, Bethal RA, Ueki IF, Holtzman MJ, Nadel JA. Leukotriene B_4 induces airway hyperresponsiveness in dogs. J Appl Physiol 1985; 59:1941–1946.
47. Martin TR, Pistorese BP, Chi EY, Goodman RB, Matthay MA. Effects of leukotriene B_4 in the human lung. J Clin Invest 1989; 94:1609–1619.
48. Chavis C, Godard P, Michel FB, Crastes de Paulet A, Damon M. Sulfidopeptide leukotrienes contribute to human alveolar macrophage activation in asthma. Prostaglandins Leukotrienes Essential Fatty Acids 1991; 42:95–100.
49. Smith LJ, Shamsuddin M, Houston M. Effect of leukotriene D_4 and platelet activating factor on human alveolar macrophage eicosanoid and PAF synthesis. Am Rev Respir Dis 1993; 148:682–688.
50. Smith LJ, Houston M, Anderson J, Shamsuddin M. Leukotriene D_4 increases alveolar macrophage LTB_4 synthesis in patients with asthma. Am Rev Respir Dis 1993; 147: A311.
51. Balter MS, Eschenbacher WL, Peters-Golden M. Arachidonic acid metabolism in cultured alveolar macrophages from normal, atopic and asthmatic subjects. Am Rev Respir Dis 1988; 138:1134–1142.
52. Restrick LJ, Sampson AP, Piper PJ, Costello JF. Reduction in leukotriene B_4 generation by bronchoalveolar lavage cells in asthma. Thorax 1995; 50:67–73.
53. Laitinen LA, Laitinen A, Haahtela T, Vilkka V, Spur BW, Lee TH. Leukotriene E_4 and granulocytic infiltration into asthmatic airways. Lancet 1993; 341:989–990.
54. Martin TR, Raugi G, Merritt TL, Henderson WR. Relative contribution of leukotriene B_4 to the neutrophil chemotactic activity produced by resident human alveolar macrophages. J Clin Invest 1987; 80:1114–1124.
55. Palmer RM, Stepney RJ, Haggs GA, Eakins KE. Chemokinetic activities of arachidonic and lipoxygenase products in leukocytes of different species. Prostaglandins 1980; 20:411–418.
56. Israel E, Rubin P, Kemp J, et al. The effect of inhibition of 5-lipoxygenase by zileuton in mild to moderate asthma. Ann Intern Med 1993; 119:1059–1066.
57. Israel E, Cohn J, Dube L, Drazen J. Effect of treatment with zileuton, a 5-lipoxygenase inhibitor, in patients with asthma. JAMA 1996; 275:931–936.
58. Smith LJ, Glas M, Minkwitz MC. Inhibition of leukotriene D_4-induced bronchoconstriction in subjects with asthma: concentration effect study of ICI 204,219. Clin Pharmacol Ther 1993; 54:430–436.
59. Kips JC, Joos GF, DeLepeleire I, Margolskee DJ, Buntinx A, Pauwels RA, van der Straeten ME. MK-571, a potent antagonist of leukotriene D_4-induced bronchoconstriction in the human. Am Rev Respir Dis 1991; 144:617–621.
60. Spada CS, Nieves AL, Krauss AH-P, Woodward DF. Comparison of leukotriene B_4

and D_4 effects on human eosinophil and neutrophil motility in vitro. J Leukocyte Biol 1994; 55:183–191.
61. Joris I, Majno G, Corey EJ, Lewis RA. The mechanism of vascular leakage induced by leukotriene E_4. Am J Pathol 1987; 126:19–24.
62. Stewart AG, Thompson DC, Fennessy MR. Involvement of capsaicin-sensitive afferent neurons in a vagal-dependent interaction between leukotriene D_4 and histamine on bronchomotor tone. Agents Actions 1984; 15:500–508.

10

Analysis of Leukotrienes and Lipoxins

GRAHAM W. TAYLOR

Imperial College School of Medicine
Hammersmith Hospital
London, England

I. Introduction

There is a vast family of eicosanoids, and a great number of the compounds exhibit a wide range of biological actions at low concentrations. Many eicosanoids are produced in humans in vivo. In order to understand their functions in health and disease, it is necessary to know how, where, and why they are produced and, in particular, if the compounds may be found in vivo at concentrations sufficient to be able to exert biological effects. Studies of the mechanism of action and efficacy of drugs that act directly or indirectly on eicosanoid production also require quantitative measurements of eicosanoid levels. Assays are thus an essential tool for understanding the biological roles of the eicosanoids. There are a number of reviews on analysis of lipid mediators (1,2), and two volumes of *Methods in Enzymology* have been dedicated to these compounds (3,4).

This chapter outlines the general principles and main methods the author has found useful when measuring leukotrienes and lipoxins. Particular attention will be paid to a number of potential errors and pitfalls, which may produce incorrect and unreliable results.

II. General Analytical Principles

There are a number of principles applicable to every assay, in particular, the information now required for assay validation (e.g., good laboratory practice, or GLP). Guidelines have been published (5,6) establishing criteria for the accuracy, precision, and limits of detection of an assay.* Some of the main characteristics of an assay are discussed below.

A. Specificity Versus Sensitivity

Clearly, assays are designed to be quantitative and to give an accurate value of the amount of analyte present. There is a second and perhaps more important aspect, however—that of knowing exactly what the assay measures under the conditions of its use. This latter aspect is very natural to the analytical chemist but may not always be appreciated by scientists or clinicians with less experience in assay development and validation. For example, the clinical laboratories using high-throughput autoanalyzers often create the impression that it is possible to perform very accurate measurements of a wide range of biochemical parameters. This may, however, vary considerably. The problem is particularly highlighted by the large number of commercially available kits for assay of eicosanoids and other mediators. Although the label may claim that the assay is "specific," there are many examples of how uncritical application of commercial kits may give false results. One prominent example is that of prostacyclin, where the application of inappropriate assays led to erroneously high estimates of circulating levels of the mediator. Plasma levels of 6-oxo-$PGF_{1\alpha}$ determined by RIA [and even GC-MS (7)] at 10–20 pg/ml were 10- to 20-fold higher than the true circulating level at 1–2 pg/ml (8,9). Thus, over 80% of the immunoreactivity was due to cross-reactive material other than 6-oxo-$PGF_{1\alpha}$, i.e., impurities.

Complete structural identification of an analyte is out of the question for mediators present at normal physiological levels. A full characterization using NMR spectroscopy and mass spectrometry would require microgram amounts of analyte. On the other hand, methods such as immunoassays which are sensitive enough to detect picogram amounts of materials may not be able to differentiate between the compound to be assayed and impurities. It is rarely possible to obtain RIA or EIA assays where the antibody used will recognize *only* the analyte and *nothing else*. Such a high degree of specificity and selectivity is seldom obtained in assays for eicosanoids. There is thus a balance between the requirements for sensitivity and those of specificity, which requires a judgment to be made about the overall confidence of both qualitative and quantitative aspects of any assay (Fig. 1). For example, a chromatography or extraction step can be used before the assay to afford an extra degree of confidence to the specificity of the assay.

---

*Accuracy is the closeness of the determined value to the true value; precision is the closeness of replicate determinations and can be subdivided into inter- and intra-assay precision; limit of detection is the lowest level of analyte that can be reliably differentiated from background; limit of quantitation is the lowest concentration that can be measured with a stated level of confidence (e.g., an S.D. $<10\%$ for replicate values). (5,6)

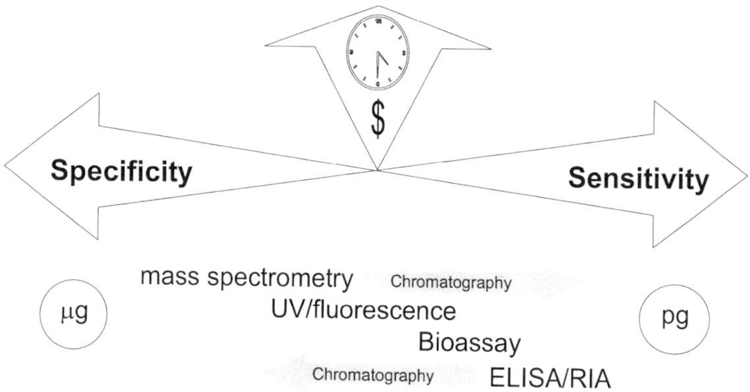

Figure 1 Every assay is a structure elucidation program in miniature. For each assay, there is a balance between sensitivity and specificity. Full structure elucidation can be achieved with the many MS techniques available, but they may not have the required sensitivity for picogram analysis. The specificity of antibody-based techniques such as RIA or EIA require that the antibody recognize only the analyte and nothing else. Chromatography can be used to increase specificity. Other factors such as capital and running costs, the requirements for trained staff, and time taken for each assay must also be taken into consideration.

However, as soon as a purification step is introduced, the risk of variable losses during handling of the samples is increased and must be dealt with (see Sec. II. D). Indeed, the greatest sources of quantitative error probably occur during sample workup, where losses due to poor and variable extraction or chemical breakdown can occur.

B. Assay Limits

Every assay has a limit of detection, a limit of quantitation, and a usable range. This is exemplified by one radioimmunoassay for LTE_4 investigated in the author's laboratory (Fig. 2). In principle, amounts of less than 5 pg of LTE_4 can be detected with this assay, which is the limit of detection. However, as the binding curve flattens out in this range, a small difference in B/B_0 can represent a relatively large difference in measured LTE_4. The quantitative error then becomes significant. The limit of quantitation is 5 pg, and the usable range of the assay is therefore between 5 and 160 pg. Over 160 pg, the curve again flattens out, and the errors again become significant. Regrettably, one of the most common errors encountered when uncritical investigators apply immunoassays arises from extrapolating beyond the usable range of the assay. There is a further consideration that determines the true detection limit of the assay. When small amounts

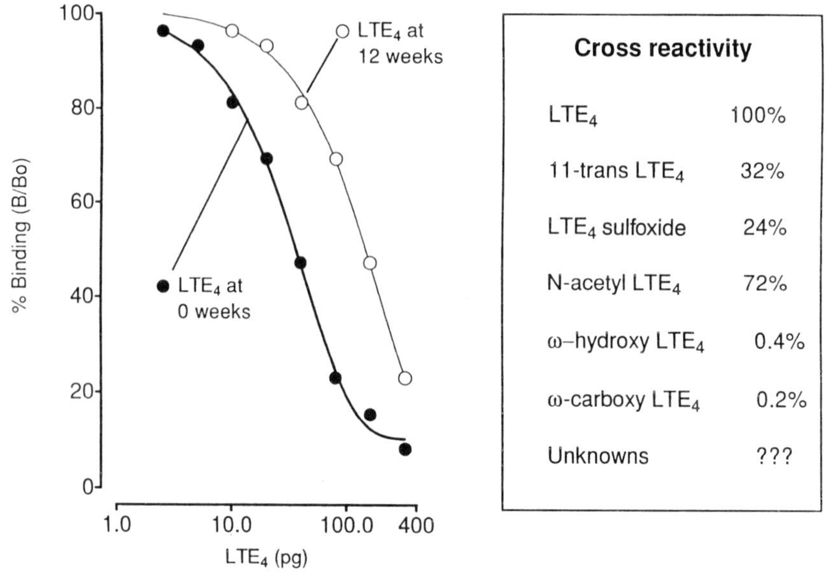

Figure 2 Binding curve for LTE_4 (-●-) and "aged" (12-week storage) LTE_4 (-○-). The usable range of the curve is 5–160 pg; although LTE_4 immunoreactivity can be detected outside this range, the errors in measurement become unacceptable. LTE_4 is converted to weakly immunoreactive species on storage. Increased amounts of aged LTE_4 were required to displace the radiolabeled ligand resulting in an apparent rightward shift in the binding curve and an overestimate in the measured LTE_4. The relative cross-reactivities of LTE_4 and its metabolites are shown in the right panel. The potential cross-reactivity with unknowns is stressed.

of analyte are present in complex matrices, the effects of nonspecific binding to glass surfaces during extraction can result in a complete loss of material. Thus, an assay with a detection limit of 5 pg for the analyte when added from a pure chemical solution may not at all detect 5 pg of the analyte when it is present in a biological sample such as plasma, lavage fluids, or urine.

C. Other Sources of Errors

Standards are required for all quantitative assays. It may seem trite, but any errors in the measurement of the standards will appear in the final data. With analytes such as LTE_4, there is always the danger of isomerization and oxidation on storage. This is exemplified in Figure 2, which shows the sigmoidal binding curves in an RIA carried out using fresh and "aged" LTE_4 to displace the ^{3}H-LTE_4 ligand. As LTE_4 breaks down on storage to the less immunoreactive sulfoxide, the binding curve shifts to the right, and the apparent B_{50} increases fourfold with the consequent (incorrect) increase in measured LTE_4 values.

Occasionally, there will also be problems with the equipment used in an assay. For example, in our laboratory, a simple RIA for TXB_2 began to give problems. For no obvious reason apparent binding varied from sample to sample. After changing everything from solvents to the antibody, the problem was traced to the plastic tubes; some tubes in each batch were found to bind TXB_2. The manufacturing process had changed and tubes from different batches had been mixed, leading to differential binding from sample to sample and totally unusable data. We observed a similar problem in our gas chromatography–mass spectrometry (GC-MS) assay for mevalonic acid (10), where two different batches of glass tubes affected the derivatization of the sample.

D. Extraction and Recovery

If extraction is required before assay to remove contaminating impurities, the method used should be simple, reproducible, and rapid, and with a good extraction yield. It is essential that the extraction procedure not lead to a modification of the analyte. Extremes of pH should be avoided to minimize hydrolysis of labile bonds, the elimination of water from alcohols, or isomerization. Solvents should be removed at low temperatures (<30°C) using a stream of nitrogen or under vacuum wherever possible to prevent oxidation. The possibility of chemical interactions of the solvents or modifiers with the analyte should also be considered: the presence of acidic methanol can result in some esterification. At every stage of an extraction, some impurities are added to the sample (such as phthalate plasticizers), and these may interfere with the final result. The most common methods for extracting eicosanoids are solid phase extraction (with cartridges such as Sep-Paks® or Bond Eluts®), immunoaffinity chromatography, and high-performance liquid chromatography (HPLC).

Solid Phase Extraction

The use of reverse-phase solid phase cartridges has almost completely replaced solvent extraction. There are numerous high-yield methods based on ODS Sep Paks or Bond Eluts designed for eicosanoid purification (11–13). One difficulty with ODS cartridge extraction is the loss caused during solvent removal and resuspension, particularly if HPLC is then applied. This can be overcome by coupling the extraction cartridge directly to HPLC; the number of separate handling steps (each with some loss of sample) may thus be minimized (14–16). Another benefit of on-line extraction/HPLC systems is that they allow for full automation, which is essential when high throughput is required (17,18).

Immunoaffinity Purification

The specificity of antibodies can also be exploited in a clean-up step for urine before assay. Immunoaffinity columns may be prepared by coupling suitable antibodies to CNBr-activated sepharose (19,20). We have used these columns in our laboratory for the purification LTE_4 (21). They are easy to use and produce a remarkably clean sample in good yield for further purification and assay. The columns can be reused, but the possibility of cross-contamination from one sample to another must be kept in mind. Recently, Wescott and colleagues (22) applied immunoaffinity purification as part of a urinary LTE_4 assay. LTE_4 is eluted from the immunoaffinity filter in >85% yield and measured using an ELISA with a different LTE_4 antibody. The procedure is rapid and cannot result in intersample contamination. Cross-reactivity with LTE_4 metabolites is low, therefore, the method can be extremely useful for urinanalysis where the only immunoreactive LT present is LTE_4. The only potential drawback, inherent in all assays that do not use high-resolution chromatography, is that immunoreactive impurities may bind to both the immunoaffinity antibody and the ELISA antibody, giving a false positive.

High-Performance Liquid Chromatography

The problems of interfering compounds can best overcome by using HPLC. The combined benefits of high resolution, good recovery, and invariant retention times (adding a further degree of specificity to many assays) make HPLC an ideal extraction method in an assay system. The excellent resolving power of the technique can be seen in the separation of a number of closely related leukotriene metabolites (Fig. 3). Although a number of normal phase HPLC procedures are used in eicosanoid research, the vast majority of HPLC separations of lipid mediators used in eicosanoid research (including assay protocols) are now carried out in the reverse-phase mode, particularly on the wide range of C18 or ODS columns (14–18,23–26). It should be noted that the characteristics of the ODS packing can vary between manufacturers, and this can markedly affect chromatography (2). The physical size, pore size, and shape of the packings affect resolution and loading capacity, the carbon load determines retention time, and the degree of end capping can affect tailing. These differences have been exploited in the online extraction/HPLC procedure now used in a number of laboratories to analyze cysLTs in urine (15–18,27). In our laboratory (15), we use a rheodyne injector, which is connected to a solid phase Brownlee cartridge containing MCH10 packing (Varian) and also to a HPLC column. Urine (or other fluids) is pumped onto the Brownlee cartridge and washed with water; the cartridge is switched on-line, and the HPLC solvent elutes the LTs directly onto the HPLC column, where chromatography is carried out. Cysteinyl-leukotrienes bind onto a precolumn packed with Varian MCH10 ODS and are eluted as a sharp band in 35% methanol. At this solvent concentration, LTs bind to a Hypersil ODS HPLC column

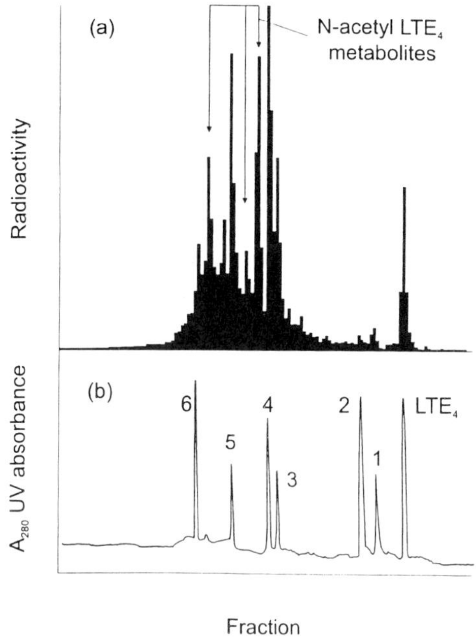

Figure 3 (a) HPLC of radiolabeled metabolites of LTE_4 produced in an isolated perfused pig kidney. (b) Identity of the metabolites was determined by co-chromatography with authentic standards. 1:LTE_4 sulfoxide; 2:*N*-acetyl LTE_4; 3:20-hydroxy LTE_4; 4:20-carboxy LTE_4; 5: 18-carboxy dinor LTE_4; 6: 16-carboxy tetranor LTE_3. The elution position of the *N*-acetyl metabolites of 20-hydroxy, 20-carboxy, and 18-carboxy dinor LTE_4 are indicated by arrows.

and are eluted as a sharp peak in a methanol : water gradient. HPLC fractions are then assayed by RIA. With this system, there is a single stage where solvent is removed before the sample is resuspended in RIA buffer. Extraction yields are good (but can still be low in some cases), and the chances of sample deterioration are minimized.

A poor choice of packings leads either to peak broadening or the cysLTs eluting in the void volume of the column. Further control of chromatography can be achieved with a careful choice of both solvents and modifiers such as trifluoroacetic acetic acid (TFA) or ammonium acetate, with alterations in concentration or pH leading to markedly different chromatographic characteristics. This can be seen in the HPLC of LTE_4 and LTD_4, where the relative elution positions are reversed as the concentration of TFA in the elution solvent is increased (25). A number of groups also include chelators such as EDTA in the elution buffer to sharpen up HPLC peaks (less necessary with an ion pair reagent such as TFA or HFBA) and to reduce cation-mediated decomposition (28).

Estimation of Handling Losses

The extraction and chromatography of trace amounts of eicosanoids from complex biological mixtures can result in variable, and often poor, recovery. This will of course materially affect any quantitative data. It is essential that an estimate of extraction losses be made by use of standards.

External Standards

With an external standard, the analyte is taken through the extraction protocol a number of times and the mean recovery determined; all further analyses are then corrected for this mean recovery. This option relies on good recovery (>85%) with little variation (±5%). Problems arise if the recovery is poor and the variation is large. In our laboratory, the extraction/HPLC of [^{3}H]-LTE_4 from human urine resulted in a recovery of 40.8 ± 2.6% (mean ± SEM). The data expressed in this way (with a small SEM) appear to be tightly controlled and thus suitable for use as an external standard correction. Recovery actually varied from 24.1 to 67.8% (n = 16). At the two extremes of recovery, a sample of 1 ng LTE_4 could be reported as 241 pg (based on the minimum recovery) or 678 pg (maximum recovery). Quantitative data generated by applying a mean recovery of 40.8% (i.e., 408 pg) would obviously be very misleading.

Internal Standards

The most accurate method of accounting for variable extraction yields is to include an internal standard to every analyzed sample. This not only determines the recovery of analyte in each sample (and, if added on sample collection, the degree of sample deterioration on storage), but also defines the elution position on GC or HPLC. Analogs of similar structure may be used as internal standards: 19-hydroxy PGB_2 has been used in the HPLC-UV assay for LTB_4 (14). The ideal internal standard is one that is essentially of identical chemical structure—labeled with heavy isotopes (e.g., ^{2}H, ^{3}H, ^{14}C) which behave indistinguishably from the analyte and thus confer a sample-dependent marker of extraction yield. In most laboratories, trace amounts of ^{3}H-LTE_4 are used as internal standards in HPLC-RIA assays of LTE_4, and ^{2}H- or ^{18}O-labeled analogs for GC-MS and HPLC-MS assays of LTE_4 and hydroxylated eicosanoids. Although a number of radiolabeled and deuterium-labeled eicosanoids are available commercially, others must be synthesized from $^3H_8$- and $^2H_8$-arachidonic acid or by ^{18}O incorporation (29–32).

E. Where to Assay

Ideally, eicosanoid concentrations should be determined at or near their site of production or action. The more distal the sampling site, the greater the degree of correction required and the greater care needed when expressing data in a meaningful way.

Exhaled Air

There has been a report of leukotriene B_4 immunoreactivity appearing in the breath of asthmatics (41): LTB_4 is presumably carried on water droplets in the breath. The method has, however, not been validated, and the relevance of measuring LTB_4 in breath condensates is not clear.

The Airways

Sampling of eicosanoids in the epithelial lining fluid (ELF) of the airways is carried out by bronchoalveolar lavage (BAL). Lavage mediator levels represent a single time point during a study, with the danger of missing short-lived changes in mediator production. There is also a greater difficulty in deciding how to express the data (33). Mediator levels can be expressed as total amount of mediator recovered or normalized in terms of ng/ml of recovered lavage fluid, ng/10^6 recovered cells, or by correcting for protein [particularly albumin (34,35)]. Because lavage fluid recovery as well as the degree of dilution of the secretions are both variable and there may be marked differences in the protein concentration and cell number, quantitative comparisons between two recovered lavage fluids may not be valid. A number of groups use the urea dilution method and correct for ELF concentration (27,34). This assumes that there is no alteration in the plasma/ELF urea equilibrium during the lavage, and this may not hold in damaged airways. There are two benefits of lavage studies. First, BALF may routinely be available for clinical reasons. A number of groups have reported BALF mediator levels, which, if nothing else, shows that the leukotrienes and lipoxins are actually present in the lungs (36–39). Second, it is possible to use a different lobe of the lung as a control; we have compared allergen challenge and sham (saline) challenge in human volunteers in vivo and shown that only the active challenge leads to the formation of cysLTs (40).

The nose is a readily accessible tissue to investigate mediator production, under both basal condition and also following challenge (42,43). Mediators produced within the nose are relatively easy to collect for assay by washing with 5 ml normal saline. By including ^{3}H-inulin in the wash, correction can be made for dilution of the nasal secretions and the 30–50% loss (by swallowing) of the nasal perfusate. Mediator levels can then be expressed in terms of ng/ml of secretions or, if protein content is also determined, as ng/mg of secreted protein. Presumably because of the limited size of the nose, nasal production of mediators is, however, generally low.*

*The volume of nasal secretions (V_n) can be determined from the equation $P_1/P_2 = (V_n + 5)/V_n$. The dilution factor (P_1/P_2) is determined from the concentration of ^{3}H-inulin in 5 ml of the perfusing fluid (P_1) and the recovered nasal wash (P_2). This assumes that dilution of the nasal secretions occurs before any loss of the perfusing fluid.

Plasma

Plasma eicosanoids are normally expressed as concentrations (ng/ml) and none of the problems associated with interpreting BAL data are evident. Venapuncture is only mildly invasive in comparison to BAL, and multiple samples can be obtained giving a time-dependent variation of mediator production. Venous plasma levels of many eicosanoids are, in many cases, extremely low due to the rapid clearance and dilution into the blood pool, and this makes detection and assay difficult. It is, however, often possible to detect immunoreactivity at levels where confidence in the quantitation is low. There have been several reports on plasma levels of leukotrienes (44–48). Some care must be taken in the interpretation of high normal levels of immunoreactive LT levels in plasma. It has been calculated from urinary excretion of LTE_4 and the renal clearance (determined from ^3H-LTC_4 infusions) that the normal circulating levels of cysteinyl-leukotrienes are less than 10 pg/ml, and of this the majority is LTE_4 with less than 5% accounted for by LTC_4 (49). Published values of immunoreactive LTC_4 above 100 pg/ml, therefore, raise serious questions as to the specificity of the assay. Arterial sampling (50,51) can be used to measure local production of mediators, however, the significant risks involved mean that arterial samples are normally only taken when there is a sound clinical reason for introducing an arterial line (e.g., during balloon angioplasty) (52) (Fig. 4a).

As whole blood contains all the factors required to produce most eicosanoids, the potential dangers of ex vivo generation on collection must be considered and suitable inhibitors may be included in the collection syringe. Controlled ex vivo production is, however, another alternative. The stimulated production of LTB_4 or the cysLTs from whole blood or leukocyte preparations by ionophore or other stimuli (53–55) has been used to monitor the presence (and efficacy) of 5-lipoxygenase inhibitors in vivo (Fig. 4b) and to delineate the roles of the LTs in disease.

Urine

Urinary mediator measurements are noninvasive and offer a time-integrated assessment of endogenous mediator production (40,56–58). In the absence of renal synthesis, urinary mediator (or metabolite) levels will reflect plasma levels and, importantly, are generally much higher. It has been suggested that, as ω-oxidation products are produced by the liver, measurement of these metabolites in urine will reflect the plasma load of the parent eicosanoid. However, the kidney also has the capacity for ω-oxidation (21) and can convert LTC_4 through to ω-hydroxy-LTE_4 and other metabolites (Fig. 3). Urinary mediator levels are expressed in terms of concentration (ng/ml), excretion rate (ng/h), or as a ratio with creatinine excretion (nmol/mmol creatinine). The latter takes into account

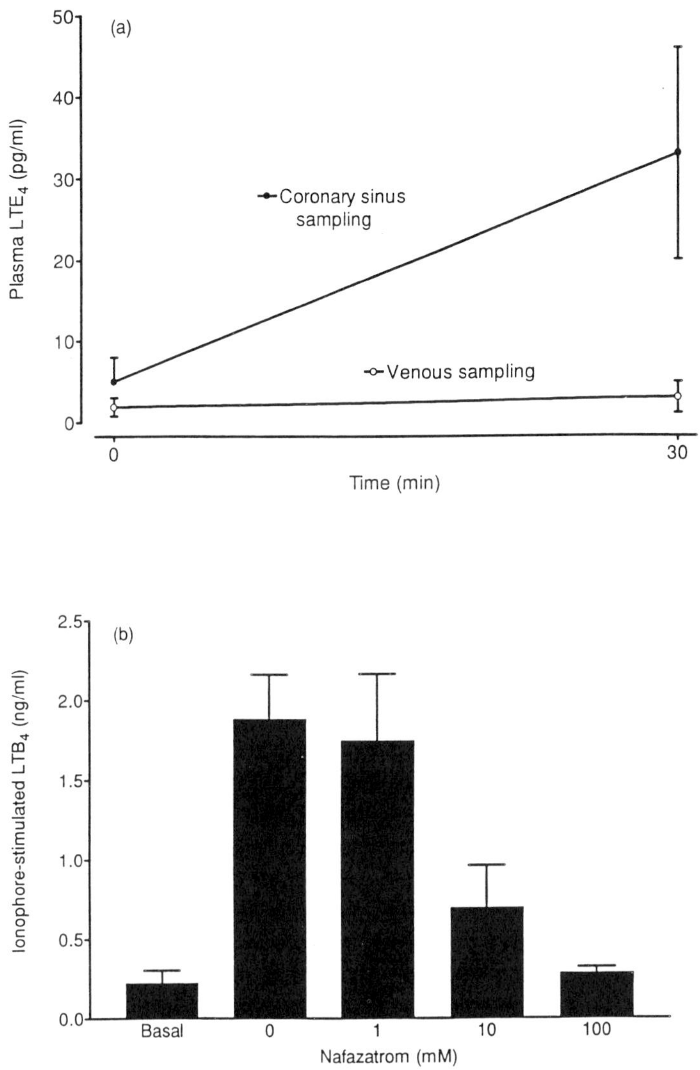

Figure 4 (a) Plasma LTE_4 was determined by HPLC-RIA in patients following balloon angioplasty. There is a marked increase in plasma LTE_4 sampled locally from the coronary sinus with no measurable change in venous LTE_4. Although the low basal levels of LTE_4 ($\leq$5 pg/ml) can be detected by this method, confidence in the accuracy of the measurement is low. (b) Ionophore-stimulated LTB_4 (measured by HPLC-RIA) was reduced in a dose-dependent manner in the presence of the lipoxygenase inhibitor nafazatrom. A significant proportion of the LTB_4 immunoreactivity did not coelute with LTB_4 on HPLC.

the variation in excretion volume and is most suitable for spot collections from patients, where it is not always possible to obtain accurate timed collections. It is assumed that creatinine is produced continuously within the body and that the production rate is similar between subjects. Thus, creatinine concentration acts as marker of GFR and can be used to normalize urinary metabolite excretion in normal subjects. The effect of renal and hepatic function on excretion rate is important and must also be considered. This can best be seen by comparing urinary LTE_4 excretion in patients with liver and kidney disease. In renal failure, urinary LTE_4 is decreased (concomitant on a fall in renal clearance), whereas in decompensated liver disease urinary LTE_4 is raised due to a reduction in biliary clearance and an associated increase in systemic synthesis consequent upon endotoxemia (Fig. 5a). Clearly, in any condition where renal dysfunction occurs, it is no longer acceptable to use creatinine to normalize mediator levels: here, correction for creatinine clearance (CrCl) may be made and eicosanoid excretion expressed as ng/ml CrCl (59) (Fig. 5b). The value of correction for creatinine clearance is exemplified in patients with hepatorenal syndrome (HRS) where renal failure occurs following liver damage: the increased production of cysLTs in these patients is masked by the reduced excretion rate.

III. Assays for the Leukotrienes and Lipoxins

Having considered some of the general problems with assays in this field, I will outline the current techniques used for these eicosanoids. Many of the methods are applicable to both the cysteinyl leukotrienes and the hydroxylated eicosanoids.

A. Cysteinyl Leukotrienes

The specificity of the 5-lipoxygenase and LTC_4 synthase enzyme system has led to the formation of only a limited number of cysteinyl leukotrienes. Although other glutathione conjugates have been reported (60–63), they seem to have little biological importance. The rapid metabolism of LTC_4, and the constant proportion ($\sim$5%) excreted as LTE_4 in urine simplifies the assay requirements for determining cysLYT production in vivo. Internal standards added on collection can account for storage and handling losses, however, the possibility of *cis-trans* isomerization should be kept in mind when assaying for these compounds.

Bioassays

The guinea pig ileum bioassay was instrumental in the purification and characterization of the cysLTs. The cysLTs cause a dose-dependent contraction of the

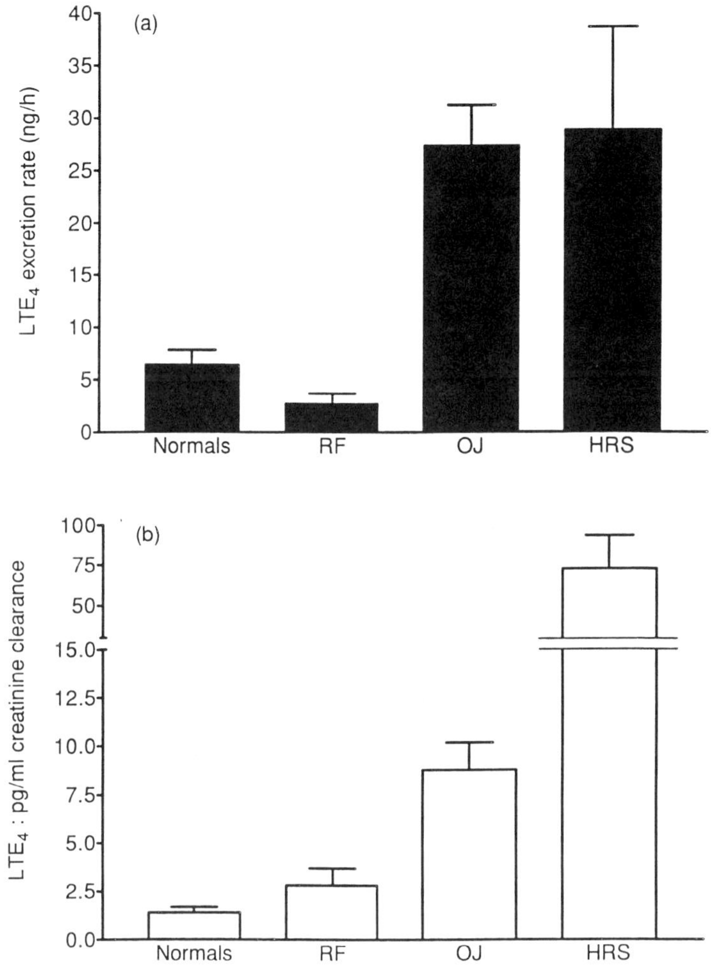

Figure 5 (a) Urinary LTE_4 excretion rates in normal subjects and patients with renal failure (RF), obstructive jaundice (OJ), and hepatorenal syndrome (HRS). Renal failure leads to a fall in LTE_4 excretion, whereas hepatic impairment results in increased synthesis of cysLT and an increased excretion rate of LTE_4. The increased synthesis of cysLTs in HRS consequent on liver damage is masked by the accompanying renal failure. (b) By correcting for the effects of renal failure (using creatinine clearance), the true production of cysLTs in HRS becomes apparent. Here, the corrected excretion in patients with renal failure is not significantly different from normals, but is higher in OJ and (markedly) in HRS.

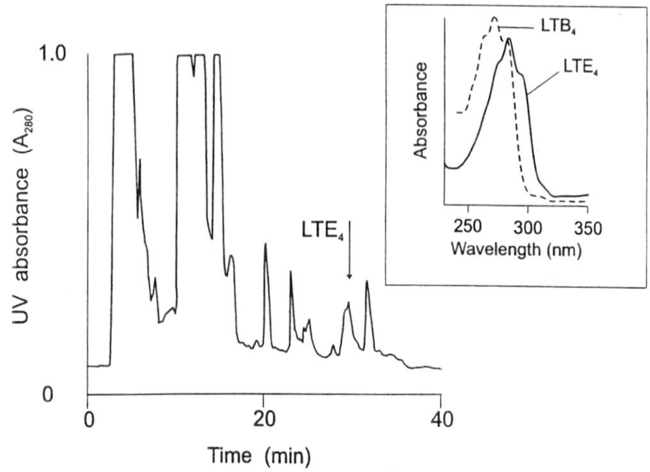

Figure 6 HPLC-UV profile of plasma spiked with 10 ng LTE_4. Although there is a UV-absorbing peak at the elution position of LTE_4, the absorbance is 1000-fold higher than can be accounted for by the presence of LTE_4. The full UV spectra of LTB_4 and LTE_4 are inset.

tissue ($LTD_4 > LTC_4 > LTE_4$); specificity was achieved by preincubating the tissue with indomethacin and histamine antagonists and using the Fisons antagonist, FPL55712, to differentiate the cysLTs from a wide range of other spasmogens (64). Differential assay on a number of tissues in the cascade system can also be used to differentiate LTD_4 from LTB_4 (65). One major drawback of the bioassay is that unless HPLC purification is employed, it is only possible to quantify LTC_4 in the presence of LTD_4 or LTE_4. Neither is the assay sufficiently sensitive to LTE_4 and its metabolites. Such in vitro assays, although vital in the early days of cysLT research, are of little value nowadays for measuring these compounds.

Spectrophotometric Assays

The characteristic triene chromophore of the cysteinyl leukotrienes (λ_{max} 280nm, ε_{max} 40,000; Fig. 6) (66,67) can be employed to quantify synthetic standards. HPLC purification can add specificity to the assay, and, where cysLT levels are high enough, can be used to quantify these compounds in simple biological matrices. The limit of detection for HPLC-UV–based assays is ~5 ng on column. Further specificity can be added by using multiwavelength (or diode array) monitoring. For a given analyte, the ratio of two (or more) wavelengths is constant: for example, the A_{280}/A_{254} ratio for LTE_4 (2.6:1) differs from that of LTB_4 and the other DHETEs (~1.3:1). Even with analytes with intense UV absorbances, such as the leukotrienes, there are dangers of using UV detection for trace amounts in complex biological matrices where there may be many UV-absorbing impurities present. As shown in Figure 6, plasma containing leukotriene E_4 (10 ng/ml) was extracted and subjected to reverse-phase HPLC: there is a UV-absorbing species with the retention time of LTE_4, but the absorbance is equivalent to a concentration of >10 μg/ml. Clearly, any LTE_4 present was hidden by the presence of a co-eluting impurity.

Antibody-Based Assays

The development of the first immunoassays (IA) for the cysLTs (68,69) revolutionized the measurement of these compounds. Kits soon became available, and data on picogram levels of immunoreactive cysLTs began to appear in the literature (70–73). The development of enzyme immunoadsorbant assays such as EIA (ELISA) (74–76) simplified the assay procedures, lowered the limits of detection (<1 pg), and did away for the need for radiolabeled ligands, and there are numerous reports on the application of EIA/ELISA for cysLT analysis. Although many groups would assert that their antibodies are specific (77–80), it is my opinion that the evidence points to a need for chromatography before assay. For example, an EIA that always gives higher values than a similar HPLC-immunoassay (HPLC-IA) should be treated with some caution. Even where known compounds of minimal cross-reactivity are present, there is the potential for error. The cross-reactivity of arachidonic acid with the antibody used in our laboratory is low (<0.1%), however, in the not uncommon situation where there is a vast excess (1000-fold) of this substrate over product, the excess substrate may be identified incorrectly as ''immunoreactive'' LTE_4. This situation is not uncommon in many experimental systems challenged with exogenous arachidonic acid. As a minimum, prepurification on C18 cartridges before immunoassay or the approach of Wescott and colleagues (22) using immunoaffinity adsorption followed by EIA using a different antibody seems to offer a good compromise between the specificity of HPLC-IA and the convenience and speed of EIA.

Perhaps the most specific IA method for measuring the cysLTs, particularly in urine, is HPLC-RIA/EIA (70–73,78,79) following either C18 solid phase or immunoaffinity cartridge extraction (Sec. II. D). Immunoreactivity is measured at the elution position of authentic LTE_4, and correction made for background immunoreactivity. The use of HPLC-IA is exemplified in the assay for urinary LTE_4 used in our department (40,59). Trace amounts of ^3H-LTE_4 (5000 dpm) are included in the urine on collection and act as an internal standard. The urine is purified by either LTE_4-immunoaffinity column chromatography or on-line extraction/HPLC. To increase specificity and determine accurately background immunoreactivity, 10 HPLC fractions are analyzed for radioactivity and immuno-

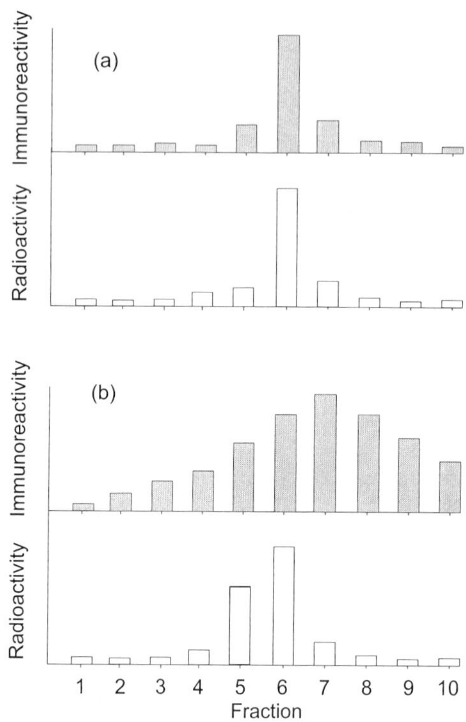

Figure 7 (a) HPLC-immunochromatogram of urine from a patient with acute asthma (■). The elution position of LTE_4 is defined by the co-eluting ^3H-LTE_4 internal standard (□). The presence of LTE_4 is only accepted when there is a concomitant rise and fall of immunoreactivity and radioactivity. (b) In another urine sample from a patient with hepatorenal syndrome, immunoreactivity (■) did not coelute with the radioactivity (□), and it was not possible to be confident that LTE_4 was present.

reactivity (Fig. 7a). The retention time of LTE_4 is defined by the radiolabeled internal standard. Although LTE_4 is well separated from other immunoreactive species such as *N*-acetyl LTE_4, it is only accepted when there is a concomitant rise and fall of immunoreactivity and radioactivity (internal standard). This allows us to determine recovery in each sample (which, as we have already seen is variable) and to estimate the background immunoreactivity. This is of particular importance when dealing with dirty matrices, where there may be interfering cross-reacting species co-eluting with LTE_4 (Fig. 7b). Using the rise-and-fall approach, we can often detect immunoreactivity at very low levels where confidence in the quantitation is low. The time required for HPLC-IAs is the main drawback. A variation on this theme has been reported by Oosterkamp and colleagues, who have developed an automated, on-line HPLC-immunochemical detection system for measuring cysLTs (81). Samples are chromatographed on a Kromasil C4 column at pH 7.4 followed by postcolumn mixing of the HPLC eluate with a cysLT antibody and the fluorophore labeled (BODIPY) LTE_4. The antibody complex is separated from the labeled ligand and monitored in a fluorescence detector. In principle, the procedure should be applicable to routine sampling for LTC_4 and its immunoreactive metabolites, but it remains to be seen whether this method ever leaves the realms of developing laboratory to compete with commercially available LT kits.

Immunoassays can only detect immunoreactive species. As metabolites often possess only poor cross-reactivity compared to the parent eicosanoid, it becomes necessary to raise a new antibody for each metabolite. This is rarely worthwhile. There is one report of an immunoassay that can be used for the ω-oxidized metabolites of LTE_4 (82), although the antibody is not commercially available. A universal detector for all cysLTs and their metabolites such as the mass spectrometer is preferred.

Mass Spectrometric Assays

Mass spectrometry was instrumental in the structure elucidation of the $LTC_4/D_4/E_4$, although until recently it had not played a major role in measuring these compounds.

Gas Chromatography–Mass Spectrometry

Although GC-MS has been widely used for the analysis of a wide range of eicosanoids from prostaglandins to Trioxilins, it has not been possible to chromatograph intact $LTC_4/D_4/E_4$ on GC. This was overcome in part by Murphy and colleagues (83), who demonstrated that hydrogenation of the cysLTs was accompanied by desulfurization to generate 5-hydroxyeicosanoic acid (5-HE) (Fig. 8). 5-HE chromatographs as the O-TMS ether pentafluorobenzyl (PFB) ester and is quantified by the electron capture (EC) mode (cf. Fig. 12). The base peak in the EC mass spectrum of derivatized 5-HE is the M-PFB$^-$ ion at *m/z* 399, and this fragments to generate ions at *m/z* 309 and 253. Care must be taken with the choice of internal standard as ^1H-^2H scrambling can occur during hydrogenation. The 20,20,20 $^2H_3$ analog or $^{18}O_2$ analog appear to be the most suitable internal standards (29). This approach, now used in other laboratories (84,85), requires prior HPLC separation to differentiate 5-HETE, LTC_4, LTD_4, LTE_4, and *N*-acetyl LTE_4, their 11-*trans* isomers, and the 3 and 5 series eicosanoids, and this increases the time required for assay. The hydrogenation/desulfurization approach is also applicable to ω-oxidized LTE_4 metabolites, where the formation of 5-hydroxy eicosa-1,20-dioic acid can be used to measure ω-COOH LTE_4 (84,86). The increased specificity of tandem MS (GC-MS/MS) has been applied to reduced-desulfurized LTE_4

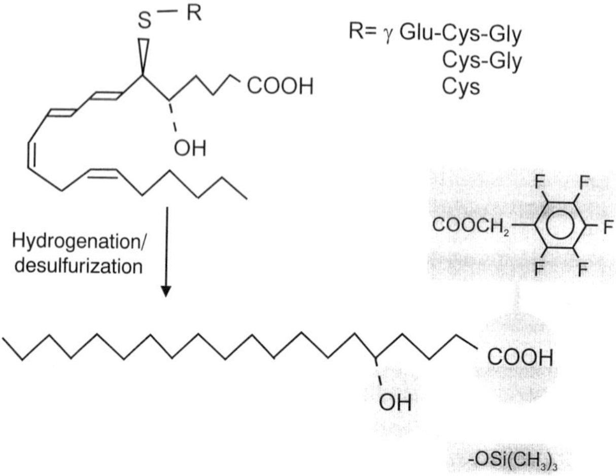

Figure 8 Catalytic hydrogenation of the cysLTs leads to the formation of 5-hydroxy-eicosanoic acid. On conversion to the *O*-trimethylsilyl ether pentafluorobenzyl ester, 5-hydroxyeisanoic acid is quantified by GC-ECMS using the major (M-PFB)− fragment ion at *m/z* 399 (see Fig. 12). HPLC purification is required to differentiate LTC_4, LTD_4, and LTE_4.

(29,87), where multiple reaction monitoring of the 399/309 or 399/253 transitions (and the equivalent transitions in the ^{2}H-labeled internal standard) is used.

HPLC–Mass Spectrometry

The introduction of LC-thermospray mass spectrometry in the early 1980s coincided with the wave of development in cysLT assays. Thermospray MS was not a user-friendly technique, and, although the cysLTs generated thermospray mass spectra post HPLC (88), the chromatograms were extremely noisy (Fig. 9) and unsuitable for assay purposes. The development of the electrospray (or ionspray) interface revolutionized HPLC-MS. The cysLTs generate positive ion and negative ion ESP mass spectra with little fragmentation (Fig. 10). Although HPLC-ESP MS with selected ion monitoring can be applied for cysLT analysis, HPLC-tandem MS offers the best scope for rapid sample throughput because the second mass spectrometer acts as a mass filter and there is far less need for extensive prepurification. Short HPLC columns can be used with low retention times for the analytes, and the system is ideally suited for automation. Yu and colleagues have reported the first HPLC-MS-MS assay for LTE_4 (89) using the transition *m/z* 438 (M-H$^-$) → *m/z* 333. The assay has a lower level of quantitation (LOQ) of 50 pg/ml (for a 5-ml sample), which makes it ideal for urinary LTE_4 analyses.

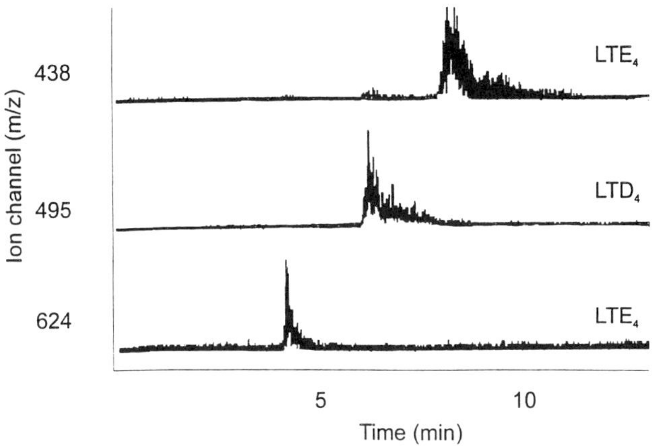

Figure 9 HPLC-thermospray negative ion profiles for LTC_4, LTD_4, and LTE_4. Samples were chromatographed on a Hypersil ODS column at 1.2 ml/min using a methanol:ammonium acetate gradient. Full spectra could be generated on 50–100 ng. The poor quality of the data arises from the instability of the early thermospray ion sources.

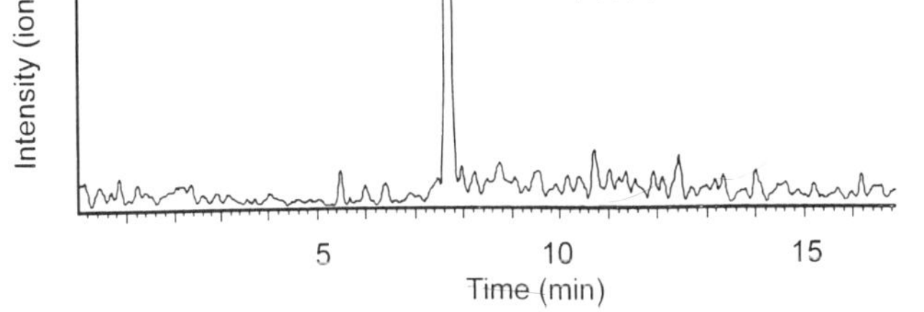

Figure 10 HPLC-electrospray positive ion profile of LTE_4 using an RPB microbore column and eluting in an acetonitrile:aqueous TFA gradient at 50 μl/min. Full mass spectra (inset) could be generated on 5–10 ng.

Other Assays

Radioreceptor assays have been developed for the cysLTs but have not found widespread application (90,91). There have been two reports of capillary electrophoretic (CE) techniques applied for the separation of the cysLTs (92,93). Detection post-CE is through UV (including diode array detection), conductivity, fluorescence, and, in principle, mass spectrometry. Although CE is becoming more common in the pharmaceutical industry for drug analysis, it has not found wide application yet in the eicosanoid field and may follow techniques such as supercritical flow chromatography into obscurity.

B. Lipoxins, LTB_4, and Other Hydroxylated Eicosanoids

It was originally thought that the cysLTS were the most difficult eicosanoids to assay; after all, fatty acids and their derivatives had been amenable to GC and GC-MS analysis for years, whereas routine measurement of the cysLTs (particularly LTE_4) awaited the development of the first RIA. The cysLTs possess one major benefit over the lipoxins, LTB_4, and other hydroxylated eicosanoids—there are only a limited number of cysteinyl-containing species, whereas there are numerous hydroxylated, unsaturated arachidonic acid metabolites (Fig. 11). Many of these compounds have similar mass, UV spectra, or chromatographic properties compounding the difficulties of measuring the compounds in the (potential) presence of a large number of isomers. The list in Figure 11 does not include eicosanoids arising from C18 and C22 polyunsaturated fatty acids, which markedly increases the potential number of interfering compounds.

There is also the possibility of producing nonenzymically generated eicosanoids on storage. In 1990 Morrow and colleagues (94) reported that storage of plasma led to a marked increase in prostaglandin $F_{2\alpha}$–like material. This was ascribed to the generation, from membrane phospholipids, of a series of isomeric iso (or epi) prostaglandins by nonenzymic routes and helped to explain some of the anomalously high prostanoid measurements reported over the past 20 years. More recently, a similar phenomenon has been observed with the nonenzymic (Cu^{2+}-mediated) oxidation of glycerophospholipids to form a large number oxygenated eicosanoids including the LTB_4 isomer, isoleukotriene B_4 (a 5,12-dihydroxy-6,8,10,14-eicosatetraenoic acid) (95). The relative cross-reactivity of the isomers to LTB_4 antibodies has not been reported, raising the specter of assay interference, particularly where the origin of LTB_4 has not been proven to be entirely through the 5-LO pathway. Similarly, with GC-MS assays there is the danger of coelution of LTB_4 with nonenzymically generated DHETEs.

Bioassays

The actions of a whole range of hydroxylated eicosanoids have been measured on isolated tissues, although much of this work has been for pharmacological

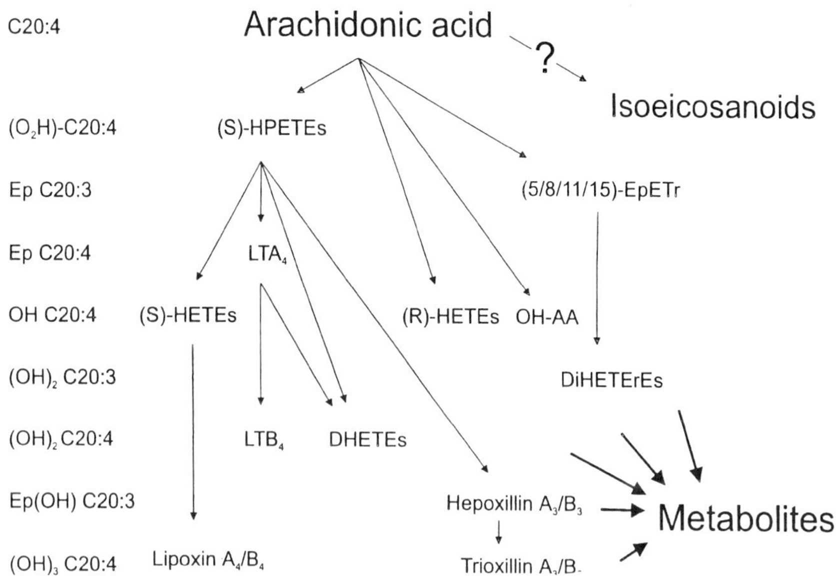

Figure 11 The analysis of hydroxylated eicosanoids is bedeviled by the vast number of similar compounds that can be generated from arachidonic acid. A number of these compounds will possess similar UV or mass spectrometric characteristics or may cross-react with ''specific'' immunoassays, requiring high-resolution HPLC or GC analysis to guarantee specificity.

rather than assay reasons. The most convenient bioassay for LTB_4 is the neutrophil chemotaxis assay. Human neutrophils are readily available, and the potent chemotactic effects of LTB_4 can easily be demonstrated in a Boyden chamber (96). Chemotaxins generally exhibit a bell-shaped dose-response curve, and it is important to carry out the assay at multiple dilutions. Other DiHETEs also exhibit chemotaxis against blood-derived cells (97). Both LxA_4 and LxB_4 also exhibit a range of activities against tissues (98–101), although these are not used routinely for assay purposes. As with the cysteinyl leukotrienes, there is little need nowadays for bioassays, which have now been superseded by RIA/EIA and GC-MS methods.

Antibody-Based Assays

Both radioimmunoassays (102,103) and EIAs (104,105) for LTB_4 have been developed and are now commercially available. Prepurification with HPLC should be used to confer specificity (106,107). An antiserum to LxA_4 has been generated

Table 1 UV Characteristics of Eicosanoids

Eicosanoid	λ_{max} (nm)	ε_{max}	Notes
$LTC_4/D_4/E_4$	280	40,000	Characteristic triplet spectrum; bathochromic shift (2–3 nm) for the 11-*trans* compound.
LTB_4	270	50,000	Characteristic triplet spectrum
DiHETEs	268–272	40,000	Over 10 common DiHETEs with the conjugated triene structure. Note that 8,15 DHETE (6, 8,11,13) is a conjugated diene (λ_{max} 243 nm)
HETEs	236–237	23,000	Diene absorbance common to all lipoxygenase products
LXA_4	301	50,000	Characteristic tetraene spectrum
LXB_4	301	50,000	
Arachidonic acid, EpETEs, DiHETrEs, hepoxillins, trioxillins	$<$220 nm		Single double bond absorbs ~180 nm; not normally suitable for HPLC-UV detection

Metabolism or chemical inactivation that does not lead to a change in the degree or conjugation will have little effect on the UV spectrum. Thus, ω-oxidation of LTs will not alter the λ_{max}, whereas a simple *cis-trans* transition in the cysLTs causes a 2- to 3-nm bathochromic shift.

by Levy and colleagues and used to develop an EIA (108). Similar qualifications as to specificity apply to these assays as to the cysLT assays.

HPLC–UV Assays

Many of the hydroxylated eicosanoids possess characteristic UV spectra (Table 1). HPLC-UV detection is used routinely for LTB_4 (109–113) and lipoxin (114–117) detection and assay. Multiwavelength monitoring can be employed to increase specificity.

Mass Spectrometic Assays

GC-MS is still often used to identify hydroxylated eicosanoids (118,119). Derivatization is required to increase the lipophobicity and stability of polar, thermally labile functional groups such as carbonyl, hydroxyl, and carboxyl. As with prostanoids, GC-ECMS (with selected ion monitoring) offers greater sensitivity over EIMS methods for the analysis of oxygenated arachidonic acid metabolites such as LTB_4 and lipoxins; esterification with pentafluorobenzyl (PFB) or *bis*-trifluoromethyl-benzyl groups leads to the formation of an intense M-PFB ion under electron capture ionization, which normally carries >50% of the ion cur-

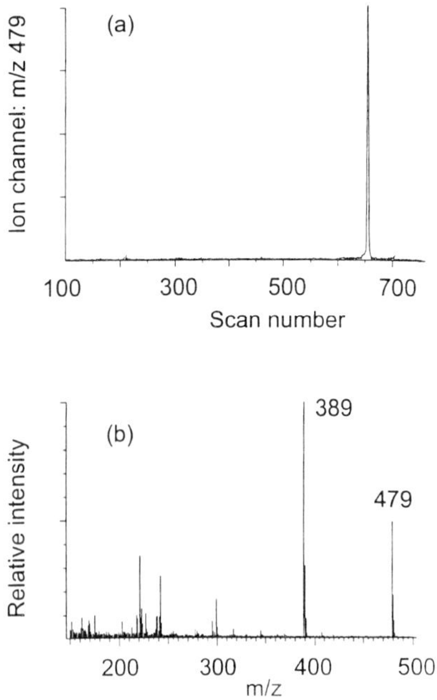

Figure 12 (a) GC-ECMS profile (*m/z* 479 ion channel) of the *O*-trimethylsilyl ether, *bis*-(trifluoromethyl)benzyl ester of LTB_4. (b) Electron capture mass spectrum of the *O*-trimethylsilyl ether, *bis*-(trifluoromethyl)benzyl ester of LTB_4. There are two major ions in the mass spectrum: *m/z* 479 (loss of the *bis*-(trifluoromethyl)benzyl radical) and *m/z* 389 (sequential loss of trimethylsilanol). GC-ECMS offers unrivaled sensitivity for the picogram analysis of eicosanoids.

rent and results in picogram sensitivity (52,55,120,121) (Fig. 12). Tandem MS can be used to increase specificity (122,123), using the transition $M\text{-}PFB^- \rightarrow (M\text{-}PFB\text{-}TMSOH)^-$ to monitor for LTB_4. The detection limits for LTB_4 in plasma using GC-MS-MS are ~10 pg/ml. A recent report indicated that catalytic hydrogenation of LTB_4 can be used to optimize both chromatographic and MS/MS transition parameters in the GC-MS-MS assay or leukotrienes (87). Thermospray LC-MS been applied to measure LTB_4 and metabolites in blood (88), however, as with the cysLTs, electrospray (or ionspray) ionization offers greater ease of use. The hydroxylated eicosanoids all generate intense deprotonated ($M\text{-}H^-$) ions, which undergo collisional deactivation (Fig. 13). Tandem MS can be applied to increase specificity (124,125), with the collision-induced mass spectra used to differentiate isomers (126). In the pharmaceutical industry there is a trend toward replacing GC-MS with HPLC-MS; however, there is still a place for GC-MS,

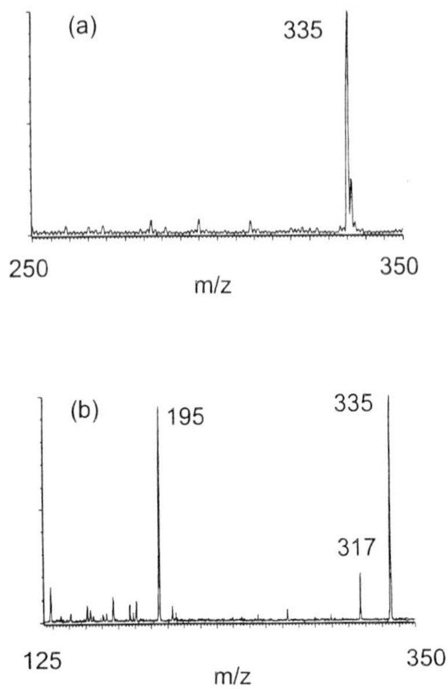

Figure 13 (a) Electrospray ionization of 5(*S*),12(*S*)DHETE leading to the formation of an intense M-H^- ion at *m/z* 335. (b) The collision-induced dissociation spectrum of *m/z* 335 (using the tandem MS facility). Multiple reaction monitoring of the 335 → 195 transition post-HPLC could be used to monitor for this eicosanoid.

particularly for the hydroxy eicosanoids. Capillary GC-ECMS offers greater sensitivity than HPLC-MS, and, through the use of different GC phases and derivatization groups, offers the option of altering the selectivity for the large number of isomeric hydroxy eicosanoids.

Other Assays

HPLC with electrochemical detection (127,128) and HPLC-fluorescence detection following precolumn derivatization with 9-anthryldiazomethane (129,130) have also been employed to identify LTB_4 in biological fluids. The overriding benefit of using fluorophores is for the detection of non–UV-absorbing eicosanoids such as the hepoxillins (131). Radioreceptor assays for LTB_4 have been reported (132,133) but do not appear to be in general use.

IV. Summary

The choice of assay is not just a question of technically balancing specificity and sensitivity. There are three other important practical considerations—costs, staffing, and time. The low capital costs, high throughput, and lack of requirement for highly trained staff make immunoassays a compelling choice for many laboratories, particularly since a number of commercial kits are now available. As discussed, a simple assay may also be a poor assay if not applied appropriately. On the other hand, increasing specificity by adding extraction, HPLC, internal standards, and two mass spectrometric steps may create a very complicated procedure where the chance of something going (often expensively) wrong increases. The capital costs of HPLC-MS-MS are high and, although the assays once set up are simple to manage, highly trained staff are required when machines misbehave. At the end of the day, we all want be sure that we are measuring what we think we are measuring, however, confidence costs money. The best compromise for most laboratories is to use a ''specific'' immunoassay with a simple high-yield extraction step to reduce the level of impurities. The greatest problems arise when a normally robust assay is used inappropriately, particularly in a new biological model where the assay problems may not be immediately obvious. Laboratories with GC-MS and HPLC-MS/(MS) will still have the edge in assay methodology, particularly as automation can be used to increase throughput. As the price of these instruments continues to fall and the machines become far more user-friendly, it is felt that more laboratories may employ mass spectrometric methods to measure eicosanoids.

References

1. Benedetto C. Prostaglandins and Related Substances: A Practical Approach. Oxford, UK: IRL Press, 1987.
2. Taylor GW. Quantification of lipid mediators in the respiratory tract. In: Robinson C, ed. Lipid Mediators in Allergic Diseases of the Respiratory Tract. Boca Raton, FL: CRC Press, 1994:159–189.
3. Lands WE, Smith WL. Prostaglandins and Arachidonate Metabolites: Methods in Enzymology. San Diego, CA: Academic Press, 1982.
4. Murphy RC, Fitzpatrick FA. Arachidonic Acid and Related Lipid Mediators: Methods in Enzymology. San Diego, CA: Academic Press, 1990.
5. Shah VP, Midha KK, Dighe S, McGilveray IJ, Skelly JP, Yacobi A, Layloff T, Viswanathan CT, Cook CE, McDowall RD. Analytical methods validation: bioavailability, bioequivalence and pharmacokinetic studies. Conference report. Eur J Drug Metab Pharmacokinet 1991; 16:249–255.
6. Karnes HT, Shiu G, Shah VP. Validation of bioanalytical methods. Pharm Res 1991; 8:421–426.
7. Blair IA, Barrow SE, Waddell KA, Lewis PJ, Dollery CT. Prostacyclin is not a circulating hormone in man. Prostaglandins 1982; 23:579–589.
8. FitzGerald GA, Brash AR, Falardeau P, Oates JA. Estimated rate of prostacyclin secretion into the circulation of normal man. J Clin Invest 1981; 68:1272–1275.

9. Dollery CT, Hensby CN. Is prostacyclin a circulating anti-coagulant? Nature 1978; 273:706.
10. Naoumova RP, Marais AD, Mountney J, Firth JC, Rendell NB, Taylor GW, Thompson GR. Plasma mevalonic acid, an index of cholesterol synthesis in vivo, and responsiveness to HMG-CoA reductase inhibitors in familial hypercholesterolaemia. Atherosclerosis 1996; 119:203–213.
11. Ramis I, Rosello Catafau J, Artigot M, Bulbena O, Picado C, Gelpi E. Simultaneous reversed-phase extraction of lipoxygenase and cyclooxygenase metabolites of arachidonic acid in nasal secretions: methodological aspects. J Chromatogr 1990; 532: 217–225.
12. Salari H, Steffenrud S. Comparative study of solid phase extraction techniques for isolation of leukotrienes from plasma. J Chromatogr 1986; 378:35–44.
13. Eskra JD, Pereira MJ, Ernest MJ. Solid-phase extraction and high-performance liquid chromatography analysis of lipoxygenase pathway products. Anal Biochem 1986; 154:332–337.
14. Borgeat P, Picard S. 19-Hydroxyprostaglandin B_2 as an internal standard for on-line extraction-high-performance liquid chromatography analysis of lipoxygenase products. Anal Biochem 1988; 171:283–289.
15. Richmond R, Turner NC, Maltby N, Heavey D, Vial J, Dollery CT, Taylor GW. Single-step procedure for the extraction and purification of leukotrienes B_4, C_4 and D_4. J Chromatogr 1987; 417:241–251.
16. VanAlstyne EL, Spaethe SM. Rapid method for automated on-line extraction and fractionation of plasma leukotrienes and 12-hydroxy-5,8,10,14-eicosatetraenoic acids by reversed-phase high-performance liquid chromatography. J Chromatogr 1992; 579:37–43.
17. Hsieh JY, Lin C, Matuszewski BK. Robotic sample preparation and high-performance liquid chromatographic analysis of verlukast in human plasma. J Chromatogr B Biomed Appl 1994; 661:307–312.
18. Ramis I, Hotter G, Rosello Catafau J, Bulbena O, Picado C, Gelpi E. Application of totally automated on-line sample clean up system for extraction and high-performance liquid chromatography separation of peptide leukotrienes. J Pharm Biomed Anal 1993; 11:1135–1139.
19. Vrbanac JJ, Eller TD, Knapp DR. Quantitative analysis of 6-keto-prostaglandin $F_{1\alpha}$ using immunoaffinity purification and gas chromatography-mass spectrometry. J Chromatogr 1988; 425:1–9.
20. Matsumoto S, Hayashi Y, Kinoshita I, Ikata T, Yamamoto S. Immunoaffinity purification of prostaglandin E_2 and leukotriene C_4 prior to radioimmunoassay: application to human synovial fluid. Ann Clin Biochem 1993; 30:60–68.
21. Moore KP, Taylor GW, Gove C, Wood J, Tan KC, Eason J, Williams R. Synthesis and metabolism of cysteinyl leukotrienes by the isolated pig kidney. Kidney Int 1992; 41:1543–1548.
22. Wescott JY, Sloan S, Wenzell SE. Immunofiltration purification for urinary leukotriene quantitation. Anal Biochem 1997; 248:202–210.
23. Mathews WR, Rokach J, Murphy RC. Analysis of leukotrienes by high-pressure liquid chromatography. Anal Biochem 1981; 118:96–101.
24. Osborne DJ, Peters BJ, Meade CJ. The separation of leukotrienes and hydroxyeico-

satetraenoic acid metabolites of arachidonic acid by high performance liquid chromatography (HPLC). Prostaglandins 1983; 26:817–832.
25. Yu W, Powell WS. Analysis of leukotrienes, lipoxins, and monooxygenated metabolites of arachidonic acid by reversed-phase high-pressure liquid chromatography. Anal Biochem 1995; 226:241–251.
26. Surette ME, Odeimat A, Palmantier R, Marleau S, Poubelle PE, Borgeat P. Reverse-phase high-performance liquid chromatography analysis of arachidonic acid metabolites in plasma after stimulation of whole blood ex vivo. Anal Biochem 1994; 216:392–400.
27. Ward C, Duddridge M, Fenwick J, Williams S, Gardiner PV, Hendrick DJ, Walters EH. The origin of water and urea sampled at bronchoalveolar lavage in asthmatic and control subjects. Am Rev Respir Dis 1992; 146:444–447.
28. Anderson FS, Westcott JY, Zirrolli JA, Murphy RC. Ethylenediaminetetraacetic acid in liquid chromatography of leukotrienes. Anal Chem 1983; 55:1837–1839.
29. Tsikas D, Fauler J, Gutzki FM, Roder T, Bestmann HJ, Frolich JC. Gas chromatographic-mass spectrometric determination of leukotriene E_4 in human urine using deuterium-labelled leukotriene E_4 standards. J Chromatogr 1993; 622:1–7.
30. Bestmann HJ, Roder T. Syntheses of leukotriene-derivatives. Eicosanoids 1992; 5(supp):S1–3.
31. Nicoll Griffith D, Zamboni R. N-acetyl(3H)leukotriene D_4: a stable internal standard for automated BIO-FAST HPLC extraction and separation of LTE_4 from human urine. Prostaglandins 1992; 43:523–532.
32. Tsikas D, Fauler J, Frolich JC. Enzymic preparation of dioxygen-18 labelled leukotriene E_4 and its use in quantitative gas chromatography-mass spectrometry. J Chromatogr 1992; 574:181–187.
33. Walters EH, Gardiner PV. Bronchoalveolar lavage as a research tool. Thorax 1991; 46:613–618.
34. McGorum BC, Dixon PM, Halliwell RE, Irving P. Evaluation of urea and albumen as endogenous markers of dilution of equine bronchoalveolar lavage fluid. Res Vet Sci 1993; 55:52–56.
35. Ward C, Duddridge M, Fenwick J, Gardiner PV, Fleetwood A, Hendrick DJ, Walters EH. Evaluation of albumin as a reference marker of dilution in bronchoalveolar lavage fluid from asthmatic and control subjects. Thorax 1993; 48:518–522.
36. Oosterhoff Y, Overbeek SE, Douma R, Noordhoek JA, Postmaa DS, Hoogsteden HC, Zijlstra FJ. Lower leukotriene C_4 levels in bronchoalveolar lavage fluid of asthmatic subjects after 2.5 years of inhaled corticosteroid therapy. Mediators Inflamm 1995; 4:426–430.
37. Lee TH, Crea AE, Gant V, Spur BW, Marron BE, Nicolaou KC, Reardon E, Brezinski M, Serhan CN. Identification of lipoxin A_4 and its relationship to the sulfidopeptide leukotrienes C_4, D_4, and E_4 in the bronchoalveolar lavage fluids obtained from patients with selected pulmonary diseases. Am Rev Respir Dis 1990; 141:1453–1458.
38. Wenzel SE, Larsen GL, Johnston K, Voelkel NF, Westcott JY. Elevated levels of leukotriene C_4 in bronchoalveolar lavage fluid from atopic asthmatics after endobronchial allergen challenge. Am Rev Respir Dis 1990; 142:112–119.

39. Oda H, Kadota J, Kohno S, Hara K. Leukotriene B_4 in bronchoalveolar lavage fluid of patients with diffuse panbronchiolitis. Chest 1995; 108:116–122.
40. Taylor GW, Taylor I, Black P, Maltby NH, Turner N, Fuller RW, Dollery CT. Urinary leukotriene E_4 after antigen challenge and in acute asthma and allergic rhinitis. Lancet 1989; 1:584–588.
41. Becher G, Winsel K, Beck E, Stresseman E. Leukotriene B_4 in breathing condensate of patients with bronchopulmonary diseases and of normal patients. ACP Appl Cardiopulmon Pathophysiol 1995; 5:215–219.
42. Wihl JA, Baumgarten CR, Petersson G. Contralateral differences among biomarkers determined by a modified nasal lavage technique after unilateral antigen challenge. Allergy 1995; 50:308–315.
43. Wang D, Clement P, Smitz J, Derde MP. Concentrations of chemical mediators in nasal secretions of patients with hay fever during natural allergen exposure. Acta Otolaryngol Stockh 1994; 114:552–555.
44. Seggev JS, Wiessner JH, Thornton WH, Jr., Edes TE. Comparison of serum and plasma leukotriene B_4 levels in normal and asthmatic subjects. Ann Allergy Asthma Immunol 1995; 75:365–368.
45. Shiratsuki N, Uyama O, Kitada O, Suenaga N, Nakamura H, Sugita M, Hayashi Y, Yamamoto S. Effects of hydrocortisone and aminophylline on plasma leukotriene C_4 levels in patients during an asthmatic attack. Prostaglandins Leukot Essent Fatty Acids 1990; 40:285–289.
46. Iwasaki E. Leukotriene C_4 in children with atopic asthma. II. Plasma levels in bronchial challenge with specific allergen. Acta Paediatr Jpn 1989; 31:295–302.
47. Schwartzberg SB, Shelov SP, Van Praag D. Blood leukotriene levels during the acute asthma attack in children. Prostaglandins Leukot Med 1987; 26:143–155.
48. Shindo K, Miyakawa K, Fukumura M. Plasma levels of leukotriene B_4 in asthmatic patients. Int J Tissue React 1993; 15:181–184.
49. Maltby NH, Taylor GW, Ritter JM, Moore K, Fuller RW, Dollery CT. Leukotriene C_4 elimination and metabolism in man. J Allergy Clin Immunol 1990; 85:3–9.
50. Shindo K, Fukumura M, Miyakawa K. Leukotriene B_4 levels in the arterial blood of asthmatic patients and the effects of prednisolone. Eur Respir J 1995; 8:605–610.
51. Takase B, Kurita A, Maruyama T, Uehata A, Nishioka T, Mizuno K, Nakamura H, Katsura K, Kanda Y. Change of plasma leukotriene C_4 during myocardial ischemia in humans. Clin Cardiol 1996; 19:198–204.
52. Brezinski DA, Nesto RW, Serhan CN. Angioplasty triggers intracoronary leukotrienes and lipoxin A_4. Impact of aspirin therapy. Circulation 1992; 86:56–63.
53. Israel E, Dermarkarian R, Rosenberg M, Sperling R, Taylor GW, Rubin P, Drazen JM. The effects of a 5-lipoxygenase inhibitor on asthma induced by cold, dry air. N Engl J Med 1990; 323:1740–1744.
54. Spaethe SM, Snyder DW, Pechous PA, Clarke T, Van Alstyne EL. Guinea pig whole blood 5-lipoxygenase assay: utility in the assessment of potential 5-lipoxygenase inhibitors. Biochem Pharmacol 1992; 43:377–382.
55. Brezinski DA, Serhan CN. Characterization of lipoxins by combined gas chromatography and electron-capture negative ion chemical ionization mass spectrometry:

formation of lipoxin A_4 by stimulated human whole blood. Biol Mass Spectrom 1991; 20:45–52.
56. Manning PJ, Rokach J, Malo JL, Ethier D, Cartier A, Girard Y, Charlson S, O'Byrne PM. Urinary leukotriene E_4 levels during early and late asthmatic responses. J Allergy Clin Immunol 1990; 86:211–220.
57. Westcott JY, Smith HR, Wenzel SE, Larsen GL, Thomas RB, Felsien D, Voelkel NF. Urinary leukotriene E_4 in patients with asthma. Effect of airways reactivity and sodium cromoglycate. Am Rev Respir Dis 1991; 143:1322–1328.
58. Christie PE, Tagari P, Ford Hutchinson AW, Charlesson S, Chee P, Arm JP, Lee TH. Urinary leukotriene E_4 concentrations increase after aspirin challenge in aspirin-sensitive asthmatic subjects. Am Rev Respir Dis 1991; 143:1025–1029.
59. Moore KP, Taylor GW, Maltby NH, Siegers D, Fuller RW, Dollery CT, Williams R. Increased production of cysteinyl leukotrienes in hepatorenal syndrome. J Hapatol 1990; 11:263–271.
60. Pace Asciak CR, Laneuville O, Su WG, Corey EJ, Gurevich N, Wu P, Carlen PL. A glutathione conjugate of hepoxilin A3: formation and action in the rat central nervous system. Proc Natl Acad Sci USA 1990; 87:3037–3041.
61. Spearman ME, Prough RA, Estabrook RW, Falck JR, Manna S, Leibman KC, Murphy RC, Capdevilla J. Novel glutathione conjugates formed from epoxyeicosatrienoic acids (EETs). Arch Biochem Biophys 1985; 242:225–230.
62. Laneuville O, Corey EJ, Couture R, Pace Asciak CR. Hepoxilin A3 (HxA3) is formed by the rat aorta and is metabolized into HxA3-C, a glutathione conjugate. Biochim Biophys Acta 1991; 1084:60–68.
63. Inamura T, Pardridge WM, Kumagai Y, Black KL. Differential tissue expression of immunoreactive dehydropeptidase I, a peptidyl leukotriene metabolizing enzyme. Prostaglandins Leukot Essent Fatty Acids 1994; 50:85–92.
64. Piper PJ, Samhoun MN. The mechanism of action of leukotrienes C_4 and D_4 in guinea-pig isolated perfused lung and parenchymal strips of guinea pig, rabbit and rat. Prostaglandins 1981; 21:793–803.
65. Samhoun MN, Piper PJ. The combined use of isolated strips of guinea-pig lung parenchyma and ileum as a sensitive and selective bioassay for leukotriene B_4. Prostaglandins 1984; 27:711–724.
66. Murphy RC, Hammarstrom S, Samuelsson B. Leukotriene C: a slow-reacting substance from murine mastocytoma cells. Proc Natl Acad Sci USA 1979; 76:4275–4279.
67. Morris HR, Taylor GW, Piper PJ, Sirois P, Tippins JR. Slow-reacting substance of anaphylaxis: purification and characterisation. FEBS Lett 1978; 87:203–206.
68. Hayes EC, Lombardo DL, Girard Y, Maycock AL, Rokach J, Rosenthal AS, Young RN, Egan RW, Zweerink HJ. Measuring leukotrienes of slow reacting substance of anaphylaxis: development of a specific radioimmunoassay. J Immunol 1983; 131:429–433.
69. Levine L, Morgan RA, Lewis RA, Austen KF, Clark DA, Marfat A, Corey EJ. Radioimmunoassay of the leukotrienes of slow reacting substance of anaphylaxis. Proc Natl Acad Sci USA 1981; 78:7692–7696.
70. Asano K, Lilly CM, O'Donnell WJ, Israel E, Fischer A, Ransil BJ, Drazen JM. Diurnal variation of urinary leukotriene E_4 and histamine excretion rates in normal

subjects and patients with mild-to-moderate asthma. J Allergy Clin Immunol 1995; 96:643–651.

71. Israel E, Fischer AR, Rosenberg MA, Lilly CM, Callery JC, Shapiro J, Cohn J, Rubin P, Drazen JM. The pivotal role of 5-lipoxygenase products in the reaction of aspirin-sensitive asthmatics to aspirin. Am Rev Respir Dis 1993; 148:1447–1451.
72. Frolich JC, Fauler J, Tsikas D. Assessment of cysteinyl leukotriene synthesis in man. J Lipid Mediat Cell Signal 1994; 9:75–78.
73. Fauler J, Tsikas D, Holch M, Seekamp A, Nerlich ML, Sturm J, Frolich JC. Enhanced urinary excretion of leukotriene E_4 by patients with multiple trauma with or without adult respiratory distress syndrome. Clin Sci Colch 1991; 80:497–504.
74. Miller DK, Sadowski S, DeSousa D, Maycock AL, Lombardo DL, Young RN, Hayes EC. Development of enzyme-linked immunosorbent assays for measurement of leukotrienes and prostaglandins. J Immunol Methods 1985; 81:169–185.
75. Furukawa K, Tengler R, de Weck AL, Maly FE. Simplified sulfidoleukotriene ELISA using LTD_4-conjugated phosphatase for the study of allergen-induced leukotriene generation by isolated mononuclear cells and diluted whole blood. J Investig Allergol Clin Immunol 1994; 4:110–115.
76. Volland H, Vulliez Le Normand B, Mamas S, Grassi J, Creminon C, Ezan E, Prazelles P. Enzyme immunometric assay for leukotriene C_4. J Immunol Methods 1994; 175:97–105.
77. Qiu DW, Hui KP, Lee CW, Lim TK, Tan WC. Simplified method for measuring urinary leukotriene E_4. J Chromatogr B Biomed Appl 1996; 677:152–155.
78. Kumlin M, Stensvad F, Larsson L, Dahlen B, Dahlen SE. Validation and application of a new simple strategy for measurements of urinary leukotriene E_4 in humans. Clin Exp Allergy 1995; 25:467–479.
79. Sala A, Armetti L, Piva A, Folco G. An improved assay for urinary LTE_4. Prostaglandins 1994; 47:281–292.
80. Kumlin M. Analytical methods for the measurement of leukotrienes and other eicosanoids in biological samples from asthmatic subjects. J Chromatogr 1996; 725: 29–40.
81. Oosterkamp AJ, Irth H, Heintz L, Markovarga G, Tjaden UR, Vandergreef J. Simultaneous determination of cross reactive leukotrienes in biological matrices using on line liquid chromatography immunochemical detection. Anal Chem 1996; 68: 4101–4106.
82. Tagari P, Rasmussen JB, Delorme D, Girard Y, Eriksson LO, Charleson S, Ford-Hutchinson AW. Comparison of urinary leukotriene E_4 and 16-carboxytetranordihydro leukotriene E_4 excretion in allergic asthmatics after inhaled antigen. Eicosanoids 1990; 3:75–80.
83. Balazy M, Murphy RC. Determination of sulfidopeptide leukotrienes in biological fluids by gas chromatography/mass spectrometry. Anal Chem 1986; 58:1098–1101.
84. Mayatepek E, Lehmann WD. Defective hepatobiliary leukotriene elimination in patients with the Dubin-Johnson syndrome. Clin Chim Acta 1996; 249:37–46.
85. Fauler J, Thon A, Tsikas D, von der Hardt H, Frolich JC. Enhanced synthesis of

cysteinyl leukotrienes in juvenile rheumatoid arthritis. Arthritis Rheum 1994; 37: 93–97.

86. Mayatepek E, Lehmann WD, Fauler J, Tsikas D, Frolich JC, Schutgens RB, Wanders RJ, Keppler D. Impaired degradation of leukotrienes in patients with peroxisome deficiency disorders. J Clin Invest 1993; 91:881–888.
87. Tsikas D, Fauler J, Velasquez RD, Gutzki FM, Frolich JC. Catalytic hydrogenation of leukotriene B_4 enhances sensitivity and specificity of gas chromatography tandem mass spectrometry techniques and enables simultaneous analysis with cysteinyl leukotrienes in biological fluids. Anal Biochem 1996; 236:175–178.
88. Taylor GW, Watson D. Biomedical applications of thermospray liquid chromatography-mass spectrometry. J Chromatogr 1987; 394:135–146.
89. Wu Y, Li LY, Henion JD, Krol GJ. Determination of LTE_4 in human urine by liquid chromatography coupled with ionspray tandem mass spectrometry. J Mass Spectrom 1996; 31:987–993.
90. Kohi F, Agrawal DK, Cheng JB, Bewtra AK, Townley RG. A simple and sensitive radioreceptor assay for leukotrienes. Prostaglandins 1987; 33:121–136.
91. Tamura N, Agrawal DK, Townley RG. A specific radioreceptor assay for leukotriene C4 and the measurement of calcium ionophore-induced leukotriene C4 production from human leukocytes. J Pharmacol Methods 1987; 18:327–333.
92. Tsikas D, Fauler J, Bracht S, Brunner G, Frolich JC. Analysis of leukotrienes, prostaglandins, thromboxane B_2 and their metabolites by capillary isotachophoresis. Electrophoresis 1993; 14:664–666.
93. Tsikas D, Fauler J, Brunner G, Frolich JC. Capillary isotachophoretic determination of cysteinyl leukotrienes. J Chromatogr 1991; 545:375–378.
94. Morrow JD, Harris TM, Roberts LJ, 2d. Noncyclooxygenase oxidative formation of a series of novel prostaglandins: analytical ramifications for measurement of eicosanoids [published erratum appears in Anal Biochem 1990; 186(1):184–185]. Anal Biochem 1990; 184:1–10.
95. Harrison KA, Murphy RC. Isoleukotrienes are biologically active free radical products of lipid peroxidation. J Biol Chem 1995; 270:17273–17278.
96. Ford Hutchinson AW, Bray MA, Doig MV, Shipley ME, Smith MJ. Leukotriene B, a potent chemokinetic and aggregating substance released from polymorphonuclear leukocytes. Nature 1980; 286:264–265.
97. Sehmi R, Cromwell O, Taylor GW, Kay AB. Identification of guinea pig eosinophil chemotactic factor of anaphylaxis as leukotriene B_4 and 8(S), 15(S)-dihydroxy-5,9,11, 13(Z,E,Z,E)-eicosatetraenoic acid. J Immunol 1991; 147:2276–2283.
98. Maddox JF, Serhan CN. Lipoxin A_4 and B_4 are potent stimuli for human monocyte migration and adhesion: selective inactivation by dehydrogenation and reduction. J Exp Med 1996; 183:137–146.
99. Lee TH, Horton CE, Kyan Aung U, Haskard D, Crea AE, Spur BW. Lipoxin A_4 and lipoxin B_4 inhibit chemotactic responses of human neutrophils stimulated by leukotriene B_4 and N-formyl-L-methionyl-L-leucyl-L-phenylalanine. Clin Sci 1989; 77:195–203.
100. Serhan CN, Hamberg M, Samuelsson B. Lipoxins: novel series of biologically active compounds formed from arachidonic acid in human leukocytes. Proc Natl Acad Sci USA 1984; 81:5335–5339.

101. Lee TH. Lipoxin A_4: a novel anti-inflammatory molecule? (editorial). Thorax 1995; 50:111–112.
102. Lewis RA, Mencia Huerta JM, Soberman RJ, Hoover D, Marfat A, Corey EJ, Austen KF. Radioimmunoassay for leukotriene B_4. Proc Natl Acad Sci USA 1982; 79: 7904–7908.
103. Salmon JA, Simmons PM, Palmer RM. A radioimmunoassay for leukotriene B_4. Prostaglandins 1982; 24:225–235.
104. Quinn JV, Bilgrami S, Seidel GJ, Slotman GJ. Evaluation of enzyme linked immunosorbent assays for quantitation of eicosanoid mediators of sepsis syndrome. Shock 1996; 6:142–149.
105. Antoine C, Lellouche JP, Maclouf J, Pradelles P. Development of enzyme immunoassays for leukotrienes using acetylcholinesterase. Biochim Biophys Acta 1991; 1075:162–168.
106. Celardo A, Dell'Elba G, Eltantawy ZM, Evangelista V, Cerletti C. Simultaneous determination of leukotrienes B_4 and E_4 in whole blood and of leukotriene E_4 in urine of rabbit by reversed-phase high-performance liquid chromatography. J Chromatogr B Biomed Appl 1994; 658:261–269.
107. Fuller RW, Maltby N, Richmond R, Dollery CT, Taylor GW, Ritter W, Phillip E. Oral nafazatrom in man: effect on inhaled antigen challenge. Br J Clin Pharmacol 1987; 23:677–681.
108. Levy BD, Bertram S, Tai HH, Israel E, Fischer A, Drazen JM, Serhan CN. Agonist-induced lipoxin A_4 generation: detection by a novel lipoxin A_4-ELISA. Lipids 1993; 28:1047–1053.
109. Strasser T, Fischer S, Weber PC. Leukotriene B_5 is formed in human neutrophils after dietary supplementation with icosapentaenoic acid. Proc Natl Acad Sci USA 1985; 82:1540–1543.
110. Lee TH, Mencia Huerta JM, Shih C, Corey EJ, Lewis RA, Austen KF. Effects of exogenous arachidonic, eicosapentaenoic, and docosahexaenoic acids on the generation of 5-lipoxygenase pathway products by ionophore-activated human neutrophils. J Clin Invest 1984; 74:1922–1933.
111. Clancy RM, Dahinden CA, Hugli TE. Oxidation of leukotrienes at the omega end: demonstration of a receptor for the 20-hydroxy derivative of leukotriene B_4 on human neutrophils and implications for the analysis of leukotriene receptors. Proc Natl Acad Sci USA 1984; 81:5729–5733.
112. Lee CW, Lewis RA, Tauber AI, Mehrotra M, Corey EJ, Austen KF. The myeloperoxidase-dependent metabolism of leukotrienes C_4, D_4, and E_4 to 6-trans-leukotriene B_4 diastereoisomers and the subclass-specific S-diastereoisomeric sulfoxides. J Biol Chem 1983; 258:15004–15010.
113. Yamane M, Shimizu S, Abe A, Sugiura H, Miyaoka M, Saitoh T. High-performance liquid chromatography-thermospray mass spectrometry of omega-carboxyleukotriene B_4 and omega-hydroxyleukotriene B_4 from an incubation mixture of human colonic well-differentiated adenocarcinoma homogenate. J Chromatogr B Biomed Appl 1995; 666:197–202.
114. Chavis C, Vachier I, Chanez P, Bousquet J, Godard P. 5(s), 15(s) dihydroxyeicosatetraenoic acid and lipoxin generation in human polymorphonuclear cells: dual

specificity of 5 lipoxygenase towards endogenous and exogenous precursors. J Exp Med 1996; 183:1633–1643.

115. Nert K, Virk SM, Hegrorman CA. Thrombocytes are the predominant source of endogenous sulfidopeptide leukotrienes in the american bullfrog (rana catesbeiana). Biochim Biophys Acta 1995; 125:203–210.
116. Serhan CN. On the relationship between leukotriene and lipoxin production by human neutrophils: evidence for differential metabolism of 15-HETE and 5-HETE. Biochim Biophys Acta 1989; 1004:158–168.
117. Stenke L, Edenius C, Samuelsson J, Lindgren JA. Deficient lipoxin synthesis: a novel platelet dysfunction in myeloproliferative disorders with special reference to blastic crisis of chronic myelogenous leukemia. Blood 1991; 78:2989–2995.
118. Wheelan P, Murphy RC, Simon FR. Gas chromatographic/mass spectrometric analysis of oxo and chain-shortened leukotriene B_4 metabolites. Leukotriene B_4 metabolism in Ito cells. J Mass Spectrom 1996; 31:236–246.
119. Stromberg F, Hamberg M, Rosenzvist U, Dahlen SE, Haegstrom JZ. Formation of a novel enzymatic metabolite of leukotriene A_4 in tissues of *Xenopus laevis*. Eur J Biochem 1996; 238:599–605.
120. Westcott JY, Stenmark KR, Murphy RC. Analysis of leukotriene B_4 in human lung lavage by HPLC and mass spectrometry. Prostaglandins 1986; 31:227–237.
121. MacDermot J, Kelsey CR, Waddell KA, Richmond R, Knight RK, Cole PJ, Dollery CT, Landon DN, Blair IA. Synthesis of leukotriene B_4, and prostanoids by human alveolar macrophages: analysis by gas chromatography/mass spectrometry. Prostaglandins 1984; 27:163–179.
122. Takamoto M, Yano T, Shintani T, Hiraku S. A highly sensitive and selective method for the determination of leukotriene B_4 in human plasma by negative ion chemical ionization gas chromatography tandem mass spectrometry. J Pharm Biomed Anal 1995; 13:1465–1472.
123. Hughes H, Nowlin J, Gaskell SJ, Parr VC. Selected reaction monitoring during gas chromatography/mass spectrometry of eicosanoids. Biomed Environ Mass Spectrom 1988; 16:409–413.
124. Wheelan P, Murphy RC. Quantitation of 5 lipoxygenase products by electrospray mass spectrometry: effect of ethanol on zymosan stimulated production of 5 lipoxygenase products by human neutrophils. Anal Biochem 1997; 244:110–115.
125. Wheelan P, Murphy RC. Metabolism of leukotriene B_4 in cultured hepatoma cells. Arch Biochem Biophys 1995; 321:381–389.
126. Griffiths WJ, Yang Y, Sjovall J, Lindgren JA. Electrospray-collision-induced dissociation mass spectrometry of mono-, di- and tri-hydroxylated lipoxygenase products, including leukotrienes of the B-series and lipoxins. Rapid Commun Mass Spectrom 1996; 10:183–196.
127. Herrmann T, Steinhilber D, Roth HJ. Determination of leukotriene B_4 by high-performance liquid chromatography with electrochemical detection. J Chromatogr 1987; 416:170–175.
128. Shirali P, Teissier E, Marez T, Hildebrand HF, Haguenoer JM. Effcct of alpha Ni3S2 on arachidonic acid metabolites in cultured human lung cells (L132 cell line). Carcinogenesis 1994; 15:759–762.

129. Yamaki K, Oh ishi S. Comparison of eicosanoids production between rat polymorphonuclear leukocytes and macrophages: detection by high-performance liquid chromatography with precolumn fluorescence labeling. Jpn J Pharmacol 1992; 58: 299–307.
130. Yamaki K, Oh ishi S. Release of leukotriene B_4 and 6-keto-prostaglandin $F_{1\alpha}$ from rat leukocytes in response to platelet-activating factor or Ca-ionophore A23187. J Lipid Mediat 1990; 2:317–327.
131. Reynaud D, Demin P, Pace Asciak CR. Hepoxilin A3 formation in the rat pineal gland selectively utilizes (12S)-hydroperoxyeicosatetraenoic acid (HPETE), but not (12R)-HPETE. J Biol Chem 1994; 269:23976–23980.
132. Simmet T. Radioreceptor assay for leukotriene B_4 and its use for the determination of leukotriene B_4 production by clotting human blood. Prog Clin Biol Res 1989; 301:119–124.
133. Kohi F, Agrawal DK, Cheng JB, Bewtra A, Townley RG, Olesch JW. The development of a sensitive and specific radioreceptor assay for leukotriene B_4. Life Sci 1988; 42:2241–2248.

11

Measurement of Leukotrienes from Human Biological Fluids

JAY Y. WESTCOTT

National Jewish Medical and Research Center
Denver, Colorado

IAN K. TAYLOR

Sunderland Royal Hospital
Sunderland, England

The cysteinyl-leukotrienes (LTC_4, LTD_4, and LTE_4) are peptido-lipid conjugates formed following lipoxygenation of arachidonic acid. These eicosanoids have received much attention for their potential role in inflammatory diseases, especially asthma (for review, see Refs. 1–7). Recently, the development of potent leukotriene synthesis and receptor antagonists has further linked leukotrienes with asthma. This has generated an interest in the measurement of leukotrienes in a variety of biological fluids in humans, as a means both to verify the presence of the leukotrienes and to monitor the effectiveness of inhibitors. The aim of this chapter is to discuss important considerations and potential problems of measuring leukotrienes in human fluids. The focus will be primarily on the peptidoleukotrienes because of their tight linkage with asthma and other inflammatory disease, but LTB_4 and other lipoxygenase products have been measured in fluids and many of the general considerations apply to these metabolites as well. This chapter will briefly review many of the studies that have measured peptidoleukotrienes in fluids. Since urine has been the major fluid utilized for leukotriene measurement, greater emphasis will be placed on reviewing studies utilizing this fluid. Studies examining urine LTE_4 have been subdivided into those concerned with basal levels, levels in asthmatics stimulated spontaneously or clinically, levels following pharmacological manipulation, and levels measured in inflammatory diseases other than asthma.

I. General Considerations for the Measurement of Leukotrienes In Vivo

The level of leukotriene (or any substance) in a biological fluid is the difference between the addition to the fluid (often synthesis) and the removal of the substance (metabolic or oxidative catabolism or transfer out of a compartment). The processes that control the synthesis and removal of leukotrienes from specific fluids are crucial factors in determining in what fluids leukotrienes should be measured, what methods should be utilized, and how the results should be interpreted.

Basal leukotriene synthesis is typically very low and is triggered by stimuli that elevate intracellular calcium levels and activate phospholipases (which release arachidonic acid) and 5-lipoxygenase (5-LO). LTA_4 is the initial leukotriene produced, and this unstable endoperoxide can be released from cells making it accessible for transcellular metabolism or converted to LTB_4 or LTC_4. Regardless of the leukotriene produced, the leukotriene is rapidly exported out of the cell. The export process for LTC_4 utilizes a specific export process similar to that of other glutathione conjugates and requires ATP (8).

After export from the cell, the leukotriene enters an extracellular fluid compartment. In many instances this fluid is blood or an interstitial fluid that mixes with blood with no distinct barrier. However, in other instances the leukotriene enters a fluid, which is removed from the blood. Some of these fluids that have not been extensively studied include tears (9), skin blister fluids (9,10), gastric fluids (11), joint fluid (12,13), middle ear fluid (14), cerebral spinal fluid (15), and bile (16). These fluids will not be further discussed in this chapter. Other fluids studied more extensively include lung and nasal fluids. These fluids have the advantage of conveying information on metabolic events that are occurring in a specific tissue at a specific time. The final route of elimination of much of the leukotrienes synthesized throughout the body is urine. Urine is thus an index of total body leukotriene synthesis over a period of time.

LTC_4 is readily metabolized in many biological fluids by extracellular enzymes present on cells or in fluids (17). γ-Glutamyl transpeptidase cleaves the glutamic acid residue off LTC_4, producing LTD_4 (18). The metabolism of LTD_4 is usually even faster than LTC_4 as a specific dipeptidase cleaves off another amino acid residue, resulting in LTE_4 (19). LTE_4 is generally a stable metabolite in many fluids. However, in some cases LTE_4 can be taken up by cells and *N*-acetylated to *N*-acetyl LTE_4. LTE_4 is not *N*-acetylated in the human hepatocyte, so urinary *N*-acetyl LTE_4 may represent products of renal metabolism (20,21).

Following collection of samples, the fluids are usually frozen prior to quantitation. Either -20 or $-70°C$ is adequate, and most samples are stable for at least a short period of time. Urine samples have been shown to be stable for months when frozen (22). In some instances, 1–10 volumes of methanol or ethanol is added to a fluid to remove proteins, stabilize samples (and halt further synthesis or metabolism), and allow for some sample concentration. Although in some cases repeated freeze-thawing of samples is without effect, with other samples there can be marked decomposition. In most samples and conditions, freeze-thawing has not been well studied and should in general be avoided.

A variety of methods have been utilized for the quantitation of leukotrienes in biological fluids. GC/MS analysis has been utilized in some cases, but the time and expensive equipment required for these assays have kept these procedures from becoming routine (23). HPLC purification coupled with UV absorbance has been utilized in some cases (24,25), but low sensitivity and the requirement of very clean samples makes this procedure unsuitable for most samples. Immunoassays have been the most often utilized methods for quantitation because they are simple, sensitive, and inexpensive. It is important that antibodies utilized for quantitation be appropriate for the fluid utilized. LTE_4 is often the major in vivo metabolite, and it is not appropriate to use LTC_4 specific antibodies for most fluids. Although some fluids are suitable for direct analysis by immunoassay, most procedures have some concentration or purification steps. Solid phase extraction is routinely performed using octadecylsilyl cartridges. This procedure accomplishes a crude purification, but primarily functions as a convenient method for sample concentration. For many samples (e.g., BALF), this procedure is all that is required. For other samples (most notably urine), further purification is required, and this is usually accomplished by HPLC.

II. The Measurement of Leukotrienes in Blood

LTC_4 and LTD_4 are readily metabolized in blood or in plasma. In blood (ex vivo) the half-life of LTC_4 was 11.5 minutes and the half-life of LTD_4 5 minutes (26). The survival of LTC_4 was compared in blood of asthmatics and healthy subjects, and no difference was found. Since leukotriene metabolism is so rapid in blood, neither LTC_4 nor LTD_4 is a good candidate to measure in plasma.

In addition to the rapid metabolism of leukotrienes in blood, the liver rapidly takes up the peptidoleukotrienes from blood and metabolizes them by β and ϖ oxidation (27). These metabolites are primarily excreted into the bile, although some metabolites reenter the circulation as very polar metabolites. Maltby et al. (28) performed calculations of maximal plasma LTE_4 levels based on renal clearance estimations following leukotriene infusion. These investigators calculated that the maximal plasma LTE_4 concentration should be less than 7 pg/ml. This extremely low level has been a major factor for plasma LTE_4 levels not being utilized as an index of LTC_4 synthesis.

Other considerations have limited the applicability for quantitation of LTE_4 in plasma as an index of endogenous levels. The major concern is that leuko-

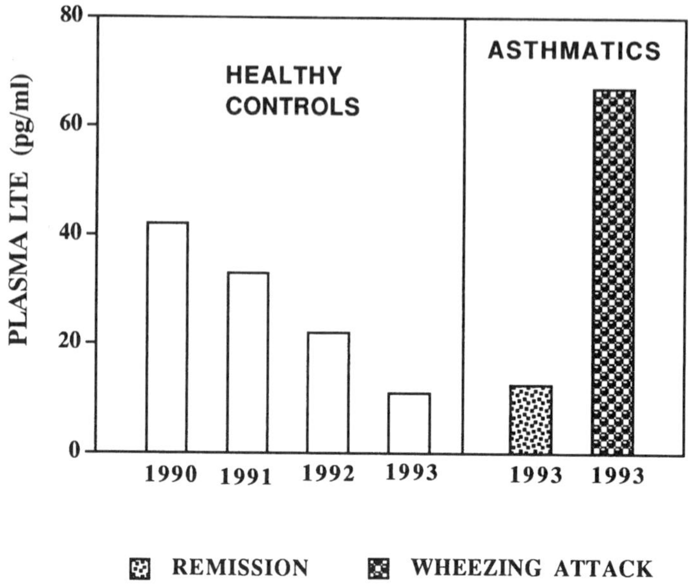

Figure 1 Plasma LTE_4 levels measured in healthy subjects and asthmatics. Measurements were made by the same research group over several years.

trienes could be synthesized by blood cells stimulated by the collection or storage/purification of the blood. This is especially important considering the low maximal level possible in blood, which would cause even low levels produced during collection to be an important interference. A similar problem with interference from TXB_2 platelet production was experienced when utilizing TXB_2 as an index of endogenous in vivo thromboxane levels in blood (29). Analysis of blood leukotrienes (especially LTB_4) ex vivo can be useful in studies where stimulated levels of leukotrienes are utilized as an index of synthetic capability or effectiveness of synthesis inhibitors.

In spite of these potential problems, several studies have measured plasma LTE_4 levels as an index of endogenous leukotrienes. Shindo et al. published seven papers between 1990 and 1994 (30–36) in which plasma LTE_4 was measured in healthy subjects or asthmatics (Fig. 1). These authors reported plasma LTE_4 levels of 79 ± 42 pg/ml (mean $\pm$ SD) in wheezing asthmatics compared to 42 ± 17 in healthy control subjects in 1990 (30). In later studies the LTE_4 plasma concentration in healthy subjects was reported to be 33 ± 12 (32), 22 ± 8 (33), and 11 ± 4 (35,36). These progressively decreasing values may indicate improvements in methodology with time. These authors did consistently find elevated levels of LTE_4 in plasma of asthmatics during wheezing attacks. Several other studies have measured LTC_4 instead of or in addition to LTE_4. These include studies of chronic obstructive pulmonary disease (37), sickle cell disease (38), and asthma (39,40). Very high levels of LTC_4 were reported, ranging from 168 to 74,000 pg/ml. These levels should be regarded with skepticism since LTC_4 is not usually appropriate for quantitation in plasma.

III. The Measurement of Leukotrienes in Lung Fluids

In asthmatics, it is generally believed that increased leukotrienes are produced in the airways in response to allergen. At least some of the LTC_4 produced is released into the epithelial lining fluid. This alveolar space inside the airways is distinct in that it is surrounded by a tight layer of epithelial cells, which acts as a barrier for substances moving in or out of the airways (41). A variety of studies have been performed to investigate levels of leukotrienes present in these airway fluids.

The majority of studies in humans have utilized fiberoptic bronchoscopy coupled with bronchoalveolar lavage to sample the fluids from the lower airways. Although this is an invasive procedure, it has been shown to be relatively safe and well tolerated (42). However, there are still controversies as to how best to express levels of substances in these fluids, and common methods for lavage fluid are as pg/ml, pg/mg protein, or pg/μg albumin (43). Some studies have tried to estimate the dilution of epithelial lining fluid that occurs during the lavaging process by comparing urea levels in lavage fluid to the level in plasma (44). There are also different methods of lavaging procedure, so it is difficult to directly compare levels obtained by different research groups.

Many of the first reports of leukotrienes in airway fluids were performed in small numbers of patients. Purification was usually by HPLC and quantitation by UV absorbance of compounds eluting from the HPLC or by GC/MS. One of the first reports of leukotrienes in airway fluids came from Stenmark et al., who found LTC_4 and LTD_4 in the airways of newborn infants with hypoxemia and hypertension (45). Westcott et al. also reported LTD_4 (46) and LTB_4 (47) in lung lavages from newborns with lung disease, and this was confirmed in later studies (48,49). Other early studies found increased leukotrienes in lung lavage or edema fluid of patients with ARDS (50,51) and pulmonary alveolar proteinosis (52).

The majority of studies examining leukotrienes in lavage fluid have focused on asthma. Murray et al. (53) performed one of the first studies, which examined BALF for leukotrienes in asthmatics. This study is especially noteworthy because, although PGD_2 and 15-HETE were detected, no leukotrienes were found by the methods utilized. During the next 3 years, several studies reported leukotrienes in BALF from unchallenged asthmatics (24,54,55) or challenged asthmatics (25,56). These studies were novel, but the methodology and small sample size limited interpretation. Two 1989 studies that examined BALF after antigen challenge are noteworthy. Chan-Yeung et al. (25) lavaged the lung 10 minutes after antigen challenge and found LTE_4 utilizing HPLC. No LTE_4 was observed in nonasthmatics or after challenge with an inappropriate antigen. This finding of rapid synthesis of leukotrienes following challenge has been confirmed in later studies. In contrast, Diaz et al. (57) examined BALF before and 6 hours after antigen provocation and found that LTC_4 was not notably different at the two time periods.

In 1990, Wenzel et al. (58) published a study in which asthmatics and nonasthmatics received endobronchial challenge with allergen. Lavage fluid was collected prior to challenge and 5 minutes postchallenge. Peptidoleukotriene levels were very low or not detectable in nonasthmatics, even after challenge. In atopic asthmatics, the baseline level of peptidoleukotrienes was 64 ± 18, which increased to 616 ± 193 pg/ml after allergen challenge. These investigators utilized methodology involving quantitation by immunoassay utilizing an antibody that detected all three of the major peptidoleukotrienes and thus bypassed HPLC. HPLC was utilized in several samples to examine the leukotriene metabolic profile, and LTC_4, LTD_4, and LTE_4 were all detected. LTC_4 appeared to be the major leukotriene following challenge, which could reflect the early (5-minute) time point examined. The results of this study as well as other studies measuring BALF leukotrienes are summarized in Figure 2.

There have been several other studies concerned with the measurement of leukotrienes in BALF of asthmatics under basal conditions. Crea et al. (59) measured leukotrienes in BALF collected from 11 unchallenged mild asthmatics and 11 healthy nonasthmatics and found no significant differences in LTC_4, LTD_4, or LTE_4. This is in contrast to the results reported earlier by Wenzel et al. (58), which suggested elevated basal levels in asthmatics compared to healthy subjects. Subsequent studies by Wenzel et al. confirmed elevated levels of peptidoleukotrienes in BALF of asthmatics compared to levels in nonasthmatics, although the time of BALF collection was important (60). Dworski et al. (61) examined BALF of unchallenged asthmatics and reported a level of LTE_4 of 35 pg/ml but had no healthy controls for comparison.

Two recent studies have examined the effect of time of day on BALF levels of peptidoleukotrienes in asthmatics who experience nocturnal worsening. Oosterhoff et al. (62) reported LTC_4 was increased in BALF collected at 4 A.M. in asthmatics with nocturnal worsening compared to nonasthmatics and asthmatics with no nocturnal worsening. However, as a group, the level of LTC_4 in BALF was not higher in these asthmatics at 4 A.M. compared to 4 P.M. Part of the problem could be due to LTC_4 being specifically measured rather than LTE_4, which would be the predominant peptidoleukotriene in BALF. Wenzel et al. (60) also performed a study in which BALF leukotrienes were measured at 4 P.M. and 4 A.M. in nocturnal asthmatics and normal controls. At 4 P.M., asthmatic BALF

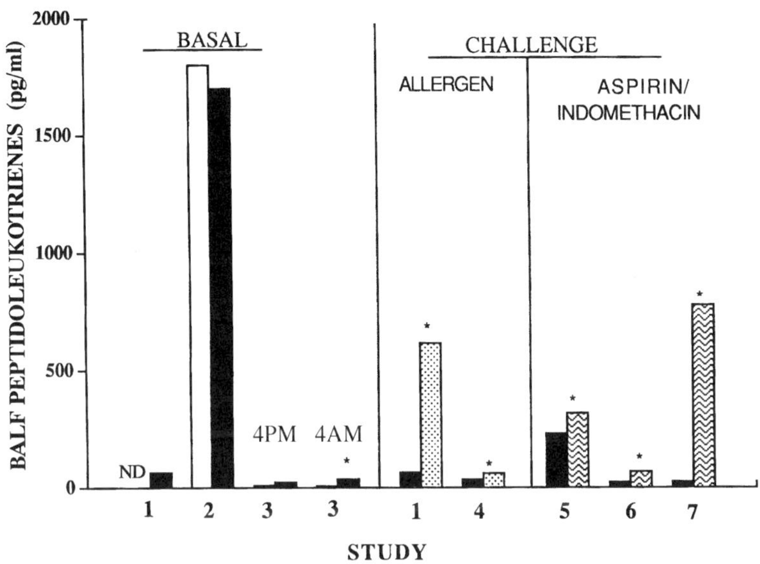

Figure 2 Reported levels of BALF peptidoleukotrienes in humans. Basal levels were obtained from healthy subjects or asthmatics. Asthmatic subjects were challenged with allergen or aspirin/indomethacin and lavaged before the challenge (Pre) and 5–30 minutes later (Post). The study numbers refer to the following references: Study 1 (58), 2 (59), 3 (60), 4 (104), 5 (61), 6 (64) and 7 (65). In Study 2, results are for LTE_4 only. In Study 3, BALF was collected at 4 P.M. and 4 A.M. as noted. ND refers to not detected. *refers to $p < 0.05$.

peptidoleukotrienes were 23 ± 6 pg/ml, which increased to 36 ± 12 pg/ml at 4 A.M. In contrast, nonasthmatic controls had 10 ± 3 pg/ml leukotrienes in BALF at 4 P.M., and the level was not increased at all at 4 A.M. Thus, the level of leukotrienes in asthmatic airways was increased compared to controls at a time (4 A.M.) during which pulmonary function was impaired.

In addition to allergen challenge, other studies have examined BALF after either exercise or aspirin challenge. Broidie et al. (56) collected BALF from asthmatics before and after exercise challenge. These authors reported no detectable BALF LTC_4 in either condition. Potential problems with quantitation of peptidoleukotrienes may have been an important issue in this study, since the immunoassay utilized would detect LTC_4 and LTD_4 in a sensitive fashion, but not LTE_4. The timing utilized in this study suggests that LTE_4 would have been the predominant leukotriene present in the airways during both lavages.

Three studies have examined BALF collected from aspirin-intolerant asthmatics. Polish and American researchers collaborated in 1994 and 1996 on two studies, which measured BALF eicosanoids (63,64). LTE_4 was measured in BALF following HPLC purification and immunoassay quantitation in both cases. The first study (63) reported basal LTE_4 levels in BALF from aspirin-intolerant asthmatics of 221 ± 48 pg/ml ($n = 6$, mean ± sem), which increased to 315 ± 67 pg/ml 30 minutes following aspirin inhalational challenge. The second study (64) reported a basal level of peptidoleukotrienes of 22 ± 16 pg/ml, which increased to 68 ± 65 pg/ml 15 minutes after aspirin challenge. These results demonstrate the potential difficulty of performing these studies, as the same researchers utilizing the same methods can obtain very different absolute values of leukotrienes in similar subjects. A third study was performed by Warren et al. (65), who reported a large increase in BALF peptidoleukotrienes 15 minutes after challenge of aspirin-intolerant asthmatics with indomethacin (24–775 pg/ml). This dramatic increase was not observed in aspirin-tolerant asthmatics or healthy nonasthmatics. In all three studies basal BALF leukotrienes were not higher in aspirin-intolerant asthmatics compared with aspirin-tolerant asthmatics.

Although collection of lavage fluid has been the primary means by which samples from lung have been directly obtained, induced sputum and exhaled condensate fluids have been utilized to a limited extent. Procurement of induced sputum involves the administration of hypertonic saline via inhalation (66). The subject is then asked to cough up this induced sputum. Cellular and mediator composition can be analyzed in this fluid. This procedure has the advantage of being much less invasive than bronchoscopy and lavage. Although this fluid should be appropriate for the analysis of leukotrienes, little has been reported on these measurements. However, leukotrienes have been measured directly in sputum from patients with cystic fibrosis (67). These patients naturally have enough sputum so that sputum induction is not required. Concentrations of both LTB_4 and peptidoleukotrienes were in the range of 30–40 ng/g of sputum, which are extremely high levels. It is not clear whether these measurements are valid or how such high levels are to be interpreted in regard to the disease. A final method of lung fluid collection involves breathing through an instrument in which fluids are condensed by travel through a long tube at very low temperatures (68). Although elevated levels of leukotrienes have been reported in asthmatics utilizing this procedure, further studies are required to show its utility.

The studies reviewed to this point have focused on the measurement of leukotrienes in lavage fluid as an index of the levels in the airways. None of the studies have extensively examined metabolism or removal of leukotrienes from the lung. Westcott et al. (69) examined metabolism in BALF after removal of cellular components and found that metabolism occurred as in other fluids. The rate of metabolism was dependent in part on the protein concentration of the fluid such that higher total protein was associated with faster metabolism.

Westcott et al. (69) also examined pulmonary metabolism and clearance of exogenously administered [^{3}H]LTC_4 in nonasthmatics, asthmatics, and asthmatics challenged with instilled allergen. BALF was obtained 15 minutes after instillation of the radiolabeled leukotriene which was instilled with [^{14}C] dextran as a reference for estimation of the recovery. This study found that 77% of the radiolabeled leukotriene had been specifically removed from the airways by 15 minutes in nonasthmatics, whereas 72% was removed from unchallenged asthmatics. In contrast, following allergen challenge in asthmatics, a 26% decrease in the airway removal of leukotrienes occurred, which would potentially augment the physiological effects of leukotrienes in the lung. The metabolic composition of the radiolabeled leukotriene metabolites recovered in BALF was determined by HPLC purification and scintillation spectrophotometry. LTE_4 was the predominant metabolite in all cases, with lesser amounts of LTC_4 and LTD_4. The authors speculate that LTC_4 is metabolized to LTD_4 and then to LTE_4 in the airways and that LTE_4 is then specifically transferred out of the airways. This metabolic sequence followed by transport into cells is very similar to that of the antioxidant tripeptide glutathione, which is a component of LTC_4.

IV. The Measurement of Leukotrienes in Nasopharyngeal Fluids

The role of leukotrienes in allergic rhinitis is likely similar to allergic asthma and has been extensively reviewed (7,70). In a manner similar to that utilized in allergic asthmatics, nasal lavages have been performed in subjects with rhinitis and normal controls. Shaw et al. (71) reported that peptidoleukotrienes and LTB_4 were elevated in nasal washings of subjects with allergic rhinitis after challenge with nasal allergen but not after methacholine. In a similar fashion, Miadonna et al. (72) found elevated LTC_4 in nasal washings collected from subjects with hay fever who were challenged with antigen. Subsequent studies by Georgitis et al. (73) and Wihl et al. (74) confirmed that increased levels of peptidoleukotrienes could be recovered in nasal secretions in subjects with allergic rhinitis following a clinical antigen challenge. The release and the biological response to nasal allergen challenge was abrogated by prior treatment with a 5-lipoxygenase inhibitor (75). Two studies have also examined leukotriene levels in nasal secretions after natural exposure to ragweed or hay in sensitive individuals, and both studies found increased levels of leukotrienes (76,77). This suggests that during the active season allergic rhinitis reflects a chronic state of inflammation of the nasal mucosa.

Leukotrienes have also been measured in nasal secretions in children with and without respiratory disease. Little or no LTC_4 was detected in nasopharyngeal secretions from healthy children (78). In contrast, LTC_4 was elevated in wheezing children without viral infection (709 pg/0.1 ml) and further elevated in children with evidence of respiratory viruses (1520 pg/0.1 ml). A second study found that severe bronchiolitis due to respiratory syncytial virus was also associated with high levels of LTC_4 in nasopharyngeal secretions (79). It was suggested that this release of LTC_4 was due to IgE-mediated hypersensitivity reactions to viral antigens.

Two studies utilized aspirin as a challenge in aspirin-intolerant asthmatics. In the first study, ingestion of aspirin in aspirin-intolerant asthmatics, but not in healthy subjects, increased the release of inflammatory mediators, including leukotrienes in nasal lavage fluid (80). In a second study, aspirin was administered by local instillation, which was also effective in increasing leukotrienes into nasal secretions of aspirin-intolerant asthmatics (81).

V. Leukotriene Synthesis by Isolated Cells and Tissue Homogenates

Although not really an in vivo fluid, a variety of studies have examined leukotriene synthesis in supernatants of isolated cells. These studies have the advantages that the cells are relatively pure and experimental conditions can be more easily controlled. The supernatants are relatively clean and the products are at a high enough concentration after stimulation that the supernatants can be analyzed without purification. The data obtained from these studies can be utilized as evidence of total synthetic capacity of cells to produce leukotrienes. Most of these studies have examined blood leukocytes or eosinophils in asthmatics and healthy subjects following stimulation with A23187. Two studies reported increased levels of LTB_4 in supernatants of neutrophils from atopic asthmatics compared to healthy controls (82,83). One study examined cells collected after bronchoalveolar lavage (mostly macrophages) and found that these cells from asthmatics produced less LTB_4 and identical LTC_4 as cells from healthy controls after A23187 stimulation (84). Five studies have looked at stimulated eosinophils in asthmatics and healthy controls, and all found increased LTC_4 synthesis in cells from asthmatics after A23187 stimulation (85–89). Finally, one study looked at basophils and found no difference in LTC_4 synthesis in asthmatics compared to controls (90). These studies all suggest that the ability of cells to synthesize leukotrienes may be affected differentially by a disease condition. In this regard, peripheral eosinophils from asthmatics appear to be characterized by an increased capability to generate leukotrienes.

At times, investigators have studied leukotriene synthesis in one specific tissue rather than just one cell type. Tissue slices or homogenates were utilized for this purpose. Early studies utilized lung tissue from asthmatics and challenged it with appropriate antigen to observe leukotriene synthesis (91). A more recent study (92) found that homogenized lung tissue from patients with idiopathic pulmonary fibrosis had 5–15 times more LTB_4 and LTC_4 than did homogenates obtained from uninvolved nonfibrotic lung tissue from patients undergoing resectional surgery for bronchogenic carcinoma. The authors in this latter paper speculate that leukotrienes participate in the pathogenesis of idiopathic pulmonary fibrosis.

VI. The Measurement of Leukotrienes in Urine

For the collection of many of the fluids previously described, invasive methods for sampling were required which could have resulted in ex vivo generation of leukotrienes. Another problem is that repeated measurements are required to give a dynamic perspective of leukotriene production over time. In contrast, urine is one fluid that can be easily collected by noninvasive procedures, is essentially free of cells circumventing potential problems of ex vivo production, and has a stable metabolite (LTE_4) that can be quantified by sensitive immunological techniques.

Numerous studies have now evaluated the metabolism, elimination, and pharmacokinetics of LTE_4 excretion in urine following intravenous infusion of LTC_4 and LTE_4, inhalation of LTD_4, or airways instillation of LTC_4 (28,69,93–95). Orning et al. (93) performed the initial study examining LTC_4 elimination in humans. [^{3}H] LTC_4 was administered to three subjects and urine and feces monitored for elimination of radioactivity. Forty-eight percent of the administered radioactivity was excreted in the urine and 8% in the feces over 3 days. In the urine 44% of the urinary radioactivity was excreted within the first hour with LTE_4 being the predominant metabolite. Huber et al. (21) also studied the elimination of [^{3}H] LTC_4 in two humans and also reported LTE_4 being a major metabolite that was rapidly excreted. Maltby et al. (28) infused three different doses of [^{3}H] LTC_4 into three healthy subjects and found 4.1 to 6.3% of the administered radiolabel was excreted as LTE_4 within 4 hours. Sala et al. (94) found similar results in their study with infusion of radiolabeled LTE_4.

Few studies have examined potential differences in leukotriene metabolism or elimination with respect to specific disease. Westcott et al. (69) examined the excretion of leukotriene metabolites to determine if excretion was altered in asthmatics compared to healthy subjects. This study found a rapid excretion of tritiated metabolites in urine following instillation of tritiated LTC_4 into the airways of healthy subjects, unchallenged asthmatics and asthmatics challenged with allergen. There was no difference in the excretion of tritiated LTE_4 (5–7% of the administered leukotriene after 6 hours) in these three groups. Mayatepek et al. (96) examined leukotriene elimination in patients with Dubin-Johnson syndrome, which is characterized by conjugated hyperbilirubinemia. These patients have an eightfold increase in LTE_4 in urine as well as increased levels of other metabolites. The authors suggest that defective leukotriene elimination into bile could be responsible for this enhanced leukotriene elimination in urine. The authors further propose that analysis of urinary leukotrienes could be utilized as a diagnostic indicator for this disease.

The stability of leukotrienes in urine has been investigated in several studies. Urine has been shown to have high levels of γ-glutamyl transpeptidase and dipeptidase, so it is not surprising that LTC_4 is metabolized in urine. Beyer et al. (97) showed that LTC_4 added to urine was converted to LTD_4 (50% in about 30 minutes) and then to LTE_4. In a similar fashion, Westcott et al. (98) showed that metabolism of [^{3}H] LTC_4 added to urine resulted in LTE_4 as a stable metabolite. Since there is increased interest in measuring LTE_4 in urine samples, the stability of LTE_4 has been tested by several investigators. Kumlin et al. (29) found that LTE_4 was stable in frozen urine samples at −20°C for months without additional preservatives. Fauler et al. (99) found that over 90% of [^{3}H] LTE_4 remained intact following 6 hours at 37°C. Westcott et al. (100) recently studied the stability of LTE_4 in urine left at 4 or 21°C for up to 24 hours. This study showed that 80–90% of the immunoreactive LTE_4 could be recovered from urine samples even after 24 hours at room temperature.

These findings of a rapid excretion of LTE_4 into urine, its stability there, and its excretion rate being similar in healthy subjects and asthmatics have caused many researchers to focus on urinary LTE_4 as a general index of total peptidoleukotriene synthesis. However, there are at least two caveats that must be considered. First, the kidney must be performing normally. If the kidney is inflamed it is conceivable that leukotrienes will be directly excreted into the urine and give a falsely exaggerated level of leukotrienes. This is because normal elimination of leukotrienes synthesized outside the kidney as urinary LTE_4 is only 5–7%. The second assumption is that liver function is normal. Leukotrienes are rapidly removed from the blood by the liver and then metabolized. If the liver is dysfunctional, the leukotrienes are not removed from the circulation so readily and the excretion by the kidney is increased. The net result is an increased level of urinary LTE_4 that is not reflective of total body synthesis.

Due to the importance of urinary LTE_4 as an indicator of total body leukotriene synthesis, appropriate methodology for its quantitation is crucial. LTE_4 levels are typically normalized to urine creatinine to allow a better comparison of samples. It is not appropriate to express levels as pg LTE_4/ml urine because of the high variability of urine volume. Occasionally, urine will be collected for specific time periods and excretion of LTE_4 expressed per some unit of time. The most commonly utilized methodology utilizes concentration over an octadecylsilyl cartridge, HPLC purification, and quantitation by immunoassay. Radiolabeled LTE_4 is added as an internal standard to facilitate detection of elution off the HPLC column and allows for correction for any losses that commonly occur throughout purification. This methodology is time consuming and prone to potential errors. However, purification is necessary because of the high amounts of substances in urine which interfere with the immunoassay. It has been suggested that LTE_4 can be directly quantified in urine without purification (22), but again the presence of interfering components does not allow this method to give accurate measurement. Recently an immunofiltration purification of urinary LTE_4 has been developed, which provides an easier yet accurate method of purification (100).

A. Basal Levels of Urinary LTE_4

LTE_4 has been measured in urine in healthy subjects by at least 13 research groups, and these studies have recently been summarized (101). A widespread of mean values have been reported. Much of the variability reported between groups is likely due to differences in methodology, although all utilized HPLC purification and immunoassay. One of the first published reports of urinary LTE_4 in healthy subjects (102) found 211 pg/mg creatinine (geometric mean, $n = 29$). Other published reports of urinary LTE_4 levels have ranged from 33 (103) to 200 pg LTE_4/mg creatinine (104) in healthy humans.

Studies with leukotriene receptor antagonists and synthesis inhibitors suggest that basal airway tone in asthmatics and their persistent bronchoconstriction is influenced by endogenous cysteinyl-leukotrienes. These leukotriene receptor antagonists and synthesis inhibitors have shown significant bronchodilatory effects in moderately severe asthmatics (105–107). However, Westcott et al. (108) and Smith et al. (109) found no correlation between baseline FEV_1 and urinary LTE_4 levels. This is consistent with the idea that different asthmatics have different sensitivity to leukotrienes, which is likely to change with time in any one person. It is also likely that much of the basal level of urinary LTE_4 is not reflective of leukotrienes synthesized in the airways.

Comparisons of basal urine LTE_4 in asthmatics and nonasthmatics have been evaluated as potential ''predictors'' of asthma. Several studies have found no difference in basal LTE_4 levels in urine in stable asthmatics and nonasthmatics (102,108). However, Asano et al. (101) did find significantly elevated LTE_4 in the urine of asthmatics under basal conditions. This report stressed that the variability of urinary LTE_4 in asthmatics was great and overlapped levels in healthy subjects to a large degree. It is important to remember that urine LTE_4 represents leukotriene produced throughout the body and that a significant increase in a small portion of the body may be enough to cause local physiological effects without producing a significant increase in urinary metabolites.

Asthma typically begins in childhood. In spite of this, there have been few studies to determine the role of leukotrienes in childhood asthma. One study (67) utilized 12 normal healthy children (mean = 9.2 years) and 11 atopic asthmatic children (mean = 10.2 years). The urinary LTE_4 level in the healthy children was 105 pg/mg creatinine, while the asthmatic children had a geometric mean of 759 pg/mg creatinine. These asthmatic children had been clinically stable for at least one month, had peak flows in excess of 90%, and were receiving no anti-inflammatory medicines. This same research group was involved in a second study of asthmatic children and again found increased levels of LTE_4 during and 1 month after an acute attack (110). High levels of urinary LTE_4 in these children suggest that ongoing chronic inflammation is occurring despite the lack of a pronounced lung decrement. However, a second study in asthmatic children (age 14 $\pm$ 0.5, $n = 8$) in the Netherlands found urinary LTE_4 to be just 17 pg/mg creatinine (111). No nonasthmatic children were utilized for comparison. A Japanese study (112) found basal urine LTE_4 levels to be the same in nonasthmatic and asthmatic children (122 vs. 109 pg/mg creatinine, respectively). More studies in children are needed to determine the role of leukotrienes in pediatric asthma.

A small group of asthmatics are sensitive to aspirin and other nonsteroidal anti-inflammatory drugs. At baseline, aspirin-intolerant asthmatics have higher urinary LTE_4 than other asthmatics [257 vs. 45 pg/mg creatinine (113)]. Others have confirmed this finding: Kumlin et al. (114), 435 pg/mg creatinine in AIA versus 144 in other asthmatics; Sladek et al. (104), 163 pg/mg creatinine AIA, no control group; Israel et al. (115), 469 $\pm$ 141 pg/mg creatinine in AIA, no healthy control group; Nasser et al. (116), 391 $\pm$ 72 pg/mg creatinine, no control group. The reason for this increased urinary LTE_4 concentration is unknown, but it suggests that certain cells (mast cells?) in aspirin-sensitive asthmatics are activated under normal circumstances, which is enhanced in the presence of NSAIDs. Even following aspirin desensitization, urinary LTE_4 excretion was elevated in aspirin-intolerant asthmatics under basal conditions and further increased after allergen challenge (117).

B. Urinary LTE_4 Excretion During Spontaneous Disease Exacerbations and Clinical Challenges

Several studies have examined asthmatics after severe asthmatic attacks requiring treatment in an emergency room. Taylor et al. (102) examined LTE_4 levels in 20 asthmatics who presented to emergency rooms. Mean urinary LTE_4 was three times higher than levels in healthy subjects, but there was substantial overlap between the two groups. Westcott et al. (98) examined three patients treated at an emergency room for airways obstruction due to asthma and found elevated LTE_4 levels, which quickly normalized following treatment. Drazen et al. (118) performed a larger study on patients presenting for emergency room treatment of airways obstruction. The authors created subgroups of these patients according to their response to nebulized albuterol. The group of patients that responded to albuterol treatment with at least a doubling of peak flow rates were also the patients with a higher LTE_4 excretion. The authors suggested that in this subgroup the airways obstruction could be primarily caused by elevated leukotrienes in the airways, while nonresponders may have most of the airways obstruction caused by other factors. These data provide strong evidence for a bronchoconstrictor role for cysteinyl-leukotrienes in acute severe asthma, particularly in those patients in whom bronchoconstriction per se is a major component of their airflow obstruction. Such data emphasize the likely heterogeneity of airway biological response to antileukotriene therapy not only acutely, but also chronically, between patient groups.

There are also situations in which a less dramatic spontaneous exacerbation of disease severity occurs. One such instance is associated with normal diurnal variation. A significant percentage of asthmatics show a worsening of asthma symptoms during the night. Two studies (60,119) have examined urinary LTE_4 measurements at the time of these nocturnal worsenings and compared them to earlier times or to patients that did not have nocturnal worsening. These studies both found an increase in urinary LTE_4 at 4 A.M. compared to 4 P.M., such that the increase correlated with the decrement in lung function. Bellia et al. (119) further showed that no diurnal variation occurred in urinary LTE_4 excretion in healthy controls or asthmatics without nocturnal worsening.

To further link leukotrienes and airways pathology, asthmatics have been brought into a clinical situation and challenged in a variety of ways to reproduce symptoms of the disease. Leukotrienes have been measured in BALF (see above) and urine in an attempt to better understand the relationship between leukotriene production and airways physiology. The challenges have included allergen, exercise, PAF, and nonsteroidal anti-inflammatory drugs.

Inhalation of an allergen to sensitized asthmatics has been one of the primary challenges utilized in clinical surroundings. Activation of mast cells by IgE-dependent mechanisms results in the release of inflammatory mediators such as histamine, PGD_2, and LTC_4. It is the end organ response to these mediators, including smooth muscle contraction, enhanced mucus secretion, and changes in pulmonary vascular permeability, that account for many features of the immediate bronchial response to inhaled allergen. Taylor et al. (102) first reported increased urinary LTE_4 excretion within the first 3 hours following allergen challenge of asthmatics. The magnitude of the increase in LTE_4 was variable among asthmatics, varying between a less than twofold increase and a 60-fold increase. Since this preliminary report, a number of studies have confirmed these initial findings, consistently demonstrating elevations in urinary LTE_4 during early allergen-induced bronchoconstriction (Fig. 3) (104,108,114,120–122). The magnitude of the increase in urinary LTE_4 excretion is variable between studies, likely due in part to variable durations of urinary collections, dissimilar protocols of allergen administration and different populations of asthmatics. This universal

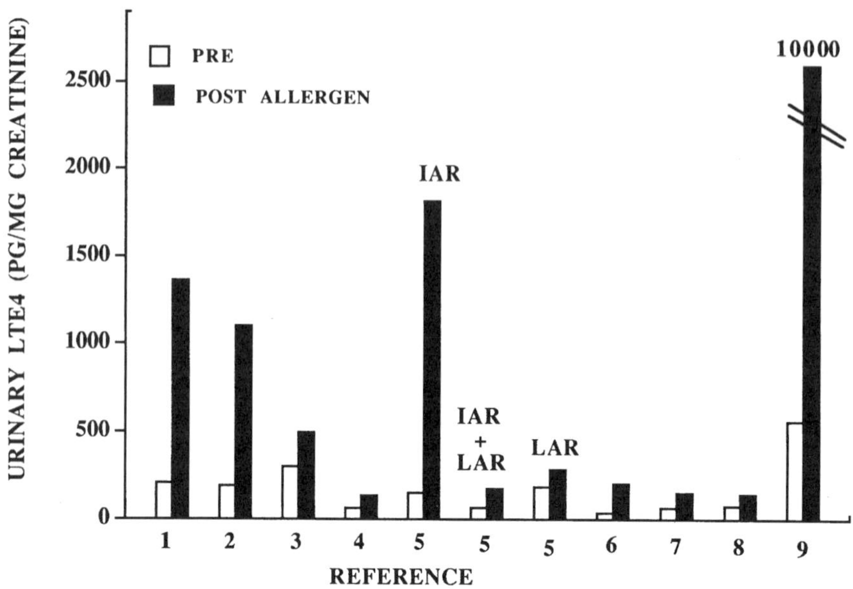

Figure 3 Published values of urine LTE_4 levels in asthmatics before and after allergen challenge. Urine was collected for 3–4 hours postallergen in all studies except Study 4, in which urine was collected for 12 hours. All studies except Study 3 (direct immunoassay of urine) utilized HPLC purification and immunoassay quantification in their methodology. Study 5 separated subjects into three groups based on the airway response to the allergen. IAR refers to subjects having an isolated immediate response only, LAR refers to asthmatics having an isolated late response only, and IAR + LAR refers to subjects having both an immediate and late response. In all cases, urinary LTE_4 levels were significantly higher post– compared to pre– allergen challenge. The study numbers refer to the following references: Study 1 (102), 2 (104), 3 (114), 4 (108), 5 (120), 6 (122), 7 (149), 8 (154), and 9 (156).

finding of elevated LTE_4 excretion in urine following allergen challenge nicely complements similar studies which have found elevated leukotrienes in BALF or nasal secretions following allergen challenge.

Many of these studies examined the potential relationship between the magnitude of the bronchoconstriction after allergen challenge and the magnitude of the increase in urinary LTE_4 excretion. Taylor et al. (123) found no significant correlation between urinary LTE_4 and airflow obstruction. Similar findings have been reported by other research groups. Such a lack of correlation may be misleadingly false considering the time-integrated nature of urinary collection, which may not be reflective of lung function at a single time. It is also important to realize that each person has a specific sensitivity to leukotrienes which will influence the relationship of airways FEV_1 and the amount of lung leukotrienes. Westcott et al. (108) showed that when airways reactivity was factored in, there was a significant correlation between the fall in FEV_1 and the increase in urinary LTE_4 following allergen challenge. Other research groups (120) have also found a positive relationship between these events.

In contrast to the well-characterized increase in urinary LTE_4 in the first few hours after allergen challenge, there does not appear to be a large increase in urinary LTE_4 associated with bronchoconstriction occurring during the late response. Westcott et al. (108) found that late urinary excretion of LTE_4 (12–24 hours after allergen challenge) was marginally increased in those asthmatics that had the largest late asthmatic responses. Manning et al. (120) found that urinary LTE_4 6–7 hours after allergen challenge was still elevated, but to a much smaller degree than during the early response. O'Sullivan et al. (124) reported increased urinary LTE_4 excretion during the late asthmatic response, but it was not apparent how the increase compared to airways physiology. This later allergen invoked bronchoconstriction is characterized by eosinophil and T-lymphocyte infiltration and activation and the development of heightened airway reactivity. It is not clear whether de novo leukotriene synthesis occurring in cells such as eosinophils recruited to the airways is responsible for late airways responses or whether it is an end organ response to leukotrienes produced earlier from mast cell activation.

Exercise is a common stimulus of bronchoconstriction in asthmatic subjects, although the exact pathogenic sequence of events remains unclear. One proposed mechanism involves mast cell mediator release secondary to respiratory water loss and hyperosmolar provocation. Bronchoconstriction invoked by hyperventilation of cold dry air is believed to share the same mechanism. Data relating to the participation of leukotrienes in either the maintenance or induction of the bronchoconstriction evoked by exercise are conflicting. Two studies have shown no increase in urinary LTE_4 following exercise challenge (122,125). In contrast, a study in children did show a modest (less than twofold) increase in urine LTE_4 after exercise (126). However, the most compelling evidence for a role of leukotrienes in exercise-induced asthma are studies showing amelioration of the airflow limitation either by selective blockade of the 5-lipoxygenase enzyme (127) or the leukotriene receptors (128–131).

The role of the ether-linked alkyl phospholipid platelet-activating factor (PAF) in asthma has attracted much attention, although its precise role in asthma pathogenesis is unclear. PAF is capable of reproducing many of the functional and histological features seen in asthma both in vivo and in vitro including microvascular leakage, bronchoconstriction, and inflammatory cell activation. Despite causing bronchoconstriction following inhalation in humans (132,133), PAF does not possess direct contractile effects on human airway smooth muscle strips in cell-free media in vitro (134), suggesting that this function in vivo may be mediated indirectly through the release of other bronchoconstricting agents. Leukotriene synthesis in response to PAF has been described from a number of animal preparations and purified human cells in vitro. Inhalational challenge with PAF has been shown to increase urinary LTE_4 10-fold in comparison to methacholine or isotonic saline (135). In addition, the oral PAF receptor antagonist UK 74505 significantly attenuated PAF-invoked rises in urinary LTE_4 excretion (136). Further support for a direct contributory role of cysteinyl-leukotrienes in the airway response to PAF is that leukotriene receptor antagonists decreased PAF-induced bronchoconstriction (137,138).

Some asthmatics are intolerant of aspirin and other nonsteroidal anti-inflammatory drugs, with the induction of asthma symptoms typically being related to the dose and potency of the inhibitors (113,114). A large increase in urinary LTE_4 excretion has been observed in aspirin-sensitive asthmatic subjects following either oral or inhalational challenge. The etiology of this phenomena remains obscure. One historic hypothesis is that inhibition of cyclooxygenase provokes bronchoconstriction via shunting of arachidonic acid toward metabolism by lipoxygenase. However, the study by Sladek et al. (104) found that allergen challenge in the presence of indomethacin did not further enhance allergen-invoked bronchoconstriction or urinary LTE_4 excretion, making ''shunting'' less likely. Furthermore, Knapp et al. (139) found that the magnitude of the increase in urinary LTE_4 following aspirin was not correlated with the degree of inhibition of platelet TXB_2 or the duration and magnitude of airflow obstruction.

Histological evidence following endobronchial provocation with lysine-aspirin suggests that susceptible aspirin-sensitive asthmatics have increased numbers of activated eosinophils and degranulated mast cells within the airway mucosa in comparison to aspirin-tolerant subjects (116). Since these cells are abundant sources of cysteinyl-leukotrienes, they may be the sources of the leukotrienes generated following aspirin challenge. It is also likely that the cells that generate leukotrienes are activated not only in the lung, but throughout the body (115). The mechanism of activation remains unclear, but may in some way involve decreases in levels of PGE_2. PGE_2 administration prior to allergen challenge has been shown to diminish the resulting airway obstruction as well as the increase in urinary LTE_4. Whatever the mechanism, in these aspirin-intolerant asthmatics administration of a nonsteroidal anti-inflammatory drug causes cellular activation, which stimulates PLA_2 to release arachidonic acid and stimulates 5-LO to generate leukotrienes. This release of large amounts of arachidonic acid may also result in a paradoxical increase in synthesis of PGD_2. Evidence of this has been observed in BALF collected following indomethacin challenge of aspirin-intolerant asthmatics where both cysteinyl leukotrienes and PGD_2 (but not other cyclooxygenase products) were increased (64,65).

Methacholine, a direct-acting cholinergic agonist, has been utilized to cause bronchoconstriction for comparative purposes in studies involving allergen (108), exercise (125), PAF (135), or adenosine (140) challenges. Without exception, methacholine administration did not significantly perturb urinary LTE_4 excretion when compared to either negative bronchoconstrictor challenges such as isotonic saline or prechallenge basal levels. Similarly, bronchial challenge of asthmatic patients with histamine did not increase urinary LTE_4 levels (114). This suggests that activation of cells, such as mast cells and eosinophils, is necessary for leukotrienes to be produced rather than only bronchoconstriction itself.

C. Pharmacological Modulation of Endogenously Synthesized Leukotrienes

A variety of drugs have been utilized in traditional asthma therapy, with β_2 agonists and steroids being the most widely used. There are also new pharmacological agents that directly affect leukotriene synthesis or actions that have proven useful in modulating the symptoms of asthma. Some of the studies utilizing these drugs and comparing the effects on leukotriene levels and asthma symptoms are reviewed below.

β_2-Selective agonists are by far the most effective bronchodilators in clinical use and are ubiquitous functional antagonists to all direct and indirect spasmogens delivered to the human airway. Although reversal of airway smooth muscle contraction represents their principal mode of action, considerable in vitro evidence suggests additional properties including attenuation of inflammatory cell mediator release (141). In a placebo-controlled comparative study in atopic subjects, the effects of single-dose inhalation of salbutamol (200 μg) or salmetrol (50 μg) were evaluated on allergen-induced bronchoconstriction, hyperreactivity, and increase in urinary LTE_4 excretion (141). Although there were clearly beneficial effects on airway physiology and airway reactivity over the 4-hour period of study by both β_2 agonists, neither drug attenuated the rise in urinary LTE_4 when compared to placebo. The authors concluded that while β_2 agonists are potent inhibitors of cysteinyl-leukotriene generation in vitro, this inhibition may not occur to a significant extent after single-dose inhalation in vivo. Furthermore, although pulmonary mast cells do possess β_2 adrenergic receptors, functionally and quantitatively the most important action of inhaled β_2 agonists in asthmatics is relaxation of airway smooth muscle rather than inhibition of mast cell degranulation.

Glucocorticoids represent the mainstay of current asthma therapy. Current guidelines (142) recommend their use as first-line disease-modifying therapy in all but the mildest of asthmatics. Steroids have potent anti-inflammatory properties on cells in vitro and in vivo and consistently attenuate heightened bronchial reactivity, a surrogate marker of airway inflammation and a cardinal feature of the asthmatic condition. With regards to leukotriene synthetic cells involved in asthma, glucocorticoids do not appear to inhibit leukotriene synthesis but instead cause a reduction in pulmonary mast cells with chronic administration. The net effect is a reduction of the local concentration of mast cell mediators in the airways. Similarly, steroids inhibit adherence and chemotaxis of eosinophils ex vivo without affecting the ability of these cells to synthesize LTC_4 after stimulation with ionophore.

Several studies have examined the effects of steroid administration on urinary LTE_4 excretion in both healthy volunteers and asthmatics. In two studies in healthy subjects (143,144) the administration of dexamethasone (8 mg/day for 2 days), inhaled budesonide (1.6 mg/day for 7 days), or prednisolone (60 mg/day for 7 days or 30 mg/day for 3 days) had no effect on urinary LTE_4 excretion. However, budesonide did reduce ex vivo thromboxane generation in zymosan-stimulated peripheral monocytes, and prednisolone administration decreased all eicosanoids in macrophage-rich BAL cells, suggesting a possible effect on arachidonate metabolism in these cells. Two additional placebo-controlled studies in asthmatics evaluated the modulating effect of chronically administered steroids on the allergen-invoked rise in urinary LTE_4 excretion. In the first (I.K. Taylor, unpublished data), pretreatment for one week prior to allergen challenge with 1.6 mg/day of budesonide derivatives attenuated the early and late allergen-induced bronchoconstriction without decreasing urinary LTE_4 excretion. In the second study (145), inhalational administration of 1 mg/day fluticasone dipropionate for 2 weeks prior to allergen challenge predictably reduced baseline airway reactivity, acute allergen-induced hyperreactivity, and early- and late-phase bronchoconstriction. Similar to the first study, steroid treatment had no inhibitory effect on the allergen-induced increase in urinary excretion of LTE_4. These in vivo data complement the ex vivo data and suggest that the disease modifying anti-inflammatory properties of the steroids relate to their modulation of cytokine networks rather than a direct action upon the metabolism of arachidonic acid.

Mechanistic strategies for inhibition of leukotriene synthesis have included inhibition of 5-lipoxygenase–activating protein (FLAP) or inhibition of 5-lipoxygenase. The activation of both enzymes are required for leukotriene synthesis in vivo (146,147). Although clinical trials utilizing FLAP inhibitors have been discontinued, early studies with MK-886 (148) and MK-0591 (149) showed that these drugs were effective in decreasing early and late allergen-induced bronchoconstriction as well as decreasing urinary LTE_4 excretion. However, the FLAP inhibitors were ineffective in attenuating the allergen-induced airway hyperresponsiveness.

Early efforts to examine the efficacy of 5-lipoxygenase inhibitors failed to show any therapeutic benefit (150–152), but they also failed to provide evidence of adequate enzyme blockade. Two recent studies have also failed to find beneficial effects of 5-lipoxygenase inhibitors (153,154). Both studies used only a single administration of inhibitor (zileuton or ZD2138) given 3–4 hours prior to allergen challenge, and both studies reported a 50% decrease in urine LTE_4 concentration. The lack of clinical effect of these inhibitors may have related to insufficient inhibition of 5-lipoxygenase.

Most recent studies utilizing 5-lipoxygenase inhibitors in asthmatics have shown therapeutic benefit. Zileuton (A64077), an oral *N*-hydroxamic 5-lipoxygenase inhibitor, was recently approved by FDA for the treatment of asthma (155). Zileuton treatment has been shown to ameliorate the bronchoconstriction produced by cold dry air (127), to produce acute bronchodilatory effects in moderately severe asthmatics (107), and to almost entirely prevent the effects of aspirin challenge in aspirin-intolerant asthmatics (115). Kane et al. (156) reported that 8 days of zileuton treatment prior to segmental allergen challenge resulted in an 86% decrease in urinary LTE_4 excretion and a reduction of eosinophil migration into the airways. This magnitude of urinary LTE_4 inhibition is higher than what is normally found, and it should be noted that the urinary LTE_4 values both pre- and postsegmental allergen challenge were also 10-fold higher than what is typically reported. In another small study with asthmatics, zileuton decreased LTB_4 levels in lavage fluid and urinary LTE_4 levels while showing a trend for improving nocturnal FEV_1 and reducing BAL and blood eosinophils (153).

Studies similar to those utilizing 5-lipoxygenase inhibitors have been performed with peptidoleukotriene receptor antagonists. Numerous recent studies have demonstrated their inhibition of bronchoconstriction induced by aspirin (157,158), PAF (137,138), allergen (157–162), and exercise challenge (128–131). It is not clear whether these drugs attenuate the allergen-invoked bronchial hyperresponsiveness, as conflicting results have been found (158,162). Several studies have examined urinary LTE_4 excretion following bronchial provocation following leukotriene receptor antagonist administration. O'Shaughnessy et al. (158), Rasmussen et al. (161), and Rasmussen et al. (163) predictably found no decrease in the enhanced urinary LTE_4 excretion following allergen challenge in the presence of leukotriene receptor antagonists.

D. Urinary Leukotrienes in Other Diseases

Although the main focus of many studies has been on leukotrienes and asthma, leukotrienes have been measured in other allergic diseases, pulmonary diseases, and nonpulmonary inflammatory diseases. Urinary LTE_4 was measured in patients with atopic dermatitis and found to be 4.5-fold higher than in healthy control patients (99). Urinary LTE_4 and *n*-acetyl LTE_4 were also measured in nine patients with anaphylaxis, a systemic life-threatening allergic reaction (164). These patients had maximum urinary leukotrienes of 68–324 nmol/mol creatinine compared to 7–25 in healthy subjects. After recovery from anaphylaxis, urinary LTE_4 returned to the normal range. Taylor et al. (102) measured LTE_4 excretion in 24-hour urine collections from allergic rhinitic patients studied in the grass pollen season and found no increase in LTE_4 compared to a period out of pollen season. However, other researchers have reported increased levels of LTC_4 in nasopharyngeal secretions of children during seasonal exposure to ragweed allergen (77). Thus, transient high local concentrations of peptidoleukotrienes in the nose following appropriate challenge do not perturb whole body LTE_4 excretion, particularly if assessed over long periods. These disparate findings in urinary LTE_4 excretion between rhinitis and acute severe asthma may simply reflect differences in the magnitude of the inflammatory insult and the inflammatory cell burden in the nose compared to the lower airways of the lung.

Urinary leukotrienes have also been measured in other nonasthma lung diseases including chronic lung disease in premature newborns, upper respiratory tract infections in infants, acute respiratory distress syndrome (ARDS), and mountain sickness/hypoxia. In babies with chronic lung disease associated with extreme prematurity, urinary LTE_4 levels were elevated more than fivefold compared with premature infants without lung disease (165). In wheezy infants or infants with upper respiratory tract infections, urinary LTE_4 excretion was not elevated (166). In patients with ARDS, very high levels of urinary LTE_4 were found (167,168). However, elevated levels may be due to a variety of factors in addition to increased synthesis. These factors include liver and renal dysfunction, both of which will alter metabolism of leukotrienes. Roach et al. (169) measured urinary LTE_4 before and after exposure to high altitude. Urinary LTE_4 excretion doubled after 1.5 days at 4300 m, and the authors hypothesized a potential role of leukotrienes in acute mountain sickness. Kaminsky et al. (170) measured urinary LTE_4 in healthy control patients and patients experiencing high-altitude pulmonary edema at low altitude and moderate altitude ($\geq$2727 m). This study found increased urinary leukotrienes in patients with high-altitude pulmonary edema compared to the same patients after returning to low altitude or to healthy subjects at high altitude. These authors speculate that physical exertion and use of nonsteroidal inflammatory drugs may have contributed to the increased leukotrienes and the observed symptoms of high-altitude sickness.

Leukotrienes have been associated with a variety of nonpulmonary diseases through measurement of high urinary LTE_4 levels. Hackshaw et al. (171) found that urinary LTE_4 levels in patients with systemic lupus erythematosus (SLE) were elevated two- to fourfold compared to healthy controls. These high urine LTE_4 levels were associated with active disease, while persons with inactive disease had normal LTE_4 levels. In a second study (172), patients with lupus received 600 mg of zileuton qid or placebo for 8 weeks. At the end of 8 weeks, patients on zileuton showed a small clinical improvement as determined by a significant decrease in the Systemic Lupus Activity Measure compared to initial measurements. However, urinary LTE_4 levels only decreased 20–40% in the patients on zileuton, which may not have been large enough to allow more significant improvement of symptoms. It is not clear why inhibition of urinary LTE_4 was not greater, but this finding stresses the importance of actually measuring urinary LTE_4 to demonstrate the effectiveness of an inhibitor. Juvenile rheumatoid arthritis is another disease that affects joints. A threefold elevation in urinary LTE_4 was found in children with this disease compared to healthy children (173). There was a slight nonsignificant positive relationship between urinary LTE_4 levels and the number of affected joints ($r = 0.49$, $p = 0.15$).

Altered urinary LTE_4 excretion has also been observed in several other pathological conditions. Kim et al. (174) reported a three- to fourfold increase in LTE_4 levels in children with active Crohn's disease, with the magnitude of the urinary LTE_4 elevation correlating with clinical markers of mucosal inflammation. Carry et al. (175) reported that urinary LTE_4 excretion was increased four- to fivefold in patients with acute myocardial infarction or unstable angina. Allen et al. (176) also found increased urinary LTE_4 excretion in patients with coronary artery disease, which increased further 2 days following coronary bypass surgery. Fauler et al. (177) found a fourfold increase in patients with psoriasis. Mayatepek et al. (178) examined LTE_4 excretion in children with a variety of pathologies. They reported a greater than 10-fold increase in urinary LTE_4 excretion in patients with mevalonate kinase deficiency, although this increase could largely be caused by associated hepatosplenomegaly altering leukotriene excretion rather than increased leukotriene synthesis (178). A similar increase in urinary LTE_4 excretion was found in children with kwashiorkor in which protein energy malnutrition is manifested as edema and skin lesions (179). Children with Kawasaki disease, an acute multisystem vasculitis, also had urinary LTE_4 levels five times higher than healthy children (180). Finally, two children with glutathione synthetase deficiency were studied and found to have only 2% of the urinary LTE_4 excretion as healthy children (181).

In connection with the treatment of diseases rather than diseases themselves, several recent studies have investigated the role of cytokine therapy or dietary modification on urinary LTE_4 excretion. Urinary LTE_4 excretion was measured in 21 healthy subjects treated with 0.7 nmol/kg body weight of human recombinant GM-CSF (103). This is a cytokine that has been utilized in recent clinical trials involving myelosuppression and impaired host defense. Investigations in vitro have shown that this cytokine stimulates leukotriene synthesis in eosinophils and neutrophils. In this in vivo study, GM-CSF increased urinary LTE_4 excretion over 24 hours 1.3- to 44-fold. These data suggest that leukotrienes may play a significant role in GM-CSF action in vivo, especially regarding the untoward effects of this cytokine. In contrast, the cytokine G-CSF given in vivo to tumor patients actually decreased urinary LTE_4 levels (182). Dietary supplementation with fish oil or vitamin E was also found to reduce urinary LTE_4 excretion in healthy subjects (183).

VII. Conclusions

The cysteinyl-leukotrienes are thought to play a role in a wide variety of inflammatory diseases. The evidence for leukotriene involvement usually begins with their being able to reproduce many of the functional and histological features of the disease. Further involvement of leukotrienes is indicated by increased levels of leukotrienes found in biological fluids either at the site of origin or at the site of elimination from the body (urine). Recent development of pharmaceutical tools such as receptor antagonists and synthesis inhibitors have also been important in linking leukotrienes with diseases. It should be emphasized that in most cases, there is no single inflammatory mediator responsible for all the clinical and pathological manifestations of a disease and that the leukotrienes are but one of several important contributors.

One strategy adopted to clarify the role of leukotrienes in disease has been the extensive utilization of urinary measurements of LTE_4, and much of these data have been reviewed in this chapter. There is little doubt that urinary measurements for the in vivo assessment of leukotriene release possess inherent advantages over more invasive means of evaluation. However, a number of disadvantages are apparent and should be considered. First, urine is a complex mixture, therefore analytical methodology is very crucial in generating good data. This means that in most instances, urine must be concentrated and purified prior to quantitation by immunoassay. Second, it is important to interpret the data correctly. Urinary leukotriene measurements are made distal from the site of production and their putative end organ site of action. Indeed, the nature of urinary measurements is by inference an assessment of whole body production and may not necessarily relate to or be exclusively derived from that part of the body where a physiological response is observed. It should be remembered that only a small percentage (5–7%) of leukotrienes produced in the body is excreted as LTE_4 in urine, so anything that significantly changes metabolism can affect urinary levels of LTE_4. Similarly, increased kidney production of leukotrienes can result in elevated levels of urinary LTE_4 that do not accurately relate to total body synthesis of leukotrienes.

Correct interpretation of data is also fundamentally important when invoking mechanistic roles of leukotrienes in mediating specific symptoms. Often a physiological response is a result of multiple mediators or other independent events and not just solely due to leukotrienes. It is also not just the amount of leukotriene synthesized that is important, but also the responsiveness of a person to the leukotriene. For example, asthmatics have enhanced airways sensitivity to a wide variety of compounds and stimuli. But even among asthmatics there is a large variability in the sensitivity of the airways to leukotrienes such that a given amount of leukotrienes may produce extensive bronchoconstriction in some but little effect in others.

Measurement of urinary LTE_4 has been and will continue to be important in clinical studies with 5-lipoxygenase inhibitors, where it is utilized to demonstrate the effectiveness of inhibition. It has been a common feature of inhibitor studies that stimulated LTB_4 synthesis in blood is often inhibited by more than 90%, while urinary LTE_4 is inhibited by only 40–60%. The reason for this discrepancy is not clear but may involve problems with the inhibitors getting into the body compartments that synthesize peptidoleukotrienes. If this is true, it suggests that the role of leukotrienes has been underestimated and that increased bioavailability of inhibitors could further reduce leukotrienes synthesized at the sites where they produce pathological actions. This has also given rise to the suggestion that a combination of a synthesis inhibitor and a receptor antagonist might provide more benefit than either drug given alone.

The usefulness of urinary LTE_4 measurements in asthma for predicting potential responders for antileukotriene therapy is unclear. Asthma is a heterogeneous disease which includes a variety of subgroups in which the extent of leukotriene participation can differ. It is possible that the presence of such subgroups could be established and described by utilizing urinary LTE_4 levels. For example, aspirin-intolerant asthmatics have increased basal synthesis of leukotrienes, which appear to substantially mediate the symptoms observed following ingestion of nonsteroidal anti-inflammatory drugs. Most of the studies utilizing pharmacological intervention with leukotriene receptor antagonists or inhibitors have utilized mild asthmatics, and it is unclear how beneficial these inhibitors will prove to be with more severe asthmatics and steroid-resistant asthmatics. Finally, the role of leukotrienes in the initiation and progression of asthma in children has not been well studied and could be further illuminated by measurements of urinary leukotrienes.

Leukotrienes could conceivably mediate symptoms in a wide variety of inflammatory diseases. The potential involvement of leukotrienes in psoriasis, juvenile rheumatoid arthritis, systemic lupus, and Crohn's disease has been studied by measurement of urinary LTE_4. It is likely that other diseases will also be detected that involve elevated leukotriene synthesis by utilizing the determination of levels of urinary LTE_4.

References

1. Barnes PJ, Chung KF, Page CP. Inflammatory mediators and asthma. Pharmacol Rev 1988; 40:49–84.
2. Lewis RA, Austen KF, Soberman RJ. Leukotrienes and other products of the 5-lipoxygenase pathway. Biochemistry and relation to pathobiology in human diseases. N Engl J Med 1990; 323:645–655.
3. Arm JP, Lee TH. Sulphidopeptide leukotrienes in asthma. Clin Sci 1993; 84:501–510.

4. Henderson WR, Jr. The role of leukotrienes in inflammation. Ann Intern Med 1994; 121:684–697.
5. Pauwels RA, Joos GF, Kips JC. Leukotrienes as therapeutic target in asthma. Allergy 1995; 50:615–622.
6. Holgate ST, Bradding P, Sampson AP. Leukotriene antagonists and synthesis inhibitors: new directions in asthma therapy. J Allergy Clin Immunol 1996; 98:1–13.
7. Busse WW. The role of leukotrienes in asthma and allergic rhinitis. Clin Exp Allergy 1996; 26:868–879.
8. Lam BK, Owen WF, Jr., Austen KF, Soberman RJ. The identification of a distinct export step following the biosynthesis of leukotriene C4 by human eosinophils. J Biol Chem 1989; 264:12885–12889.
9. Bisgaard H, Ford-Hutchinson AW, Charleson S, Taudorf E. Production of leukotrienes in human skin and conjunctival mucosa after specific allergen challenge. Allergy 1985; 40:417–423.
10. Atkins PC, Zweiman B, Littman B, Presti C, von Allmen C, Moskovitz A, Eskra JD. Products of arachidonic acid metabolism and the effects of cyclooxygenase inhibition on ongoing cutaneous allergic reactions in human beings. J Allergy Clin Immunol 1995; 95:742–747.
11. Hommes DW, Meenan J, de Haas M, ten Kate FJ, von dem Borne AE, Tytgat GN, van Deventer SJ. Soluble Fc gamma receptor III (CD 16) and eicosanoid concentrations in gut lavage fluid from patients with inflammatory bowel disease: reflection of mucosal inflammation. Gut 1996; 38:564–567.
12. Koshihara Y, Isono T, Oda H, Karube S, Hayashi Y. Measurement of sulfidopeptide leukotrienes and their metabolism in human synovial fluid of patients with rheumatoid arthritis. Prostaglandins Leukotrienes Essential Fatty Acids 1988; 32:113–119.
13. Moilanen E. Prostanoids and leukotrienes in rheumatoid synovitis. Pharmacol Toxicol 1994; 75:4–8.
14. Jung TT. Prostaglandins, leukotrienes, and other arachidonic acid metabolites in the pathogenesis of otitis media. Laryngoscope 1988; 98:980–993.
15. Haupts M, Smektala K, Finkbeiner T, Simmet T, Gehlen W. Immunoreactive leukotriene C4 levels in CSF of MS patients. Acta Neurol Scand 1992; 85:365–367.
16. Richter L, Hesselbarth N, Eitner K, Bosseckert H, Krell H. Increased biliary secretion of cysteinyl-leukotrienes in human bile duct obstruction. J Hepatol 1996; 25: 725–732.
17. Kuo CG, Lewis MT, Jakschik BA. Leukotriene D4 and E4 formation by plasma membrane bound enzymes. Prostaglandins 1984; 28:929–938.
18. Anderson ME, Allison RD, Meister A. Interconversion of leukotrienes catalyzed by purified gamma-glutamyl transpeptidase: concomitant formation of leukotriene D4 and gamma-glutamyl amino acids. Proc Natl Acad Sci USA 1982; 79:1088–1091.
19. Campbell BJ, Baker SF, Shukla SD, Forrester LJ, Zahler WL. Bioconversion of leukotriene D4 by lung dipeptidase. Biochim Biophys Acta 1990; 1042:107–112.
20. Uemura M, Buchholz U, Kojima H, Keppler A, Hafkemeyer P, Fukui H, Tsujii T, Keppler D. Cysteinyl leukotrienes in the urine of patients with liver diseases. Hepatology 1994; 20:804–812.
21. Huber M, Muller J, Leier I, Jedlitschky G, Ball HA, Moore KP, Taylor GW, Wil-

liams R, Keppler D. Metabolism of cysteinyl leukotrienes in monkey and man. Eur J Biochem 1990; 194:309–315.

22. Kumlin M, Stensvad F, Larsson L, Dahlen B, Dahlen SE. Validation and application of a new simple strategy for measurements of urinary leukotriene E4 in humans. Clin Exp Allergy 1995; 25:467–479.
23. Fauler J, Tsikas D, Holch M, Seekamp A, Nerlich ML, Sturm J, Frolich JC. Enhanced urinary excretion of leukotriene E4 by patients with multiple trauma with or without adult respiratory distress syndrome. Clin Sci (Colch) 1991; 80:497–504.
24. Lam S, Chan H, LeRiche JC, Chan-Yeung M, Salari H. Release of leukotrienes in patients with bronchial asthma. J Allergy Clin Immunol 1988; 81:711–717.
25. Chan-Yeung M, Chan H, Tse KS, Salari H, Lam S. Histamine and leukotriene release in bronchoalveolar fluid during plicatic acid-induced bronchoconstriction. J Allergy Clin Immunol 1989; 84:762–768.
26. Zakrzewski JT, Sampson AP, Evans JM, Barnes NC, Piper PJ, Costello JF. The biotransformation in vitro of cysteinyl leukotrienes in blood of normal and asthmatic subjects. Prostaglandins 1989; 37:425–444.
27. Ishikawa T, Muller M, Klunemann C, Schaub T, Keppler D. ATP-dependent primary active transport of cysteinyl leukotrienes across liver canalicular membrane. Role of the ATP-dependent transport system for glutathione S-conjugates. J Biol Chem 1990; 265:19279–19286.
28. Maltby NH, Taylor GW, Ritter JM, Moore K, Fuller RW, Dollery CT. Leukotriene C4 elimination and metabolism in man. J Allergy Clin Immunol 1990; 85:3–9.
29. Kumlin M. Analytical methods for the measurement of leukotrienes and other eicosanoids in biologic samples from asthmatic subjects. J Chromatogr A 1996; 725: 29–40.
30. Shindo K, Matsumoto Y, Matsumura M, Okubo T. Leukotriene E4 levels in the arterial blood of asthmatic patients during an attack of wheezing. Current Ther Res 1990; 47:285–291.
31. Shindo K, Matsumoto Y, Sumitomo M, Matsumura M, Okubo T. Measurement of leukotriene C4 and D4 in arterial blood of asthmatic patients during remission. Ann Allergy 1991; 66:405–410.
32. Shindo K, Matsumoto Y, Matsumura M, Sumitoma M, Okubo T. Leukotriene E4 in arterial blood of asthmatic patients during remission. Current Ther Res 1991; 50:1–9.
33. Shindo K, Fukumura M. Effect of oral prednisolone on plasma levels of leukotriene E4 in asthmatic patients during a wheezing attack. A pilot study. Current Ther Res 1992; 52:916–921.
34. Shindo K, Fukumura M, Miyakawa K. Plasma levels of leukotriene E4 during clinical course of bronchial asthma and the effect of oral prednisolone. Chest 1994; 105:1038–1041.
35. Shindo K, Fukumura M. Relationship between plasma levels of leukotriene E4 and arterial partial pressure of carbon dioxide in asthmatic patients. Current Ther Res 1993; 54:366–370.
36. Shindo K, Fukumura M. Relationship between plasma levels of leukotriene E4 and FEV1 in asthmatic patients. Current Ther Res 1993; 53:285–290.
37. Piperno D, Pacheco Y, Hosni R, Moliere P, Gharib C, Lagarde M, Perrin-Fayolle

M. Increased plasma levels of atrial natriuretic factor, renin activity, and leukotriene C4 in chronic obstructive pulmonary disease. Chest 1993; 104:454–459.
38. Ibe BO, Kurantsin-Mills J, Raj JU, Lessin LS. Plasma and urinary leukotrienes in sickle cell disease: possible role in the inflammatory process. Eur J Clin Invest 1994; 24:57–64.
39. Isono T, Koshihara Y, Murota S, Fukuda Y, Furukawa S. Measurement of immunoreactive leukotriene C4 in blood of asthmatic children. Biochem Biophys Res Commun 1985; 130:486–492.
40. Schwartzberg SB, Shelov SP, Van Praag D. Blood leukotriene levels during the acute asthma attack in children. Prostaglandins Leukotrienes Med 1987; 26:143–155.
41. Kilburn KH. Alveolar microenvironment. Arch Intern Med 1970; 126:435–449.
42. Van Vyve T, Chanez P, Bousquet J, Lacoste JY, Michel FB, Godard P. Safety of bronchoalveolar lavage and bronchial biopsies in patients with asthma of variable severity. Am Rev Respir Dis 1992; 146:116–121.
43. Walters EH, Gardiner PV. Bronchoalveolar lavage as a research tool. Thorax 1991; 46:613–618.
44. Rennard SI, Basset G, Lecossier D, O'Donnell KM, Pinkston P, Martin PG, Crystal RG. Estimation of volume of epithelial lining fluid recovered by lavage using urea as marker of dilution. J Appl Physiol 1986; 60:532–538.
45. Stenmark KR, James SL, Voelkel NF, Toews WH, Reeves JT, Murphy RC. Leukotriene C4 and D4 in neonates with hypoxemia and pulmonary hypertension. N Engl J Med 1983; 309:77–80.
46. Westcott JY, Balazy M, Stenmark KR, Murphy RC. Analysis of leukotriene D4 in human lung lavage by HPLC, RIA and mass spectrometry. Adv Prostaglandin Thromboxane Leukotriene Res 1986; 16:353–61.
47. Westcott JY, Stenmark KR, Murphy RC. Analysis of leukotriene B4 in human lung lavage by HPLC and mass spectrometry. Prostaglandins 1986; 31:227–237.
48. Mirro R, Armstead W, Leffler C. Increased airway leukotriene levels in infants with severe bronchopulmonary dysplasia. Am J Dis Child 1990; 144:160–161.
49. Dobyns EL, Westcott JY, Kennaugh JM, Ross MN, Stenmark KR. Eicosanoids decrease with successful extracorporeal membrane oxygenation therapy in neonatal pulmonary hypertension. Am J Respir Crit Care Med 1994; 149:873–880.
50. Matthay MA, Eschenbacher WL, Goetzl EJ. Elevated concentrations of leukotriene D4 in pulmonary edema fluid of patients with the adult respiratory distress syndrome. J Clin Immunol 1984; 4:479–483.
51. Stephenson AH, Lonigro AJ, Hyers TM, Webster RO, Fowler AA. Increased concentrations of leukotrienes in bronchoalveolar lavage fluid of patients with ARDS or at risk for ARDS. Am Rev Respir Dis 1988; 138:714–719.
52. Zijlstra FJ, Vincent JE, van den Berg B, Hoogsteden HC, Neyens HJ, van Dongen JJ. Pulmonary alveolar proteinosis: determination of prostaglandins and leukotrienes in lavage fluid. Lung 1987; 165:79–89.
53. Murray JJ, Tonnel AB, Brash AR, Roberts LJ, Gosset P, Workman R, Capron A, Oates JA. Release of prostaglandin D2 into human airways during acute antigen challenge. N Engl J Med 1986; 315:800–804.
54. Miadonna A, Tedeschi A, Leggieri E, Brasca C, Folco GC, Sala A, Froldi M, Za-

nussi C. Mediators and allergic inflammation of human airways. Respiration 1988; 54:78–83.

55. Wardlaw AJ, Hay H, Cromwell O, Collins JV, Kay AB. Leukotrienes, LTC_4 and LTB_4, in bronchoalveolar lavage in bronchial asthma and other respiratory diseases. J Allergy Clin Immunol 1989; 84:19–26.
56. Broide DH, Eisman S, Ramsdell JW, Ferguson P, Schwartz LB, Wasserman SI. Airway levels of mast cell-derived mediators in exercise-induced asthma. Am Rev Respir Dis 1990; 141:563–568.
57. Diaz P, Gonzalez MC, Galleguillos FR, Ancic P, Cromwell O, Shepherd D, Durham SR, Gleich GJ, Kay AB. Leukocytes and mediators in bronchoalveolar lavage during allergen-induced late-phase asthmatic reactions. Am Rev Respir Dis 1989; 139: 1383–1389.
58. Wenzel SE, Larsen GL, Johnston K, Voelkel NF, Westcott JY. Elevated levels of leukotriene C4 in bronchoalveolar lavage fluid from atopic asthmatics after endobronchial allergen challenge. Am Rev Respir Dis 1990; 142:112–119.
59. Crea AE, Nakhosteen JA, Lee TH. Mediator concentrations in bronchoalveolar lavage fluid of patients with mild asymptomatic bronchial asthma. Eur Respir J 1992; 5:190–195.
60. Wenzel SE, Trudeau JB, Kaminsky DA, Cohn J, Martin RJ, Westcott JY. Effect of 5-lipoxygenase inhibition on bronchoconstriction and airway inflammation in nocturnal asthma. Am J Respir Crit Care Med 1995; 152:897–905.
61. Dworski R, Fitzgerald GA, Oates JA, Sheller JR. Effect of oral prednisone on airway inflammatory mediators in atopic asthma. Am J Respir Crit Care Med 1994; 149:953–959.
62. Oosterhoff Y, Kauffman HF, Rutgers B, Zijlstra FJ, Koeter GH, Postma DS. Inflammatory cell number and mediators in bronchoalveolar lavage fluid and peripheral blood in subjects with asthma with increased nocturnal airways narrowing. J Allergy Clin Immunol 1995; 96:219–229.
63. Sladek K, Dworski R, Soja J, Sheller JR, Nizankowska E, Oates JA, Szczeklik A. Eicosanoids in bronchoalveolar lavage fluid of aspirin-intolerant patients with asthma after aspirin challenge. Am J Respir Crit Care Med 1994; 149:940–946.
64. Szczeklik A, Sladek K, Dworski R, Nizankowska E, Soja J, Sheller J, Oates J. Bronchial aspirin challenge causes specific eicosanoid response in aspirin-sensitive asthmatics. Am J Respir Crit Care Med 1996; 154:1608–1614.
65. Warren MS, Sloan SI, Wenzel SE. Inflammatory cells and mediators increase after endobronchial indomethacin challenge in aspirin-intolerant asthmatics. Am J Respir Crit Care Med Submitted.
66. Pizzichini E, Pizzichini MMM, Efthimiadis A, Evans S, Morris MM, Squillace D, Gleich GJ, Dolovich J, Hargreave FE. Indices of airway inflammation in induced sputum: reproducibility and validity of cell and fluid-phase measurements. Am J Crit Care Med 1996; 154:308–317.
67. Greally P, Cook AJ, Sampson AP, Coleman R, Chambers S, Piper PJ, Price JF. Atopic children with cystic fibrosis have increased urinary leukotriene E4 concentrations and more severe pulmonary disease. J Allergy Clin Immunol 1994; 93: 100–107.

68. Becher G, Beck E, Neubauer G, Stresemann E, Norpoth K, Schutte W, Hummel S, Lichey J. Leukotrienes in breathing condensate released during bronchial challenge test. Am J Respir Crit Care Med 1996; 153:A214.
69. Westcott JY, Voelkel NF, Jones K, Wenzel SE. Inactivation of leukotriene C4 in the airways and subsequent urinary leukotriene E4 excretion in normal and asthmatic subjects. Am Rev Respir Dis 1993; 148:1244–1251.
70. Naclerio RM, Baroody FM, Togias AG. The role of leukotrienes in allergic rhinitis: a review. Am Rev Respir Dis 1991; 143:S91–95.
71. Shaw RJ, Fitzharris P, Cromwell O, Wardlaw AJ, Kay AB. Allergen-induced release of sulphidopeptide leukotrienes (SRS-A) and LTB4 in allergic rhinitis. Allergy 1985; 40:1–6.
72. Miadonna A, Tedeschi A, Leggieri E, Lorini M, Folco G, Sala A, Qualizza R, Froldi M, Zanussi C. Behavior and clinical relevance of histamine and leukotrienes C4 and B4 in grass pollen-induced rhinitis. Am Rev Respir Dis 1987; 136:357–362.
73. Georgitis JW, Stone BD, Gottschlich G. Nasal inflammatory mediator release in ragweed allergic rhinitis: correlation with cellular influx into nasal secretions. Int Arch Allergy Appl Immunol 1991; 96:231–237.
74. Wihl JA, Baumgarten CR, Petersson G. Contralateral differences among biomarkers determined by a modified nasal lavage technique after unilateral antigen challenge. Allergy 1995; 50:308–315.
75. Knapp HR. Reduced allergen-induced nasal congestion and leukotriene synthesis with an orally active 5-lipoxygenase inhibitor. N Engl J Med 1990; 323:1745–1748.
76. Wang D, Clement P, Smitz J, Derde MP. Concentrations of chemical mediators in nasal secretions of patients with hay fever during natural allergen exposure. Acta Otolaryngol (Stockh) 1994; 114:552–555.
77. Volovitz B, Osur SL, Bernstein JM, Ogra PL. Leukotriene C4 release in upper respiratory mucosa during natural exposure to ragweed in ragweed-sensitive children. J Allergy Clin Immunol 1988; 82:414–418.
78. Volovitz B, Faden H, Ogra PL. Release of leukotriene C4 in respiratory tract during acute viral infection. J Pediatr 1988; 112:218–222.
79. Volovitz B, Welliver RC, De Castro G, Krystofik DA, Ogra PL. The release of leukotrienes in the respiratory tract during infection with respiratory syncytial virus: role in obstructive airway disease. Pediatr Res 1988; 24:504–507.
80. Ferreri NR, Howland WC, Stevenson DD, Spiegelberg HL. Release of leukotrienes, prostaglandins, and histamine into nasal secretions of aspirin-sensitive asthmatics during reaction to aspirin. Am Rev Respir Dis 1988; 137:847–854.
81. Picado C, Ramis I, Rosello J, Prat J, Bulbena O, Plaza V, Montserrat JM, Gelpi E. Release of peptide leukotriene into nasal secretions after local instillation of aspirin in aspirin-sensitive asthmatic patients. Am Rev Respir Dis 1992; 145:65–69.
82. Sampson AP, Thomas RU, Costello JF, Piper PJ. Enhanced leukotriene synthesis in leukocytes of atopic and asthmatic subjects. Br J Clin Pharmacol 1992; 33:423–430.
83. Pacheco Y, Hosni R, Chabannes B, Gormand F, Moliere P, Grosclaude M, Piperno

D, Lagarde M, Perrin-Fayolle M. Leukotriene B4 level in stimulated blood neutrophils and alveolar macrophages from healthy and asthmatic subjects. Effect of beta-2 agonist therapy. Eur J Clin Invest 1992; 22:732–739.

84. Restrick LJ, Sampson AP, Piper PJ, Costello JF. Reduction in leukotriene B4 generation by bronchoalveolar lavage cells in asthma. Thorax 1995; 50:67–73.
85. Tenor H, Hatzelmann A, Church MK, Schudt C, Shute JK. Effects of theophylline and rolipram on leukotriene C4 (LTC4) synthesis and chemotaxis of human eosinophils from normal and atopic subjects. Br J Pharmacol 1996; 118:1727–1735.
86. Taniguchi N, Mita H, Saito H, Yui Y, Kajita T, Shida T. Increased generation of leukotriene C4 from eosinophils in asthmatic patients. Allergy 1985; 40:571–573.
87. Schauer U, Eckhart A, Muller R, Gemsa D, Rieger CH. Enhanced leukotriene C4 production by peripheral eosinophilic granulocytes from children with asthma. Int Arch Allergy Appl Immunol 1989; 90:201–206.
88. Roberge CJ, Laviolette M, Boulet LP, Poubelle PE. In vitro leukotriene (LT) C4 synthesis by blood eosinophils from atopic asthmatics: predominance of eosinophil subpopulations with high potency for LTC4 generation. Prostaglandins Leukotriene Essential Fatty Acids 1990; 41:243–249.
89. Shindo K, Hirai Y, Koide K, Sumitomo M, Fukumura M. In vivo effect of prednisolone on release of leukotriene C4 in eosinophils obtained from asthmatic patients. Biochem Biophys Res Commun 1995; 214:869–874.
90. van der Donk EM, Blok W, Kok PT, Bruijnzeel PL. Leukotriene C4 formation by enriched human basophil preparations from normal and asthmatic subjects. Prostaglandins Leukotrienes Essential Fatty Acids 1991; 44:11–17.
91. Dahlen SE, Hansson G, Hedqvist P, Bjorck T, Granstrom E, Dahlen B. Allergen challenge of lung tissue from asthmatics elicits bronchial contraction that correlates with the release of leukotrienes C4, D4, and E4. Proc Natl Acad Sci USA 1983; 80:1712–1716.
92. Wilborn J, Bailie M, Burdick M, Strieter R, Peters-Golden M. Constitutive activation of 5-lipoxygenase in the lungs of patients with idiopathic pulmonary fibrosis. J Clin Invest 1996; 97:1827–1836.
93. Orning L, Kaijser L, Hammarstrom S. In vivo metabolism of leukotriene C4 in man: urinary excretion of leukotriene E4. Biochem Biophys Res Commun 1985; 130:214–220.
94. Sala A, Voelkel N, Maclouf J, Murphy RC. Leukotriene E4 elimination and metabolism in normal human subjects. J Biol Chem 1990; 265:21771–21778.
95. Verhagen J, Bel EH, Kijne GM, Sterk PJ, Bruynzeel PL, Veldink GA, Vliegenthart JF. The excretion of leukotriene E4 into urine following inhalation of leukotriene D4 by human individuals. Biochem Biophys Res Commun 1987; 148:864–868.
96. Mayatepek E, Lehmann WD. Defective hepatobiliary leukotriene elimination in patients with the Dubin-Johnson syndrome. Clin Chim Acta 1996; 249:37–46.
97. Beyer G, Meese CO, Klotz U. Stability of leukotrienes C4 and D4 in human urine. Prostaglandins Leukotrienes Med 1987; 29:229–235.
98. Westcott JY, Johnston K, Batt RA, Wenzel SE, Voelkel NF. Measurement of peptidoleukotrienes in biological fluids. J Appl Physiol 1990; 68:2640–2648.
99. Fauler J, Neumann C, Tsikas D, Frolich J. Enhanced synthesis of cysteinyl leukotrienes in atopic dermatitis. Br J Dermatol 1993; 128:627–630.

100. Westcott JY, Sloan S, Wenzel SE. Immunofiltration purification for urinary leukotriene quantitation. Anal Biochem 1997; 248:202–210.
101. Asano K, Lilly CM, O'Donnell WJ, Israel E, Fischer A, Ransil BJ, Drazen JM. Diurnal variation of urinary leukotriene E4 and histamine excretion rates in normal subjects and patients with mild-to-moderate asthma. J Allergy Clin Immunol 1995; 96:643–651.
102. Taylor GW, Taylor I, Black P, Maltby NH, Turner N, Fuller RW, Dollery CT. Urinary leukotriene E4 after antigen challenge and in acute asthma and allergic rhinitis. Lancet 1989; 1:584–588.
103. Denzlinger C, Tetzloff W, Gerhartz HH, Pokorny R, Sagebiel S, Haberl C, Wilmanns W. Differential activation of the endogenous leukotriene biosynthesis by two different preparations of granulocyte-macrophage colony-stimulating factor in healthy volunteers. Blood 1993; 81:2007–2013.
104. Sladek K, Dworski R, Fitzgerald GA, Buitkus KL, Block FJ, Marney SR, Jr., Sheller JR. Allergen-stimulated release of thromboxane A2 and leukotriene E4 in humans. Effect of indomethacin. Am Rev Respir Dis 1990; 141:1441–1445.
105. Gaddy JN, Margolskee DJ, Bush RK, Williams VC, Busse WW. Bronchodilation with a potent and selective leukotriene D4 (LTD4) receptor antagonist (MK-571) in patients with asthma. Am Rev Respir Dis 1992; 146:358–363.
106. Hui KP, Barnes NC. Lung function improvement in asthma with a cysteinyl-leukotriene receptor antagonist. Lancet 1991; 337:1062–1063.
107. Israel E, Rubin P, Kemp JP, Grossman J, Pierson W, Siegel SC, Tinkelman D, Murray JJ, Busse W, Segal AT, et al. The effect of inhibition of 5-lipoxygenase by zileuton in mild-to-moderate asthma. Ann Intern Med 1993; 119:1059–1066.
108. Westcott JY, Smith HR, Wenzel SE, Larsen GL, Thomas RB, Felsien D, Voelkel NF. Urinary leukotriene E4 in patients with asthma. Effect of airways reactivity and sodium cromoglycate. Am Rev Respir Dis 1991; 143:1322–1328.
109. Smith CM, Hawksworth RJ, Thien FC, Christie PE, Lee TH. Urinary leukotriene E4 in bronchial asthma. Eur Respir J 1992; 5:693–699.
110. Sampson AP, Castling DP, Green CP, Price JF. Persistent increase in plasma and urinary leukotrienes after acute asthma. Arch Dis Child 1995; 73:221–225.
111. Christie PE, Yntema JL, Tagari P, Ysselstijn H, Ford-Hutchinson AW, Lee TH. Effect of altitude on urinary leukotriene (LT) E4 excretion and airway responsiveness to histamine in children with atopic asthma. Eur Respir J 1995; 8:357–363.
112. Kikawa Y, Miyanomae T, Inoue Y, Saito M, Nakai A, Shigematsu Y, Hosoi S, Sudo M. Urinary leukotriene E4 after exercise challenge in children with asthma. J Allergy Clin Immunol 1992; 89:1111–1119.
113. Christie PE, Tagari P, Ford-Hutchinson AW, Charlesson S, Chee P, Arm JP, Lee TH. Urinary leukotriene E4 concentrations increase after aspirin challenge in aspirin-sensitive asthmatic subjects. Am Rev Respir Dis 1991; 143:1025–1029.
114. Kumlin M, Dahlen B, Bjorck T, Zetterstrom O, Granstrom E, Dahlen SE. Urinary excretion of leukotriene E4 and 11-dehydro-thromboxane B2 in response to bronchial provocations with allergen, aspirin, leukotriene D4, and histamine in asthmatics. Am Rev Respir Dis 1992; 146:96–103.
115. Israel E, Fischer AR, Rosenberg MA, Lilly CM, Callery JC, Shapiro J, Cohn J,

Rubin P, Drazen JM. The pivotal role of 5-lipoxygenase products in the reaction of aspirin-sensitive asthmatics to aspirin. Am Rev Respir Dis 1993; 148:1447–1451.
116. Nasser SM, Bell GS, Foster S, Spruce KE, MacMillan R, Williams AJ, Lee TH, Arm JP. Effect of the 5-lipoxygenase inhibitor ZD2138 on aspirin-induced asthma. Thorax 1994; 49:749–756.
117. Nasser SM, Patel M, Bell GS, Lee TH. The effect of aspirin desensitization on urinary leukotriene E4 concentrations in aspirin-sensitive asthma. Am J Respir Crit Care Med 1995; 151:1326–1330.
118. Drazen JM, O'Brien J, Sparrow D, Weiss ST, Martins MA, Israel E, Fanta CH. Recovery of leukotriene E4 from the urine of patients with airway obstruction. Am Rev Respir Dis 1992; 146:104–108.
119. Bellia V, Bonanno A, Cibella F, Cuttitta G, Mirabella A, Profita M, Vignola AM, Bonsignore G. Urinary leukotriene E4 in the assessment of nocturnal asthma. J Allergy Clin Immunol 1996; 97:735–741.
120. Manning PJ, Rokach J, Malo JL, Ethier D, Cartier A, Girard Y, Charleson S, O'Byrne PM. Urinary leukotriene E4 levels during early and late asthmatic responses. J Allergy Clin Immunol 1990; 86:211–220.
121. Tagari P, Rasmussen JB, Delorme D, Girard Y, Eriksson LO, Charleson S, Ford-Hutchinson AW. Comparison of urinary leukotriene E4 and 16-carboxytetranordihydro leukotriene E4 excretion in allergic asthmatics after inhaled antigen. Eicosanoids 1990; 3:75–80.
122. Smith CM, Christie PE, Hawksworth RJ, Thien F, Lee TH. Urinary leukotriene E4 levels after allergen and exercise challenge in bronchial asthma. Am Rev Respir Dis 1991; 144:1411–1413.
123. Taylor IK. Release of urinary leukotriene E4 in asthmatic subjects: a review. Adv Prostaglandin Thromboxane Leukotriene Res 1994; 22:167–83.
124. O'Sullivan S, Dahlen B, Dahlen SE, Kumlin M. Increased urinary excretion of the prostaglandin D2 metabolite 9 alpha, 11 beta-prostaglandin F2 after aspirin challenge supports mast cell activation in aspirin-induced airway obstruction. J Allergy Clin Immunol 1996; 98:421–432.
125. Taylor IK, Wellings R, Taylor GW, Fuller RW. Urinary leukotriene E4 excretion in exercise-induced asthma. J Appl Physiol 1992; 73:743–748.
126. Kikawa Y, Nakai A, Shigematsu Y, Sudo M, Suehiro Y, Hirao T. Rapid and simple assay method to study the content and the biosynthesis of peptide leukotrienes in whole blood. J Chromatogr 1989; 491:193–199.
127. Israel E, Dermarkarian R, Rosenberg M, Sperling R, Taylor G, Rubin P, Drazen JM. The effects of a 5-lipoxygenase inhibitor on asthma induced by cold, dry air. N Engl J Med 1990; 323:1740–1744.
128. Manning PJ, Watson RM, Margolskee DJ, Williams VC, Schwartz JI, O'Byrne PM. Inhibition of exercise-induced bronchoconstriction by MK-571, a potent leukotriene D4-receptor antagonist. N Engl J Med 1990; 323:1736–1739.
129. Finnerty JP, Wood-Baker R, Thomson H, Holgate ST. Role of leukotrienes in exercise-induced asthma. Inhibitory effect of ICI 204219, a potent leukotriene D4 receptor antagonist. Am Rev Respir Dis 1992; 145:746–749.
130. Israel E, Juniper EF, Callaghan JT, Mathur PN, Morris MM, Dowell AR, Enas

GG, Hargreave FE, Drazen JM. Effect of a leukotriene antagonist, LY171883, on cold air-induced bronchoconstriction in asthmatics. Am Rev Respir Dis 1989; 140: 1348–1353.

131. Robuschi M, Riva E, Fuccella LM, Vida E, Barnabe R, Rossi M, Gambaro G, Spagnotto S, Bianco S. Prevention of exercise-induced bronchoconstriction by a new leukotriene antagonist (SK&F 104353). A double-blind study versus disodium cromoglycate and placebo. Am Rev Respir Dis 1992; 145:1285–1288.
132. Cuss FM, Dixon CM, Barnes PJ. Effects of inhaled platelet activating factor on pulmonary function and bronchial responsiveness in man. Lancet 1986; 2:189–192.
133. Smith LJ, Rubin AH, Patterson R. Mechanism of platelet activating factor-induced bronchoconstriction in humans. Am Rev Respir Dis 1988; 137:1015–1019.
134. Schellenberg RR. Airway responses to platelet activating factor. Am Rev Respir Dis 1987; 136:S28–S31.
135. Taylor IK, Ward PS, Taylor GW, Dollery CT, Fuller RW. Inhaled PAF stimulates leukotriene and thromboxane A2 production in humans. J Appl Physiol 1991; 71: 1396–1402.
136. O'Connor BJ, Uden S, Carty TJ, Eskra JD, Barnes PJ, Chung KF. Inhibitory effect of UK,74505, a potent and specific oral platelet activating factor (PAF) receptor antagonist, on airway and systemic responses to inhaled PAF in humans. Am J Respir Crit Care Med 1994; 150:35–40.
137. Spencer DA, Evans JM, Green SE, Piper PJ, Costello JF. Participation of the cysteinyl leukotrienes in the acute bronchoconstrictor response to inhaled platelet activating factor in man. Thorax 1991; 46:441–445.
138. Kidney JC, Ridge SM, Chung KF, Barnes PJ. Inhibition of platelet-activating factor-induced bronchoconstriction by the leukotriene D4 receptor antagonist ICI 204,219. Am Rev Respir Dis 1993; 147:215–217.
139. Knapp HR, Sladek K, Fitzgerald GA. Increased excretion of leukotriene E4 during aspirin-induced asthma. J Lab Clin Med 1992; 119:48–51.
140. Fuller RW, Taylor GW, O'Connor BJ. Cysteinyl-leukotriene production in asthma: effects of mast cell and neurally mediated bronchoconstriction. Am Rev Respir Dis 1990; 145:A290.
141. Taylor IK, O'Shaughnessy KM, Choudry NB, Adachi M, Palmer JB, Fuller RW. A comparative study in atopic subjects with asthma of the effects of salmeterol and salbutamol on allergen-induced bronchoconstriction, increase in airway reactivity, and increase in urinary leukotriene E4 excretion. J Allergy Clin Immunol 1992; 89:575–583.
142. British Thoracic Society. Guidelines on the management of asthma. Thorax 1993; 48:S1–S24.
143. Sebaldt RJ, Sheller JR, Oates JA, Roberts LJd, FitzGerald GA. Inhibition of eicosanoid biosynthesis by glucocorticoids in humans. Proc Natl Acad Sci USA 1990; 87:6974–6978.
144. Manso G, Baker AJ, Taylor IK, Fuller RW. In vivo and in vitro effects of glucocorticosteroids on arachidonic acid metabolism and monocyte function in nonasthmatic humans. Eur Respir J 1992; 5:712–716.

145. O'Shaughnessy KM, Wellings R, Gillies B, Fuller RW. Differential effects of fluticasone propionate on allergen-evoked bronchoconstriction and increased urinary leukotriene E4 excretion. Am Rev Respir Dis 1993; 147:1472–1476.
146. Dixon RA, Diehl RE, Opas E, Rands E, Vickers PJ, Evans JF, Gillard JW, Miller DK. Requirement of a 5-lipoxygenase-activating protein for leukotriene synthesis. Nature 1990; 343:282–284.
147. Miller DK, Gillard JW, Vickers PJ, Sadowski S, Leveille C, Mancini JA, Charleson P, Dixon RA, Ford-Hutchinson AW, Fortin R, et al. Identification and isolation of a membrane protein necessary for leukotriene production. Nature 1990; 343:278–281.
148. Friedman BS, Bel EH, Buntinx A, Tanaka W, Han YH, Shingo S, Spector R, Sterk P. Oral leukotriene inhibitor (MK-886) blocks allergen-induced airway responses. Am Rev Respir Dis 1993; 147:839–844.
149. Diamant Z, Timmers MC, van der Veen H, Friedman BS, De Smet M, Depre M, Hilliard D, Bel EH, Sterk PJ. The effect of MK-0591, a novel 5-lipoxygenase activating protein inhibitor, on leukotriene biosynthesis and allergen-induced airway responses in asthmatic subjects in vivo. J Allergy Clin Immunol 1995; 95:42–51.
150. Fujimura M, Sasaki F, Nakatsumi Y, Takahashi Y, Hifumi S, Taga K, Mifune J, Tanaka T, Matsuda T. Effects of a thromboxane synthetase inhibitor (OKY-046) and a lipoxygenase inhibitor (AA-861) on bronchial responsiveness to acetylcholine in asthmatic subjects. Thorax 1986; 41:955–959.
151. Mann JS, Robinson C, Sheridan AQ, Clement P, Bach MK, Holgate ST. Effect of inhaled piriprost (U-60, 257) a novel leukotriene inhibitor, on allergen and exercise induced bronchoconstriction in asthma. Thorax 1986; 41:746–752.
152. Fuller RW, Maltby N, Richmond R, Dollery CT, Taylor GW, Ritter W, Philipp E. Oral nafazatrom in man: effect on inhaled antigen challenge. Br J Clin Pharmacol 1987; 23:677–681.
153. Hui KP, Taylor IK, Taylor GW, Rubin P, Kesterson J, Barnes NC, Barnes PJ. Effect of a 5-lipoxygenase inhibitor on leukotriene generation and airway responses after allergen challenge in asthmatic patients. Thorax 1991; 46:184–189.
154. Nasser SM, Bell GS, Hawksworth RJ, Spruce KE, MacMillan R, Williams AJ, Lee TH, Arm JP. Effect of the 5-lipoxygenase inhibitor ZD2138 on allergen-induced early and late asthmatic responses. Thorax 1994; 49:743–748.
155. McGill KA, Busse WW. Zileuton. Lancet 1996; 348:519–524.
156. Kane GC, Pollice M, Kim CJ, Cohn J, Dworski RT, Murray JJ, Sheller JR, Fish JE, Peters SP. A controlled trial of the effect of the 5-lipoxygenase inhibitor, zileuton, on lung inflammation produced by segmental antigen challenge in human beings. J Allergy Clin Immunol 1996; 97:646–654.
157. Christie PE, Smith CM, Lee TH. The potent and selective sulfidopeptide leukotriene antagonist, SK&F 104353, inhibits aspirin-induced asthma. Am Rev Respir Dis 1991; 144:957–958.
158. O'Shaughnessy KM, Taylor IK, O'Connor B, O'Connell F, Thomson H, Dollery CT. Potent leukotriene D4 receptor antagonist ICI 204,219 given by the inhaled route inhibits the early but not the late phase of allergen-induced bronchoconstriction. Am Rev Respir Dis 1993; 147:1431–1435.

159. Dahlen B, Zetterstrom O, Bjorck T, Dahlen SE. The leukotriene-antagonist ICI-204,219 inhibits the early airway reaction to cumulative bronchial challenge with allergen in atopic asthmatics. Eur Respir J 1994; 7:324–331.
160. Findlay SR, Barden JM, Easley CB, Glass M. Effect of the oral leukotriene antagonist, ICI 204,219, on antigen-induced bronchoconstriction in subjects with asthma. J Allergy Clin Immunol 1992; 89:1040–1045.
161. Rasmussen JB, Eriksson LO, Margolskee DJ, Tagari P, Williams VC, Andersson KE. Leukotriene D4 receptor blockade inhibits the immediate and late bronchoconstrictor responses to inhaled antigen in patients with asthma. J Allergy Clin Immunol 1992; 90:193–201.
162. Taylor IK, O'Shaughnessy KM, Fuller RW, Dollery CT. Effect of cysteinyl-leukotriene receptor antagonist ICI 204.219 on allergen-induced bronchoconstriction and airway hyperreactivity in atopic subjects. Lancet 1991; 337:690–694.
163. Rasmussen JB, Eriksson LO, Tagari P, Margolskee DJ, Girard Y, Andersson KE. Urinary LTE4 excretion in antigen-provoked asthmatic patients treated with the inhaled LTD4 antagonist, L-648,051. Allergy 1992; 47:599–603.
164. Denzlinger C, Haberl C, Wilmanns W. Cysteinyl leukotriene production in anaphylactic reactions. Int Arch Allergy Immunol 1995; 108:158–164.
165. Davidson D, Drafta D, Wilkens BA. Elevated urinary leukotriene E4 in chronic lung disease of extreme prematurity. Am J Respir Crit Care Med 1995; 151:841–845.
166. Balfour-Lynn IM, Valman HB, Wellings R, Webster AD, Taylor GW, Silverman M. Tumour necrosis factor-alpha and leukotriene E4 production in wheezy infants. Clin Exp Allergy 1994; 24:121–126.
167. Westcott JY, Thomas RB, Voelkel NF. Elevated urinary leukotriene E4 excretion in patients with ARDS and severe burns. Prostaglandins Leukotrienes Essential Fatty Acids 1991; 43:151–158.
168. Bernard GR, Korley V, Chee P, Swindell B, Ford-Hutchinson AW, Tagari P. Persistent generation of peptido leukotrienes in patients with the adult respiratory distress syndrome. Am Rev Respir Dis 1991; 144:263–267.
169. Roach JM, Muza SR, Rock PB, Lyons TP, Lilly CM, Drazen JM, Cymerman A. Urinary leukotriene E4 levels increase upon exposure to hypobaric hypoxia. Chest 1996; 110:946–951.
170. Kaminsky DA, Jones K, Schoene RB, Voelkel NF. Urinary leukotriene E4 levels in high-altitude pulmonary edema. A possible role for inflammation. Chest 1996; 110:939–945.
171. Hackshaw KV, Voelkel NF, Thomas RB, Westcott JY. Urine leukotriene E4 levels are elevated in patients with active systemic lupus erythematosus. J Rheumatol 1992; 19:252–258.
172. Hackshaw KV, Shi Y, Brandwein SR, Jones K, Westcott JY. A pilot study of zileuton, a novel selective 5-lipoxygenase inhibitor, in patients with systemic lupus erythematosus. J Rheumatol 1995; 22:462–468.
173. Fauler J, Thon A, Tsikas D, von der Hardt H, Frolich JC. Enhanced synthesis of cysteinyl leukotrienes in juvenile rheumatoid arthritis. Arthritis Rheum 1994; 37:93–97.
174. Kim JH, Tagari P, Giffiths AM, Ford-Hutchinson A, Smith C, Sherman PM. Levels

of peptidoleukotriene E4 are elevated in active Crohn's disease. J Ped Gastroenterol Nutr 1995; 20:403–407.
175. Carry M, Korley V, Willerson JT, Weigelt L, Ford-Hutchinson AW, Tagari P. Increased urinary leukotriene excretion in patients with cardiac ischemia. In vivo evidence for 5-lipoxygenase activation. Circulation 1992; 85:230–236.
176. Allen SP, Sampson AP, Piper PJ, Chester AH, Ohri SK, Yacoub MH. Enhanced excretion of urinary leukotriene E4 in coronary artery disease and after coronary artery bypass surgery. Coronary Artery Dis 1993; 4:899–904.
177. Fauler J, Neumann C, Tsikas D, Frolich J. Enhanced synthesis of cysteinyl leukotrienes in psoriasis. J Invest Dermatol 1992; 99:8–11.
178. Mayatepek E, Hoffmann GF, Bremer HJ. Enhanced urinary excretion of leukotriene E4 in patients with mevalonate kinase deficiency. J Pediatr 1993; 123:96–98.
179. Mayatepek E, Becker K, Gana L, Hoffmann GF, Leichsenring M. Leukotrienes in the pathophysiology of kwashiorkor. Lancet 1993; 342:958–960.
180. Mayatepek E, Lehmann WD. Increased generation of cysteinyl leukotrienes in Kawasaki disease (see comments). Arch Dis Child 1995; 72:526–527.
181. Mayatepek E, Hoffmann GF, Carlsson B, Larsson A, Becker K. Impaired synthesis of lipoxygenase products in glutathione synthetase deficiency. Ped Res 1994; 35: 307–310.
182. Denzlinger C, Holler E, Reisbach G, Hiller E, Wilmanns W. Granulocyte colony-stimulating factor inhibits the endogenous leukotriene production in tumour patients. Br J Haematol 1994; 86:881–882.
183. Denzlinger C, Kless T, Sagebiel-Kohler S, Lemmen C, Jacob K, Wilmanns W, Adam O. Modulation of the endogenous leukotriene production by fish oil and vitamin E. J Lipid Mediat Cell Signal 1995; 11:119–132.

12

Cysteinyl-Leukotriene Receptor Antagonism and 5-Lipoxygenase Inhibition in Asthma

S. M. SHUAIB NASSER

Addenbrooke's Hospital
Cambridge, England

TAK H. LEE

United Medical and Dental Schools
Guy's Hospital
London, England

I. Introduction

The cysteinyl leukotrienes have biological properties consistent with a central role in asthma. These lipid mediators are found in increased amounts in both clinical asthma and in models of asthma after challenge with aspirin and allergen. Further significant evidence to support their key role in the pathophysiology of asthma has accumulated over the past 10 years and involves the pharmacological inhibition of cysteinyl leukotrienes during experimentally induced and naturally occurring symptoms in asthma. Most early work with antileukotrienes focused on a number of models of asthma and employed allergen provocation and aspirin challenge in sensitive subjects and exercise challenge, isocapnic hyperventilation, and the inhalation of cold dry air in exercise-induced asthma. This has allowed promising antileukotriene compounds to undergo further evaluation in larger-scale studies of clinical asthma.

The action of cysteinyl leukotrienes may be inhibited either by antagonism at the leukotriene (LT) D_4 (Cys-LT_1) receptor or by inhibition of their biosynthesis. Several LTD_4 receptor antagonists have been evaluated in human trials, but LTB_4 receptor antagonists are still in the early stages of development. Inhibition of 5-lipoxygenase (5-LO) is accomplished either by direct interference with its enzymatic properties or by a secondary inhibition of its interaction with the cofactor 5-lipoxygenase–activating protein (FLAP) with resultant inhibition of 5-LO activation.

II. Pharmacology of Cysteinyl-Leukotriene Receptor Antagonists

A potent LTD_4 receptor antagonist must achieve an at least 20-fold rightward shift of the dose-response curve to inhaled LTD_4 for adequate inhibition of the effects of cysteinyl leukotriene in humans. The hydroxyacetophenone FPL 55712 was the first antagonist to be evaluated, and it displayed selective activity against SRS-A even before the chemical structure of SRS-A was elucidated (1). However, because of low potency, a short half-life, and bioavailability only by inhalation, it proved disappointing in clinical trials of asthma (2). Other first-generation LTD_4 antagonists have been evaluated in humans and include LY-171,883 (3), L-649,923 (4), and YM-16638, all of which have a structure similar to that of FPL 55712. Other early cysteinyl leukotriene receptor antagonists include L-648,051 (5) and LY-170,680 (6). All these compounds were of only moderate potency with a rightward shift in the LTD_4 dose-response curve of 3- to 10-fold and demonstrated only nominal clinical efficacy in early trials.

More recently, second-generation, highly selective LTD_4 antagonists have been developed with 100-fold or greater potency than FPL 55712. SK&F 104,353 is bioavailable only by aerosol and has been extensively investigated. In a study of six subjects with asthma, after pretreatment with SK&F 104,353 the geometric mean concentration of inhaled LTC_4 and LTE_4 required to reduce specific airways conductance by 35% (PC_{35} SGaw) was increased 12-fold and 16-fold, respectively (7). Among the most potent of these compounds is the 3,5-substituted indole, ICI 204,219, which has similar potency to the related structure ICI 198,615 but superior oral bioavailability, and both antagonize the action of the cysteinyl leukotrienes on human bronchi in the nanomolar dose range. These compounds have up to 1000-fold greater potency than FPL 55712 in inhibiting contraction of guinea pig tracheal and parenchymal strips (8). When given as a single oral dose of 40 mg 2 hours before an inhaled challenge, ICI 204,219 inhibited by 117-fold the concentration of LTD_4 required to reduce specific airways conductance by 35% (9). In a dose-ranging study of between 5 mg and 100 mg, an association was found between the plasma concentration of ICI 204,219 and the protective effect against inhaled LTD_4 (10).

The recently developed cysteinyl leukotriene receptor antagonist ONO 1078 inhibited both LTC_4 and LTD_4 in isolated guinea pig lung tissue with 400- to 3300-fold greater potency than FPL 55712 (11) and demonstrated 180-fold greater potency than FPL 55712 in isolated human bronchus (12).

RG 12525 is an orally active and potent LTD_4 receptor antagonist containing a 2-quinolinylmethoxyl moiety with an additional phenyl ring to improve receptor affinity. When administered at a dose of 800 mg to eight male subjects with mild asthma, RG 12525 led to a 7.5-fold displacement of the concentration of inhaled LTD_4 required to reduce FEV_1 by 20% (PC_{20} FEV_1) (13). However,

PC_{35} SGaw and PC_{20} FEV_1 cannot be taken as equivalent measures, and because some studies have reported the effects on normal volunteers and others have used asthmatic subjects, a direct in vivo comparison of the potency of various leukotriene antagonists is not always possible.

MK-571, MK-679, and MK-476 are members of a family of quinolone-derived LTD_4 antagonists which demonstrate a 44- to 84-fold rightward shift in the LTD_4 dose-response curve in asthmatic subjects (14). From radioligand-binding studies MK-571 potently antagonized LTD_4 binding of isolated human lung and using guinea pig trachea and ileum demonstrated specific competitive inhibition of LTD_4 and LTE_4 but was essentially inactive against LTC_4 (15). In a study of six asthmatic subjects, MK-571, given intravenously at a dose of 277 mg, demonstrated an 84-fold rightward shift in the dose-response curve to inhaled LTD_4 as measured by PC_{35} SGaw (14). MK-679 (verlukast) is the orally active R enantiomer of MK-571 and displays a similar pharmacological profile to the racemic compound, but the drug has not been further evaluated because phase II clinical trials suggested that MK-679 caused liver dysfunction in some patients. MK-0476 is a highly potent, long-acting, and orally bioavailable compound which was developed as a structural modification of MK-679 and is currently undergoing clinical trials.

BAY × 7195 is a new orally active cysteinyl leukotriene antagonist in the early stages of development. In a study of normal male volunteers receiving BAY × 7195 at a dose of between 100 and 500 mg, there was an increase of between 1- and 23-fold in the concentration of inhaled LTD_4 required to shift the dose-response curve as measured by PC_{35} SGaw (16).

III. Leukotriene Biosynthesis Inhibitors

Inhibitors of leukotriene biosynthesis were postulated to be more effective than LTD_4 receptor antagonists in preventing the pathophysiological consequences of leukotriene release within the airways because of the dual inhibition of both LTB_4 and cysteinyl leukotriene generation. Current evidence suggests that 5-LO contains a nonheme iron which is normally in the dormant ferrous state (Fe^{2+}) and upon activation by hydroperoxides, adenosine triphosphate (ATP), and calcium is converted to the active ferric form (Fe^{3+}). The activated 5-LO translocates, possibly due to a change from a hydrophilic to a hydrophobic conformation, to the nuclear membrane, where it comes into contact with a membrane-spanning, 18 kDa cofactor termed 5-lipoxygenase–activating protein (FLAP), thus allowing access to the substrate. The enzyme complex then acts on arachidonic acid, which is oxidized stereoselectively by a free radical process involving removal of the 7H(S) hydrogen followed by peroxidation and then oxidation of

Fe^{2+} in 5-LO with simultaneous reduction of the hydroperoxide radical to give 5-HPETE.

There are, therefore, a number of possible mechanisms by which 5-LO may be inhibited. Direct inhibition of the enzyme can be accomplished by ''redox inhibitors,'' which may act either by chelation or reduction of the nonheme iron; examples include acetohydroxamic acids such as BW A4C, *N*-hydroxyurea derivatives such as zileuton and BW70C, benzofurans such as L-670,630 and L-650,224, and indazolinones such as ICI 207,968. Zileuton inhibits airway microvascular leakage and bronchoconstriction induced by inhaled allergen in the sensitized guinea pig model and inhibits leukocyte accumulation (17). Following oral administration to volunteers, zileuton inhibited LTB_4 biosynthesis ex vivo with a duration of action of 6 hours at doses of 600–800 mg (18). Direct inhibition of 5-LO can also be achieved by a ''nonredox'' mechanism through antioxidant/free radical scavenger activity on radical intermediates of 5-LO, for example, flavonoids, nafazatrom (BAY-G576), naphthalene derivatives such as RS-43,179 and WY-47,288, and the enantioselective, competitive, and reversible inhibitor ZD2138 (ICI D2138), a methoxyalkylthiazole. ZD2138 exhibits prolonged inhibition of ex vivo leukotriene synthesis when administered orally to volunteers with a half-life of about 12 hours. A further mechanism involves the use of substrate analogs such as eicosatetraenoic acid (ETA).

Indirect 5-LO inhibition is achieved by using compounds that bind with high affinity to FLAP and probably act by preventing arachidonic acid presentation to 5-LO, for example, the indole derivative MK-886, the quinolone/indole hybrid MK-0591, and the quinolone BAY × 1005. In normal volunteers, MK-886 at a single dose of 500 mg significantly inhibited LTB_4 synthesis by a maximum of 60% at 2 hours (19). MK-0591 inhibits LTB_4 synthesis ex vivo by up to 90% and urinary LTE_4 by more than 80% at 24 hours with a half-life of 6 hours (20). BAY × 1005 inhibits anti-immunoglobulin E challenge in human airways in vitro (21). The FLAP antagonists REV5091 and WY-50295 demonstrated activity in vitro and in animals but were inactive in inhibiting leukotriene biosynthesis in human volunteers (22,23).

The thiopyrano [2,3,4-c,d]indoles are a new class of 5-LO inhibitor that reversibly complex with the enzyme and do not involve reduction of the nonheme iron of 5-lipoxygenase. An example of these compounds is L-691,816, but so far no clinical trials in asthma have been reported with this potential drug. Some 5-LO inhibitors have more than one mode of action. At low concentrations of racemic WY-50,295, inhibition of 5-LO binding to FLAP predominates, but at higher concentrations its activity as an arachidonic acid analog becomes more significant (23). Hydroxamic acids and hydroxyureas act primarily by chelating the essential iron at the active site of the enzyme, but it is likely that they also have additional antioxidant activity (24).

The potency of new 5-LO inhibitors is usually assessed by the in vitro concentration required to produce 50% inhibition (IC50) of 5-HPETE production by both rat and human 5-LO. Inhibition of ex vivo LTB_4 synthesis by human PMN leukocytes is measured in most human studies where leukotriene biosynthesis inhibitors have been evaluated and provide a good correlation with plasma drug concentration. However, a more useful measure of efficacy in trials of asthma is the inhibitory activity against the increase in urinary LTE_4 production, as this provides a useful indirect measure of airway cysteinyl leukotriene release. Clinical trials involving 5-LO inhibitors have followed the pattern set by the cysteinyl leukotriene antagonists, with earlier studies using compounds with weak inhibitory activity, such as piriprost, which demonstrated little clinical utility (25), and later more potent compounds reported to have potential therapeutic value.

IV. Allergen-Induced Asthma

A. Cys LT_1 Receptor Antagonists

L-649,923

The first-generation LTD_4 receptor antagonist L-649,923 was evaluated in some very early clinical studies. In eight asthmatic subjects with a dual asthmatic response to specific inhaled allergen, pretreatment with 1000 mg L-649,923 resulted in a small improvement in the reduction in the mean maximal decrease in FEV_1 from 1.78 L after placebo to 1.35 L after active drug during the early asthmatic response (EAR). There was also a small reduction in peak expiratory flow rate and the maximum flow at 25% of vital capacity but not SGaw. No effect on the late asthmatic response (LAR) could be demonstrated with any of these measures of bronchoconstriction (26).

LY 171,883

In atopic asthmatic subjects the inhaled allergen dose required to produce a 40% decrease in FEV_1 at 40% of vital capacity was determined. Pretreatment with a single 400-mg dose of LY 171,883 resulted in a slight reduction in the mean maximal antigen-induced bronchoconstriction of the EAR from 54% after placebo to 35% after LY 171,883 but had no effect on baseline lung function or the LAR. Interestingly, LY 171,883 significantly shifted the intradermal LTD_4 dose-response curve for both wheal and flare to the right, an effect not reported with other LTD_4 receptor antagonists (27).

L-648,051

A study was carried out to determine the protective effect of the inhaled cysteinyl leukotriene antagonist L-648,051 in 10 asthmatic subjects known to have a dual asthmatic response to inhaled house dust mite. Either placebo or two doses of 12 mg L-648,051 were inhaled at 20 minutes before and 3 hours after allergen challenge. No difference was found between the drug and placebo periods for baseline lung function or early or late asthmatic responses, and there was no attenuation of the allergen-induced airway responsiveness, implying insufficient cysteinyl leukotriene antagonism in the airways (28). In a study of 12 asthmatic subjects, 800 μg of inhaled L-648,051 was administered 15 minutes after allergen challenge and again during the late-phase asthmatic response to determine whether reversal of bronchoconstriction could be achieved. However, the allergen-induced bronchoconstriction was not reversed either in the early or late phases compared to placebo. In the second part of the study, L-648,051 given at the same dose before allergen challenge resulted in a slight reduction of bronchoconstriction in the EAR but not in the LAR (29). In a further study the effect of more prolonged predosing with L-648,051 was examined. For a 7-day period 10 asthmatic subjects inhaled either placebo or 6 mg L-648,051 four times daily. On the eighth day, patients underwent inhaled allergen challenge after receiving a further single dose of placebo or 6 mg L-648,051 and were then given another dose 3 hours later. There was a significant attenuation of the EAR at between 20 and 60 minutes and a more modest attenuation at 5 hours post–allergen challenge during the LAR. In addition there was a significant reduction of nonspecific airway reactivity to methacholine 24 hours after inhaled allergen challenge (30).

ICI 204,219 (Accolate, Zafirlukast)

In a study of 10 asthmatic subjects, a single oral dose of 40 mg of the potent LTD_4 antagonist ICI 204,219 attenuated the EAR by 80% and the LAR by 50% (Fig. 1) and suppressed the allergen-induced rise in nonspecific bronchial reactivity by one doubling dilution as assessed by PC_{20} histamine at 6 hours postchallenge (31). In a separate study, 13 allergic asthmatic individuals were premedicated with a single oral dose of 40 mg ICI 204,219. In 8 of these subjects there was a 3- to 30-fold increase in PD_{20} FEV_1 to inhaled cat allergen with an overall shift of 10-fold in the dose-response curve compared to placebo (32). An inhaled formulation of ICI 204,219 has also been evaluated in the allergen challenge model. A group of 10 atopic subjects with mild asthma received either 1600 μg of inhaled ICI 204,219 or propellent alone. Using PD_{15} FEV_1 as a measure of bronchoconstriction, allergen was administered 30 minutes after placebo or active treatment. There was no effect on basal airway caliber, but there was a significant inhibition of the maximum decrease in FEV_1 from 38% to 21% but without a significant effect on the LAR (33). Further work is being carried out to improve the inhaled formulation. Using PD_{20} FEV_1 as a measure of the bronchoconstrictor dose of allergen, 10 male asthmatic subjects were pretreated with an oral dose of 20 mg ICI 204,219 2 hours prior to allergen challenge and the effect compared

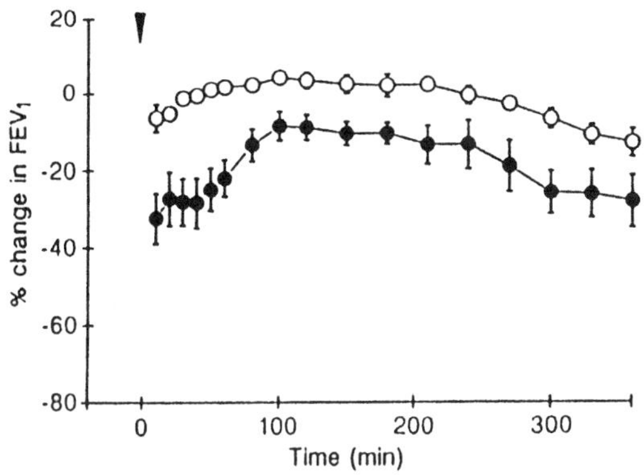

Figure 1 Percent change in FEV_1 over time following allergen challenge in eight asthmatic patients pretreated with ICI 204,219 (open circles) or placebo (solid circles). The arrow indicates the time of allergen challenge. (From Ref. 31.)

with placebo. After ICI 204,219, the group geometric mean PD_{20} FEV_1 increased 2.5-fold, and there was also a shortening of the recovery time after the immediate bronchoconstrictor response from 60 to 40 minutes (34).

MK 571 (L660,711)

In a study of asthmatic subjects, the quinolone derivative MK 571 was administered as an infusion of either 450 or 37.5 mg to two groups prior to inhalation of allergen. With the higher dose there was an 88% inhibition of the EAR and 63% inhibition of the LAR as assessed by AUC of FEV_1 versus time (35).

ONO 1078 (Pranlukast)

Asthmatic subjects were treated with 150 mg ONO 1078 or matched placebo for one week in a double-blind crossover study, after which they underwent inhaled allergen challenge. During the later part of the immediate airway response there was a significant reduction in the decrease in FEV_1 at 20–60 minutes after inhaled allergen (36).

B. Leukotriene Biosynthesis Inhibitors

Piriprost (U-60,257)

One of the very early leukotriene biosynthesis inhibitors, piriprost, was administered at a dose of 1 mg by inhalation to 12 subjects with allergic asthma. When compared to placebo, piriprost demonstrated no significant protective effect on the decrement in FEV_1 at any time point within 60 minutes of allergen challenge and had no effect on peak expiratory flow measurements for 20 hours afterward. In the four subjects who developed a late reaction at 2–12 hours, there was no significant protection with piriprost when compared to placebo (25).

Zileuton (A64077)

In a single-dose, placebo-controlled crossover study, nine asthmatic subjects received the leukotriene biosynthesis inhibitor zileuton followed by inhaled allergen challenge. Despite almost complete inhibition of ex vivo whole blood LTB_4 generation and 50% reduction of the rise in urinary LTE_4, there was no significant attenuation of the early or late asthmatic response and no decrease of the airway responsiveness to methacholine. However, there was a nonsignificant trend toward a reduction in the maximal fall in FEV_1 during the EAR, and this was most marked in patients with the greatest reduction in urinary LTE_4 (37).

ZD2138 (ICI D2138)

The potent and selective nonredox 5-LO inhibitor ZD2138 was evaluated in a study of eight asthmatic subjects undergoing specific inhaled allergen challenge. Despite an 82% reduction of ex vivo LTB_4 generation in whole blood and an overall 72% inhibition of the rise in urinary LTE_4 excretion, there was no inhibition of the allergen-induced early or late asthmatic responses (38).

MK-886

In a placebo-controlled study of eight atopic men, 500 mg of the FLAP inhibitor MK-886 was given 1 hour before and 250 mg 2 hours after allergen inhalation. Compared to placebo, MK-886 inhibited the EAR by 58% and the LAR by 44%. This was accompanied by a 54% inhibition of calcium ionophore (A23187)–stimulated whole blood LTB_4 generation with a 51% inhibition of the rise in urinary LTE_4 during the early and 80% inhibition during the late asthmatic response. However, there was no significant change in airways responsiveness to histamine at 30 hours post–allergen challenge (39).

MK-0591

In eight atopic asthmatic subjects, the FLAP inhibitor MK-0591 (250 mg) was administered at three time points: 24, 12, and 1.5 hours before house dust mite inhalation challenge. Over the 24-hour period following allergen inhalation, LTB_4 generation was inhibited by 98% and urinary LTE_4 excretion by 87%. Although there was no effect on baseline lung function, the early asthmatic response to allergen was inhibited by 79% and the late asthmatic response was inhibited by

39% and delayed by 3 hours. No effect was observed on airway responsiveness to histamine at 24 hours post–allergen challenge (40).

Both cysteinyl leukotriene receptor antagonists and FLAP inhibitors have therefore demonstrated protection against the bronchoconstrictor effect of specific inhaled allergen in susceptible asthmatics. The protection occurs predominantly during the later part of the EAR, and it is likely that the earliest bronchoconstriction is caused by other mediators such as histamine. The LAR has also been significantly inhibited by antileukotrienes but to a lesser extent, implying a greater role for noncysteinyl leukotriene inflammatory mediators in this part of the dual asthmatic response. Bronchial hyperresponsiveness using PD_{20} FEV_1 for both histamine and methacholine has also been shown to be relatively modestly inhibited by the more potent antileukotrienes in studies using both the allergen challenge model after single-dose treatment and in studies of clinical asthma using more prolonged therapy, again implying the involvement of other mediators such as the prostaglandins.

V. Aspirin-Sensitive Asthma

Current evidence suggests that aspirin-induced asthma is the most leukotriene-dependent model presently available for the evaluation of antileukotriene therapy in asthma. Asthmatic subjects undergo careful incremental oral aspirin or inhaled lysine-aspirin challenge in order to determine whether they are aspirin-sensitive and to ascertain the dose of aspirin resulting in a decrease in FEV_1 of 15–20%. This dose is designated the threshold dose. After a washout period of at least 10–14 days, because of the post–aspirin refractory period during which further doses do not lead to symptoms, a subsequent aspirin challenge can be performed after pretreatment with placebo or active compound.

A. Cys LT_1 Receptor Antagonists

SK&F 104,353

The LTD_4 antagonist SK&F 104,353 administered at a mean nebulized dose of 893 μg inhibited the bronchoconstrictor response to ingested aspirin by a mean 47% and range of 40–70% in five out of six subjects. There was no effect in one patient (41).

MK-0679

In a study of eight subjects with aspirin-sensitive asthma and with mean baseline FEV_1 of 78%, a single dose of 825 mg MK-0679 was shown to improve baseline pulmonary function for 9 hours postdose with a mean peak improvement in FEV_1 of 18% (range 5–34%) (42). In the same subjects, the dose of inhaled lysine-aspirin required to decrease FEV_1 by 20% (PD_{20} FEV_1) was determined. One hour after oral administration of 750 mg MK-0679 or matched placebo, the PD_{20} FEV_1 for lysine-aspirin was again determined. Compared to placebo, MK-0679 significantly attenuated the airway obstruction produced by inhaled lysine-aspirin in all eight subjects, with a median 4.4-fold rightward shift in the dose-response curve with three subjects failing to produce a 20% decrease in FEV_1 on inhaling the highest dose of lysine-aspirin (43).

ONO-1078

In a study of six aspirin-sensitive subjects, the inhaled threshold concentration of the nonsteroidal anti-inflammatory drug dipyrone (a pyrazalone derivative), leading to a 20% decrease in FEV_1, was determined. There was a 14-fold increase in PC_{20} FEV_1 after ingestion of 225 mg ONO 1078 compared to placebo. In four subjects there was no reduction in FEV_1 even at the maximum inhaled concentration of dipyrone, and this correlated with drug plasma levels (44).

B. Leukotriene Biosynthesis Inhibitors

Zileuton

Eight subjects with aspirin-sensitive asthma and hyperexcretion of urinary LTE_4 were treated with either placebo or zileuton at a dose of 600 mg for 7 days and the effect of aspirin ingestion examined. Compared to placebo, zileuton reduced the increase in urinary LTE_4 excretion by 68% and prevented the fall in FEV_1 in response to aspirin challenge. In addition, there was protection against reported nasal, gastrointestinal, and dermal symptoms in response to aspirin (45).

ZD2138

In a separate study, seven subjects with aspirin-induced asthma were premedicated with a single dose of 350 mg ZD2138. In response to oral aspirin challenge, the mean maximum fall in FEV_1 was 20% after placebo and less than 5% after premedication with ZD2138 (Fig. 2), and this was associated with a reduction in systemic symptoms. The active treatment resulted in a 72% inhibition of ex vivo whole blood LTB_4 generation and a 74% inhibition of the rise in urinary LTE_4 excretion at 6 hours after aspirin ingestion (46).

VI. Exercise Challenge and Isocapnic Hyperventilation

The release of cysteinyl leukotrienes after exercise-induced bronchoconstriction is supported (47) by some studies and refuted (48,49) by others. Despite this conflicting evidence, pharmacological studies indicate an important role for cysteinyl leukotrienes in exercise-induced bronchospasm. Our inability to detect

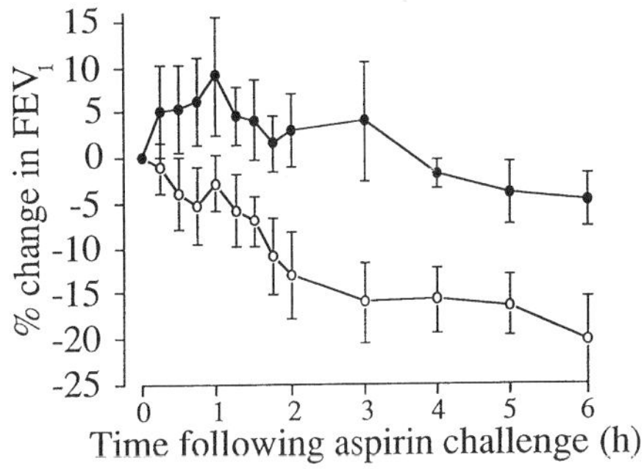

Figure 2 Bronchoprotection by ZD2138 (5-LO inhibitor) against the decrease in FEV_1 induced by aspirin challenge in 7 subjects with aspirin-sensitive asthma. ZD2138 (solid circles); placebo (open circles). (From Ref. 46.)

these mediators consistently in biological fluids after exercise may be due to a relatively modest rise in cysteinyl leukotriene release and because currently employed detection systems are insufficiently sensitive. Further confounding variables to hinder detection of leukotriene generation also come into play after exercise, which are not present after other forms of asthma, such as changes in bronchial and pulmonary blood flow in response to airway cooling and local changes in pH and osmolarity, which may lead to alterations in leukotriene metabolism and elimination.

Bronchospasm occurs in exercise-induced asthma after several minutes of strenuous exercise and generally 8–15 minutes after the patient has stopped exercising. The mechanism by which bronchospasm occurs is not certain, although respiratory water loss, changes in osmolality, or airway cooling have been proposed as triggers of mast cell degranulation. The degree of bronchospasm achieved by exercise can be mimicked by controlled isocapnic hyperventilation, which is considered to stimulate similar if not identical pathological effector mechanisms for the initiation of bronchoconstriction, provided respiratory heat exchange is matched in a time-dependent manner.

A. Cys LT_1 Receptor Antagonists

SK&F 104,353

A randomized crossover study of 18 asthmatic subjects compared SK&F 104,353 with disodium cromoglycate (DSCG) and placebo. Both 800 μg of inhaled SK&F 104,353 and 20 mg DSCG attenuated the exercise-induced decrease in FEV_1 from 29 to 20%, with a more pronounced effect with SK&F 104,353 at 20 minutes after completion of exercise (50).

ICI 204,219

In eight asthmatic subjects respiring cold dry air, an oral 20-mg dose of ICI 204,219 was given 2 hours before treadmill exercise challenge. There was no significant effect on baseline airway caliber, but compared to placebo, ICI 204,219 reduced the mean maximum fall in FEV_1 from 36 to 21%, with greatest protection occurring over the latter part of the assessment period (51). In a study of nine asthmatic subjects undergoing exercise challenge using a cycle ergometer, an inhaled dose of 400 μg ICI 204,219 or matched placebo was given 30 minutes before exercise. Although there was no significant effect on baseline airway caliber, ICI 204,219 reduced the exercise-induced decrease in FEV_1 from 30 to 14% with a significant reduction in the area under the curve (AUC) for FEV_1 during the first 30 minutes after exercise. The active treatment also reduced the time to recovery of FEV_1 to within 5% of baseline from a median of 60 minutes to 20 minutes. However, it was notable that the protection against exercise-induced asthma was variable with complete or partial inhibition in only six of nine subjects and no protection in three subjects (52).

MK-571

In a placebo-controlled study of 12 asthmatic subjects, MK-571 was given at an intravenous dose of 160 mg 20 minutes before an exercise challenge predetermined to produce a decrease in FEV_1 of 20%. After active treatment, there was a 70% attenuation of the exercise-induced decrease in FEV_1 (Fig. 3) and a marked reduction in recovery time from 33 to 8 minutes (53).

B. Leukotriene Biosynthesis Inhibitors

Piriprost

In a study of 12 asthmatic subjects the amount of exercise required to decrease FEV_1 by 25% was determined. On separate days either 1 mg piriprost or vehicle placebo alone was inhaled 15 minutes before treadmill exercise challenge. The leukotriene biosynthesis inhibitor piriprost demonstrated no significant protective effect at any time point within 60 minutes of exercise when compared to placebo (25).

Zileuton

Twenty-four subjects with mild asthma were premedicated for 2 days with zileuton 2.4 g/day prior to exercise challenge. There was no bronchodilation at baseline, but zileuton pretreatment produced a 40% inhibition of bronchospasm post-exercise compared to placebo. The mean time required for FEV_1 to return to baseline values was significantly reduced after zileuton pretreatment from 40 to

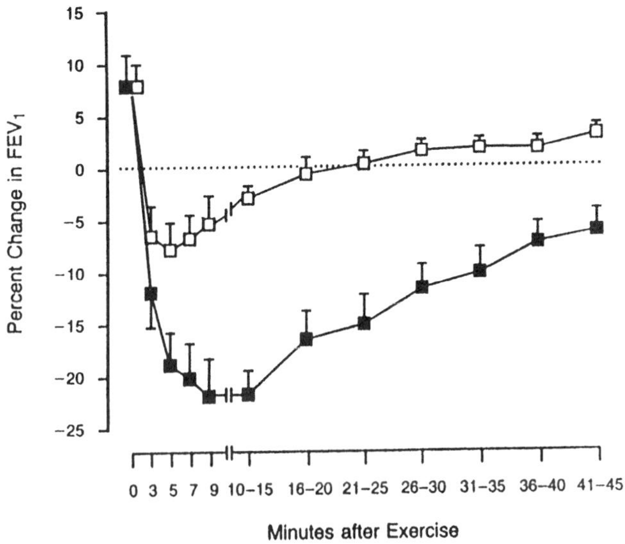

Figure 3 Percent change in FEV_1 over time following exercise in 12 patients pretreated with MK-571 (open squares) or placebo (solid squares). (From Ref. 53.)

21 minutes. This study also demonstrated a significant protection against the fall in forced vital capacity (FVC) compared to placebo at 5 minutes after exercise (54).

Despite their potency, antileukotriene formulations have only demonstrated partial protection against the bronchoconstrictor response to exercise. The results are similar to those seen in the EAR of the allergen challenge model, with protection most marked in the later stages of immediate phase bronchoconstriction. This suggests that other mediators such as mast cell–derived histamine or prostaglandins are also implicated in the pathogenesis of exercise-induced asthma.

VII. Effect of Antileukotrienes on Other Inhaled Challenges in Asthma

A. Cys LT_1 Receptor Antagonists

LY-171,883

In a crossover study, 20 asthmatic subjects were treated for 2 weeks with either LY-171,883 at a dose of 600 mg twice daily or matched placebo. The subjects then underwent isocapnic hyperventilation with cold air to induce a 20% decrease in FEV_1. There was a significant increase in the $PD_{20}FEV_1$ for the amount of cold dry air as calculated from the geometric mean respiratory heat loss from 1.0 kcal/min with placebo to 1.24 kcal/min with active treatment. In this study the most reactive subjects demonstrated greatest protection (55).

ICI 204,219

A single 80-mg dose of ICI 204,219 was administered to 10 asthmatic subjects in a placebo-controlled crossover study. Cold air challenges were carried out at 30 minutes, 4 hours, and 24 hours after treatment. $Log_{10}PD_{20}FEV_1$ respiratory heat exchange and $log_{10}PD_{20}FEV_1$ minute ventilation were used as measures of the amount of cold air required to induce bronchoconstriction, and both were significantly greater at 24 hours after treatment with ICI 204,219 compared to placebo. However, there was no difference between treatment groups at the two earlier time points. Interestingly, treatment with ICI 204,219 shortened recovery times from cold-air challenges at 30 minutes and 4 hours but not at 24 hours after dosing (56). In a similar study, 24 asthmatic subjects undergoing cold air challenges received either placebo or ICI 204,219 at doses of 20 or 40 mg in a three-period study. Bronchoprovocation with cold air was carried out at 2 and 8 hours postdose. At 8 hours after dosing, $log_{10}PD_{10}FEV_1$ minute ventilation was significantly greater with either dose of ICI 204,219 compared to placebo representing a 29 and 32% increase in the amount of cold air required to reduce FEV_1 by 10% with 20 and 40 mg ICI 204,219, respectively. There were no significant differences between the three treatment arms at 2 hours (57).

Zileuton

A single 800-mg dose of zileuton administered to 13 asthmatic subjects inhibited ex vivo whole blood LTB_4 generation by 74% without affecting thromboxane $(TX)B_2$ levels. This produced a 47% increase in the amount of cold dry air required to reduce FEV_1 by 10% with an increase in minute ventilation from 27 to 40 L/min (Fig. 4) (58).

B. Platelet Activating Factor

SK&F 104,353

A number of studies have identified a link between PAF and leukotriene synthesis. PAF inhalation stimulates increased biosynthesis of the bronchoconstrictor eicosanoid TXA_2 and the cysteinyl leukotrienes (59). LTD_4 receptor antagonists have been shown to reduce the bronchoconstrictor response to inhaled PAF in normal volunteers. The cysteinyl leukotriene antagonist SK&F 104,353 was given to eight healthy volunteers to evaluate whether the effect of PAF on the airways may be due to the secondary generation of cysteinyl leukotrienes. A single nebulized dose of SK&F 104,353 significantly inhibited the bronchoconstrictor response to an inhaled dose of PAF with a decrease in SGaw of 22% after active treatment compared to 34% after placebo pretreatment (60).

ICI 204,219

In a similar study the more potent and orally active, LTD_4 antagonist ICI 204,219 administered at a single dose of 40 mg in a study of eight healthy men inhibited PAF-induced bronchoconstriction by 59% as assessed by a comparison of the maximum fall in SGaw (61). By contrast, thromboxane receptor antagonists demonstrate little effect on PAF-induced bronchoconstriction (62), suggesting that the secondary generation of cysteinyl leukotrienes plays a key role in this response.

C. Sulfur Dioxide

The concentration of sulfur dioxide required to induce an 8-unit increase in specific airway resistance (PC_8SRaw) was measured in a study of 12 asthmatic subjects at 2 and 12 hours after administration of 20 mg ICI 204,219 or matched placebo. Compared to placebo there was a significant increase in PC_8SRaw at 2 hours after ICI 204,219 from 1.5 to 3.1 ppm which remained higher at 10 hours

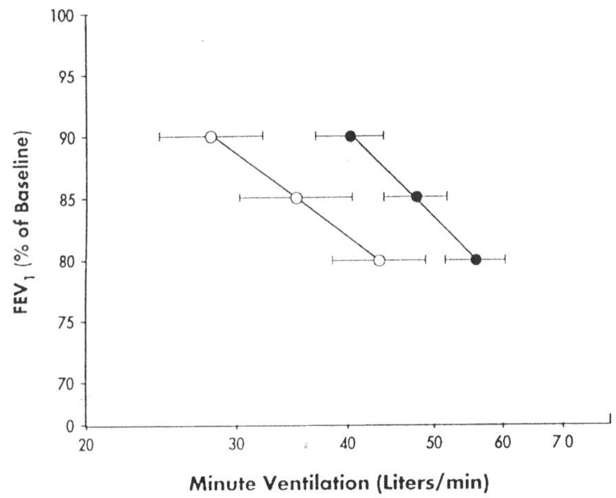

Figure 4 Composite dose-response curves demonstrating the decrease in FEV_1 in relation to minute ventilation after subjects received placebo (open circles) or zileuton (closed circles). The minute ventilation is plotted on a log proportional scale. (From Ref. 58.)

Table 1 Clinical Data on Cysteinyl-Leukotriene Receptor Antagonists

Compound	*Effect on allergen-induced bronchoconstriction*			Ref.
	EAR	LAR	BHR	
LY 649,923				
1000 mg oral	24% decrease	No effect	—	26
LY 171,883				
400 mg oral	35% decrease	No effect	—	27
L 648,051				
12 mg inhaled	No effect	No effect	No effect	28
800 μg inhaled	16% decrease	No effect	—	29
6 mg Q.I.D. inhaled 7 d	18% decrease	No effect	Decrease (1 × DD)	30
ICI 204,219				
40 mg oral	80% decrease	50% decrease	Decrease (1 × DD)	31
40 mg oral	$PD_{20}FEV_1$ cat-allergen increased 10-fold			32
1.6 mg inhaled	45% decrease	No effect	—	33
20 mg oral	$PD_{20}FEV_1$ increased 2.5-fold			34
MK-571				
450 mg infusion	88% decrease	63% decrease	—	35
ONO 1078				
150 mg B.I.D. for 7 d oral	29% decrease	—	—	36

	Effect on aspirin-induced bronchoconstriction	
SK&F 104,353		
893 μg inhaled	47% inhibition in 5/6 subjects	41
MK-0679		
750 mg oral	Baseline lung function improved	42,43
	4.4-fold increase in aspirin dose	
ONO 1078		
225 mg oral	14-fold increase in dipyrone dose	44
	Effect on exercise-induced bronchoconstriction	
MK-571		
160 mg I.V.	70% inhibition	53
	Recovery time reduced from 33 to 8 minutes	
SK&F 104,353		
800 μg inhaled	31% inhibition	50
ICI 204,219		
20 mg oral	39% inhibition	51
400 μg inhaled	50% inhibition	52
	Recovery time reduced from 60 to 20 minutes	
	Effect on PAF-induced bronchoconstriction	
SK&F 104,353		
1.2 mg inhaled	35% inhibition	60
ICI 204,219		
40 mg oral	59% inhibition	61
	Effect on sulfur dioxide–induced bronchoconstriction	
ICI 204,219		
20 mg oral	PC_8SRaw increased by 51%	63

EAR = Early asthmatic response; LAR = late asthmatic response; BHR = bronchial hyperreactivity; DD = doubling dose.

Table 2 Clinical Data on Leukotriene Biosynthesis Inhibitors

Compound	*Effect on allergen-induced bronchoconstriction* EAR	LAR	BHR	Ref.
Piriprost				
1 mg inhaled	No effect	No effect	—	25
Zileuton				
800 mg oral	No effect	No effect	—	37
ZD2138				
350 mg oral	No effect	No effect	—	38
MK-886				
500 mg & 250 mg oral	58% decrease	44% decrease	No change	39
MK-0591				
250 mg oral, 24, 12 & 1.5 h before	58% decrease	Delayed by 3 hours	No change	40
	Effect on aspirin-induced bronchoconstriction			
ZD2138				
350 mg oral	Complete inhibition of bronchoconstriction/symptoms			46
Zileuton				
7 d 600 mg QID	Complete inhibition of bronchoconstriction/symptoms			45
	Effect on exercise-induced bronchoconstriction			
Piriprost				
1 mg inhaled	No inhibition			25
Zileuton				
800 mg oral	40% inhibition			54
	Effect on cold dry air–induced bronchoconstriction			
Zileuton				
800 mg oral	47% increase in $PD_{10}FEV_1$ cold-dry air			58

EAR = Early asthmatic response; LAR = late asthmatic response; BHR = bronchial hyperreactivity; DD = double dose.

postdose (from 1.9 to 2.7 ppm). There was a correlation between plasma concentrations of ICI 204,219 and PC_8SRaw at 10 hours (63).

VIII. Conclusion

Antileukotriene therapy will be most effective in subjects in whom leukotriene-dependent bronchospasm and inflammation play a major role (Tables 1 and 2). Examples of such patients include those with acute severe asthma or aspirin-sensitive asthma. We require further information from larger-scale clinical studies to accurately predict the future role of antileukotrienes in asthma therapy in order to ascertain whether their major role is as bronchodilators, anti-inflammatory agents, or if they can replace existing treatments such as inhaled corticosteroids or theophyllines. There is already preliminary evidence from reported studies to suggest that antileukotriene drugs may provide additional anti-inflammatory effects in patients taking inhaled corticosteroids (64,65). This is supported by two studies which demonstrate that even high doses of oral or inhaled steroids are unable to inhibit the increased leukotriene production in asthma (66,67).

References

1. Augstein J, Farmer JB, Lee TB, Sheard P, Tattersall ML. Selective inhibitor of slow reacting substance of anaphylaxis. Nature N Biol 1973; 245:215–217.
2. Lee TH, Walport MJ, Wilkinson AH, Turner-Warwick M, Kay AB. Slow reacting substance of anaphylaxis antagonist FPL 55712 in chronic asthma. Lancet 1981; 2: 304–305.
3. Phillips GD, Rafferty P, Robinson C, Holgate ST. Dose-related antagonism of leukotriene D_4-induced bronchoconstriction by p.o. administration of LY-171883 in non-asthmatic subjects. J Pharm Exp Ther 1988; 246:732–738.
4. Barnes N, Piper PJ, Costello J. The effect of an oral leukotriene antagonist L-649,923 on histamine and leukotriene D_4-induced bronchoconstriction in normal man. J Allergy Clin Immunol 1987; 79:816–821.
5. Jones TR, Young R, Champion E, Charette L, Denis D, Ford-Hutchinson AW, Frenette R, Gauthier JY, Guindon Y, Kakushima M, et al. L-649,923 sodium (beta S*, gamma R*)-4-(3-(4-acetyl-3-hydroxy-2-propylphenoxy)-propylthio)-gamma-hydroxy-beta-methylbenzenebutanoate, a selective, orally active leukotriene receptor antagonist. Can J Physiol Pharmacol 1986; 64:1068–1075.
6. Wood-Baker R, Phillips GD, Lucas RA, Turner GA, Holgate ST. The effect of inhaled LY-170,680 on leukotriene D_4-induced bronchoconstriction in healthy volunteers. Drug Invest 1991; 3:239–247.
7. Joos GF, Kips JC, Pauwels RA, Van Der Straeten ME. The effect of aerosolized SK&F 104353-Z2 on the bronchoconstrictor effect of leukotriene D_4 in asthmatics. Pulm Pharmacol 1991; 4:37–42.

8. Krell RD, Aharony D, Buckner CK, Keith RA, Kusner EJ, Snyder DW, Matassa VG, Yee YK, Brown FJ, et al. The preclinical pharmacology of ICI 204,219. A peptide leukotriene antagonist. Am Rev Respir Dis 1990; 141:978–987.
9. Smith LJ, Geller S, Ebright L, Glass M, Thyrum PT. Inhibition of leukotriene D_4-induced bronchoconstriction in normal subjects by the oral LTD_4 receptor antagonist ICI 204,219. Am Rev Respir Dis 1990; 141:988–992.
10. Smith LJ, Glass M, Minkwitz MC. Inhibition of leukotriene D_4-induced bronchoconstriction in subjects with asthma: a concentration-effect study of ICI 204,219. Clin Pharmacol Ther 1993; 54:430–436.
11. Obata T, Okada Y, Motoishi M, Nakagawa N, Terawaki T, Aishita H. In vitro antagonism of ONO-1078, a newly developed anti-asthma agent, against peptide leukotrienes in isolated guinea pig tissues. Jpn J Pharmacol 1992; 60:227–237.
12. Yamaguchi T, Kohrogi H, Honda I, Kawano O, Sugimoto M, Araki S, Ando M. A novel leukotriene antagonist, ONO-1078, inhibits and reverses human bronchial contraction induced by leukotrienes C_4 and D_4 and antigen in vitro. Am Rev Respir Dis 1992; 146:923–929.
13. Wahedna I, Wisniewski AS, Tattersfield AE. Effect of RG 12525, an oral leukotriene D_4 antagonist, on the airway response to inhaled leukotriene D_4 in subjects with mild asthma. Br J Clin Pharmacol 1991; 32:512–515.
14. Kips JC, Joos GF, De Lepeleire I, Margolskee DJ, Buntinx A, Pauwels RA, Van Der Straeten ME. MK-571, a potent antagonist of leukotriene D_4-induced bronchoconstriction in the human. Am Rev Respir Dis 1991; 144:617–621.
15. Jones TR, Zamboni R, Belley M, Champion E, Charette L, Frenette R, Gauthier JY, Leger S, Masson P. Pharmacology of L-660,711 (MK-571): a novel potent and selective leukotriene D_4 receptor antagonist. Can J Physiol Pharmacol 1989; 67:17–28.
16. Wensing G, Heinig R, Priesnitz M, Kuhlmann J. Effect of BAY × 7195, an oral receptor antagonist of cysteinyl-leukotrienes, on leukotriene D_4-induced bronchoconstriction in normal volunteers. Eur J Clin Pharmacol 1994; 47:227–230.
17. Hui KP, Lotvall J, Chung KF, Barnes PJ. Attenuation of inhaled allergen-induced airway microvascular leakage and airflow obstruction in guinea pigs by a 5-lipoxygenase inhibitor (A-63162). Am Rev Respir Dis 1991; 143:1015–1019.
18. Rubin P, Dube L, Braeckman R, Swanson L, Hansen R, Albert D, Carter G. Pharmacokinetics, safety, and ability to diminish leukotriene synthesis by zileuton, an inhibitor of 5-lipoxygenase. Agents Actions Suppl 1991; 35:103–116.
19. Depre M, Friedman B, Tanaka W, Van Hecken A, Buntinx A, DeSchepper PJ. Biochemical activity, pharmacokinetics, and tolerability of MK-886, a leukotriene biosynthesis inhibitor, in humans. Clin Pharmacol Ther 1993; 53:602–607.
20. Prasit P, Belley M, Blouin M, Brideau C, Chan C, Charleson S, Evans JF, Frenette R, Gauthier JY, Guay J. A new class of leukotriene biosynthesis inhibitor: the development of MK-0591. J Lipid Mediators 1993; 6:239–244.
21. Gorenne I, Labat C, Gascard JP, Norel X, Muller Peddinghaus R, Mohrs KH, Taylor WA, Gardiner PJ, Brink C. (R)-2-[4-(Quinolin-2-yl-methoxy)phenyl]-2-cyclopentyl] acetic acid (BAY × 1005), a potent leukotriene synthesis inhibitor: effects on anti-IgE challenge in human airways. J Pharmacol Exp Ther 1994; 268:868–872.
22. Grimes D, Sturm RJ, Marinari LR, Carlson RP, Berkenkopf JW, Musser JH, Kreft AF, Weichman BM. WY-50,295 Tromethamine, a novel, orally active 5-lipoxyge-

nase inhibitor: biochemical characterization and antiallergic activity. Eur J Pharmacol 1993; 236:217–228.

23. Evans JF, Leville C, Mancini JA, Prasit P, Therien M, Zamboni R, Gauthier JY, Fortin R, Charleson P, MacIntyre DE, Luell S, Bach TJ, Meurer R, Guay J, Vickers PJ, Rouzer CA, Gillard JW, Miller DK. 5-Lipoxygenase-activating protein is the target of a quinolone class of leukotriene biosynthesis inhibitors. Mol Pharmacol 1991; 40:22–27.
24. Garland LG, Salmon JA. Hydroxamic acids and hydroxyureas as inhibitors of arachidonate 5-lipoxygenase. Drugs Future 1991; 16:547–558.
25. Mann JS, Robinson C, Sheridan AQ, Clement P, Bach MK, Holgate ST. Effect of inhaled piriprost (U-60, 257) a novel leukotriene inhibitor, on allergen and exercise induced bronchoconstriction in asthma. Thorax 1986; 41:746–752.
26. Britton JR, Hanley SP, Tattersfield AE. The effect of an oral leukotriene D_4 antagonist L-649,923 on the response to inhaled antigen in asthma. J Allergy Clin Immunol 1987; 79:811–816.
27. Fuller RW, Black PN, Dollery CT. Effect of the oral leukotriene D_4 antagonist LY171883 on inhaled and intradermal challenge with antigen and leukotriene D_4 in atopic subjects. J Allergy Clin Immunol 1989; 83:939–944.
28. Bel EH, Timmers MC, Dijkman JH, Stahl EG, Sterk PJ. The effect of an inhaled leukotriene antagonist, L-648,051, on early and late asthmatic reactions and subsequent increase in airway responsiveness in man. J Allergy Clin Immunol 1990; 85: 1067–1075.
29. Rasmussen JB, Eriksson LO, Andersson KE. Reversal and prevention of airway response to antigen challenge by the inhaled leukotriene D_4 antagonist (L-648,051) in patients with atopic asthma. Allergy 1991; 46:266–273.
30. Rasmussen JB, Eriksson LO, Tagari P, Stahl EG, Andersson KE. Reduced nonspecific bronchial reactivity and decreased airway response to antigen challenge in atopic asthmatic patients treated with the inhaled leukotriene D_4 antagonist, L-648,051. Allergy 1992; 47:604–609.
31. Taylor IK, O'Shaughnessy KM, Fuller RW, Dollery CT. Effect of cysteinyl-leukotriene receptor antagonist ICI 204,219 on allergen-induced bronchoconstriction and airway hyperreactivity in atopic subjects. Lancet 1991; 337:690–694.
32. Findlay SR, Barden JM, Easley CB, Glass M. Effect of the oral leukotriene antagonist, ICI 204,219, on antigen-induced bronchoconstriction in subjects with asthma. J Allergy Clin Immunol 1992; 89:1040–1045.
33. O'Shaughnessy KM, Taylor IK, O'Connor B, O'Connell F, Thomson H. Potent leukotriene D_4 receptor antagonist ICI 204,219 given by the inhaled route inhibits the early but not the late phase of allergen-induced bronchoconstriction. Am Rev Respir Dis 1993; 147:1431–1435.
34. Dahlen B, Zetterstrom O, Bjorck T, Dahlen SE. The leukotriene-antagonist ICI-204,219 inhibits the early airway reaction to cumulative bronchial challenge with allergen in atopic asthmatics. Eur Respir J 1994; 7:324–331.
35. Rasmussen JB, Eriksson LO, Margolskee DJ, Tagari P, Williams VC. Leukotriene D_4 receptor blockade inhibits the immediate and late bronchoconstrictor responses to inhaled antigen in patients with asthma. J Allergy Clin Immunol 1992; 90:193–201.

36. Taniguchi Y, Tamura G, Honma M, Aizawa T, Maruyama N, Shirato K, Takishima T. The effect of an oral leukotriene antagonist, ONO-1078, on allergen-induced immediate bronchoconstriction in asthmatic subjects. J Allergy Clin Immunol 1993; 92:507–512.
37. Hui KP, Taylor IK, Taylor GW, Rubin P, Kesterson J, Barnes NC. Effect of a 5-lipoxygenase inhibitor on leukotriene generation and airway responses after allergen challenge in asthmatic patients. Thorax 1991; 46:184–189.
38. Nasser SM, Bell GS, Hawksworth RJ, Spruce KE, MacMillan R, Williams AJ, Lee TH, Arm JP. Effect of the 5-lipoxygenase inhibitor ZD2138 on allergen-induced early and late asthmatic responses. Thorax 1994; 49:743–748.
39. Friedman BS, Bel EH, Buntinx A, Tanaka W, Han YH, Shingo S, Spector R, Sterk P. Oral leukotriene inhibitor (MK-886) blocks allergen-induced airway responses. Am Rev Respir Dis 1993; 147:839–844.
40. Diamant Z, Timmers MC, van der Veen H, Friedman BS, De Smet M, Tanaka W, Depre M, Bel EH, Dijkman JH, Sterk PJ. The effect of MK-0591, a potent oral leukotriene biosynthesis inhibitor, on allergen-induced airway responses in asthmatic subjects. Am Rev Respir Dis 1993; 147:A446.
41. Christie PE, Smith CM, Lee TH. The potent and selective sulfidopeptide leukotriene antagonist, SK&F 104353, inhibits aspirin-induced asthma. Am Rev Respir Dis 1991; 144:957–958.
42. Dahlen B, Margolskee DJ, Zetterstrom O, Dahlen SE. Effect of the leukotriene receptor antagonist MK-0679 on baseline pulmonary function in aspirin sensitive asthmatic subjects. Thorax 1993; 48:1205–1210.
43. Dahlen B, Kumlin M, Margolskee DJ, Larsson C, Blomqvist H, Williams VC, Zetterstrom O, Dahlen SE. The leukotriene-receptor antagonist MK-0679 blocks airway obstruction induced by inhaled lysine-aspirin in aspirin-sensitive asthmatics. Eur Respir J 1993; 6:1018–1026.
44. Yamamoto H, Nagata M, Kuramitsu K, Tabe K, Kiuchi H, Sakamoto Y, Yamamoto K, Dohi Y. Inhibition of analgesic-induced asthma by leukotriene receptor antagonist ONO-1078. Am J Respir Crit Care Med 1994; 150:254–257.
45. Israel E, Fischer AR, Rosenberg MA, Lilly CM, Callery JC, Shapiro J, Rubin P, Drazen JM. The pivotal role of 5-lipoxygenase products in the reaction of aspirin-sensitive asthmatics to aspirin. Am Rev Respir Dis 1993; 148:1447–1451.
46. Nasser SM, Bell GS, Foster S, Spruce KE, MacMillan R, Williams AJ, Lee TH, Arm JP. Effect of the 5-lipoxygenase inhibitor ZD2138 on aspirin-induced asthma. Thorax 1994; 49:749–756.
47. Kikawa Y, Hosoi S, Inoue Y, Saito M, Nakai A, Shigematsu Y, Hirao T. Exercise-induced urinary excretion of leukotriene E_4 in children with atopic asthma. Ped Res 1991; 29:455–459.
48. Broide DH, Eisman S, Ramsdell JW, Ferguson P, Schwartz LB, Wasserman SI. Airway levels of mast cell-derived mediators in exercise-induced asthma. Am Rev Respir Dis 1990; 141:563–568.
49. Smith CM, Christie PE, Hawksworth RJ, Thien F, Lee TH. Urinary leukotriene E_4 levels after allergen and exercise challenge in bronchial asthma. Am Rev Respir Dis 1991; 144:1411–1413.
50. Robuschi M, Riva E, Fuccella LM, Vida E, Barnabe R, Rossi M, Gambaro G, Spag-

notto S, Bianco S. Prevention of exercise-induced bronchoconstriction by a new leukotriene antagonist (SK&F 104353). A double-blind study versus disodium cromoglycate and placebo. Am Rev Respir Dis 1992; 145:1285–1288.
51. Finnerty JP, Wood-Baker R, Thomson H, Holgate ST. Role of leukotrienes in exercise-induced asthma. Inhibitory effect of ICI 204219, a potent leukotriene D_4 receptor antagonist. Am Rev Respir Dis 1992; 145:746–749.
52. Makker HK, Lau LC, Thomson HW, Binks SM, Holgate ST. The protective effect of inhaled leukotriene D_4 receptor antagonist ICI 204,219 against exercise-induced asthma. Am Rev Respir Dis 1993; 147:1413–1418.
53. Manning PJ, Watson RM, Margolskee DJ, Williams VC, Schwartz JI. Inhibition of exercise-induced bronchoconstriction by MK-571, a potent leukotriene D_4-receptor antagonist. N Engl J Med 1990; 323:1736–1739.
54. Meltzer SS, Rechsteiner EA, Johns MA, Cohn J, Bleecker ER. Inhibition of exercise-induced asthma by zileuton, a 5-lipoxygenase inhibitor. Am J Respir Crit Care Med 1994; 149:A215.
55. Israel E, Juniper EF, Callaghan JT, Mathur PN, Morris MM, Dowell AR, Hargreave FE, Drazen JM. Effect of a leukotriene antagonist, LY171883, on cold-air-induced bronchoconstriction in asthmatics. Am Rev Respir Dis 1989; 140:1348–1353.
56. Boulet LP, Bai TR, Miller CJ, Lavins BJ, Cohn J, Turcotte H, Atton L. Effect of zafirlukast on cold-air-induced bronchoconstriction in patients with asthma. Eur Respir J 1996; 9(suppl 23):273S.
57. Israel E, Lavins BJ, Miller CJ, Cohn J. Effect of zafirlukast 20 and 40 mg on cold-air-induced bronchoconstriction in patients with bronchial asthma. Eur Respir J 1996; 9(suppl 23):51S.
58. Israel E, Dermarkarian R, Rosenberg M, Sperling R, Taylor G, Rubin P. The effects of a 5-lipoxygenase inhibitor on asthma induced by cold, dry air. N Engl J Med 1990; 323:1740–1744.
59. Taylor IK, Ward PS, Taylor GW, Dollery CT, Fuller RW. Inhaled PAF stimulates leukotriene and thromboxane A_2 production in humans. J Appl Physiol 1991; 71: 1396–1402.
60. Spencer DA, Evans JM, Green SE, Piper PJ, Costello JF. Participation of the cysteinyl leukotrienes in the acute bronchoconstrictor response to inhaled platelet activating factor in man. Thorax 1991; 46:441–445.
61. Kidney JC, Ridge SM, Chung KF, Barnes PJ. Inhibition of platelet-activating factor-induced bronchoconstriction by the leukotriene D_4 receptor antagonist ICI 204,219. Am Rev Respir Dis 1993; 147:215–217.
62. Stenton SC, Ward C, Duddridge M, Harris A, Palmer JB, Hendrick DJ. The actions of GR32191B, a thromboxane receptor antagonist, on the effects of inhaled PAF on human airways. Clin Exp Allergy 1990; 20:311–317.
63. Lazarus SC, Lavins BJ, Wong HH, Watts MJ, Minkwitz MC. Effect of Accolate (zafirlukast) on sulfur dioxide (SO_2)-induced bronchoconstriction in patients with asthma. Am J Respir Crit Care Med 1995; 151:A41.
64. Wahedna I, Wisniewski AFZ, Wong CS, Tattersfield AE. Effect of multiple doses of RG 12525, an oral leukotriene D_4 antagonist, in chronic asthma. Am Rev Respir Dis 1992; 145:A16.
65. Chapman KR, Friedman BS, Shingo S, Heyse J, Reiss T, Spector R. The efficacy

of an oral inhibitor of leukotriene synthesis (MK-0591) in asthmatics treated with inhaled steroids. Am J Respir Crit Care Med 1994; 149:A215.

66. Dworski R, Fitzgerald GA, Oates JA, Sheller JR. Effect of oral prednisone on airway inflammatory mediators in atopic asthma. Am J Respir Crit Care Med 1994; 149: 953–959.

67. O'Shaughnessy KM, Wellings R, Gillies B, Fuller RW. Differential effects of fluticasone propionate on allergen-evoked bronchoconstriction and increased urinary leukotriene E_4 excretion. Am Rev Respir Dis 1993; 147:1472–1476.

13

Leukotriene Receptor Antagonism and Synthesis Inhibition in Chronic Stable Asthma

ELLIOT ISRAEL and JEFFREY M. DRAZEN

Harvard Medical School
and Brigham and Women's Hospital
Boston, Massachusetts

Numerous studies have demonstrated that leukotriene receptor antagonism and synthesis inhibition can blunt the bronchospastic response to allergen, exercise, and aspirin; all are forms of induced asthma rather than spontaneous asthma. Currently only six studies published in the archival literature describe the effects of these agents in chronic stable asthma. We will describe these studies and then comment on the implications of these studies vis-à-vis the role of these agents in the treatment of asthma.

I. Leukotriene Antagonists

Three studies have been published utilizing agents that antagonize the effects of the leukotrienes at the $CysLT_1$ receptor. These studies examine the effects of LY171883, zafirlukast, and montelukast. These agents have been shown to block the bronchoconstrictive effects of inhaled LTD_4. The former two shift the dose-response curve to inhalation of LTD_4 as measured by bronchoconstriction by 5- to 6-fold and by about 100-fold, respectively.

A. LY171883

Cloud and colleagues reported the first study in chronic stable asthma utilizing agents active on products of the 5-lipoxygenase pathway. The $CysLT_1$ antagonist LY171883, which shifts the inhaled LTD_4 $PD_{12}FEV_1$ dose response by 4.6-fold

Table 1 Patients and Study Characteristics in Leukotriene Antagonist Studies

Characteristic	LY171883	ICI 204,219 (Zafirlukast)	Montelukast
Doses	600 mg bid	40 mg, 20 mg, 10 mg bid	200 mg bid
Design	Parallel	Parallel	Crossover
Duration of active arm	6 weeks	6 weeks	10⅓ d
Average no. of patients/arm	69	69	29
Mean age (yr)	31	36	34[a]
Males (% of study)	79	71	79[a]
Baseline FEV_1 (% predicted)	78%	67%	68%[a]
Mean baseline FEV_1 (L)	~3.10[b]	—	2.48[a]
Mean AM PEFR (L/min)	385	—	—
Mean PM PEFR (L/min)	409	—	—
Weekly puffs β-agonist	34*	42	38

[a]Median.
[b]Derived from figures or statistics.
Source: Refs. 3 and 4.

and the $PD_{30}V_{p30}$ by 6.1-fold was utilized in a 6-week, randomized, parallel design study (1).

Design

This was a double-blind, placebo-controlled, randomized parallel group study. Patients participated in a 1-week run-in during which they used inhaled metaproterenol as needed. Those patients who satisfied the entry criteria were randomized to treatment with oral LY171883, 1200 mg per day (600 mg twice daily), or placebo for 6 weeks.

Entry Criteria

Nonsmoking asthmatics were enrolled in this study. All patients used no other antiasthma medications except for inhaled β-agonists. All patients demonstrated a $\geq$15% improvement in FEV_1 following inhalation of bronchodilator and had a baseline FEV_1 $\geq$50% of predicted. Patients who used metaproterenol daily and had stable pulmonary function were randomized to treatment.

Subjects

One hundred and thirty-eight patients entered the study after the run-in. The characteristics of the subjects randomized are shown in Table 1. Of note, the subjects' baseline FEV_1 was 76.5–78.8% of predicted.

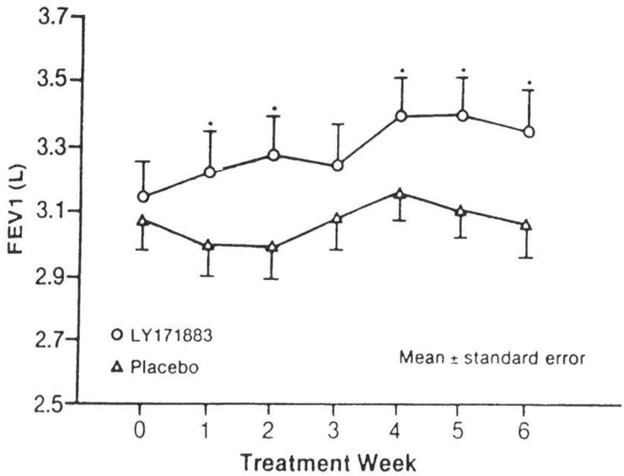

Figure 1 Effect of LY171883 on FEV_1. Mean change ± SEM in FEV_1. $*p \leq 0.05$ compared with placebo.

Outcomes

At the end of the study (last data point for people who left the study) the FEV_1 improved 0.3 L in the active treatment group and declined 0.1 L in the placebo-treated group ($p = 0.003$) (Fig. 1); calculated from the graphic data, this appears to be about a 9% improvement in the FEV_1 expressed as a percentage of baseline. Expressed as a percent of the predicted FEV_1, the LY171883-treatment group improved from 78.8 to 83.3%, whereas the placebo-treated group declined from 76.5 to 73.9%. No differences in diurnal peak flows occurred during treatment or at the end of the study.

Metaproterenol use decreased in the active treatment group from 36 inhalations per week to 22 inhalations per week versus a decline from 31 inhalations per week to 23 inhalations per week in the placebo group ($p = 0.089$). An analysis of a subset of the patients who utilized at least the median amount of metaproterenol per week (36 inhalations or 23 mg) showed that there was a 22.2 inhalation per week decrease in the LY171883-treatment group versus a 6.0 inhalation per week increase in the placebo-treatment group.

Nighttime and daytime asthma attacks were not significantly decreased. Daytime wheezing decreased ($p = 0.016$) as did breathlessness ($p = 0.023$). Wheezing ($p = 0.0323$) and breathlessness ($p = 0.015$) scores at night were reduced as well.

Adverse Events

One active treatment and three placebo-treated patients discontinued due to adverse events. Five LY171883- and nine placebo-treated patients withdrew early because of lack of efficacy. Persistent diarrhea occurred in four LY171883-treated patients and none of the placebo-treated patients ($p = 0.037$). Seven active-treatment patients and two placebo-treated patients developed self-limited headaches ($p = 0.070$).

Summary

This relatively weak $CysLT_1$ antagonist, studied in a mild group of asthmatics, produced almost a 9% improvement in FEV_1. There was a trend toward decreased inhaler use, which became more evident in the subgroup of asthmatics who exceeded the median inhaler use at baseline.

B. Zafirlukast (Accolate™)

Zafirlukast, formerly known as ICI204,219, shifts the $PD_{20}FEV_1$ to inhaled LTD_4 by 90- to 100-fold (2). Spector and colleagues examined the effects of administration of three different doses of zafirlukast administered twice daily for 6 weeks (3).

Design

This was a double-blind, placebo-controlled, randomized parallel group study. After a 2-week placebo run-in, patients who had a daytime asthma score (based on a self-rating scale) above a predetermined threshold for the last 7 days of the placebo run-in were randomized. Patients received placebo, 10 mg, 20 mg, or 40 mg of zafirlukast per day administered in two divided doses for 6 weeks.

Entry Criteria

All patients were using no other antiasthma medications at the time of entry into the trial except inhaled β-agonists. Patients demonstrated a ≥15% improvement in FEV_1 or a positive response to methacholine bronchoprovocation challenge. Baseline FEV_1 had to be between 40 and 75% of predicted.

Subjects

Two hundred and seventy-six subjects were randomized after the run-in. The available characteristics are shown in Table 1. The baseline FEV_1 at the time of randomization was 66–69% of predicted.

Outcomes

Although all zafirlukast treatment groups tended to do better than placebo for the outcome measures reported, these improvements only reached statistical significance in the 40 mg/day group. FEV_1 improved 0.23 L in the 40 mg zafirlukast

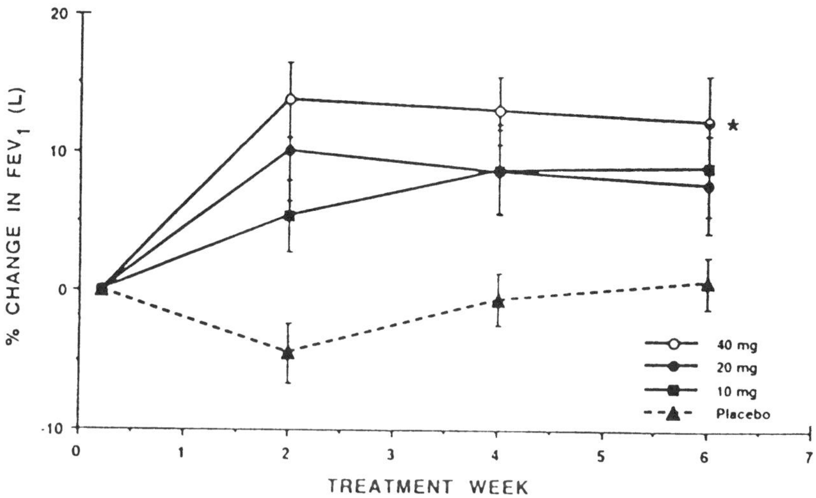

Figure 2 Effect of zafirlukast on percentage change in FEV_1. Percentage change ± SEM in FEV_1 from week 0 (randomization) through week 6 (endpoint). $*p \le 0.01$ between 40 mg and placebo.

group compared to the placebo ($p < 0.05$) (Fig. 2). The improvement in FEV_1 represented an 11% improvement from baseline. Data in the discussion of this paper note that when the subset of patients with an FEV_1 45–65% of predicted was examined the improvement was 0.37 L versus 0.19 L in the placebo group. Although there were only six patients with an $FEV_1 \le 45\%$ of predicted, these patients had a mean 0.8 L improvement versus four similarly grouped placebo patients, who had an 0.10 L improvement.

In the zafirlukast 40 mg/day group, morning peak flow improved 6% (22 L/min) ($p = 0.07$) from baseline. Evening peak flow improved 4% vs. placebo (16 L/min vs. 2 L/min) ($p = 0.04$). Inhaled albuterol use decreased 31% from 39.2 puffs per week at baseline to 26.2 puffs per week ($p = 0.02$).

The frequency of nighttime awakenings decreased by 2.6 events per week compared to placebo ($p = 0.001$) and represented a 46% decrease compared to the baseline frequency of these events. Asthma symptom scores (first morning and daytime) decreased compared to placebo as well ($p \le 0.05$ and $p \le 0.01$, respectively).

Although statistically significant salutary effects were not noted with the doses of zafirlukast below 40 mg per day, there was a negative correlation between an increasing dose of zafirlukast and decreasing inhaler use (correlation coefficient −0.16, $p < 0.01$). Linear trends (correlation coefficients absolute values of 0.14–0.25) were also noted between dose and evening PEF and asthma symptoms. Similar levels of correlation were seen with plasma levels of zafirlukast and FEV_1.

Treatment failures (additional medications required for control of asthma) occurred significantly less frequently in the zafirlukast-treatment groups (2%) than in placebo (10%) ($p = 0.015$).

Adverse Events

Two patients withdrew due to adverse events. Two, three, and eight patients on zafirlukast 20 mg, 10 mg, and placebo, respectively, withdrew due to asthma exacerbations. Adverse events occurring in more than 5% of any treatment group occurred no more frequently in the zafirlukast-treated groups than with placebo except for rhinitis. Rhinitis occurred in 7, 9, 3, and 1% of the 40 mg, 20 mg, 10 mg, and placebo groups, respectively. Four percent of subjects in the 40-mg zafirlukast-treatment group and in the placebo group were reported to have developed an elevated SGPT.

Summary

Zafirlukast was studied in a moderate group of asthmatics with a mean FEV_1 66–69% of predicted. The highest dose (40 mg/day) of this potent $CysLT_1$ antagonist improved FEV_1 by 11%. Albuterol use decreased by 31%, and nighttime awakenings decreased 46%. The percentage of patients who required additional asthma treatment of any kind was only 2% in the combined active treatment groups and 10% in the placebo group.

C. Montelukast

Montelukast, a $CysLT_1$ antagonist, was studied by Reiss and colleagues in a crossover study in 29 patients (4).

Design

This was a randomized, placebo-controlled, double-blind crossover study. After a 2-week open-label observation period, patients who met symptom and compliance criteria were randomized. At randomization patients received 600 mg of montelukast (200 mg tid) or placebo for 10 1/3 days. All morning doses were administered in the clinic under observation. Patients were crossed over after an interval of at least 48 hours.

Entry Criteria

Asthmatics who were not on inhaled corticosteroids, as well as those on inhaled corticosteroids who continued a stable dose of inhaled corticosteroids, were accepted into this study. All patients were required to demonstrate a 15% improvement in the absolute FEV_1. Baseline FEV_1 had to be between 50 and 80% of predicted.

Subjects

Twenty-nine asthmatics were randomized. Thirteen were using inhaled corticosteroids and one was using theophylline. An additional patient was using both inhaled corticosteroids and theophylline. The baseline FEV_1 was 68% of predicted (2.48 L).

Outcomes

No clinically significant differences in outcome were noted between patients receiving and those not receiving inhaled corticosteroids. The maximum improvement in FEV_1 occurred at 3 hours after drug administration on day 11. The FEV_1 increased slightly more than 16% from baseline ($p \leq 0.05$) (Fig. 3).

Peak flow data were not reported. Inhaled albuterol use decreased from a baseline of 37.7 puffs per week, but the absolute decrease was not reported. The difference compared to placebo was 7.0 puffs per week. Decreases in nighttime awakening scores approached statistical significance. Daytime symptoms decreased significantly.

Adverse Events

Two patients withdrew due to adverse events during montelukast treatment—an upper respiratory infection and a rash that occurred during concurrent use of ciprofloxacin. One placebo patient required hospitalization due to worsening asthma. Two patients experienced mild elevations in liver function tests with treatment.

Summary

In a study of moderate asthmatics (FEV_1 68% predicted) almost 11 days of montelukast increased FEV_1 by 16% at the maximum point of observation. Albuterol use decreased (degree unclear), as did daytime symptoms.

II. Synthesis Inhibitors

While inhibition of synthesis of the cysteinyl leukotrienes alone could occur by inhibition of the effects of LTC_4 synthase, pharmacological agents have been

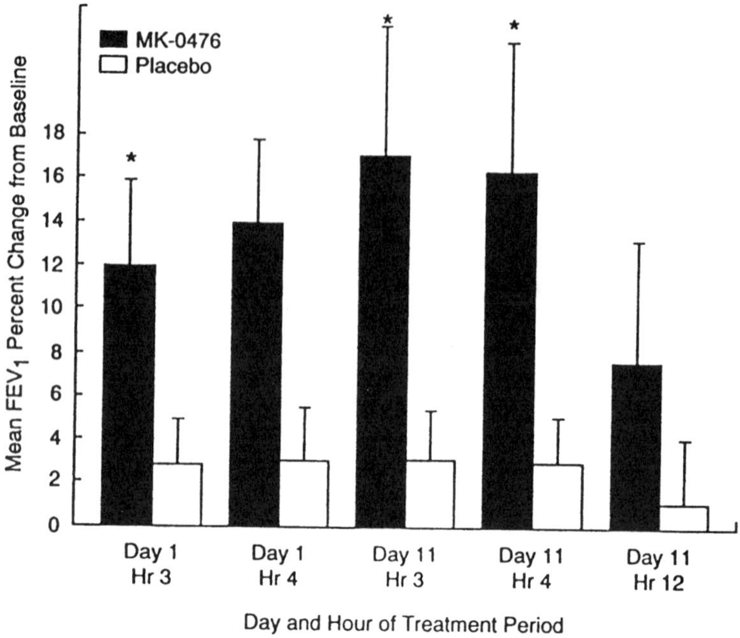

Figure 3 Effect of montelukast (MK-0476) on FEV_1. Increase in FEV_1 (mean ± SEM on days 1 and 11 of each treatment period) as a percentage improved from the period-specific, day 1 predosing baseline value. Hours represent hours after dosing.

developed that antagonize the effects of critical enzymes more proximally in the metabolic pathway by which arachidonic acid is transformed into the cysteinyl leukotrienes (see previous chapters). The primary targets have been 5-lipoxygenase (5-LO) and the 5-LO–activating protein (FLAP). Agents that interfere with either aspect of this pathway inhibit the production of the cysteinyl leukotrienes. However, such agents also interfere with the synthesis of other products of this pathway, which may have a pathophysiological role in asthma. These products include the 5-HETEs (mucus secretogogues) and LTB_4 (a potent neutrophil chemotactic agent). While both FLAP antagonists and 5-LO antagonists have been tested in induced models of asthma (see previous chapters), clinical outcomes in trials of chronic use have been reported only for a drug that targets 5-LO—zileuton (Zyflo™). The results of the three reported trials utilizing this drug are summarized below.

Table 2 Characteristics of Patients in Synthesis Inhibition Studies

Characteristic	Zileuton—4 weeks	Zileuton—13 weeks	Zileuton—6 months
Doses	600 mg qid, 800 mg bid	600 mg, 400 mg qid	600 mg, 400 mg qid
Design	Parallel	Parallel	Parallel
Average no. of patients/arm	46	134	121
Mean age (yr)	35	32	34
Males (% of study)	79	47	44
Baseline FEV_1 (% predicted)	58%	60%	63%
Mean baseline FEV_1 (L)	2.30	2.24	2.30
Mean AM PEFR (L/min)	386	366	365
Mean PM PEFR (L/min)	427	412	410
Weekly puffs β-agonist	~42[a]	41.5	40

[a]Derived by 1.8 times occasions of use.
Source: Refs. 5, 6, and 9.

A. 4-Week Trial of Zileuton

The earliest of the studies with zileuton examined its effects in a 4-week trial (5).

Design

This was a double-blind, placebo-controlled parallel group trial. After a one-week, single-blind, placebo lead-in, patients with ≥7 occasions of β-agonist use who had an asthma score above a predetermined threshold were randomized. Patients received zileuton 2.4 g/d (600 mg qid), 1.6 g/d (800 mg bid), or placebo for 4 weeks.

Entry Criteria

Patients could only be using β-agonists for the control of their asthma. Patients demonstrated a ≥15% improvement in FEV_1. Baseline FEV_1 had to be between 40 and 75% of predicted.

Subjects

One hundred and forty-three patients were randomized after the run-in. Subject characteristics are shown in Table 2. The baseline FEV_1 for the evaluated patients was 57–60% of predicted.

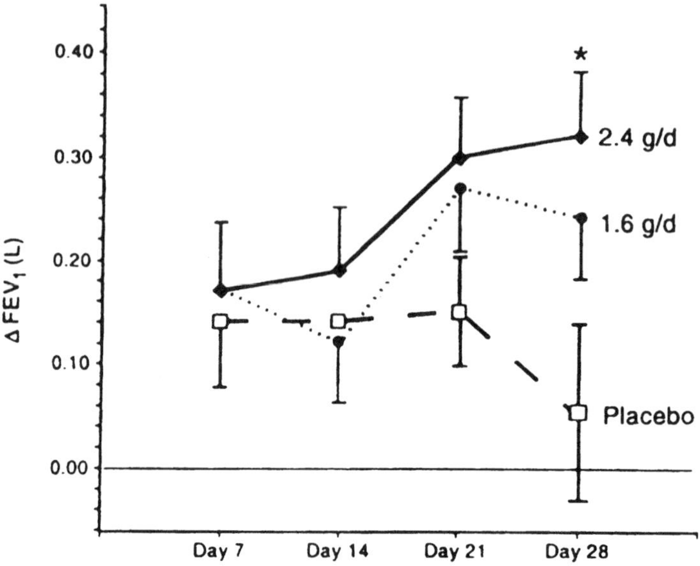

Figure 4 Effect of 4 weeks of zileuton on FEV_1. Mean change in weekly FEV_1 (± SEM) compared with values at the end of the dummy lead-in. $*p = 0.02$.

Outcomes

Although both active treatment groups tended to do better than placebo, the statistically significant improvements were by and large restricted to the zileuton 2.4 g/d group. FEV_1 improved 0.32 L in the zileuton 2.4 g/d group ($p = 0.02$ vs. placebo). This improvement in FEV_1 represented a 13.4% improvement in FEV_1 from baseline (Fig. 4).

In the zileuton 2.4 g/d group the morning peak expiratory flow improved 10% (39.5 L/min) at week three ($p \leq 0.001$). Evening peak flow improved 7% from baseline (30.5 L/min) ($p = 0.004$). Inhaled β-agonist use decreased by 24% from 22.1 occasions per week to 15.7 occasions per week ($p < 0.001$).

Asthma symptoms decreased more in both treatment groups than they did in the placebo group. Leukotriene synthesis was inhibited as determined by examining urinary LTE_4 excretion. Zileuton 2.4 g/d decreased urinary LTE_4 excretion by 39% compared to baseline ($p = 0.007$ vs. placebo).

Adverse Effects

One patient in the 1.6 g/d group withdrew during the first week of the study due to worsening asthma. There was no difference in the occurrence of adverse effects among the study groups. Three patients each in the zileuton 2.4 and 1.6 g/d groups reported dyspepsia versus none in the placebo group. Hives and increased liver function tests occurred in one patient on 1.6 g/d. Both resolved after discontinuation of therapy.

Summary

Zileuton was studied in a group of moderate-to-severe asthmatics (mean FEV_1 57–60% predicted). The higher dose (2.4 g/d), which inhibited urinary LTE_4 production by 39%, produced a 13.4% improvement in FEV_1 at a time when inhaled β-agonist use decreased 24%.

B. 13-Week Trial of Zileuton

Zileuton was subsequently studied in a 13-week trial; in this trial asthma exacerbations were also used as an outcome indicator (6).

Design

This was a double-blind, placebo-controlled, randomized parallel group study. After a 10-day single-blind lead-in, patients who had used their albuterol inhaler ≥20 times in the lead-in and who had asthma symptom scores above a predetermined threshold were randomized. Patients received zileuton 2.4 g/d (600 mg qid), 1.6 g/d (400 mg qid), or placebo for 13 weeks.

Entry Criteria

Antiasthma medications were restricted to inhaled β-agonists. Patients demonstrated a ≥15% improvement in FEV_1 post–β-agonist inhalation. Baseline FEV_1 had to be between 40–80% of predicted.

Subjects

Four hundred and one patients were randomized after the run-in. Subject characteristics are shown in Table 2. The baseline FEV_1 of these patients ranged from 58 to 62% of predicted.

Outcomes

While both doses produced salutary effects, the 2.4 g/d produced greater and more frequent positive outcomes. Zileuton 2.4 g/d improved the FEV_1 2–4 hours after ingestion by an average of 15.7% over the entire study period (0.36 L)

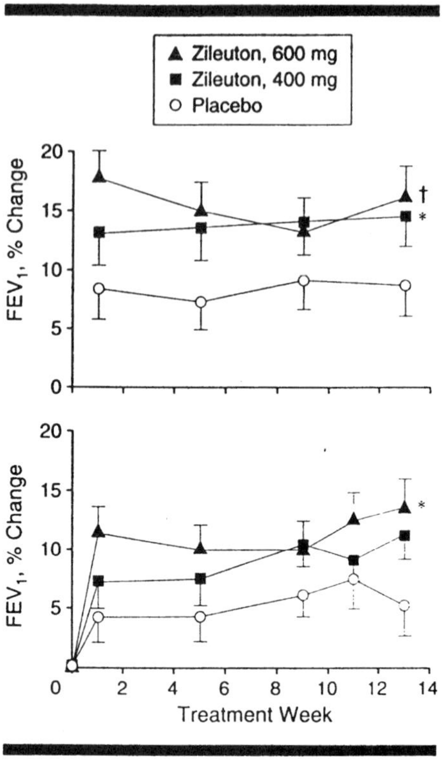

Figure 5 Effect of 13 weeks of zileuton treatment on FEV_1. (Top) Peak effects—average FEV_1 2 to 4 hours after drug ingestion (expected time of peak drug levels). (Bottom) Trough effects—FEV_1 before ingestion of morning dose of drug (expected time of low drug levels). $*p < 0.05$ vs. placebo; $\dagger p < 0.01$ vs. placebo.

(p = 0.006 vs. placebo) (Fig. 5). Trough FEV_1 levels (AM levels 8–12 hours after zileuton administration) improved an average of 11.5% through the entire study in the 2.4 g/d group (p = 0.02 vs. placebo) (Fig. 5).

The average morning peak flow improved 18.2 L/min in the zileuton 2.4 g/d group (5%, p = 0.02). Evening peak flow improved 18.7 L/min (4.5%, p = 0.004). Inhaled β-agonist use decreased 26% from 41 puffs per week at baseline (p = 0.03).

Patients treated with zileuton 2.4 g/d experienced more symptom-free nights than placebo-treated patients (39.5 vs. 29.0, p = 0.009). Average daytime symptom scores decreased with zileuton 2.4 g/d treatment versus placebo (p =

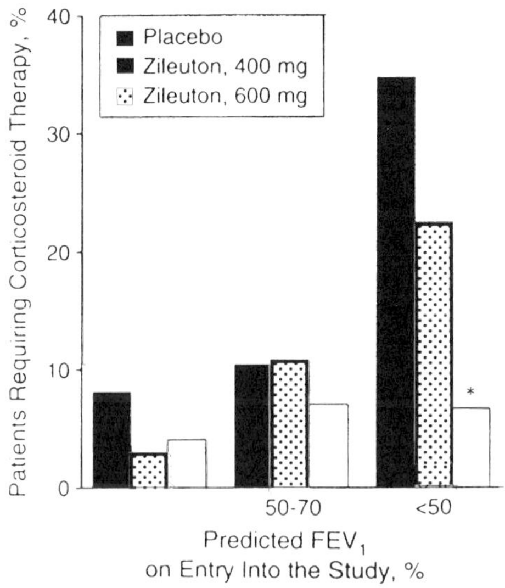

Figure 6 Effect of 13 weeks of zileuton treatment on percentage of patients requiring corticosteroid therapy. Groups are stratified by FEV_1 as a percentage of predicted on entry into the study. A total of 111 patients had an FEV_1 greater than 70%, 187 had an FEV_1 of 50–70%, and 103 had an FEV_1 less than 50%. Before stratification, zileuton 2.4 g/d decreased the percentage of patients requiring corticosteroid treatment by 60% ($p = 0.02$). $^*p < 0.05$ vs. placebo.

0.003). Zileuton 2.4 g/d produced significant improvements in all domains of a validated Asthma Quality of Life Questionnaire (7,8).

Zileuton 2.4 g/d decreased asthma exacerbations requiring corticosteroids by more than 60% ($p = 0.02$). More than 15% of the placebo-treated patients experienced such exacerbations versus a little more than 6% of patients receiving zileuton 2.4 g/d. When patients were stratified based on their baseline FEV_1, as a percent of predicted on entry into study, the risk of experiencing such asthma exacerbations was reduced from 34.4 to 6.7% ($p = 0.01$) (Fig. 6).

Adverse Events

Withdrawals associated with asthma exacerbations occurred less frequently in the zileuton 2.4 g/d group (4 vs. 15 in placebo group [$p = 0.02$]). Withdrawals for reasons other than asthma occurred in 10, 7, and 4 patients in the zileuton 2.4 g/d, zileuton 1.6 g/d, and placebo groups, respectively. Five patients, three patients, and no patients developed elevations in liver enzymes three times greater than the upper limit of normal ($p = 0.03$ zileuton 2.4 g/d vs. placebo). All returned to 2 times normal or baseline while receiving treatment or after withdrawal of study drug.

Summary

Zileuton 2.4 g/d was studied in a group of moderate to severe asthmatics with a mean FEV_1 60% of predicted. Over the 13 weeks of this study, this dose produced an average 15.7% improvement 2–4 hours after ingestion of drug. Albuterol use decreased 26%. The percentage of patients requiring oral corticosteroid bursts was 15.6% in the placebo group vs. 6.1% in the zileuton 2.4 g/d group. About 3% of patients developed self-limited elevations in liver function tests.

C. 6-Month Study with Zileuton

The effects of zileuton were also studied in a 6-month study reported below (9).

Design

This was a double-blind, placebo-controlled, randomized parallel group study. After a 10-day lead-in, patients who had used a β-agonist inhaler ≥20 times in the lead-in and who had asthma symptom scores above a predetermined threshold were randomized. Patients received zileuton 2.4 g/d (600 mg qid), 1.6 g/d (400 mg qid), or placebo for 25 weeks.

Entry Criteria

Antiasthma medications were restricted to inhaled β-agonists. Patients demonstrated a ≥15% improvement in FEV_1 after β-agonist inhalation. Baseline FEV_1 had to be between 40 and 80% of predicted.

Subjects

Three hundred and seventy-three patients were randomized after the run-in. Subject characteristics are shown in Table 2. The baseline FEV_1 of these subjects was approximately 63% of predicted.

Outcomes

While both zileuton doses produced salutary effects, as occurred in the prior two zileuton studies cited, the 2.4 g/d dose produced improvements of greater

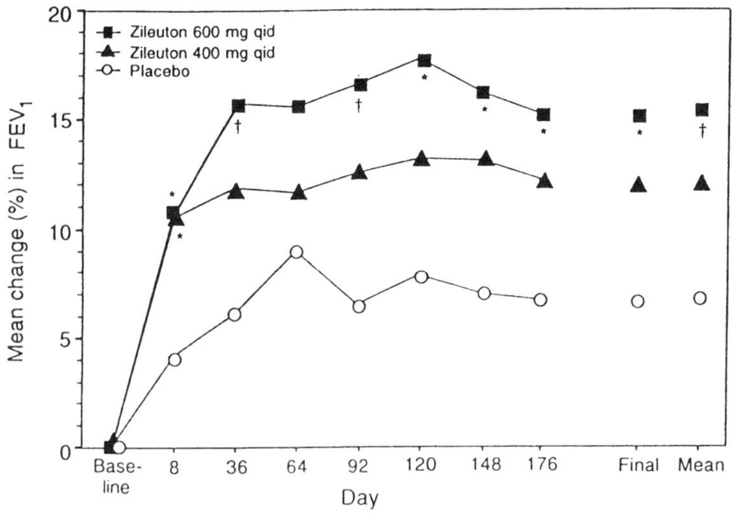

Figure 7 Comparison of chronic trough effects of on FEV_1 over 6 months. The chronic trough effect was determined by measurement of FEV_1 before the first daily dose of zileuton at each of eight visits during the 26-week trial. $*p \leq 0.05$; $\dagger p \leq 0.01$.

magnitude, which were more frequently of statistical significance. Zileuton 2.4 g/d improved the trough FEV_1 an average of 15% ($p = 0.004$ vs. placebo) through the entire study with the maximum improvement reaching 18% (Fig. 7). In patients who entered the study with a FEV_1 less than 50% of the predicted value, the mean increase in FEV_1 was 38% compared to 13% in the placebo group ($p \leq 0.005$).

The average morning peak flow improved ~30 L/min in the zileuton 2.4 g/d group (8.3%, $p \leq 0.01$). Inhaled β-agonist use for the periods reported declined 24–30% in patients receiving zileuton 2.4 g/d and only 7% in those on placebo ($p \leq 0.001$).

Zileuton 2.4 g/d significantly decreased daytime and nighttime symptom scores. Acute asthma exacerbations (33% increase in bronchodilator use or 20% decrease in FEV_1 or 25% drop in AM peak flow) occurred in 27% of the zileuton 2.4 g/d group versus 38% of the placebo group ($p = 0.043$). Zileuton 1.6 g/d and 2.4 g/d reduced the number of patients requiring corticosteroids for treatment of their exacerbations by 50% and 62%, respectively.

Of interest, these investigators reported that eosinophil counts decreased significantly in both treatment groups. Baseline percentages of eosinophils ranged from 3.5 to 5% and decreased ~1% during treatment.

Adverse Effects

The number of patients discontinuing due to adverse events was equivalent across all study groups. A total of 11 patients who received zileuton at either dose developed elevated liver enzyme levels greater than three times normal; these levels normalized while patients continued in the study or with discontinuation of active drug. No such elevations occurred in the placebo group.

Summary

Zileuton 2.4 g/d, studied in a group of moderate to severe asthmatics (FEV_1 63% of predicted) improved the trough FEV_1 15%. Inhaled β-agonist use decreased 24–30%. The percentage of patients requiring oral corticosteroid bursts decreased from 22 to 8%. About 3% of patients developed self-limited elevations in liver function tests.

III. Overview

A summary of the major outcomes reported in the studies we have reviewed is shown in Table 3. Although the data suggest differences among these agents in terms of effect on outcome indicators, some of these differences should be consid-

Table 3 Comparison of Improvement in Outcomes

	LY171883	Zafirlukast	Montelukast	Zileuton (6-month study)
Doses	600 mg bid	40 mg bid	600 mg tid	600 mg qid
Trough FEV_1 (L)[a]	0.3L	0.23L[b]	—	0.34L
% Trough FEV_1[a,c]	9(9)[b]	11(13–14)[b]	—	15(18)
% Peak FEV_1[c,d]	—	—	16	20[e](23)[b]
β-Agonist use reduction[c]	39%[f]	31%	>18.5%	(30%)
AM PEFR	No Δ	6% (?)	—	7.1% (8.3%)
Adverse events/ corticosteroid bursts[g]	—	10% vs. 2%	—	21.5% vs. 8.3%

[a]Trough values are values immediately prior to next dose or those values not reported as obtained at times of expected peak concentrations or effects.
[b]Derived from figures or statistics.
[c]Figures not in parentheses represent means over the study period or endpoint analyses. Figures in parentheses represent maximum effect among the study observation intervals reported.
[d]Peak values are values recorded at time of agent's expected peak concentration or effects.
[e]Endpoint value. NS vs. placebo at week 26.
[f]$p = 0.089$ vs. placebo.
[g]Adverse events for zafirlukast, corticosteroid bursts for zileuton.

ered in the context of the differing baseline characteristics of the cohorts studied. Secondary analyses of the zafirlukast cohort and the zileuton 13-week and 6-month cohorts suggest that more severe asthmatics (as defined by FEV_1) have a greater response to these agents than their less severely affected counterparts. This may explain part of the lesser degree of effect seen with LY171883. Of interest, the zafirlukast, montelukast, and 6-month zileuton studies are quite similar in terms of baseline FEV_1 and may therefore permit more direct comparisons. While the trend in these data suggests greater improvements with the use of the synthesis inhibitors than the antagonists, as indicated by FEV_1 and PEF, it would be premature to draw definitive conclusions in regard to differential effectiveness of these agents. Such conclusions require direct comparative studies utilizing appropriately randomized populations.

An examination of these outcomes and review of these papers reveal that these agents produce clinically important ameliorative effects in asthma. These drugs produced about 15% improvement in FEV_1 in the populations studied. Of note, as mentioned above, the magnitude of improvement in FEV_1 was even more apparent in patients with a low baseline FEV_1, suggesting that leukotriene-mediated mechanisms may play a greater role in these patients.

In these studies, zileuton and montelukast have been shown to produce bronchodilation within several hours of ingestion. Zafirlukast was not reported to produce this effect, although a smaller study suggested that it is possible such an effect may occur with this drug (10).

In addition to the effects on the physiological indices of asthma severity, all accompanying indices of asthma control improved with the use of these drugs. Thus β-agonist use usually fell by more than 25%, and daytime and nighttime symptoms and nighttime awakenings fell as well. Validated quality of life scores reinforced these findings as well. The salutary effects on these physiological indices and symptoms were reflected in real-life outcomes. Three of the studies (3,6,9) demonstrated that use of these agents markedly reduced the number of patients requiring additional therapy for treatment of asthma exacerbations. Zafirlukast was reported to decrease the need for theophylline or other therapy during the 6-week study from 10 to 2%. Zileuton decreased the percentage of patients requiring corticosteroids for treatment of asthma exacerbations by 50% to more than 60% (6,9). When the population was characterized based on FEV_1, it could be seen that the majority of this effect was occurring in the more severe patients (Fig. 6). In these severe patients, corticosteroid requiring events were reduced by 60–80% (6,9) and the incidence of exacerbations was reduced to the incidence in patients who had mild disease ($FEV_1 \geq 70\%$ predicted) (Fig. 6). Finally, one study (9) noted a decrease in peripheral eosinophil counts, suggesting that additional antiasthmatic effects may be mediated by these agents.

Review of these papers also allows us to draw some general conclusions regarding the time course of the effects of these drugs. Although it was not our purpose to review the acute effects of the leukotriene antagonists and synthesis inhibitors, four of the papers reviewed demonstrate that FEV_1 increases of approximately 15% occurred within the first few hours after the first dose (4–6,9). While there is ample evidence that some of these agents produce acute effects, additional positive effects accrue with chronic use. It appears that it can take 2–3 weeks for >80% of the FEV_1 effects of these drugs to become evident. Additionally, even after chronic effects have plateaued, additional acute improvements are still noted after administration of the drug (Fig. 5). Peak flow continues to rise for a longer period of time, generally approaching a plateau at 4–6 weeks. The full effect on asthma symptoms appears to peak even later. Symptoms continue to fall and appear to begin to approach a plateau after more than 2 months of treatment. The persistence of salutary effects after withdrawal of these agents has not been fully explored. In one study, the bronchospastic response to inhalation of cold, dry air was blunted after withdrawal of zileuton for a period of time that exceeded its pharmacokinetic ability to inhibit 5-lipoxygenase (11).

The slow onset of the improvements seen with these chronic studies, separate from the acute improvements seen in these studies and others, as well as the decrease in asthma exacerbations noted suggest that properties other than the smooth muscle constrictor actions of the leukotrienes are targets of these agents. While it is possible that in the case of 5-lipoxygenase inhibitors prevention of formation of other agents that contribute to the asthmatic response may be responsible for these outcomes, recent data demonstrating a broad array of inflammatory effects resulting from the cysteinyl leukotrienes themselves suggest that agents targeted at the actions of these biomolecules alone may be able to produce these effects. As reviewed elsewhere in this book, cysteinyl leukotrienes have been shown to mediate recruitment of eosinophils into the airways (12). Inhibition of cysteinyl leukotriene synthesis has been shown to decrease the influx of inflammatory cells into asthmatic airways (13), and leukotrienes have been shown to possess possible cytokinelike activity (14). The decrease in peripheral eosinophils noted in patients receiving zileuton is consistent with inhibition of such putative cytokinelike activity (9). It is possible that this "anti-inflammatory" activity may be responsible for the time course of these chronic effects.

The role of the leukotriene antagonists and synthesis inhibitors vis-à-vis currently available asthma treatments is a subject for speculation since there are no published studies in which such direct comparisons have occurred. The magnitude of the effects noted in the chronic studies we have reviewed compare favorably with the effects seen with theophylline (15) or inhaled steroids (16–19) (Table 4). For example, Dutoit and coworkers noted a 15.5% improvement in FEV_1 after 10 weeks of therapy with 800 μg/d of beclomethasone dipropionate in patients with a baseline FEV_1 70% of predicted (16). In a group of similar severity, 1000 μg of the high-potency inhaled corticosteroid fluticasone produced a 10% improvement in FEV_1 (18). In a group with an FEV_1 63% of predicted 200

Table 4 Inhaled Corticosteroid Studies

Rx	Duration (weeks)	Base FEV_1	FEV_1 (%)	Δ FEV_1 (%)	Ref.
FLU 50–1000 μg	8	~2.66	72	3–10	18
BDP 800 μg	10	N/A	70	15.5	16
BUD 1600 μg	3	2.71	68	20	19
FLU 50–200 μg	12	2.42	63	16.5–21.4	17

μg of fluticasone produced a 17% improvement in FEV_1 while 100 μg produced a 21% improvement (17). A study of high-dose budesonide (1600 μg/d) did produce a 20% increase in FEV_1 in patients with an FEV_1 of 68% predicted at baseline (19).

In summary, chronic treatment with leukotriene antagonists and synthesis inhibitors produces clinically important improvements in the physiological impairments noted in asthma, decreases medication use, decreases symptoms, and in some cases improves asthma control as reflected in a decrease in the need for additional medications for asthma exacerbations. Depending on the outcome measured, these effects approach a steady state within about 2 months. Patients with more severe disease appear to benefit to an even greater extent than those with mild disease. The precise role of these agents in a step-care approach to asthma treatment will require more extensive experience with these agents. A delineation of clinical differences, if any, between these agents will require direct comparison studies.

References

1. Phillips GD, Rafferty P, Robinson C, Holgate ST. Dose-related antagonism of leukotriene D4-induced bronchoconstriction by p.o. administration of LY-171883 in nonasthmatic subjects. J Pharmacol Exp Ther 1988; 246:732–738.
2. Smith LJ, Glass M, Minkwitz MC. Inhibition of leukotriene D4-induced bronchoconstriction in subjects with asthma: a concentration-effect study of ICI 204,219. Clin Pharmacol Ther 1993; 54:430–436.
3. Spector SL, Smith LJ, Glass M, Accolate Asthma Trialists Group. Effects of 6 weeks of therapy with oral doses of ICI 204,219, a leukotriene D4 receptor antagonist, in subjects with bronchial asthma. Am J Respir Crit Care Med 1994; 150:618–623.
4. Reiss TF, Altman LC, Chervinsky P, Bewtra A, Stricker WE, Noonan GP, et al. Effects of montelukast (MK-0476), a new potent cysteinyl leukotriene (LTD4) receptor antagonist, in patients with chronic asthma. J Allergy Clin Immunol 1996; 98: 528–534.
5. Israel E, Rubin P, Kemp J, Grossman J, Pierson W, Siegel S, et al. The effect of

inhibition of 5-lipoxygenase by zileuton in mild to moderate asthma. Ann Intern Med 1993; 119:1059–1066.
6. Israel E, Cohn J, Dube L, Drazen J, for the Zileuton Clinical Trial Group. Effect of treatment with zileuton, a 5-lipoxygenase inhibitor, in patients with asthma. JAMA 1996; 275:931–936.
7. Juniper EF, Guyatt GH, Willan A, Griffith LE. Determining a minimal important change in a disease-specific Quality of Life Questionnaire. J Clin Epidemiol 1994; 47:81–87.
8. Juniper EF, Guyatt GH, Ferrie PJ, Griffith LE. Measuring quality of life in asthma. Am Rev Respir Dis 1993; 147:832–838.
9. Liu MC, Dube LM, Lancaster J, and the Zileuton Study Group. Acute and chronic effects of a 5-lipoxygenase inhibitor in asthma: a 6-month randomized multicenter trial. J Allergy Clin Immunol 1996; 98:859–871.
10. Hui KP, Barnes NC. Lung function improvement in asthma with a cysteinyl-leukotriene receptor antagonist. Lancet 1991; 337:1062–1063.
11. Fischer AR, McFadden CA, Frantz R, Awni WM, Cohn J, Drazen JM, et al. Effect of chronic 5-lipoxygenase inhibition on airway hyperresponsiveness in asthmatic subjects. Am J Respir Crit Care Med 1995; 152:1203–1207.
12. Laitinen LA, Laitinen A, Haahtela T, Vilkka V, Spur BW, Lee TH. Leukotriene E4 and granulocytic infiltration into asthmatic airways. Lancet 1993; 341:989–990.
13. Kane GC, Pollice M, Kim C, Cohn J, Dworski RT, Murray JJ, et al. A controlled trial of the effect of the 5-lipoxygenase inhibitor, zileuton, on lung inflammation produced by segmental antigen challenge in human beings. J Allergy Clin Immunol 1996; 97:646–654.
14. Johnson HM, Russell JK, Torres BA. Second messenger role of arachidonic acid and its metabolites in interferon-gamma production. J Immunol 1986; 137:3053–3056.
15. Pierson WE, LaForce CF, Bell TD, MacCosbe PE, Sykes RS, Tinkelman D. Long-term, double-blind comparison of controlled-release albuterol versus sustained-release theophylline in adolescents and adults with asthma. J Allergy Clin Immunol 1990; 85:618–626.
16. Dutoit JI, Salome CM, Woolcock AJ. Inhaled corticosteroids reduce the severity of bronchial hyperresponsiveness in asthma but oral theophylline does not. Am Rev Respir Dis 1987; 136:1174–1178.
17. Sheffer AL, LaForce C, Chervinsky P, Pearlman D, Schaberg A, and the Fluticasone Propionate Asthma Study Group. Fluticasone propionate aerosol: efficacy in patients with mild to moderate asthma. J Fam Pract 1996; 42:369–375.
18. Chervinsky P, van As A, Bronsky EA, Dockhorn R, Noonan M, LaForce C, et al. Fluticasone propionate aerosol for the treatment of adults with mild to moderate asthma. J Allergy Clin Immunol 1994; 94:676–683.
19. Wempe JB, Postma DS, Breederveld N, Alting-Hebing D, van der Mark TW, Koeter GH. Separate and combined effects of corticosteroids and bronchodilators on airflow obstruction and airway hyperresponsiveness in asthma. J Allergy Clin Immunol 1992; 89:679–687.

14

Montelukast—An Antileukotriene Treatment for Asthma

Changing the Asthma-Treatment Paradigm

BETH C. SEIDENBERG and THEODORE F. REISS

Merck & Co., Inc.
Rahway, New Jersey

I. Introduction

Montelukast (SINGULAIR®, Merck & Co., Rahway, NJ) is an oral, potent, specific cysteinyl leukotriene ($CysLT_1$) receptor antagonist. As a once-daily treatment in patients (adults and children 6–14 years old) with asthma, montelukast has advantages over, and is an important addition to, currently available therapies.

In large, double-blind, placebo-controlled clinical trials in patients with chronic persistent asthma, once-daily montelukast produces statistically significant and clinically important improvements in symptoms, pulmonary function, and disease outcomes (episodes of worsening asthma). Improvement occurs within the first day of therapy and persists with long-term administration. Montelukast has additive effects with inhaled corticosteroids (provides additional asthma control and allows tapering of inhaled corticosteroid), decreases the dose of "as-needed" inhaled β-agonist, and benefits patients with aspirin-sensitive and exercise-induced asthma. In clinical trials, montelukast controls asthma in patients across a broad spectrum of baseline disease severity and demographic characteristics, with the convenience of once-daily oral administration and a good tolerability profile in both adult and pediatric patients.

Montelukast and other leukotriene blockers will provide critical insights into asthma pathophysiology and help redefine the treatment paradigm of asthma.

II. Description

Montelukast sodium, an orally active, specific cysteinyl leukotriene ($CysLT_1$) receptor antagonist, is [R-(E)]-1-[[[1-[3-[2-(7-chloro-2-quinolinyl)ethenyl]phenyl]-3-[2-(1-hydroxy-1-methylethyl)phenyl]-propyl]thio]methyl]cyclopropaneacetic acid sodium salt. The molecular formula of montelukast is $C_{35}H_{35}ClNO_3S$-Na. Its molecular weight is 608.2.

III. Pharmacology of Montelukast

A. In Vitro Pharmacology

Montelukast is a highly potent, competitive, and selective $CysLT_1$ receptor antagonist. The effects of montelukast on receptor binding in guinea pig and human lung membrane are summarized below.

Effects of Montelukast on [3H]Leukotriene Binding in Receptor-Binding Studies

Montelukast is a competitor of the specific binding of [^{3}H]leukotriene D_4 in homogenized guinea pig lung membranes, membranes from human DMSO differentiated U937 (dU937) cells, and sheep lung with respective IC_{50} values of 0.61 $\pm$ 0.09 nM (n = 16), 0.78 nM $\pm$ 0.2 (n = 7), and 6.0 nM (n = 2) (1). Montelukast also effectively competes for specific binding of [^{3}H]leukotriene D_4 to guinea pig lung membrane in the presence of 0.05% (w/v) human serum albumin, with an IC_{50} of 0.42 $\pm$ 0.089 (n = 7). Montelukast has an IC_{50} of 1.2 $\pm$ 0.36 nM (n = 5) with 1% (v/v) and 2.5 nM with 4% (v/v) squirrel monkey plasma and 16 nM (n = 2) with 1% (v/v) sheep plasma. Montelukast had little or no effect on the binding of either [^{3}H]leukotriene C4 to dU937 membranes or [^{3}H]leukotriene B_4 to THP-1 cell membranes or [^{3}H]leukotriene B_4 to THP-1 cell membranes (1). Synthetic metabolites of montelukast had comparable affinity to montelukast versus [^{3}H]leukotriene D_4 binding in guinea pig lung membranes (in the absence and presence of 0.05% (w/v) human serum albumin) but had similar or less affinity than montelukast in dU937 cell membranes (Table 1).

Effects of Montelukast on Agonist-Induced Contraction of Isolated Tissues

Montelukast was shown to be a potent and competitive antagonist of contractions of nontotal guinea pig trachea induced by leukotriene D_4 (pA_2 value 9.3; slope 0.8) (1). The selectivity of montelukast for $CysLT_1$ receptor has been demonstrated on guinea pig trachea as indicated by nonsignificant shifts in the dose-response curves to LTC_4 (45 nM serine borate present), U-44069, PGD_2, serotonin, acetylcholine, histamine, and PGF_{2a} (1). Montelukast also failed to inhibit

Table 1 Biological Activities of Montelukast

Assay	Montelukast
Guinea pig lung membranes (IC_{50}—nM)	
IC_{50} vs. [^{3}H]-LTD_4	0.61 ± 0.09 (*n* = 16)
IC_{50} vs. [^{3}H]-LTD_4 (+0.05% HSA)	0.42 ± 0.08 (*n* = 7)
IC_{50} vs. [^{3}H]-LTD_4 (+1% human plasma)	1.2 ± 0.36 (*n* = 5)
(+2% human plasma)	1.3
(+4% human plasma)	2.3
(+1% squirrel monkey plasma)	0.99 and 0.84
(+2% squirrel monkey plasma)	2.4
(+4% squirrel monkey plasma)	2.5
(+1% sheep plasma)	13.3 and 18.8
Human receptor (U937 cell membranes) (IC_{50})	
IC_{50} vs. [^{3}H]-LTD_4	0.78 ± 0.2 nM (*n* = 7)
IC_{50} vs. [^{3}H]-LTC_4	10 μM (*n* = 1)
Sheep lung membranes (IC_{50}—nM)	
IC_{50} vs. [^{3}H]-LTD_4	6 (*n* = 2)
THP-1 cell (IC_{50}—μM)	
IC_{50} vs. [^{3}H]-LTB_4	40 (*n* = 2)
Guinea pig trachea (pA_2)	
(vs. LTD_4-induced contraction)	
(1.6 × 10_8M to 1.6 × 10_6M)	9.3 (*n* = 14) (slope 0.8)

cholinergic contractions of isolated guinea pig tracheal rings to electrical field stimulation (1).

B. In Vivo Pharmacology in Animal Models

Effects of Montelukast on LTD_4-Induced Bronchoconstriction In Vivo

Intravenous administration of montelukast to anesthetized guinea pigs produced a potent inhibition of bronchoconstriction induced by intravenous leukotriene D_4 (ED_{50} I.V. 0.001 mg/kg) (1). Ongoing bronchoconstriction to a continuous infusion of leukotriene D_4 (0.16 μg/kg/min) in anesthetized guinea pigs was rapidly reversed by intravenous montelukast (0.1 and 1.0 mg/kg). (1) Montelukast also produced shifts in the leukotriene D_4 dose-response curve in anesthetized guinea pigs when administered intravenously and in conscious guinea pigs and sheep (1) when administered by aerosol. Montelukast, administered at doses up to 10 mg/kg I.V. to anesthetized guinea pigs, demonstrated pharmacological selectivity by failing to significantly inhibit the bronchoconstriction induced by the intravenous administration of histamine, arachidonic acid, serotonin, and acetylcholine (1). In conscious squirrel monkeys, montelukast, (0.003 and 0.001 mg/kg administered orally 4 hours pretreatment), significantly reduced the increase in pulmonary resistance and the decrease in dynamic compliance produced by an aerosol challenge with leukotriene D_4 (1). Montelukast (0.01 mg/kg 4 hours oral pretreatment and 0.03 mg/kg 24 hours oral pretreatment) inhibited the increase in specific airway resistance induced by an aerosol of leukotriene D_4 in conscious squirrel monkeys in another study (1).

Effects of Montelukast on Antigen-Induced Bronchoconstriction In Vivo

Montelukast (oral) significantly inhibited antigen-induced dyspnea in inbred hyperreactive rats (1) pretreated with methysergide (ED_{50} of 0.03 mg/kg, 4 hours pretreatment). Montelukast in conscious squirrel monkeys produced inhibition of antigen-induced acute bronchoconstriction (0.03 mg/kg; 4 hours pretreatment) and antigen-induced early and late-phase response (0.1 mg/kg; 4 hours pretreatment) (1). Montelukast inhibited antigen-induced bronchoconstriction in guinea pigs when administered intravenously at 10 mg/kg (1). Intravenous infusion of 8 μg/kg/min montelukast in ascaris-challenged sheep produced a 70% and 75% inhibition of the early- and late-phase bronchoconstriction, respectively (1). This regimen achieved a steady-state plasma level of approximately 10 μM of the parent drug.

Ancillary Pharmacology

Ancillary pharmacology studies (1) showed that montelukast had no deleterious effects on cardiovascular, autonomic, renal, gastrointestinal, or respiratory functions in dogs in doses up to 10 mg/kg i.v. or 20 mg/kg/administered orally or via fistula. No significant behavioral changes were observed in mice treated with montelukast, 100 mg/kg, orally.

C. In Vivo Pharmacology in Humans

Results of inhalational LTD_4 challenges in asthmatic patients demonstrate montelukast's potent and long-lasting antagonism of LTD_4-induced bronchoconstriction. In a double-blind, placebo-controlled, crossover study of six patients with mild asthma, the degree and duration of leukotriene receptor blockade by montelukast was assessed following bronchial inhalation challenge with LTD_4 (2,3). Montelukast 40 and 200 mg or placebo administered orally once daily for 2 days were compared with respect to their bronchoprotective effects 20–24 hours after dosing. All patients showed inhibition of LTD_4-induced bronchoconstriction up to the highest challenge dose of LTD_4 (approximately 100 times that of baseline) following treatment with 200 mg. In addition, four of six patients with montelukast 40 mg demonstrated similar inhibition of bronchoconstriction. In the other two patients, substantial shifts (~20-fold) of the dose-response were also observed.

IV. Dosage and Administration of Montelukast

The previously described inhalational LTD_4 challenge studies suggested that montelukast had pharmacodynamic properties sufficient for once-daily dosing. The chronobiology of asthma implied that dosing at bedtime might be optimal and was chosen to provide maximum plasma concentrations in the early morning hours (~4–5 hours postdose) when asthmatics' airway function is at its nadir. The efficacy of once-daily dosing of montelukast was evaluated in (1) exercise challenge (at the end of the once daily dosing interval) and (2) chronic asthma.

Two chronic asthma and two exercise-challenge studies evaluated montelukast at doses ranging from 0.4 to 200 mg once daily. These studies demonstrated that montelukast 10 mg once daily at bedtime was equally effective as higher doses. The clinical studies conducted demonstrate that efficacy is maintained throughout the dosing interval. Twice-daily dosing did not produce additional clinical effects (4–7). A lower dose (2 mg once daily) was less effective. No dose-limiting toxicity has been observed in any of these dose-response studies (7).

The recommended adult (≥ 15 years of age) daily dose of montelukast is 10 mg administered once daily at bedtime. In pediatric patients (6–14 years of age), the recommended daily dose is 5 mg once daily at bedtime.

V. Pharmacokinetic Properties of Montelukast

Montelukast is administered to adults and children orally as either a film-coated or a chewable tablet, respectively. These formulations have linear pharmacokinetics over the range of clinical doses. In pharmacokinetic analyses, the plasma concentrations of montelukast have been assayed by high-performance liquid chromatography (8,9).

A. Absorption

Montelukast was rapidly and well absorbed following oral administration in healthy volunteers. In a study of males and females receiving a single 10-mg oral tablet under fasting conditions, the oral bioavailability was 66% in men and 58% in women (10).

Maximum plasma concentrations are achieved within approximately 3–5 hours of oral administration of a 10-mg film-coated tablet and range between 0.33

and 0.54 μg/ml (10). The absorption of montelukast is not appreciably affected by coadministration with food.

B. Distribution

Montelukast is extensively bound to plasma proteins (approximately 99.5%). The steady-state volume of montelukast distribution is ~10 L (10). Following administration of a radiolabeled dose to rats, concentrations were minimal in all tissue, including the brain. This suggests that the lack of accumulation in any tissue and minimal distribution of montelukast across the blood-brain barrier may contribute to its favorable safety profile.

C. Metabolism

Montelukast is extensively metabolized; however, only minor amounts of the metabolites are found in plasma. The two predominant metabolites in plasma are diastereomers of the 21- and 36-hydroxylated acid and the dicarboxylic acid species. These metabolites are present in the steady-state plasma samples of adults and children in concentrations at least 10-fold lower than those of the parent compound. Additional metabolites of montelukast, found only in bile, include the acyl glucuronide conjugate, and sulfoxide, phenolic, and dicarboxylic acid derivatives (12).

In vitro studies indicate that the hepatic cytochrome P450 CYP3A4 isoenzyme system is responsible for the formation of the 21-hydroxylated and sulfoxide montelukast metabolites (13). These studies also indicate that CYP2C9 is involved in the formation of the 36-hydroxylated metabolite. Despite its hepatic metabolism, montelukast is not anticipated to inhibit the metabolism of other hepatically metabolized drugs.

D. Elimination

Montelukast and its metabolites are almost exclusively excreted in the bile. Negligible quantities (i.e., less than 0.2%) are excreted in the urine (12).

Clinical studies have demonstrated the plasma half-life of montelukast to be between 2.7 and 5.5 hours (10,11). In healthy individuals the plasma clearance of montelukast averaged approximately 45 ml/min. Following once-daily administration of 10 mg, an accumulation of approximately 14% was noted at steady state (10,11).

E. Montelukast Pharmacokinetics in Special Populations

Renal Function Impairment

Montelukast and its metabolites are not excreted in the urine to any appreciable extent (12). Therefore, no significant differences are expected in the pharmacokinetic parameters in renally impaired patients.

Elderly Patients

The mean bioavailability, AUC, C_{max}, and T_{max} for montelukast are similar in elderly (>65 years of age) and young (6–14 years of age) subjects following administration of a 10-mg oral tablet. Following a single 7-mg intravenous dose in healthy elderly volunteers (65–73 years of age), the mean plasma clearance averaged 31 ml/min compared to 46.8 ml/min in healthy younger subjects (11). Elderly patients also demonstrated a slightly prolonged mean plasma half-life, 6.7 hours, compared to 4.9 hours in healthy younger subjects.

F. Summary of Pharmacokinetic Parameters

Montelukast displays linear pharmacokinetic properties in the range of clinical doses. Food has no important effect on the absorption of montelukast; therefore, patients can take it irrespective of meals. The drug is metabolized by the hepatic P450 enzyme system and eliminated primarily in the bile. Montelukast is well tolerated in both adult and pediatric patients. No dosage adjustment is necessary in elderly patients or anticipated in those with renal insufficiency.

VI. Montelukast: Clinical Efficacy Trials

The clinical efficacy of montelukast was determined in placebo-controlled studies involving ~3000 adult and ~500 pediatric patients with asthma. These chronic asthma studies were conducted in patients (1) requiring chronic (''controller'') therapy in addition to inhaled β-agonists alone, (2) with mild asthma and exercise-induced bronchoconstriction, and (3) receiving inhaled corticosteroids, including aspirin-sensitive asthma.

In studies in adults with chronic asthma, 10 mg montelukast administered once daily at bedtime provided statistically and clinically significant benefits in parameters of asthma control, including forced expiratory volume in one second (FEV_1), daytime symptoms, ''as-needed'' inhaled β-agonist, asthma-related quality of life, asthma-free days, and asthma outcomes (episodes of asthma worsening). In separate studies, administration of montelukast significantly reduced inhaled corticosteroid doses and attenuated exercise-induced bronchoconstriction compared to placebo.

A. Adult Studies—Patients Treated with Inhaled β-Agonist Alone

In these studies, protocol-specified inclusion criteria included chronic asthmatic patients who were nonsmokers demonstrating a 15% increase in FEV_1 (absolute value) following β-agonist administration and baseline % predicted FEV_1 of approximately 66% (range 45–90%). Patients required approximately 5.3 puffs (range 3–5 puffs) of inhaled β-agonist per day.

Two endpoints measuring the effect of montelukast on airway obstruction were FEV_1 and PEFR. FEV_1 was measured 8–10 hours after bedtime dosing and performed using a standard spirometer with centralized quality control, according to American Thoracic Society (ATS) standards (14,15). PEFR, an objective measure of airway obstruction capturing the day-to-day variability of asthma, was measured after withholding β-agonist therapy for at least 4 hours. Daytime and nocturnal symptom scores and the amount of "as-needed" inhaled β-agonist use were recorded daily on a diary card using a validated questionnaire (16).

Placebo Comparison in Chronic Asthma

Two large placebo-controlled 12-week, double-blind efficacy (with an optional one-year extension period) studies investigated the ability of montelukast to improve the signs and symptoms of chronic asthma in patients who were receiving only "as-needed" β-agonist therapy (17). Compared with placebo, montelukast significantly ($p < 0.001$) improved FEV_1 to a similar extent in the two studies (mean percent change from baseline ~10% more compared with placebo). The effect of montelukast on FEV_1 was consistent over the 12-week study, and persisted for up to one year in patients who continued in the montelukast extension phase of the trial (Fig. 1) (18). In addition to a lack of tolerance developing with the continued use of montelukast, no rebound worsening in airway obstruction occurred during the placebo washout period.

Compared with placebo, montelukast had a statistically significant decrease of the use of "as-needed" β-agonist therapy (Fig. 2). The decrease in the amount

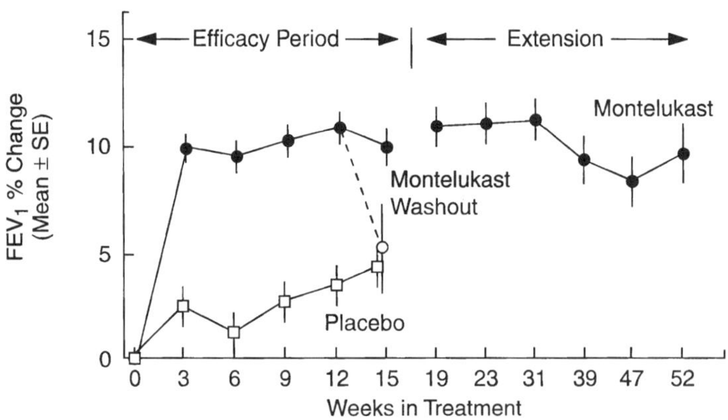

Figure 1 Effect of montelukast on FEV_1 (percent change from baseline) in two placebo-controlled trials of adult patients with chronic asthma.

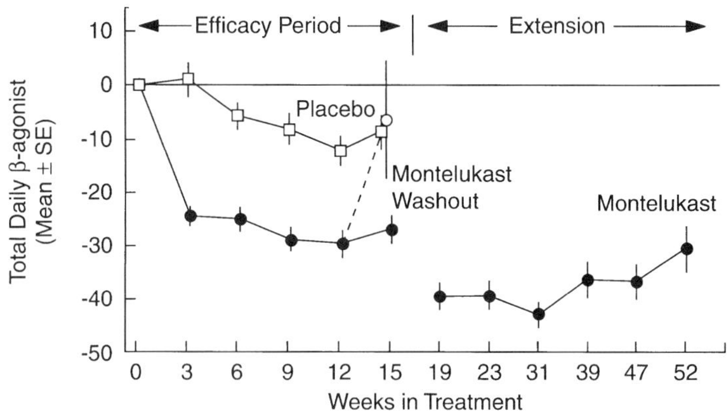

Figure 2 Effect of montelukast on "as-required" β-agonist use in adult patients with chronic asthma enrolled in two placebo-controlled trials.

of inhaled β-agonist use remained constant throughout the one-year extensions of both trials. Similar statistically significant effects were observed on daytime and nighttime asthma symptoms (18).

Asthma outcomes are important measures of overall asthma control. The effects of montelukast compared with placebo in the pooled data of these two studies included a decrease in the number of mild asthma exacerbations by 38% (defined as a significant fall in daily PEFR and an increase in β-agonist use and nocturnal awakening without a need for oral corticosteroids or additional provider care), an increase in the number of asthma-free days by 42% (defined as days without asthma attacks or nocturnal awakenings and minimal β-agonist use), and a decrease in asthma attacks by 37% (need for additional provider care and/or oral corticosteroids). All these effects of montelukast therapy were statistically significant at the $p < 0.05$ level (19).

The impact of montelukast on asthma-specific quality of life was also measured by a validated questionnaire evaluating the following: the activity limitations resulting from the patient's asthma (activity), the patient's asthma symptoms (symptoms), emotional problems caused by the patient's asthma (emotions), and the influence of environmental stimuli on the patient's asthma (environment). As illustrated in Figure 3, montelukast demonstrated significant ($p < 0.001$) improvement in all asthma-specific quality-of-life domains (19).

Protection Against Exercise-Induced Bronchoconstriction

Subjects with mild asthma may have normal pulmonary function and few symptoms; however, they frequently suffer from EIB, which may be a manifestation

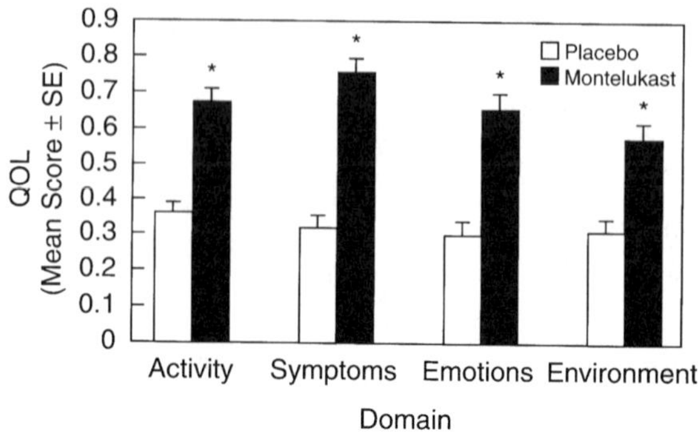

Figure 3 Effect of montelukast on asthma-specific quality-of-life parameters in adult patients with chronic asthma.

of inadequate asthma control. EIB provides a good endpoint to determine the effects of asthma therapy. Short-term treatment with leukotriene receptor antagonists protects against EIB. Montelukast produces a dose-dependent inhibition of exercise-induced bronchoconstriction (EIB) (treadmill challenge × 6 minutes) at the end of a once-daily dosing interval. In an initial short-term, crossover study, montelukast 100 mg produced significant protection against EIB (50% inhibition of the FEV_1 area under the postexercise curve) (20). In a second randomized, incomplete block placebo-controlled crossover study, 50, 10, 2, and 0.4 mg montelukast were administered once daily to 25 patients with mild asthma (defined as baseline FEV_1 >80% of predicted). Reproducible EIB prerandomization was required (mean postexercise fall in FEV_1 33%). Montelukast 10 and 50 mg once daily similarly protected against EIB 20–24 hours postdose; 0.4 and 2 mg produced significantly less protection (6).

Long-term protection against EIB with a leukotriene receptor antagonist has not been established. Montelukast was evaluated after 12 weeks of continuous treatment in patients with mild asthma and EIB.

Chronic protection against EIB was demonstrated in a 12-week study of adult patients with mild asthma (15 and 46 years of age, baseline FEV_1 83% of predicted), minimal inhaled β-agonist use, and EIB. Exercise was performed at the end of the once-daily dosing interval (mean prerandomization maximum percent fall FEV_1 36% postexercise) (21).

Compared with placebo, montelukast demonstrated a significant (p = 0.001) improvement in the week 12 $AUC_{0\text{–}60\ min}$. Protection by montelukast was consistent over the 12 weeks of continuous treatment (Fig. 4), without any evidence of tolerance. Following 12-week active treatment, there was no rebound

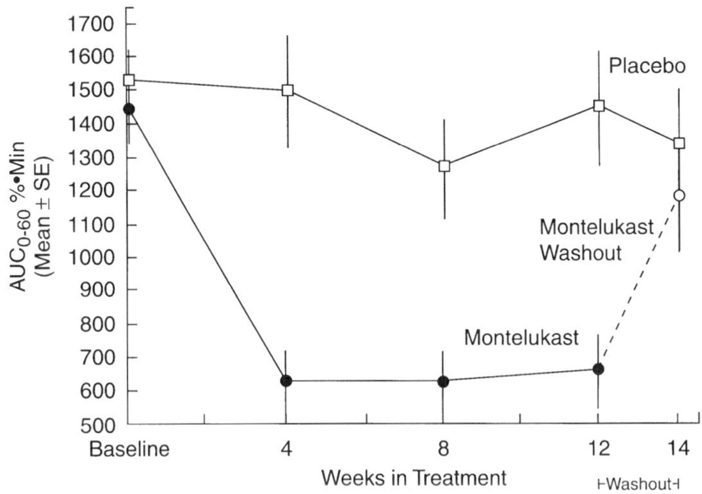

Figure 4 Effect of montelukast on exercise-induced bronchoconstriction over a 12-week treatment period as measured by postexercise $AUC_{0\text{-}60\ min}$.

worsening of asthma during a 2-week single-blind placebo washout period (Fig. 4).

Montelukast therapy was considered beneficial, measured by global assessments, by this cohort of mild asthmatics. Significantly ($p < 0.05$) more montelukast patients (71.2%) rated themselves as better at the end of the 12-week treatment period compared with those who had received placebo (44.4%). There was a significant difference ($p < 0.05$) between the montelukast and placebo groups in the proportion of patients requiring rescue medication (β-agonist) after exercise challenges at each visit during the 12-week treatment period, with a 65% reduction attributed to montelukast.

These studies demonstrate that montelukast improves asthma control in this group of patients with mild asthma. Protection against EIB was seen at the end of the dosing interval, suggesting benefit over the course of an entire day. Importantly, no tolerance to EIB developed to the protection provided by montelukast. Thus, montelukast therapy adds an important option for the treatment of mild asthmatic patients and EIB.

B. Inhaled Corticosteroid Studies—Adult Patients

Montelukast provides additive benefit to patients treated with inhaled corticosteroids, demonstrated by its ability to reduce the dose of inhaled corticosteroids.

Further, montelukast improves asthma control for patients with aspirin-sensitive asthma requiring high doses of inhaled and/or oral corticosteroids.

Inhaled Corticosteroid Tapering

In a study of patients with stable asthma (defined as a predicted $FEV_1 \geq 70\%$, minimal asthma symptoms, and inhaled β-agonist use) maintained on moderate-to-high doses (~1600 μg per day) of inhaled corticosteroids, the addition of montelukast resulted in the ability to taper the dose of corticosteroids without compromising asthma control (22,23).

During the 12 weeks of active treatment, montelukast allowed statistically significant tapering of inhaled corticosteroid doses, compared with placebo (46.7% decrease of prerandomization dose in patients treated with montelukast versus 30.3% dose decrease in patients treated with placebo). At the end of the trial, the mean last tolerated dose of corticosteroid was 727 μg in the placebo group versus 526 mcg in the montelukast group (Table 2). Forty percent of montelukast patients tolerated a complete tapering (i.e., removal) of their inhaled corticosteroid compared with 29% of placebo patients. This study demonstrated montelukast provides additive clinical efficacy to inhaled corticosteroid therapy.

The results that suggest one role for leukotriene receptor antagonists may be their ability to reduce exposure to high-dose inhaled corticosteroids.

Aspirin-Sensitive Asthma

The effect of montelukast was evaluated in a 4-week study of aspirin-sensitive asthmatic patients. Approximately 90% of patients were receiving high-dose inhaled and/or oral corticosteroids at baseline that were not adequately controlling their asthma (baseline mean FEV_1 was 69% of predicted, with at least a 12% reversibility post–inhaled β-agonists). Montelukast produced significant improvements in airway obstruction (as measured by FEV_1 and PEFR), "as-needed" β-agonist use, and nocturnal symptoms (24,25). In addition, improvements in asthma outcomes compared with placebo were noted; specifically, the number of asthma exacerbation days, the number of asthma-free days increased, and patient global and quality-of-life assessments improved. Montelukast provides clinical benefit to this more severe group of asthmatics with aspirin sensitivity who are incompletely controlled on corticosteroids, further supporting the additive benefit of montelukast and its potential therapeutic role across the entire spectrum of asthma.

C. Pediatric Studies

Asthma is the most common chronic disease in children (25). Current options for therapy are limited and often compromised by side effects or dosing adminis-

Table 2 Last Tolerated Inhaled Corticosteroid Dose in the Inhaled Corticosteroid Taper Study

Treatment	N[a]	Prestudy dose (μg/day) (mean ± SD)	Prerandomization dose (μg/day) (mean ± SD)	Last tolerated dose (μg/day) (mean ± SE)	Percent change from prerandomization baseline (mean ± SE)	Difference in LS mean[b] MNT-PBO (95% CI)
Placebo	113	1681 ± 670	1079 ± 557	727 ± 70	30.27 ± 6.34	
Montelukast	112	1588 ± 646[c]	976 ± 553	526 ± 68	46.73 ± 5.88	17.58* (0.32, 34.84)

[a]Number of patients included in intention-to-treat analysis.
[b]Least square mean.
[c]Based on the 113 randomized patients.
*$p < 0.050$, compared with placebo.
MNT = Montelukast; PBO = placebo.

tration challenges (inhaled formulations). Therefore, a clinical development program was undertaken evaluating montelukast in children 6–14 years old. The efficacy of montelukast in pediatric patients has been assessed in placebo-controlled chronic asthma and exercise-induced bronchoconstriction trials.

Placebo Comparison in Chronic Asthma

A placebo-controlled 8-week double-blind efficacy study in patients aged 6–14 years with chronic asthma (mean baseline FEV_1 77% predicted, improvement in $FEV_1 \geq 15\%$ post–inhaled β-agonist) was performed. The objective was to evaluate the ability of montelukast to improve the signs and symptoms of chronic asthma in patients who were receiving only ''as-needed'' β-agonist therapy. Patients received a 5-mg chewable montelukast tablet or placebo once daily at bedtime. Compared with placebo, patients receiving montelukast demonstrated a statistically significant improvement in FEV_1, which was consistent throughout the extension period ($p < 0.001$) (26,27). Patients also had significant improvement in secondary efficacy endpoints including total daily ''as-needed'' β-agonist use, incidence of asthma exacerbations, and asthma-specific quality of life. Parent and physician global assessment of patients' asthma also showed improvement (28).

Exercise-Induced Asthma

EIB is especially problematic for children, who tend to be very active. Montelukast is the first leukotriene receptor antagonist shown to provide protection against EIB in pediatric patients (6–14 years old). A two-period crossover study assessed the effects of a 5-mg montelukast chewable tablet at bedtime in patients 6–14 years of age with EIB. Entry criteria were similar to the adult studies. Repeat exercise challenges were performed at the end of the dosing interval (20–24 hours postdose) after a 2-day treatment period. Montelukast produced a significant improvement in AUC (mean inhibition 58.8% compared to placebo, $p = 0.013$) (29). The extent of protection against EIB (58.8% inhibition) observed in children was similar to that observed in adults (approximately 40–67% inhibition). Protection against EIB was demonstrated at the end of a once-daily dosing interval (trough plasma concentrations). Therefore, it can be assumed that montelukast attenuated exercise-induced bronchoconstriction throughout the course of this dosing interval.

VII. Montelukast Effects on Asthmatic Inflammation

Evidence suggests that leukotrienes mediate parameters of asthmatic inflammation. Clinical trials examined the effect of montelukast on peripheral blood and sputum eosinophils (presently thought to be one of the major effector cells of asthmatic inflammation), as well as the effect on the early- and late-phase response to antigen challenge, a general model of asthmatic inflammation.

A. Antigen-Induced Late Asthmatic Response

Montelukast causes a protection against the early- and late-phase response due to inhalation of antigen in patients with atopic asthma. The protective effect of montelukast 10 mg at the end of the dosing interval was compared with placebo in 12 stable, atopic patients (30). In this double-blind, two-period crossover study, montelukast produced statistically significant ($p \leq 0.008$) inhibition in maximum percent decreases in the early asthmatic response (0–3 hours postexposure) of 75.4% (AUC %fall.hr) and late asthmatic response (3–8 hours postexposure) of 56.9% (AUC%fall.hr) compared with placebo.

B. Peripheral Blood Eosinophils

Peripheral blood eosinophil counts were consistently and significantly reduced (up to 29.5%) in adult and pediatric patients receiving montelukast compared with placebo (31,32). The baseline elevations of peripheral blood eosinophils reported in these studies are consistently seen in asthma (33). The changes in peripheral blood eosinophils were mildly correlated with improvements in study endpoints (FEV_1 and daytime symptoms) (31,32).

C. Sputum Eosinophils

The effect of montelukast on clinical parameters of asthma and sputum eosinophils was evaluated in a 4-week placebo-controlled trial. Forty adult asthmatics with ≥5% sputum eosinophils at baseline and clinical asthma (FEV_1 65–85% predicted, with daytime symptoms and inhaled β-agonist use) were treated with montelukast or placebo. Montelukast significantly improved airway function, symptoms, and inhaled β-agonist use and significantly lowered sputum eosinophils ($p < 0.05$) (Fig. 5) (34). These effects on blood and sputum eosinophils are consistent with other asthma therapies affecting asthmatic inflammation.

VIII. Safety of Montelukast

At the time of this publication the safety and tolerability of montelukast for the treatment of asthma has been evaluated in approximately 3000 adult patients.

A. Adverse Events in Adults

The proportion of montelukast-treated patients with any clinical adverse experience was generally similar to placebo. The most frequently reported events were

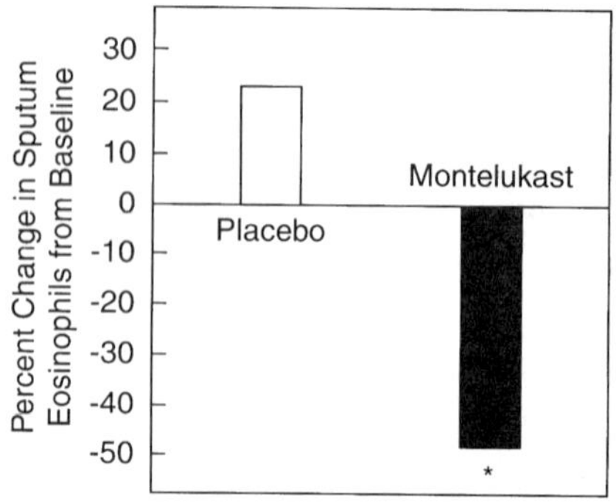

Figure 5 Effect of montelukast on sputum eosinophils in asthmatic patients after 4 weeks of treatment.

upper respiratory tract infection, asthma, and headache across studies. The incidence of these adverse events was similar to those in patients receiving placebo.

No clinically important differences in laboratory abnormalities were noted among the treatment groups. Upon specific analysis, no between-group differences (montelukast versus placebo) in blood chemistry including serum transaminase levels were found. No cases of hepatitis nor discontinuations due to the elevation of serum transaminases were reported. In summary, montelukast administered for up to 1 year to patients with chronic asthma was generally well tolerated.

B. Adverse Events in Children

At the time of this publication, approximately 500 pediatric patients received montelukast. The overall clinical and laboratory safety profile of montelukast was generally similar to placebo as found in the adult population. Adverse experiences that occurred in association with montelukast were generally transient and self-limited.

No statistically significant differences between groups in the incidence of clinical adverse experiences were noted. The individual clinical adverse experiences with the highest frequency were upper respiratory tract infection, asthma, and headache. The overall incidence was similar between placebo and montelukast treatment groups.

The laboratory safety profile was also similar between montelukast and placebo. No clinically important differences in laboratory abnormalities were noted among the treatment groups. A similar proportion of patients with laboratory values outside the predefined limits of changes was noted in both treatment groups.

Consistent with the findings in adult trials, no differences in blood chemistry including serum transaminase levels were noted between montelukast and placebo groups. There were no cases of hepatitis reported. Overall, montelukast administered to pediatric patients with chronic asthma was generally well tolerated.

IX. Summary

Asthma is a common chronic condition representing a major therapeutic challenge. Many patients remain symptomatic and poorly controlled, although many treatment options are currently available.

Montelukast is a new, highly potent, and selective $CysLT_1$ receptor antagonist. The clinical benefits of montelukast in the treatment of asthma have been demonstrated across the spectrum of asthmatic severities. In patients receiving only ''as-needed'' β-agonist treatment but requiring additional symptom control, montelukast provides an alternative to inhaled corticosteroids. In those already receiving inhaled corticosteroids, montelukast provides additional clinical benefits and allows tapering of inhaled corticosteroids. The recommended dose is 10 mg once daily at bedtime in adults and 5 mg in children.

Montelukast is generally well tolerated with an adverse event profile generally similar to that in patients receiving placebo. The significant improvement montelukast provides in clinical efficacy parameters combined with its effects on parameters of asthmatic inflammation, good tolerability, and convenience of oral once-daily dosing provides a significant advance in asthma therapy.

References

1. Jones T, et al. Pharmacology of montelukast sodium (SINGULAIR™), a potent and selective leukotriene D_4-receptor antagonist. Can J Physiol Pharmacol 1995; 73(2): 191–201.
2. Botto A, Delepeleire I, Rochette F, Reiss TF, Zhang J, Kundu S, Decramer M. MK-0476 causes prolonged, potent LTD_4 receptor antagonism in the airways of asthmatics. Am Rev Respir Dis 1994; 149:A465.
3. Delepeleire I, Rochette F, Reiss TF, Botto A, Zhang J, Kundu S, Decramer M. MK-0476 causes prolonged, potent, LTD_4 receptor antagonism in the airways of asthmatics. Eur Resp J 1994; 7(18):316S.
4. Reiss TF, Altman LC, Munk ZM, Seltzer J, Zhang J, Shingo S, Friedman B, Noonan N. MK-0476, an LTD_4 receptor antagonist, improves the signs and symptoms of asthma with a dose as low as 10 mg, once daily. Am J Respir Crit Care Med 1995; 151:A378.
5. Reiss TF, Chervinsky P, Noonan M, Prenner B, Zhang J, Hess J, Friedman B, Kundu S. MK-0476, and LTD_4 receptor antagonist, exhibits a dose related improvement in

the once daily treatment of patients with chronic asthma. Eur Respir J Suppl 1995; 289S.

6. Reiss TF, Bronsky E, Kemp J, Guerreiro D, Zhang J. Dose related protection of exercise bronchoconstriction at the end of a once daily dosing interval by montelukast, a cysteinyl leukotriene receptor antagonist. J Clin Pharm Ther. In press.
7. Reiss TF, Altman LC, Munk ZM, Seltzer J, Shingo S, Friedman B, Noonan N. MK-0476, and LTD_4 receptor antagonist improves the signs and symptoms of asthma with a dose as low as 10mg, once daily. Am J Respir Crit Care Med 1995; 151(4): A378.
8. Amin RD, Cheng H, Rogers JD. Determination of MK-0476 in human plasma by liquid chromatography. J Pharm Biomed Anal 1995; 13(2):155–158.
9. Becard S, Cheng H, Huhn R, Liu L, Hess J, Reiss T. Comparative in vitro and in vivo performance of a capsule and a tablet formulation of MK-0476. Pharm Res 1993; 10:S217.
10. Cheng H, Leff JA, Amin R, Gertz BJ, DeSmet M, Noonan N, Rogers JD, Malbecq W, Meisner D, Somers G. Pharmacokinetics, bioavailability, and safety of montelukast sodium (MK-0476) in healthy males and females. Pharm Res 1996; 13:445–448.
11. Zhao JJ, Rogers JD, Holland SD, Larson P, Amin RD, Haesen R, Freeman A, Seiberling M, Merz M, Cheng H. Pharmacokinetics and bioavailability of montelukast sodium (MK-0476) in healthy young and elderly volunteers. Biopharm Drug Disposition. In press.
12. Balani SK, Xu X, Pratha V, Koss M, Amin RD, Dufresne C, Miller RR, Arison BH, Doss GA, Chiba M, Freeman A, Holland SD, Schwartz JI, Lasseter KC, Gertz BJ, Isenberg J, Baillie TA, Lin JH. Metabolic profiles of montelukast sodium (SINGULAIR™), a potent cysteinyl $leukotriene_1$ receptor antagonist, in human plasma and bile. In press.
13. Chauret N, Yergey J, Trimble L, Nicoll-Griffith D. In vitro biotransformation of MK-0476, a new potent LTD_4 antagonist. Abstract presented at 10th International Symposium on Microsomes and Drug Oxidations, Toronto, Canada, July 18–21, 1994.
14. Botto A, Malmstrom K, Lu S, Zhang J, Reiss TF. Centralized spirometry quality control lowers the variability in multicenter asthma clinical trials. Am J Respir Crit Care Med 1997; 155(4):A893.
15. Malmstrom K, Botto A, Zhang J, Reiss TF. Centralized spriometry quality control lowers the variability in multicenter asthma clinical trials. Eur Resp J 1996; 9(23): 121S.
16. Santanello N, Barber B, Reiss T, Friedman BS, Juniper EF, Zhang J. Measurement characteristics of two asthma symptom scales for use in clinical trials. Eur Resp J 1997; 10:646–651.
17. Reiss TF, Chervinsky P, Edwards T, Dockhorn R, Nayak A, Hess J, Zhang J, Shingo S. Montelukast (MK-0476), a $CysLT_1$ receptor antagonist, improves the signs and symptoms of asthma over a 3 months treatment period. Eur Resp J 1996; 9(23): 273S.
18. Reiss TF, White R, Noonan G, Korenblat P, Hess J, Shingo S, Seidenberg B, and the Montelukast Study Group. Montelukast (MK-0476), a $CysLT_1$ receptor antagonist,

improves the signs and symptoms of asthma over one year of treatment. Eur Respir J 1997, in press.

19. Reiss TF, Chervinsky P, Edwards T, Dockhorn R, Nayak A, Hess J, Zhang J, Shingo S. Montelukast (MK-0476), a $CysLT_1$ receptor antagonist, improves asthma outcomes over a 3-month treatment period. Am J Respir Crit Care Med 1997; 155(4):A2662.
20. Reiss TF, Bronsky E, Hendeles L, et al. Increased urinary excretion of LTE_4 after exercise and attenuation of exercise-induced bronchospasm by montelukast, a CysLT receptor antagonist. Thorax. In press.
21. Leff JA, Bronsky EA, Kemp J, Pearlman DS, Hendeles L, Busse WW, Dockhorn R, Guerreiro DA, Reiss TF, Kundu S. Montelukast (MK-0476) inhibits exercise-induced bronchoconstriction (EIB) over 12 weeks without causing tolerance. Am J Respir Crit Care Med 1997; 155(4):A977.
22. Kundu S, Noonan N, Friedman BS, Reiss TF, Leff JA. Use of a composite clinical score allows safe tapering of inhaled corticosteroids (ICS) in asthmatic patients. Am J Respir Crit Care Med 1997; 155(4):A352.
23. Leff JA, Israel E, Noonan MJ, Finn AF, Godard P, Lofdahl CG, Friedman BS, Connors L, Weinland DE, Reiss TF, Kundu S. Montelukast (MK-0476) allows tapering of inhaled corticosteroids (ICS) in asthmatic patients while maintaining clinical stability. Am J Respir Crit Care Med 1997; 155(4):A976.
24. Kuna P, Malmstrom K, Dahlen SE, Nizankowska E, et al. Montelukast (MK-0476), a $CysLT_1$ receptor antagonist, improves asthma control in aspirin-intolerant asthmatic patients. Am J Respir Crit Care Med 1997; 155(4):A975.
25. Dahlen SE, Malmstrom K, Kuna P, Nizankowska E, Kowalski M, Stevenson D, Bousquet J, Dahlen B, Picado C, Lumry W, Holgate S, Pauwels R, Szczeklik A, Shahane A, Tanaka W, Reiss TF. Improvement of asthma in aspirin-intolerant patients by montelukast (MK-0476) a potent and specific $CysLT_1$ receptor antagonist: correlations with patients baseline characteristics. Eur Resp J 1997, in press.
26. National Asthma Education and Prevention Program Expert Panel Report II: Guidelines for Diagnosis and Management of Asthma, NHLBI Workshop Report, Bethesda, MD. National Heart, Lung, and Blood Institute, National Institutes of Health, 1995.
27. Knorr BA, Matz J, Bernstein J, et al. Montelukast (MK-0476) improves asthma over a 2 month treatment period in 6- to 14-year olds. Am J Respir Crit Care Med 1997; in press.
28. Knorr, BA, Matz J, Sveum, RJ, et al. Montelukast (MK-0476) improves asthma over 6 months of treatment 6- to 14-year old patients. Eur Resp J 1997, in press.
29. Kemp JP, Dockhorn RJ, Shapiro GG, Nguyen HH, Guerreiro D, Reiss TF, Friedman BS, Knorr BA. Montelukast, a leukotriene receptor antagonist, inhibits exercise-induced bronchoconstriction in 6- to 14-year old children. J Allergy Clin Immunol 1997; 99(No. 1, Part 2):S321.
30. Diamant Z, Timmers MC, Veen H, et al. Effect of oral montelukast (MK-0476, a potent leukotriene receptor antagonist, on allergen-induce airway responses in asthmatic subjects. Am J Respir Crit Care Med 1996; 153:A346.
31. Shingo S, Zhang J, Reiss TF. Relationship between peripheral blood eosinophils and asthma efficacy endpoints: FEV_1, PEFR, and daytime symptom score. Am J Respir Crit Care Med 1997, in press.

32. Zhang J, Reiss TF, Chervinsky P, Edwards T, Dockhorn R, Nayak A, Noonan G, Hess J, Shingo S. Montelukast, a $CysLT_1$ receptor antagonist, decreases peripheral blood eosinophils and improves the signs and symptoms of asthma over a 3-month period. J Allergy Clin Immunol 1997; 99(2):S268.
33. Bousquet J, Chanez P, et al. Eosinophilic inflammation in asthma. N Engl J Med 1990; 323:1033–1039.
34. Leff JA, Pizzichini E, Efthimiadis A, Boulet LP, Wei LX, Weinland DE, Hendeles L, Hargreave FE. Effect of montelukast (MK-0476) on airway eosinophilic inflammation in mildly uncontrolled asthma: a randomized placebo-controlled trial. Am J Respir Crit Care Med 1997; in press.

15

Pranlukast—The First Orally Active Cysteinyl Leukotriene Receptor Antagonist Marketed for the Treatment of Asthma

JEFFREY W. DUBB and ANTHONY S. REBUCK

SmithKline Beecham Pharmaceuticals
Collegeville, Pennsylvania

I. Introduction

Pranlukast (SB 205312, Ultair™, ONO-1078, Onon®) was launched in Japan in mid-1995 for the treatment of asthma in adults. It is the first orally active cysteinyl leukotriene receptor antagonist (LTRA) to be used in clinical practice (1). A novel, selective, and potent LTRA, pranlukast binds to the leukotriene D_4 (LTD_4) receptor, inhibiting cysteinyl leukotriene binding. The chemical formula for pranlukast is $C_{27}H_{23}N_5O_4{}^1/_2H_2O$ (Fig. 1), and its molecular weight is 490.52.

In Japan, pranlukast was selected in 1981 from among nearly 1000 promising compounds screened for their ability to antagonize leukotriene-mediated effects. After early toxicological studies determined its safety, clinical trials were initiated in Japan in 1987 and proceeded through 1992, when pranlukast was submitted to the Japanese regulatory authority (Koseisho) for marketing approval.

In 1992, SmithKline Beecham Pharmaceuticals acquired worldwide rights to develop and market pranlukast outside Japan, South Korea, and Taiwan. Phase I and IIA studies began in Europe and the United States in 1993, and Phase IIB/III clinical trials began in 1994. The results of these trials are currently undergoing analysis and are thus only briefly mentioned here. Improvements in lung function, with measurable improvements in flow rates, are seen after the first dose. In addition, use of pranlukast reduces nonspecific bronchial hyperreactivity, as measured by both histamine and methacholine challenges. On the whole, this far-reaching and broad-based worldwide clinical program is providing a picture of

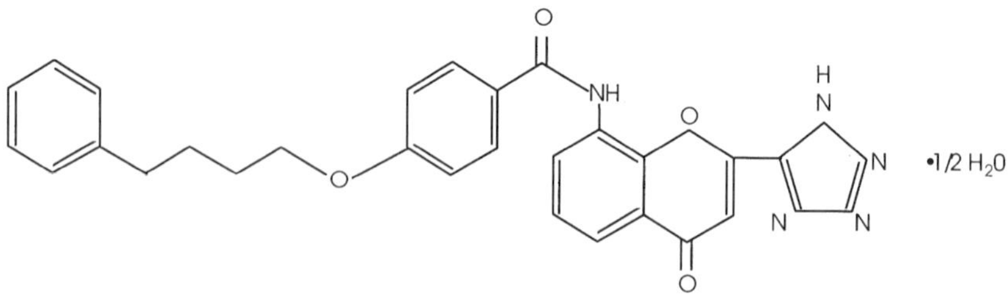

Figure 1 Structural formula of pranlukast, 4-oxo-8-[*p*-(4-phenylbutyloxy)benzoylamino]-2-(tetrazol-5-yl)-^{4}H-1-benzopyran hemihydrate. (From Ref. 22.)

the effect of pranlukast in asthma that demonstrates it is comparable to inhaled steroids on several criteria and more efficacious than nedocromil on most criteria.

II. Clinical Pharmacology

Clinical studies conducted in Japan (and subsequently in Europe and the United States) have shown that pranlukast is well tolerated and effective in reducing bronchial hyperresponsiveness, as measured by methacholine challenge (2) and histamine inhalation (3) tests. The pharmacokinetics and pharmacodynamics of pranlukast have also been studied in healthy volunteers.

In one group of healthy subjects, a study of single and repeated dosing of pranlukast under fasting conditions was conducted. Serial blood samples were taken predose and up to 14 hours postdose. After an overnight fast, pranlukast 225 mg was taken 30 minutes before breakfast and 30 minutes after breakfast. An oral absorption lag time of approximately 1–2 hours was demonstrated, with T_{max} occurring at about 3 hours (4), thus providing coverage up to 12 hours after dosing. Median T_{max} was shortened when pranlukast was dosed before breakfast; it was prolonged when dosed afterwards. Area under the curve (AUC) and C_{max} were higher following dosing before or after breakfast compared to the fasting state (4,5). Food enhances the absorption of pranlukast; thus, the product should be taken with a meal or snack. Pranlukast is highly bound to human plasma proteins (>99%). Pranlukast bioavailability is increased after evening dosing as compared to morning administration. Statistically significant ($p < 0.05$) increases were noted in $AUC_{0\text{-}t}$ (56%) and T_{max} (2.5 h) after evening administration. C_{max} was 14% higher after evening dosing (0.71, 1.84, 95% C.I.) (6).

To determine whether age has an effect on pranlukast pharmacokinetics, a trial was performed in healthy young and elderly subjects (7). The young and the elderly subjects fasted overnight, ate a light breakfast, and then 30 minutes later were given oral pranlukast 300 mg. Plasma from 24-hour serial blood samples was assayed by HPLC. Data for mean plasma concentration versus time was similar for both age groups; median T_{max} was 4.5 hours. The estimated geometric mean $AUC_{0\text{-}t}$ and C_{max} ratios for the elderly to the young were 1.00 (0.71, 1.41, 95% CI) and 0.93 (0.66, 1.33, 95% CI), respectively. It was concluded that no significant differences in the pharmacokinetics of pranlukast were observed between the young and the elderly subjects or in mean pharmacokinetic parameters with respect to gender.

A study of the effects of single oral doses of pranlukast 150, 300, and 600 mg on cardiovascular parameters including pulse rate, systolic/diastolic blood pressure, 12-lead electrocardiogram (ECG), and cardiac output was conducted in 12 healthy male subjects. The results demonstrated that the administration of pranlukast did not produce any clinically relevant effects on cardiovascular parameters (8).

Pranlukast has been safely co-administered with β_2-agonists, corticosteroids, theophylline, cromolyn sodium, nedocromil, antihistamines (including terfenadine), and antibiotics without evidence of drug interactions. No studies have been conducted in women known to be pregnant; however, animal studies have not demonstrated any fetotoxic effects.

The effect of pranlukast on LTD_4 challenge was studied in healthy male volunteers with the pharmacodynamics indicating a duration of action that should allow a b.i.d. dosing regimen. This conclusion was supported by a repeat LTD_4 challenge study. Pranlukast treatment produced a prolonged protective effect against bronchoconstriction induced by LTD_4 inhalation consistent with a twice-daily dosing regimen. In addition to demonstrating a long duration of inhibition, this study demonstrated no evidence of tachyphylaxis to pranlukast (9).

III. Asthma-Provocation Studies

A. LTD_4 Challenge

Historically, leukotriene C_4 (LTC_4), and LTD_4 challenge models have been useful in testing the clinical activity of LTRAs such as pranlukast. One study has demonstrated that in normal subjects, LTD_4 is at least 1000 times more potent than histamine in causing bronchoconstriction (10); further, it is well known that patients with asthma are more sensitive to leukotriene challenge than normal patients (11).

Pranlukast blocks bronchoconstriction induced by LTC_4 and LTD_4 in vitro (12). More importantly, in humans, O'Shaughnessy et al. (9) reported that following a single dose of pranlukast 450 mg or after 5 days of b.i.d. oral dosing with pranlukast, bronchoconstriction induced by LTD_4 inhalation was attenuated. At 3½ hours after the first dose on day 1, pranlukast produced a significant 10.6-fold shift in the LTD_4 dose-response curve, compared with placebo ($p < 0.001$).

This shift was greater at 3½ hours on day 5—25.9-fold ($p < 0.001$). Thus, the protective effect of pranlukast increased after repeat dosing for 5 days, and this effect was maintained at 9.5 hours (7.0-fold; $p < 0.001$). Compared with placebo, no significant differences were seen in histamine-induced airway reactivity in the pranlukast-treated group, expressed as change in airway conductance (PC_{35} sG_{aw}) to histamine.

The ability of pranlukast to block bronchoconstriction induced by LTD_4 inhalation, demonstrated by the shift in PC_{35}, was positively correlated with pranlukast plasma concentrations. This suggests that during oral administration, higher pranlukast plasma concentrations are associated with larger shifts in sG_{aw} PC_{35} values. Pranlukast's lack of effect on histamine inhalation–induced bronchoconstriction confirms its specificity of action as an LTRA.

A further understanding of the relationship between pranlukast exposure and inhibition of LTD_4-induced bronchconstriction was reported by Smith et al. (13). Using a double-blind, randomized, four-period crossover design, the effects of intravenous pranlukast on LTD_4 challenge in patients with mild to moderate asthma was studied. During each treatment period, patients received an intravenous infusion of pranlukast 10, 30, or 60 mg or placebo. As seen in previous studies, a shift in PC_{20} FEV_1 was increased in a dose-related fashion relative to placebo. The shift was 12.83-fold at the 10-mg dose, 27.72-fold at the 30-mg dose, and 100.02-fold at the 60-mg dose. These results demonstrate that intravenous administration of pranlukast blocks the effects of inhaled LTD_4 in a concentration-dependent manner and that pranlukast is a potent antagonist of LTD_4 in humans.

B. Effect of Pranlukast in Acute Challenge Studies

Pranlukast has been evaluated in a series of challenge studies to determine its specificity and clinical activity. It has demonstrated clinical activity in traditional challenge models, including exercise-induced asthma (14) and inhaled bronchoprovocations with allergen (15), and sulpyrine (an aspirin analog) (16). Pranlukast blocked both the early and the late asthmatic response following challenge with house dust mite antigen. This activity against the LAR suggests that pranlukast interferes with the inflammatory response. In all challenge studies, pranlukast significantly attenuated the decrease in FEV_1 induced by bronchoprovocation when compared with placebo or baseline control.

Cold Air

Strek et al. (17) studied the effect of pretreatment with pranlukast on the bronchospastic response to hyperventilation of cold air using a double-blind, randomized, two-period crossover design. Relative to placebo, pranlukast on average increased $PD_{20}V_E$ (minute ventilation causing a 20% decrease in FEV_1) 23% on day 1 and 34% on day 7 (point estimate; 95% C.I.: 4%, 44% and 2%, 75%, respectively). The investigators reported a similar effect on respiratory heat loss. These results demonstrate that pranlukast inhibits cold air–induced bronchoconstriction in patients with asthma beginning on day 1, and this protective effect was maintained for 7 days with no evidence of tolerance (17).

Allergen Challenge

Leukotrienes have been recovered from bronchoalveolar lavage fluid after both early and late airway responses following antigen challenges (18–21). Three allergen challenge studies conducted with pranlukast in Japan underscore the importance of the leukotrienes in allergen-induced immediate (early) and late airway responses as well as the ability of pranlukast to inhibit and attenuate these responses. These studies demonstrated that patients with asthma are protected by pranlukast against bronchoconstriction induced by house dust mite–antigen challenges.

The challenge studies were conducted to (1) determine the effect of a single dose of pranlukast as prechallenge treatment on the early response in asthma, (2) determine its effect when given 1 and 4 hours after house dust mite–antigen challenge, and (3) assess the effects of repeated dosing of pranlukast on early and late responses in atopic patients with asthma (22).

The first study was a single-blind, placebo-controlled, crossover trial in six patients. A single dose of oral pranlukast 300 or 450 mg or placebo was administered 3 hours prior to inhaled house dust mite–antigen challenge. Patients who weighed less than 70 kg received the 300-mg dose of pranlukast, and those who weighed 70 kg or more received the 450-mg dose. Percent change in FEV_1 was measured and was taken at 0, 10, 20, 30, 45, 60, 90, and 120 minutes postchallenge.

A mean reduction in FEV_1 from baseline greater than 40% was observed in patients exposed to house dust mite antigen. In the groups pretreated with pranlukast, FEV_1 reduction was attenuated to less than 50% of that noted in the placebo group (Fig. 2), suggesting that such treatment significantly reduced early airway response to inhaled allergen. The second trial evaluated the effect of pranlukast treatment given both 1 hour and 4 hours after house dust mite–antigen challenge. In this randomized, double-blind, placebo-controlled, crossover study, 10 patients with atopic asthma received pranlukast 300 mg (those who weighed less than 70 kg), pranlukast 450 mg (those who weighed 70 kg or more), or placebo. FEV_1 was measured each hour for up to 9 hours after house dust mite–antigen challenge.

In these 10 patients, house dust mite–antigen challenge produced early and late airway responses. When compared with placebo, pranlukast administered at both 1 and 4 hours postchallenge increased the rate and extent of recovery from the early airway response and significantly reduced the late airway response (Fig. 3).

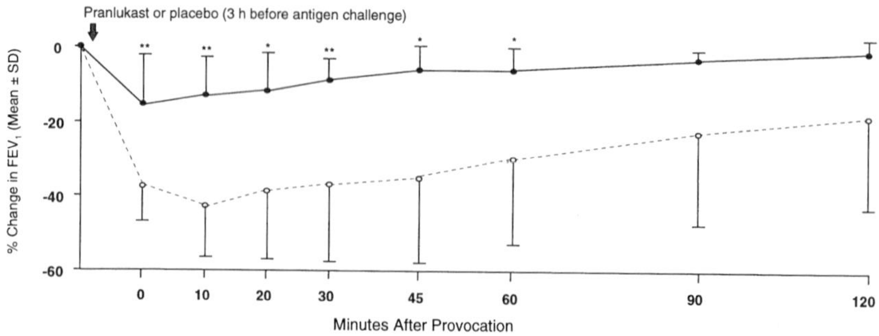

Figure 2 Pranlukast-mediated inhibition of house dust mite–antigen–induced immediate airway response. Patients were pretreated with a single dose of pranlukast (solid line) or placebo (dotted line) prior to challenge. The immediate effect on airway response to inhaled house dust mite–antigen challenge was evaluated using changes in FEV_1. Data are expressed as the mean SEM. $*p < 0.05$; $**p < 0.01$ vs. placebo. (From Ref. 22.)

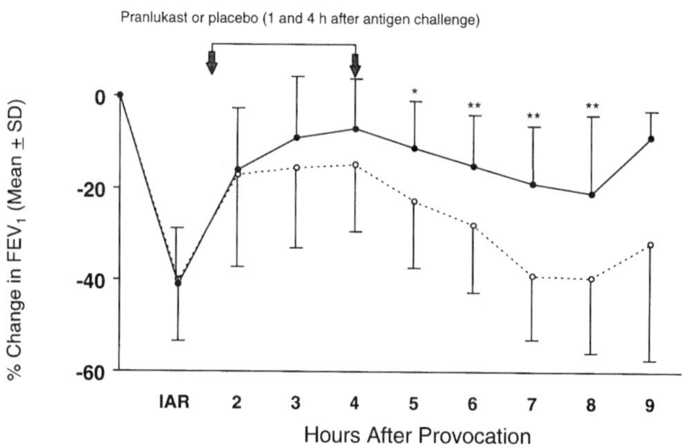

Figure 3 Effect of postchallenge pranlukast treatment on house dust mite–antigen–induced immediate and late airway responses. Two doses of pranlukast (solid line) or placebo (dotted line) were administered after challenge, and the effect on immediate and late airway response was assessed using FEV_1. Data are expressed as the mean ± SEM. $*p < 0.05$; $**p < 0.01$ vs. placebo. IAR = Immediate airway response. (From Ref. 22.)

The third study was conducted in six patients with asthma who also had a history of atopy, positive responses to house dust mite and other antigens, and radioallergosorbent test (RAST) scores of 2 or greater. This single-blind trial evaluated the effect of treatment with pranlukast for 7 days compared with baseline after house dust mite–antigen challenge–induced early and late airway responses. To establish a baseline response, FEV_1 was measured at 1, 2, 4, and 6 hours after inhalation of house dust mite antigen.

For the next 7 days, patients received pranlukast 225 mg after breakfast and dinner. Two hours after the last morning dose was administered, a house dust mite–antigen inhalation challenge was performed. Early and late airway responses were assessed by repeat FEV_1 measurements obtained 1, 2, 4, and 6 hours postchallenge. Pranlukast was found to inhibit significantly both early and late airway responses to challenge with house dust mite antigen ($p < 0.01$ at 1 hour and $p < 0.05$ at 2 and 6 hours). At baseline, all six patients demonstrated immediate (within 1 hour) and late (6 hours) airway responses to house dust mite–antigen challenge. Mean percent decreases in FEV_1 for early and late airway responses were 40.0 ± 18.2% and 36.4 ± 5.2%, respectively. After being treated with pranlukast for 7 days, patients challenged with house dust mite antigen had significant decreases in FEV_1 at the early and late airway responses (19.8 ± 17.6% and 17.8 ± 14.7%, respectively; Fig. 4). These allergen-induced reductions in FEV_1 were about 50% less than that observed in those patients treated with placebo, demonstrating that repeat dosing with pranlukast attenuates both the early and late airway responses seen following inhaled exposure to house dust mite–antigen challenge.

Aspirin-Induced Asthma

The incidence of aspirin-induced asthma varies among different communities. In the United States, approximately 5% of adult patients with asthma may suffer from aspirin-induced asthma (23,24). Leukotrienes are believed to play a role in the underlying pathophysiological mechanisms of aspirin sensitivity (25). In patients with aspirin-induced asthma, higher concentrations of LTD_4 and histamine have been found in nasal secretions, which are associated with nasal symptoms and bronchoconstriction (26). Cross-sensitivity between sulpyrine and aspirin has been noted to occur in aspirin-hypersensitive patients (27). Sulpyrine—which, unlike aspirin, is stable in solution—is thus a suitable substitute for aspirin—one that can be nebulized and administered as a bronchoprovocator.

To evaluate the protective effect of pretreatment with a single dose of pranlukast or placebo against the aspirin analog sulpyrine, six patients with a documented history of aspirin sensitivity were enrolled in a randomized, double-blind, placebo-controlled, crossover study (16). Patients inhaled saline solution as a baseline control, followed by aerosols generated from solutions of sulpyrine at

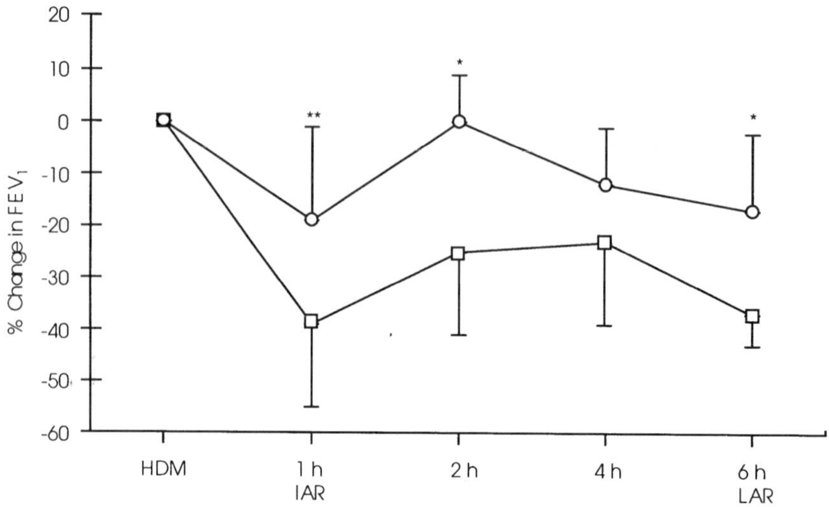

Figure 4 Effect of repeat dose treatment with pranlukast on house dust mite–antigen–induced immediate and late airway responses. The effect of pranlukast (circles) on the percent change in FEV_1 after inhaled house dust mite–antigen challenge following 225 mg b.i.d. administration of pranlukast for 7 days was compared with baseline control (prechallenge measurement; squares). Data are presented as mean ± SEM. $*p < 0.05$; $**p < 0.01$. HDM = House dust mite; IAR = immediate airway response; LAR = late airway response. (From Ref. 22.)

stepwise fivefold increasing concentrations (0.08, 0.4, 2, and 10% wt/vol). Sulpyrine concentrations were increased every 30 minutes until the maximum concentration (10%) was reached or until there was a demonstrated 20% decrease in FEV_1 from baseline. Pranlukast (225 mg) or placebo then was administered as a single oral dose 30 minutes after breakfast, and 3 hours later inhalation challenge was conducted. Sulpyrine-PC_{20} (provocation concentration that produces a 20% reduction in FEV_1) and sulpyrine-PD_{20} (provocation cumulative dose that produces a 20% reduction in FEV_1) were calculated for each patient. Using a paired *t*-test, mean sulpyrine-PD_{20} values were compared between groups. Following administration of pranlukast, the sulpyrine-PC_{20} and sulpyrine-PD_{20} values were increased in all six patients, compared with placebo. In four of six patients given the highest concentration (10%) of sulpyrine, pranlukast pretreatment blocked reduction in FEV_1. After crossover and administration of placebo in the same patients, sulpyrine-PC_{20} was 0.4% in four patients and 2% in the remaining two patients. Figure 5 illustrates a representative patient response to sulpyrine-induced bronchoconstriction after pretreatment with pranlukast and placebo.

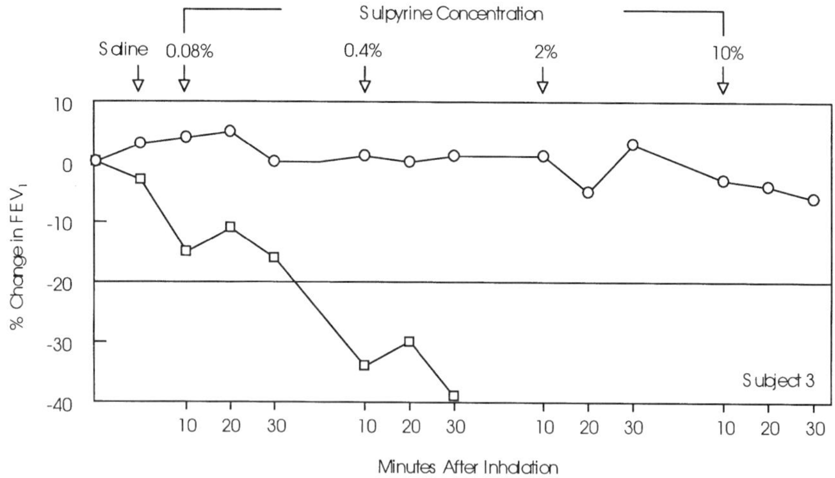

Figure 5 Pranlukast inhibition of sulpyrine-induced bronchoconstriction, shown here in a representative patient. Patients were pretreated with 225 mg pranlukast (circles) or placebo (squares) prior to sulpyrine (aspirin substitute) challenge. Sulpyrine was inhaled every 30 minutes, with stepwise increases to a maximum of 10%. (From Ref. 16.)

Sulpyrine-PD_{20} values were increased in all patients who were administered pranlukast. A statistically significant 14-fold increase in mean sulpyrine-PD_{20} values were noted in patients pretreated with 225 mg pranlukast (225 mg) compared to placebo (311.6 mg/ml vs. 21.9 mg/ml; $p < 0.001$). These results support the hypothesis that leukotrienes participate in the underlying pathophysiology of aspirin-induced asthma and that pranlukast prevents the bronchospasm associated with exposure in patients with this condition.

IV. Clinical Data for Maintenance Asthma Therapy

The worldwide clinical development program for pranlukast began with initial clinical safety and efficacy studies conducted in Japan. The design of these clinical trials allowed the use of concurrent inhaled and/or oral corticosteroids in patients with chronic stable asthma. Two Phase IIB/III trials that demonstrated the clinical efficacy of pranlukast are reviewed here. The first was a 4-week, randomized, double-blind trial comparing pranlukast, 225 mg twice daily, to placebo twice daily in 166 patients with mild to moderate asthma (28). The second study was an 8-week trial that compared pranlukast, 225 mg twice daily, to azel-

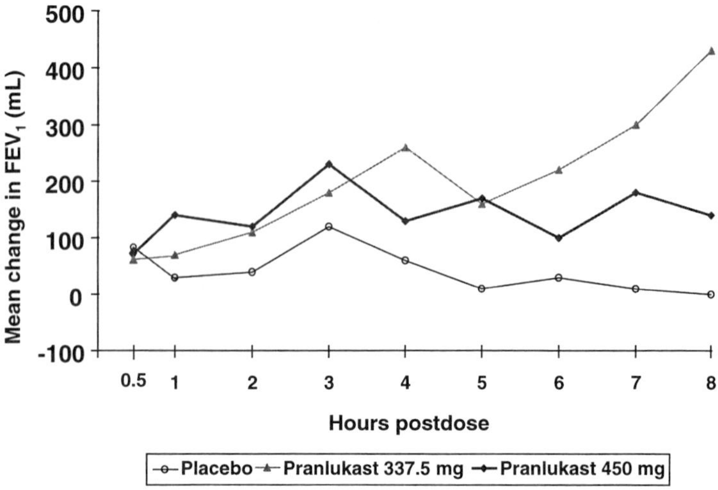

Figure 6 Effect of pranlukast on mean attack score (similar to the daily symptom score). Pranlukast reduced the mean attack score approximately 50%, from 22 to 10, versus about a 5% reduction for those receiving placebo. This difference was observed at 2 and 4 weeks and was statistically significant ($p < 0.001$). (From Ref. 28.)

astine, 2 mg twice daily, in 177 patients with mild to moderate asthma (29). Azelastine, marketed in Japan for the treatment of asthma, was chosen as the comparator because in patients with asthma it purportedly has both antihistaminic and antileukotriene activity (30,31).

In the first study, conducted in accordance with Japanese Society of Allergology guidelines, pranlukast produced a significant improvement in attack score, compared with placebo. The attack score is similar to the daily symptom score. In patients who received pranlukast, the mean attack score decreased approximately 50%, from 22 to 10, while in the patients who received placebo an approximate 5% reduction in the attack score was seen. This difference between pranlukast and placebo was observed at 2 and 4 weeks and was statistically significant ($p < 0.001$) (Fig. 6). Improved daily living scores and night sleep scores were seen, as was decreased use of bronchodilators and corticosteroids. All changes were statistically significant.

The second study of 177 patients with mild to moderate asthma, which compared pranlukast to azelastine, found that the attack score improved significantly in the pranlukast treatment group, as demonstrated by a lower mean attack score starting at week 1 and continuing through week 8. Improvement in daily living scores and nighttime scores, increased morning and evening PEFR, and decreased use of bronchodilators and corticosteroids were seen, and all changes were statistically significant (29).

Data from randomized, multicenter, placebo-controlled Phases IIB/III clinical trials that began in 1994 in the United States and Europe are currently being analyzed. Aside from one European trial, most studies in the West were conducted in patients not currently taking inhaled corticosteroids. Initial results from these studies recently were presented at the 1997 meetings of the American Academy of Allergy, Asthma and Immunology and the American Thoracic Society/American Lung Association. These trials represent a broad-based and far-reaching commitment to determine the role of pranlukast in treating asthma and allergic rhinitis and, along with results of Phase IIA studies that have already been published, are summarized in the following section.

A. Placebo-Controlled Trials

The safety and tolerability of 4 weeks of treatment with pranlukast 225 or 337.5 mg b.i.d. was evaluated in patients with asthma in a Phase IIA randomized, double-blind, placebo-controlled, parallel group, multicenter study conducted in Europe (32). Primary efficacy variables were FEV_1 and morning home peak expiratory flow rates (PEFR). An overall summary symptom score was comprised of recorded daytime and nighttime asthma symptom scores.

A total of 127 patients (age 18–70 years) completed the study. Each patient had an established diagnosis of asthma and an FEV_1 between 50 and 80% of predicted values that improved by at least 15% within 30 minutes of inhaling 200–400 μg salbutamol. During the study subjects were permitted to use inhaled steroids (≤1000 μg/day beclomethasone dipropionate or its equivalent) and on-demand salbutamol. Results demonstrated that FEV_1 was significantly increased (range 120–270 ml) within 1 hour after the first dose of either 225 or 337.5 mg pranlukast compared with baseline; this increase was maintained for 8 hours. For the pranlukast 337.5 mg group mean increase in morning home PEFR was statistically significant at all time points and, for the 225 mg group, at weeks 1 and 2 compared with placebo. At week 4, improvement in FEV_1 at the end of the dosing interval was seen for both pranlukast groups (mean increases of 210 to 340 ml; 85 to 138%) (percentages calculated on an increase from a baseline mean of 246 ml) and was statistically significant for the pranlukast 225 mg group, compared with placebo ($p < 0.05$).

In both pranlukast treatment groups, summary symptom scores and nighttime asthma scores improved. Statistically significant improvements were seen in the pranlukast 337.5 mg group versus placebo for summary symptom scores at weeks 1, 2, and endpoint ($p = 0.033$, $p = 0.048$, $p = 0.042$, respectively) and for nighttime asthma scores at all visits after baseline ($p < 0.05$) and at endpoint ($p = 0.016$). There was a similar trend for daytime asthma scores in the pranlukast treatment groups, which also reported less frequent use of on-demand salbutamol (differences not statistically significant).

No serious or unexpected adverse experiences were attributed to pranlukast. Adverse experiences that occurred in more than 2% of all patients could be identified as respiratory, gastrointestinal (abdominal pain, diarrhea), central nervous system (headache), viral infection, or pruritus. In addition, no clinically significant changes were attributed to pranlukast, as assessed by vital signs, 12-lead ECG, hematological, biochemical, and urinalysis studies, and physical examination. These results demonstrate that pranlukast is safe and well tolerated in addition to having clinical activity in patients with asthma.

The initial U.S. clinical evaluation of pranlukast was conducted in six centers to determine the safety and tolerability of 337.5 and 450 mg b.i.d. doses versus placebo in patients with mild to moderate asthma (33). Patients with a confirmed diagnosis of asthma with an FEV_1 between 50 and 90% of that predicted at baseline with a demonstrated reversibility of bronchoconstriction were eligible for the study. Reversibility was determined by a ≥15% increase in FEV_1 from baseline 30 minutes following a dose of 180 μg albuterol. Sixty-five patients between the ages of 19 and 61 years (mean age 34.1 years) were randomized to one of the two treatment groups or placebo. During the course of the study, no antiasthma medications were allowed, with the exception of on-demand inhaled albuterol and theophylline. Postrandomization, intranasal corticosteroids and short-acting antihistamines were also permitted.

After the first dose of pranlukast was administered, increases in FEV_1 compared with baseline were seen within 1 hour. These improvements were sustained throughout the 8-hour postdose observation period (Fig. 7) (34) and were maintained throughout the 4-week double-blind treatment period for both pranlukast treatment groups. In the placebo group, minimal changes in FEV_1 were observed. A greater decrease in symptoms of asthma, reflected in improvement in daytime and nighttime asthma symptom scores, was noted in the patients in the pranlukast treatment groups, compared with the placebo-treated control group. These results demonstrate that pranlukast increases FEV_1 on day 1 of treatment, and this improvement in lung function was maintained with continued dosing. The frequency and severity of adverse experiences, as assessed by adverse experience reports, vital signs, laboratory evaluation, ECG tracings, and physical and respiratory examinations, were similar in all groups.

Calhoun et al. (35) studied the efficacy and safety of oral pranlukast in a multicenter, double-blind, placebo-controlled, parallel-group, dose-ranging trial in 521 patients with asthma (FEV_1 50–85% of predicted) who were otherwise receiving only as-needed albuterol as asthma treatment. Approximately 80% of these patients also had allergic rhinitis. All doses of pranlukast (75, 150, 300, and 450 mg b.i.d.) were well tolerated and produced clinically significant im-

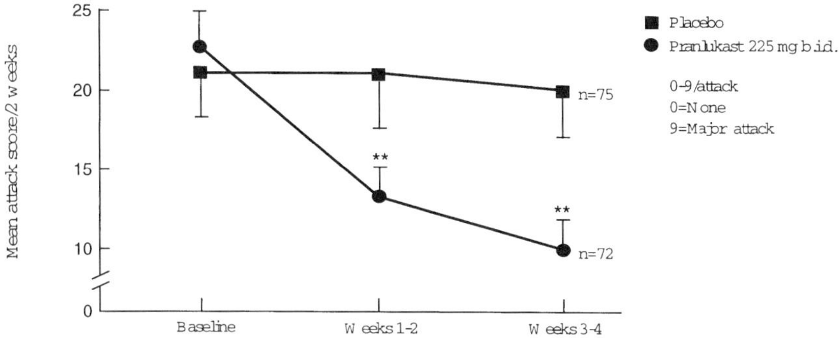

Figure 7 Effect of pranlukast over 8 hours in mean FEV_1. Mean changes from baseline in FEV_1 (ml) were measured from 0 to 8 hours after administration of a single dose of pranlukast 337.5 mg (triangles), pranlukast 450 mg (diamonds), or placebo (circles). (From Ref. 34.)

provement in symptoms of asthma, which was progressive and by week 12 had reached 31% in the 300-mg group ($p < 0.05$) compared to placebo. Improvement in symptoms of allergic rhinitis was also observed. Sustained increases in FEV_1 and PEFR and decreased use of the rescue medication albuterol were seen beginning at week 1. This study found that beginning at week 1 and compared to placebo, a broad range of pranlukast doses were effective in relieving symptoms of asthma. Thus, pranlukast is an effective oral treatment for symptoms of asthma in patients with asthma who also have allergic rhinitis (35).

B. Comparator Trials

In addition to the Japanese trial using azelastine as a comparator mentioned above, the efficacy and safety of pranlukast have been studied versus inhaled beclomethasone dipropionate (BDP) and versus nedocromil as well as versus placebo in two U.S. 12-week trials.

In the first trial, Wenzel et al. reported that in more than 400 patients with asthma, 70% of whom had a history of allergic rhinitis, pranlukast 450 mg b.i.d. is comparable to the inhaled steroid BDP in controlling asthma symptoms, clinic PEFR, and use of albuterol (36), Pranlukast 300, 450 mg b.i.d., and BPD showed statistically and clinically relevant improvements compared to placebo summary symptom scores, clinic PEFR, and decreased use of rescue medication ($p < 0.05$). FEV_1 and clinic PEFR were measured at ''trough'' (i.e., approximately 12 hours after dosing with pranlukast and 4 hours after BDP) and thus represent residual effects. Patients in the active treatment groups also experienced significantly more symptom-free nights and fewer exacerbations of asthma than those in the placebo treatment group.

In the second study, pranlukast was compared to nedocromil and placebo in a multicenter trial in 586 patients with asthma. A clinically and statistically significant improvement in FEV_1 was observed for pranlukast treated patients from week 1 ($p < 0.05$). This increase in FEV_1 was also evident at week 12. Nedocromil was not significantly different than placebo at any time point. Also from week 1, symptom scores improved in all pranlukast treatment groups and the need for albuterol rescue medication decreased significantly from baseline. Sahn et al. concluded that pranlukast is an effective and well-tolerated treatment for asthma (37).

Thus, the combined Japanese studies and trials in Europe and the United States have encompassed a broad program of asthma severity in which the majority of patients studied in Japan were taking concurrent corticosteroids and the majority studied in the West compared the effect of pranlukast with other anti-inflammatory medications. Pranlukast is also currently being studied in pediatric patients with asthma.

In clinical trials with pranlukast involving 3000 patients, adverse effects have been experienced by 7.4% of participants. Like other members of the leukotriene receptor antagonist class of drugs, transient changes in liver transaminases were observed. In no case did these elevations persist after the drug was discontinued. The most common side effects were gastrointestinal; e.g., nausea, vomiting, diarrhea, and abdominal pain occurred in about 5% of patients. Other adverse effects observed in less than 1% of patients included headache, dizziness, insomnia, urticaria, and dry mouth.

V. Allergic Rhinitis Trials

Asthma and allergic rhinitis have been found to be linked by a continuum of airway pathophysiology. As is seen with asthma, leukotrienes are at least 1000 times more potent than histamine in inducing nasal allergic responses (38). Ongoing Phase IIA/III clinical trials are assessing the effect of pranlukast on improvement of symptoms of allergic rhinitis. To date, initial results from these studies are demonstrating that pranlukast is an effective oral treatment for allergic rhinitis.

Grossman et al. (39) compared pranlukast (150 and 300 mg b.i.d.) and loratadine (10 mg, once daily) to placebo over 4 weeks in 484 patients with documented fall seasonal allergic rhinitis. Progressive decrease in mean summary symptoms scores was observed in all active treatment groups. At weeks 1, 3, and endpoint, symptoms of rhinitis (runny/stuffy nose, sneezing, itchy/watery eyes and itching nose, throat, palate, or ears) were statistically significantly reduced in patients in the pranlukast 150 mg b.i.d. treatment group compared to placebo. A trend toward symptom reduction in the pranlukast 300 mg b.i.d. and loratadine groups compared to placebo was also seen at all timepoints. The adverse experience profile was similar to that of placebo. The investigators concluded that pranlukast is an effective and well-tolerated treatment in this patient population.

VI. Summary

The current worldwide body of literature on pranlukast represents a decade of clinical experience with this orally active LTRA, the first to be used in clinical practice. The LTRAs represent the first novel therapeutic strategy for the treatment of asthma in more than 25 years. From the initial clinical trials in Japan in 1987 to ongoing, as yet unreported research in a number of trials in the United States and Europe, pranlukast is emerging as being in the vanguard of this important therapeutic advance in the treatment of asthma and the symptoms of allergic rhinitis.

References

1. Holgate ST, Bradding P, Sampson AP. Leukotriene antagonists and synthesis inhibitors: new directions in asthma therapy. J Allergy Clin Immunol 1996; 98:1–13.
2. Fujimura M, Sakamoto S, Kamio Y, Matsuda T. Effect of a leukotriene antagonist, ONO-1078, on bronchial hyperresponsiveness in patients with asthma. Respir Med 1993; 87:133–138.
3. Taki P, Suzuki R, Tori K, Mutsamoto S, Taniguchi H, Tukagi K. Reduction of the severity of bronchial hyperresponsiveness by the novel leukotriene antagonist 4-oxo-8-[4-(4-phenyl-butoxy)benzoylamino]-2(tetrazol-5-yl)-4H-1-benzopyran hemihydrate. Drug Res 1994; 44:330–333.
4. Dennis M, Minthorn E, Stelman G, Collie H, Wargenau M, Moeller M, Hust R, Georgiou P, Upward J. Effect of food on the absorption of pranlukast in healthy subjects (abstr). Pharm Res 1994; 11(10 suppl):S430.
5. Brocks DR, Upward JW, Georgiou P, Stelman G, Doyle E, Allen E, Wyld P, Dennis MJ. The single and multiple dose pharmacokinetics of pranlukast in healthy volunteers. Eur J Clin Pharmacol 1996; (51):303–308.
6. Brocks DR, Upward J, Davy M, Howland K, Compton C, McHugh C, Dennis MJ. Evening dosing is associated with higher plasma concentrations of pranlukast, a leukotriene receptor antagonist, in healthy male volunteers. Br J Clin Pharmacol. In press.
7. Brocks DR, Upward J, Hust R, Koester FE, Collie H, Qian Y, Dennis MJ. The pharmacokinetics of pranlukast in healthy young and elderly subjects. Int J Clin Pharmacol Ther 1996; 34:375–379.
8. Georgiou P, Compton C, Allen A, Hust R, Collie H. Pranlukast (Ultair™) has no

effect on cardiovascular parameters in healthy male subjects (abstr). Am J Respir Crit Care Med 1997; 155(4):A664.
9. O'Shaughnessy TC, Georgiou P, Howland K, Dennis M, Compton CH, Barnes NC. The effect of pranlukast, an oral leukotriene receptor antagonist, on leukotriene D_4 (LTD_4) challenge. Thorax 1997; 52:523–527.
10. Barnes N, Piper PJ, Costello J. The effect of an oral leukotriene antagonist L-649,923 on histamine and leukotriene D_4-induced bronchoconstriction in normal man. J Allergy Clin Immunol 1987; 79:816–821.
11. Arm JR, Lee TH. Sulphidopeptide leukotrienes in asthma. Clin Sci (Colch) 1993; 84:501–510.
12. Yamaguchi T, Kohrogi H, Honda I, Kawano O, Sugimoto M, Araki S, Ando M. A novel leukotriene antagonist, ONO-1078, inhibits and reverses human bronchial contraction induced by leukotrienes C_4 and D_4 and antigen in vitro. Am Rev Respir Dis 1992; 146:923–929.
13. Smith LJ, Jorkasky DK, Carr, A, Boike SC. Intravenous pranlukast (Ultair™) inhibits LTD_4-induced bronchoconstriction in patients with asthma (abstr). J Allergy Clin Immunol 1997; 99:S328.
14. Hirata K, Kurihara N, Kamimori T, Hikiishi F, Fujimoto S, Takeda T. Exercise-induced asthma and leukotriene antagonists. J Clin Ther Med 1993; 9;225–228.
15. Taniguchi Y, Tamura G, Honma M, Aizawa T, Maruyama N, Shirato K, Takishima T. The effect of an oral leukotriene antagonist, ONO-1078, on allergen-induced immediate bronchoconstriction in asthmatic subjects. J Allergy Clin Immunol 1993; 92:507–512.
16. Yamamoto H, Nagata M, Kuramitsu K, Tabe K, Kiushi H, Sakamoto Y, Yamamoto K, Dohi Y. Inhibition of analgesic-induced asthma by leukotriene receptor antagonist ONO-1078. Am J Respir Crit Care Med 1994; 150:254–257.
17. Strek ME, Sedy J, Solway J, Jorkasky JK, Jones B, Boike SC. Pranlukast (Ultair™) inhibits cold-air-induced bronchoconstriction in patients with asthma (abstr). J Allergy Clin Immunol 1997; 99:S329.
18. Wenzel SE, Larsen GL, Johnston K, Voelkel NF, Westcott JY. Elevated levels of leukotriene C_4 in bronchoalveolar lavage fluid from atopic asthmatics after endobronchial allergen challenge. Am Rev Respir Dis 1990; 142:112–119.
19. Wenzel SE, Westcott JY, Larsen GL. Bronchoalveolar lavage fluid mediator levels 5 minutes after allergen challenge in atopic subjects with asthma: relationship to the development of late asthmatic responses. J Allergy Clin Immunol 1991; 87:540–548.
20. Diaz P, Gonzalez MC, Galleguillos FR, Ancic P, Cromwell O, Shepherd D, Durhan SR, Gleich GJ, Kay AB. Leukocytes and mediators bronchoalveolar lavage during allergen-induced late-phase asthmatic reactions. Am Rev Respir Dis 1989; 139: 1383–1389.
21. Namba K, Takahashi K, Tada S, Simizu K, Nakato K, Okada C, Tsuji M, Oki K, Kimura I, Tanizaki Y. Studies of mechanism of late asthmatic response using bronchoalveolar lavage [in Japanese]. Arerugi 1988; 37(2):67–74.
22. Okudaira H. Challenge studies of a leukotriene receptor antagonist. Chest 1997; 111: 46S–51S.
23. Settipane GA. Adverse reactions to aspirin and related drugs. Arch Intern Med 1981; 141:328–332.
24. Speer F, Denison TR, Baptist JE. Aspirin allergy. Ann Allergy 1981; 46:123–126.

25. Stevenson DD, Lewis RA. Proposed mechanisms of aspirin sensitivity reactions. J Allergy Clin Immunol 1987; 80:788–790.
26. Ferreri NR, Howland WC, Stevenson DD, Spiegelberg HL. Release of leukotrienes, prostaglandins, and histamine into nasal secretions of aspirin-sensitive asthmatics during reaction to aspirin. Am Rev Respir Dis 1988; 137:847–854.
27. Bartoli E, Faedda in Masala R, Chiandussi L. Drug-induced asthma [letter]. Lancet 1976; 1(7973):1357.
28. Miyamoto A, Takishima T, Makino S, Shida T, Nakashima M. Therapy with cysteinyl leukotrienes C_4, D_4, and E_4: examination of the usefulness of ONO-1078 on adult bronchial asthma. Double-blind test comparing placebo [in Japanese]. J Clin Exp Med 1993; 164:225–247.
29. Miyamoto T, Takishima T, Makino S, Shida T, Nakashima M, Hanaoka K. Utility of a leukotrienes C_4, D_4, and E_4 antagonist, ONO-1078, on adult bronchial asthma in multicenter comparative double-blind clinical study with azelastine hydrochloride. J Clin Ther Med 1993; 9(suppl 1):71–107.
30. Chand N, Sofia RD. Azelastine—a novel in vivo inhibitor of leukotriene biosynthesis: a possible mechanism of action: a mini review. J Asthma 1995; 32:227–234.
31. Tinkelman DG, Bucholtz GA, Kemp JP, Koepke JW, Repsher LH, Spector SL, Storms WW, Van As A. Evaluation of the safety and efficacy of multiple doses of azelastine to adult patients with bronchial asthma over time. Am Rev Respir Dis 1990; 141:569–574.
32. Barnes NC, Pujet JC on behalf of an International Study Group. Pranlukast, a novel leukotriene receptor antagonist: results of the first European, placebo controlled, multicentre clinical study in asthma. Thorax 1997; 52:519–522.
33. Grossman J, Faiferman I, Dubb JW, et al. Results of the first U.S. double-blind, placebo-controlled multicenter clinical study in asthma with pranlukast, a novel leukotriene receptor antagonist. J Asthma 1997; 34(4):321–328.
34. Barnes NC, DeJong B, Miyamoto T. Worldwide clinical experience with the first marketed leukotriene receptor antagonist. Chest 1997; 111:52S–60S.
35. Calhoun WJ, Weisberg SC, Faiferman I, Stober PW, on behalf of the Ultair Study Group. Pranlukast (Ultair™) is effective in improving asthma: results of a 12-week, multicenter, dose-range study (abstr). J Allergy Clin Immunol 1997; 99:S318.
36. Wenzel S, Chervinsky P, Kerwin E, Silvers S, Faiferman I, Dubb J, on behalf of the Ultair Study Group. Oral pranlukast (Ultair™) vs inhaled beclomethasone: results of a 12-week trial in patients with asthma (abstr). Am J Respir Crit Care Med 1997; 155(4);A203.
37. Sahn S, Galant S, Murray J, Bronsky E, Spector S, Faiferman I, Stober P, on behalf of the Ultair Study Group. Pranlukast (Ultair™) improves FEV_1 in patients with asthma: results of a 12-week multicenter study vs nedocromil (abstr). Am J Respir Crit Care Med 1997; 155(4);A665.
38. Okuda M, Watase T, Mezawa A, Liu CM. The role of leukotriene D_4 in allergic rhinitis. Ann Allergy 1988; 60:537–540.
39. Grossman J, Ratner PH, Nathan R, Adelglass J, de Jong B. Pranlukast (Ultair™, SB 205312, ONO-1078), an oral leukotriene receptor antagonist, relieves symptoms in patients with seasonal allergic rhinitis (SAR) (abstr). J Allergy Clin Immunol 1997; 99:S443.

16

Zafirlukast

CATHERINE M. BONUCCELLI

Zeneca Pharmaceuticals
Wilmington, Delaware

TREVOR J.C. HIGGINS

Zeneca Pharmaceuticals
Cheshire, England

Zafirlukast (proprietary names—Accolate®, Vanticon®, Accoleit®) (4-(5-cyclopentyloxycarbonylamino-1-methyl-indol)-3-ylmethyl)-3-methoxy-*N*-*o*-toyl-sulfonylbenzamide) (Fig. 1). is a highly selective and potent competitive antagonist of cysteinyl leukotrienes (LTC_4, LTD_4, and LTE_4) at the cysteinyl leukotriene receptor in human airways (currently designated as CysLT-1).

I. In Vitro Pharmacology

A. Ligand-Binding Studies

Zafirlukast competes for binding to cysteinyl-leukotriene receptors derived from guinea pig lung tissue with tritiated LTD_4 and LTE_4 in a concentration-dependent fashion (1). In guinea pig lung tissue the pK_i values were 9.1 and 9.4 for LTD_4 and LTE_4, respectively. The similarity of the pK_i values for LTD_4 and LTE_4, together with the observation that LTD_4 and LTE_4 mutually compete for binding, suggests that both cysteinyl-leukotrienes bind to the same receptor and that zafirlukast competes at this same site (possibly the CysLT-1 receptor) for binding against either of these leukotrienes.

B. Antagonism of LTC_4-, LTD_4-, and LTE_4-Induced Contraction of Guinea Pig Tracheal and Parenchymal Strips

In the guinea pig trachea LTD_4 and LTE_4 interact with either the same or very similar receptors, whereas LTC_4 interacts with a distinctly different receptor (2). In isolated guinea pig tracheal strips, the concentration-response curves for LTD_4 and LTE_4 were shifted to the right in a parallel manner by zafirlukast with pA_2

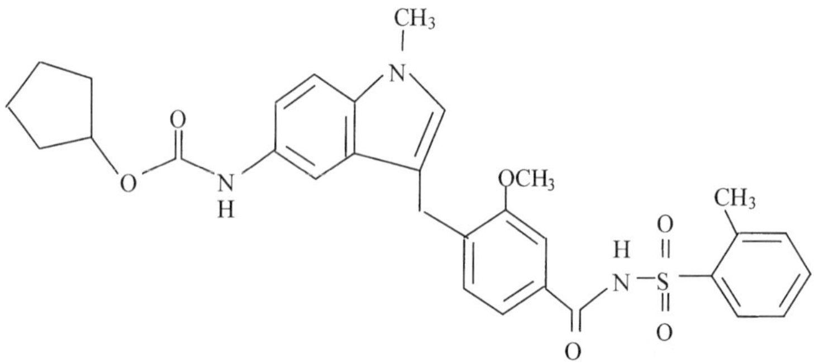

Figure 1 Chemical structure of zafirlukast, 4-(5-cyclopentyl-carbonyl-amino-1-methyl-indol-3-ylmethyl)-3-methoxy-*N*-*o*-tolylsulfonylbenzamide.

values of about 9.8 (1). The slope of the pA_2 plot versus LTD_4 concentration was slightly less than 1, reflecting the possibility that there may be multiple receptors for this agonist in guinea pig trachea. In the presence of serine-borate (a reagent that inhibits the conversion of LTC_4 to LTD_4), zafirlukast did not antagonize the response to LTC_4. When serine-borate was omitted zafirlukast blocked contractions in response to LTC_4, but pK_B values for zafirlukast were small and concentration dependent, suggesting that antagonism was related to blockade of LTD_4 which was arising from metabolism of LTC_4 to LTD_4 (1). These observations of variability of the dissociation constants for zafirlukast in the guinea pig ileum preparations, especially at higher concentrations, reflect heterogeneity in the receptors, a phenomenon described previously (3). The dissociation constants for zafirlukast appeared to be independent of both the agonist studied and concentration of antagonist. Additionally, maximum responses to all agonists were not influenced by zafirlukast. These data indicate that zafirlukast is competitive for all three cysteinyl-leukotrienes.

In guinea pig parenchymal lung strips, zafirlukast antagonized the contractile activity of LTD_4 and LTE_4 in a competitive manner with pK_B values of about 9.5 (1).

C. Antagonism of LTC_4-, LTD_4-, and LTE_4-Induced Contraction of Human Bronchus

In human isolated bronchi, the concentration-response curves for LTC_4 and LTD_4 in causing contractions were shifted to the right in a parallel manner and with similar potency by zafirlukast (1). The pK_B values for zafirlukast against LTD_4 and LTE_4 ranged from 7.98 to 8.88. This observation supports the hypothesis that LTC_4 and LTD_4 evoke contraction of human airways via a common receptor.

Table 1 Agonist Responses in the Absence (control) and Presence of 10^{-5} M Zafirlukast

Receptor	Isolated tissue	Agonist	n[a]	$-\log K_B$
α_1	Rat aorta	Phenylephrine	3	<5
α_2	Rat vas deferens	Clonidine	3	<5
β_1	Guinea pig right atrium	Isoproterenol	3	<5
β_2	Guinea pig trachea	Salbutamol	3	<5
H_1	Rabbit aorta	Histamine	3	<5
H_2	Guinea pig right atrium	Histamine	3	<5
5-HT_2	Rabbit aorta	Serotonin	3	<5
Muscarinic	Guinea pig trachea	Carbachol	3	<5
Thromboxane (TP_2)	Rabbit aorta	U46619	3	<5
Thromboxane (TP_1)	Rat aorta	U46619	3	≤5
PGE_2 (relaxation, EP_2)	Guinea pig trachea	PGE_2	4	<5
PGE_2 (contraction, EP_1)	Guinea pig ileum	PGE_2	3	5.60 ± 0.32
Ca^{2+} channel	Rabbit aorta	K^+ (80 mM)[b]	3	<5

[a]Number of tissues.
[b]Percent inhibition of 80 mM K^+ contraction at 10^{-5} M.
(Reprinted with permission from Ref. 1.)

D. Evaluation of the Activity of Zafirlukast at Other Receptor Sites

The ability of a high concentration (10^{-5} M) of zafirlukast to antagonize several receptors other than that for cysteinyl-leukotrienes was evaluated in a variety of tissues appropriately selected for the receptor type (1). Zafirlukast demonstrated virtually no affinity for most receptors (Table 1), the single exception being the guinea pig ileum EP_1 receptor, where zafirlukast was 10,000-fold less potent than on guinea pig cysteinyl-leukotriene receptors (1).

II. In Vivo Pharmacology

A. LTD_4-Induced Bronchoconstriction

Intravenous, oral, and aerosol administration of zafirlukast to guinea pigs provided dose-related protection from dyspnea induced by aerosolized LTD_4 (1). The doses or concentrations that provided 50% inhibition of the response (ED_{50}) by the three routes of administration were 0.045 and 0.52 μmol/kg and 5.1×10^{-6} M, respectively. When administered orally, activity appeared to be maximum by 3 hours and thereafter declined slowly with a pharmacodynamic half-life of >13 hours (1).

B. Effect of Zafirlukast on Impaired Lung Mechanics Following Cysteinyl-Leukotriene Administration

In anesthetized guinea pigs, LTC_4, LTD_4, and LTE_4 caused dose-dependent increases in pulmonary resistance (Rp) and decreases in dynamic lung compliance (C_{dyn}) (4). By all routes of administration zafirlukast shifted the dose-response curves rightward in a dose-dependent fashion (1).

C. Effect of Zafirlukast on Reversal of Bronchospasm Induced by LTC_4, LTD_4, and LTE_4

LTE_4 given as a bolus dose of 3 nmol/kg i.v. produced an approximately 700% increase in Rp and a 95% decrease in C_{dyn} (1). Immediately after the attainment of the maximal change in Rp, zafirlukast (0.3 μmol/kg i.v.) or vehicle was administered and the rate of return of Rp and C_{dyn} to baseline monitored. Zafirlukast produced a significant increase in the rate of return of both parameters to baseline compared with control. Qualitatively similar results were obtained with LTC_4- and LTD_4-induced bronchospasm.

D. Inhibition of Airway Edema by Zafirlukast

In anesthetized guinea pigs, zafirlukast inhibited the formation of airway edema caused by intravenously administered LTD_4. Zafirlukast, given i.v., resulted in a dose-dependent rightward shift of the LTD_4 dose-response curve for increase in extravasation of Evans blue dye (used as a marker of plasma leakage) in guinea pig trachea (5). The effective doses of zafirlukast were similar to those causing antagonism of LTD_4 in pulmonary mechanics experiments.

E. Asthma Models

Guinea pigs passively sensitized with antiovalbumin antiserum, pretreated with indomethacin, pyrilamine, and propranolol to inhibit the formation of cyclooxygenase products and the activation of H_1 and β-adrenergic receptors (1) were subsequently exposed to an aerosol of ovalbumin. This procedure produced intense bronchoconstriction in part mediated by leukotrienes (3). Pretreatment of these animals with zafirlukast (0.1 mg/kg i.v.) substantially inhibited the antigen-induced increases in Rp and C_{dyn} (1).

Similarly, administration of zafirlukast at the peak of antigen-induced bronchoconstriction produced a more rapid recovery of Rp and C_{dyn} to baseline than control. Thus, zafirlukast both inhibited and reversed ovalbumin antigen-induced bronchospasm in this model (1).

In sheep naturally allergic to *Ascaris suum*, zafirlukast inhibited antigen-induced bronchoconstrictor responses. Administration of an aerosol of *Ascaris suum* resulted in an immediate and short-lived bronchoconstriction, followed after 4–6 hours by a late phase of bronchoconstriction. These animals were also demonstrably hyperresponsive to carbachol 24 hours after antigen administration. When zafirlukast 5 mg was administered 30 minutes prior to antigen, 4 hours after antigen, and 24 hours after antigen (total dose 15 mg), there was substantial inhibition of the immediate and late phases of antigen-induced bronchoconstriction and a decrease in the sensitivity to carbachol.

F. Effect of Zafirlukast on Airway Eosinophilia

Aerosolized LTC_4, LTD_4, or LTE_4 induced eosinophil accumulation in the lungs of conscious guinea pigs, as assessed by the presence of these cells in bronchoalveolar lavage fluid (5). The presence of eosinophils was apparent at 5 hours and was still increasing 24 hours after an aerosolized dose of LTD_4. Aerosol administration of zafirlukast 5 minutes prior to LTD_4 challenge resulted in dose-dependent inhibition of eosinophil accumulation. Additionally, aerosol administration of zafirlukast 20 μM 5 minutes before agonist blocked the ability of LTC_4 and LTE_4 to increase eosinophils in bronchoalveolar lavage fluid for 24 hours. Intraperitoneal administration of zafirlukast also inhibited LTD_4-induced eosinophil recruitment to the lungs (5). These data demonstrate that zafirlukast has potential anti-inflammatory actions, especially under conditions in which animals are exposed directly to cysteinyl-leukotrienes.

The ability of zafirlukast to block responses to LTC_4 in experiments measuring pulmonary mechanics in guinea pigs in vivo may reflect rapid conversion of LTC_4 to LTD_4. However, other explanations are also possible, e.g., it could be that a metabolite of zafirlukast blocks the LTC_4 receptor. However, several metabolites of zafirlukast have been identified (6) and their pharmacology investigated. They have been found to retain less than 1% of the potency of zafirlukast.

III. Antagonism of LTD_4 Challenge in Humans

In a randomized, placebo-controlled, three-segment (each segment a two-way double-blind, crossover) study involving eight asthmatic patients (7), a single oral dose of zafirlukast 20 mg significantly increased $PC_{20}FEV_1$ compared with placebo: the mean log dose shift was 1.2 units ($p = 0.03$). Furthermore, zafirlukast significantly reduced the time required to recover from LTD_4 challenge compared with placebo (between treatment difference: 30 min; $p = 0.022$). In this study, zafirlukast had no effect on $PC_{20}FEV_1$ for histamine or methacholine or on recovery of FEV_1. Zafirlukast had no effect on platelet aggregation stimulated by either PGD_2 or the thromboxane mimetic U46619, illustrating a selective antagonism of LTD_4 (7).

In 18 healthy male subjects (aged 18–44 years) zafirlukast inhibited bronchoconstriction induced by aerosolized LTD_4 (8). On separate study days 3–7

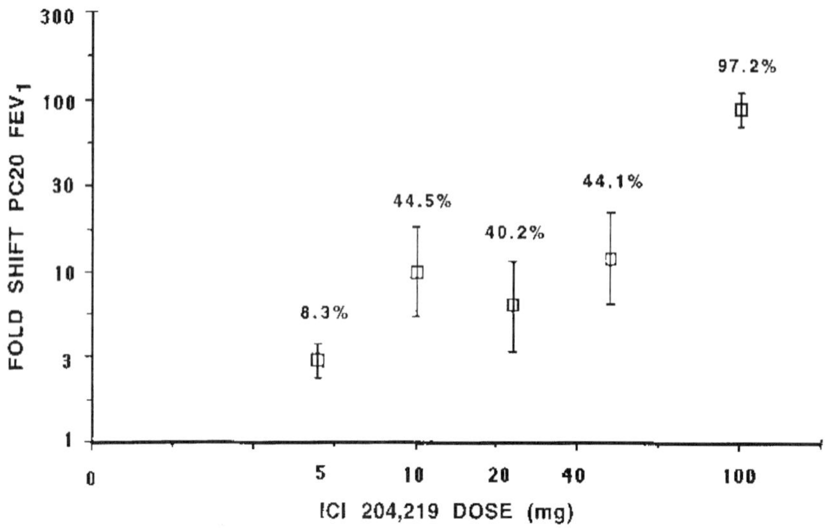

Figure 2 Relationship between the log shift in leukotriene D_4 (LTD_4) concentration that produced a 20% decrease in FEV_1 ($PC_{20}FEV_1$) and the log dose of zafirlukast. (Reprinted with permission from Ref. 9.)

days apart, subjects received either a single oral dose of 40 mg zafirlukast or placebo. At intervals of 2, 12, and 24 hours after this, the six subjects in each group were challenged with inhaled LTD_4. Zafirlukast had no effect on baseline pulmonary function, but at 2, 12, and 24 hours after dosing it had increased by 117-, 9-, and 5-fold, respectively, the concentration of LTD_4 required to reduce specific airway conductance (SGaw) by 35% (all time points $p < 0.05$). In this study plasma levels of zafirlukast correlated with effect ($r = 0.83$, $p < 0.001$).

In a double-blind, two-period crossover trial (9), 30 male subjects (aged 18–50 years) with mild asthma ($FEV_1 > 65\%$ of predicted) randomly received single oral doses of placebo and either 5, 10, 20, 40, or 100 mg zafirlukast ($n = 6$ for each dose) 12 hours before a challenge with inhaled LTD_4. Compared with placebo, zafirlukast increased the concentration ($PC_{20}FEV_1$) and dose of LTD_4 needed to reduce FEV_1 by 20% ($PD_{20}FEV_1$) ($p < 0.05$). Mean LTD_4 $PC_{20}FEV_1$ for groups that received placebo plus 10, 40, or 100 mg zafirlukast increased by 10-fold or more ($p < 0.05$). A progressive dose-response was observed for doses of zafirlukast from 5 to 100 mg (Fig. 2). There was also an association between the zafirlukast plasma concentration and its protective effect ($p < 0.01$).

Eighteen asthmatic patients underwent bronchial provocation with inhaled LTD_4 12 hours after receiving a single dose of zafirlukast 2, 5, 10, 20, 40, or 80 mg or placebo in a three-period crossover study (10). Treatments were taken 4–

10 days apart. Zafirlukast doses above 2 mg increased the amount of LTD_4 needed to produce a $PC_{20}FEV_1$ ($p < 0.01$). A linear dose-response relationship was observed ($p < 0.01$).

Single doses of zafirlukast 40 or 80 mg or placebo were given to six asthmatic patients in a double-blind, randomized, crossover study by Smith et al. (11). FEV_1 was measured before and 2 hours after dosing, before the initial challenge with LTD_4, at 2-minute intervals during the bronchoprovocation test until the $PC_{20}FEV_1$ value was reached, and thereafter at 10-minute intervals until the FEV_1 value recovered to within 5% of baseline. All estimates of treatment differences were greater than zero, indicating that, on average, compared with placebo a single dose of zafirlukast 40 or 80 mg taken 24 hours before challenge significantly increased the $PC_{20}FEV_1$ for LTD_4 ($p < 0.05$).

In all studies involving LTD_4 challenge in both normal volunteers and asthmatic patients, a positive relationship between plasma zafirlukast concentration and protection against LTD_4-induced bronchoconstriction was observed (8–11).

Smith et al. (12) examined the effect of zafirlukast on LTD_4-induced bronchoconstriction in seven asthmatic patients (aged 19–33 years) treated with inhaled corticosteroids (median dose 800 μg daily) for at least a month. Subjects were randomized to 20 mg zafirlukast 2 hours prior to LTD_4 challenge in a double-blind, placebo-controlled, two-period crossover trial. Six patients completed the study. $\log(PC_{20}FEV_1)$ and $\log(PD_{20}FEV_1)$ after placebo were -0.12 and $+0.68$ log dose units, respectively. Pretreatment with zafirlukast produced a mean log shift from placebo in $\log(PC_{20}FEV_1)$ and $\log(PD_{20}FEV_1)$ of $+1.82$ and $+1.88$ log dose units, respectively. Compared with placebo, $PC_{20}FEV_1$ and $PD_{20}FEV_1$ were increased 66- and 75-fold, respectively, after zafirlukast. These values are comparable with those obtained previously in patients not receiving inhaled corticosteroids and demonstrate that asthmatic patients, adequately treated with inhaled corticosteroids, still respond to leukotriene insult and that zafirlukast potently attenuates this.

IV. Induced Asthma

The pharmacological activity of zafirlukast in induced asthma in humans has been studied using bronchoprovocation challenges with inhaled allergen, sulfur dioxide, platelet-activating factor (PAF), cold air, or exercise. Studies of the effect of zafirlukast on aspirin-induced asthma have not been performed to date but are currently underway. These studies have used lung function (predominantly FEV_1) as the primary measure of therapeutic effect. Additionally, the effect of zafirlukast on the cellular content of bronchoalveolar lavage fluid, collected after segmental antigen bronchoprovocation has been studied.

A. Allergen Challenge

The effect of zafirlukast on the response of asthmatic patients to bronchoprovocation with inhaled allergen has been assessed in a number of studies.

Single doses of zafirlukast 20 mg or placebo have been compared in a double-blind, randomized, crossover study by Dahlén and colleagues (13). Ten atopic patients underwent cumulative bronchial challenge with specific allergen (cat, dog, or birch pollen) to establish at baseline the provocative dose of allergen resulting in a 20% decrease in FEV_1 ($PD_{20}FEV_1$). Within 4 months of this they were rechallenged with antigen 2 hours after oral administration of placebo or zafirlukast on two separate occasions separated by 2–6 weeks. After zafirlukast, the dose of allergen tolerated by the patients increased and bronchoconstriction was inhibited by 60% ($p < 0.01$). The median cumulative allergen dose was 5.5-fold higher, and the group geometric mean value for PD_{20} was increased 2.5-fold, compared with placebo ($p < 0.01$). Mean recovery time after the immediate bronchoconstriction was 40 minutes in patients on zafirlukast and 60 minutes in patients on placebo ($p < 0.05$).

In a study by Taylor and colleagues, 10 atopic patients were challenged with aerosolized allergen (birch pollen, cat, or dog dander) 2 hours after being given zafirlukast 40 mg or placebo orally (14). FEV_1 was measured over the next 6 hours. Ten minutes after allergen challenge, FEV_1 fell 32.4% on placebo versus 6.3% on zafirlukast. Up to 2 hours after a dose, zafirlukast and placebo treatments were significantly different with respect to the areas under their respective FEV_1-time curves (AUC) ($p < 0.005$). Two to six hours after the challenge, the maximum fall in FEV_1 was 27.9% for placebo and only 12.7% for the zafirlukast-treated group ($p < 0.03$) (Fig. 3). The amount of histamine needed to reduce FEV_1 by 20% (PC_{20}-histamine) decreased after allergen challenge but was significantly attenuated by zafirlukast ($p < 0.01$). Zafirlukast appears to block the late asthmatic response at least up to the period 6 hours after allergen challenge.

Findlay et al. (15) observed a similar protective effect 2 hours after a single dose of zafirlukast 40 mg in 13 subjects with asthma who had a known allergy to cats and an $FEV_1 \geq 65\%$ of predicted. Patients underwent bronchoprovocation using standardized cat dander allergen 2 hours after receiving zafirlukast or placebo. Increasing doses of allergen were given by inhalation until a $PD_{20}FEV_1$ was obtained or a maximum dose of 30000 AU (allergen units)/ml was reached. Patients who received zafirlukast has a 10-fold mean increase in the interpolated $PC_{20}FEV_1$ to cat dander compared with placebo. Areas under the curve for percent change in FEV_1 were significantly reduced ($p < 0.05$) during the 5-hour postchallenge period for the zafirlukast group compared with placebo (Fig. 4).

Studies have explored the effects of zafirlukast delivered by the inhaled route (16). Inhaled single doses of zafirlukast up to 200 μg have been shown to be potent inhibitors of bronchospasm due to inhaled ragweed pollen in reproducibly

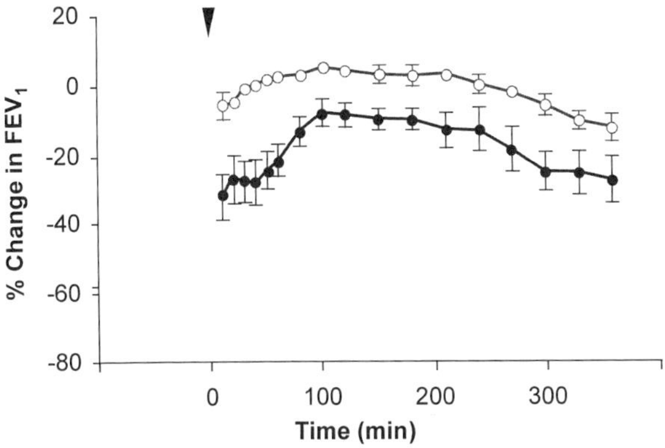

Figure 3 The effect of oral pretreatment with 40 mg zafirlukast on FEV_1 after allergen-induced bronchoconstriction in patients with atopic asthma. Zafirlukast significantly attenuated the early and late phase responses: AUC 0–2 ($p < 0.01$), AUC 2–6 ($p < 0.05$), AUC 0–6 ($p < 0.02$). (Reprinted with permission from Ref. 14.)

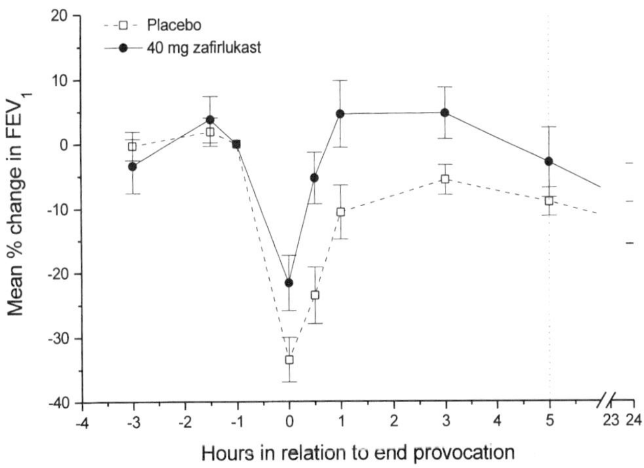

Figure 4 Mean change in FEV_1 ($n = 12$) from the bronchoprovocation endpoint to 5-hours after provocation for patients treated with zafirlukast and placebo. (Reprinted with permission from Ref. 15.)

sensitive patients (17,18) ($p < 0.05$). However, a single inhaled dose of zafirlukast (1600) μg produced a less pronounced inhibition of allergen-induced bronchoconstriction than after oral administration (16), and the effect of inhaled zafirlukast on the early portion of the late-phase response was not apparent. This is in contrast to evidence of protection in the late phase when the drug was given by the oral route (14,19) and suggests that the duration of action of the drug delivered by inhalation may be less than that by the oral route.

B. Segmental Antigen Challenge and Bronchoalveolar Lavage

Eleven mild asthmatic patients underwent segmental antigen bronchoprovocation (SBP) and broncholaveolar lavage (BAL) in a double-blind, randomized, placebo-controlled, two-period crossover study (19). Zafirlukast 20 mg twice daily or placebo was given for 7 days. SBP and BAL were performed 4 hours after dosing on day 5 of treatment. BAL was repeated 48 hours later on day 7 of treatment. Treatment periods were separated by 14–21 days. Cell counts were measured in BAL fluid and alveolar macrophages were analyzed ex vivo for phorbol myristate acetate (PMA)–driven superoxide release before and 48 hours after SBP. Forty-eight hours after SBP patients given zafirlukast showed significantly lower late-phase concentrations of basophils ($p = 0.01$), lymphocytes ($p = 0.01$), and histamine ($p < 0.05$) than patients given placebo. Late-phase superoxide production from purified alveolar macrophages was also significantly reduced following zafirlukast treatment compared with placebo treatment ($p < 0.01$). These results suggest that zafirlukast diminishes late-phase inflammatory response to inhaled antigen in patients with mild to moderate asthma.

C. Exercise Challenge

The ability of zafirlukast to attenuate exercise-induced bronchoconstriction in asthmatics has been assessed and the data presented in two publications (20,21).

Single doses of zafirlukast 20 mg or placebo were given at one-week intervals to eight nonsmoking asthmatic patients in a double-blind, crossover, placebo-controlled study by Finnerty et al. (20). The bronchoconstrictor response was analyzed as the percentage change in the AUC of the exercise-induced reduction in FEV_1 from pre-exercise baseline against time over 30 minutes. The mean baseline FEV_1 before treadmill exercise challenge breathing dry air was 4.07 L after placebo and 4.17 L after zafirlukast (N.S.). The mean maximum percentage fall in FEV_1 following exercise was significantly less after zafirlukast (21.6%) than after placebo (36.0%) ($p < 0.01$) (Fig. 5). Zafirlukast reduced the mean AUC from 834 to 331%·min ($p < 0.01$). This inhibition was most marked between 5 and 30 minutes: mean $AUC_{(5-30)}$ was reduced from 731 to 261%·min ($p < 0.01$).

In a randomized, placebo-controlled, double-blind crossover study reported by Makker and coworkers, single inhaled doses of zafirlukast 400 μg or placebo

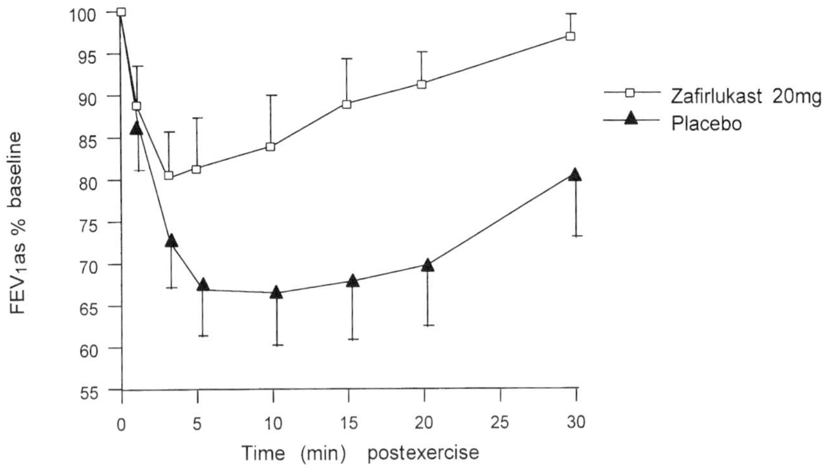

Figure 5 The effect of pretreatment with 20 mg of oral zafirlukast on FEV_1 after exercise-induced bronchoconstriction in subjects with asthma. The mean exercise-induced bronchoconstriction at each time point, expressed as a percentage of preexercise baseline FEV_1 over 30 minutes, following the oral administration of placebo and zafirlukast 20 mg. (Reprinted with permission from Ref. 20.)

were given to nine asthmatic patients 30 minutes before exercise challenge using a cycle ergometer (21). Zafirlukast had no significant effect on baseline airway caliber 20 minutes following inhalation. Bronchoconstriction (assessed as change in FEV_1 over 30 minutes) was inhibited significantly by zafirlukast compared with placebo (mean maximum percentage fall in FEV_1 14.5 and 30.2%, respectively; $p = 0.043$). The AUC for FEV_1 for the first 30 minutes postexercise was significantly reduced with zafirlukast ($p = 0.043$), as was time for recovery of FEV_1 to within 5% of the baseline value ($p = 0.018$).

D. Cold Air Challenge

Ten nonsmoking patients aged 18 through 65 years with mild to moderate asthma were enrolled in a double-blind, placebo-controlled, two-period crossover trial by Boulet et al. (22). Patients were randomized to receive a single dose of zafirlukast 80 mg or placebo and were challenged with cold, dry air 30 minutes and 4 and 24 hours after treatment. The two treatment periods were 4–10 days apart. $Log_{10}PD_{20}FEV_1RHE$ (respiratory heat exchange) and $log_{10}PD_{20}FEV_1Ve$ (minute ventilation) were both significantly greater 24 hours after treatment with zafirlukast compared with placebo treatment. No significant treatment differences were observed for challenges 30 minutes or 4 hours after treatment. Treatment with zafirlukast shortened recovery times from cold-air challenges 30 minutes and 4 hours but not 24 hours after dosing. These data suggest that zafirlukast may be capable of attenuating the response to cold air for up to 24 hours following a single 80-mg dose.

Similar data showing that lower doses of zafirlukast attenuate cold air–induced bronchoconstriction have been obtained by Israel et al. (23). In a randomized, double-blind, placebo-controlled, three-period crossover trial, 24 asthmatic patients with demonstrable reversible airway sensitivity to cold air received a single dose of zafirlukast (20 or 40 mg) or placebo, followed by bronchoprovocation with cold, dry air 2 and 8 hours after dosing. Response to bronchoprovocation was expressed as the $\log_{10}$-transformed provocative concentration of Ve that reduced FEV_1 by 10, 15, and 20% from baseline ($\log_{10}PC_{10,15,20}FEV_1Ve$). At 8 hours after dosing, this measure was significantly greater after either dose of zafirlukast than after placebo. This improvement over placebo represents mean increases of 29 and 32% in the amount of cold air required to decrease FEV_1 by 10% from baseline after 20 and 40 mg zafirlukast, respectively. There were no significant differences between the two zafirlukast dose levels at 2 or 8 hours postdose, or between either zafirlukast dose and placebo 2 hours after dosing, probably reflecting the time required for absorption of the drug.

In a randomized, placebo-controlled, double-blind, two-period crossover trial reported by Glass et al., single inhaled doses of zafirlukast 800 μg or placebo were given to 18 patients with mild to moderate asthma (24). A cold-air challenge followed 30 minutes, 6 hours, and 24 hours after zafirlukast or placebo. The interpolated respiratory heat exchange that reduced FEV_1 by 20% ($PC_{20}FEV_1RHE$) was significantly greater on zafirlukast than that on placebo 30 minutes after dosing ($p = 0.02$). FEV_1 returned to within 95% of prechallenge levels approximately 25 minutes after challenges at 30 minutes ($p = 0.03$) and 6 hours ($p < 0.01$) with zafirlukast treatment versus approximately 45 minutes with placebo.

E. Inhaled Sulfur Dioxide Challenge

Specific airway resistance (SRaw) was measured in 12 asthmatics 2 and 10 hours after the administration of zafirlukast 20 mg or placebo in a double-blind, placebo-controlled, two-period crossover study (25). SRaw was measured before and after each sulfur dioxide challenge to determine the concentration of sulfur dioxide required to induce an 8-unit increase in SRaw (PC_8SRaw). Blood was collected for the determination of zafirlukast plasma concentration. PC_8SRaw was significantly higher 2 hours after zafirlukast than placebo (3.1 vs. 1.5 ppm; $p = 0.02$) and remained higher at 10 hours postdose (2.72 vs. 1.92 ppm; $p = 0.09$). There was a relation between increases in PC_8SRaw and the zafirlukast plasma concentration 10 hours postdose ($p = 0.001$).

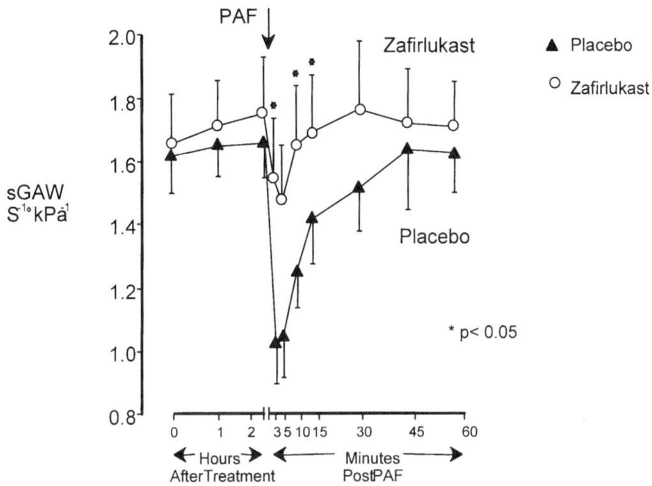

Figure 6 The effect of zafirlukast on airway-narrowing responses to inhaled PAF in normal subjects. Specific airway conductance (SGaw) after treatment with zafirlukast or placebo is shown with mean values (SEM) of eight subjects; significance of difference between placebo and drug treatment, $*p < 0.05$. (Reprinted with permission from Ref. 26.)

F. Platelet-Activating Factor

In a study reported by Kidney and colleagues, specific airway conductance (SGaw) was measured after inhalation of nebulized PAF 45 μg 2 hours after ingestion of single doses of zafirlukast 40 mg or placebo given on two study days 2 weeks apart (26). The study had a double-blind, placebo-controlled, crossover design. Zafirlukast caused significant inhibition of PAF-induced bronchoconstriction: mean SGaw 3 minutes after PAF was 1.54 units on zafirlukast compared with 1.05 on placebo ($p < 0.05$), and 1.75 and 1.66 2 hours after zafirlukast or placebo, respectively. The mean AUC for airway narrowing was 965 units on zafirlukast compared with 4178 units on placebo, representing a significant inhibition of 77% ($p < 0.05$). The mean maximum fall in SGaw was 17.5% on zafirlukast treatment and 43.1% on placebo, an inhibition of 59% ($p < 0.01$) (Fig. 6). Zafirlukast did not inhibit PAF-induced neutropenia.

V. Efficacy in Chronic Asthma

Studies of the effectiveness of zafirlukast, including those that have examined the dose-effect relationship, have used clinic-measured FEV_1 and PEFR measured by the patients in the morning and in the evening and recorded on a diary card as the primary measures of lung function. Studies have also examined efficacy using the results of symptom assessments and concomitant β_2-agonist use. Patients recorded their asthma symptoms daily on diary cards. Recorded each day were severity of daytime symptoms, the number of nighttime awakenings due to asthma, and the presence of asthma symptoms in the morning (first morning asthma). The severity of daytime symptoms was based on a 0 to 3 scale, with 0 = no asthma symptoms, 1 = mild asthma symptoms (did not interfere with patient's activity), 2 = moderate asthma symptoms (interfered with some of patient's activities), and 3 = severe asthma symptoms (interfered with many of patient's activities). Additionally, patients recorded daily β_2-agonist (albuterol) use.

A. Placebo-Controlled Studies

Several placebo-controlled studies have assessed the effect of increasing doses of zafirlukast on lung function, severity of asthma symptoms, and concomitant β_2-agonist use.

Spector et al. (27) compared three dose levels of zafirlukast (5, 10, or 20 mg twice daily) administered for 6 weeks against placebo, in a double-blind, parallel-group study involving 276 nonsmoking patients (197 male) aged 18–65 years with moderate asthma (FEV_1 40–75% predicted, daytime asthma symptoms score >10 in total over 7 consecutive days). All patients had β_2-agonist reversibility of their asthma or were demonstrated to have methacholine sensitivity. All were receiving β_2-agonist therapy with or without theophylline. The latter was withdrawn on day 1 of the 2-week placebo run-in period.

At a dose of zafirlukast 20 mg twice daily, the active treatment showed statistically significantly better results compared with placebo for all efficacy variables except morning PEFR. Over 6 weeks of treatment, zafirlukast 20 mg twice daily was more effective than placebo in reducing nighttime awakenings ($p = 0.001$), first-morning asthma ($p = 0.02$), daytime asthma symptoms scores ($p = 0.01$), and β_2-agonist use ($p < 0.02$), and in increasing evening PEFR ($p = 0.04$) and FEV_1 ($p < 0.05$). FEV_1 and morning PEFR increased 11% ($p < 0.05$) and 6% ($p = 0.07$) over baseline, respectively. Compared with baseline, zafirlukast treatment decreased nighttime awakenings by 46% ($p \leq 0.01$), β_2-agonist use by 31% ($p \leq 0.05$), and daytime asthma symptoms by 27% ($p \leq 0.01$) (Table 2).

A significant relationship between dose and response to treatment was observed for all variables except PEFR. First-morning asthma and daytime asthma symptom scores both improved linearly with increasing doses of zafirlukast. A linear trend was also observed between the reduced need for rescue medication (as assessed by inhaler use) and increasing dose of zafirlukast. A significantly linear trend has been observed between improvement in FEV_1 and plasma concentration of zafirlukast (Fig. 7).

Table 2 Percentage Change from Baseline and from Placebo for Asthma Symptoms and Lung Function Parameters After 6 Weeks of Treatment with Zafirlukast 40 mg/day

Diary card assessment	Zafirlukast 40 mg/day (n = 67) % change from baseline	Zafirlukast 40 mg/day (n = 67) % change from placebo	Placebo (n = 66); % change from baseline
Nighttime awakenings (weekly)*	−46	−2.6**	4
Morning asthma symptoms* (weekly)	−28	−1.0***	−10
Daytime asthma score* (daily)	−27	−0.24**	−13
Inhaler use (puffs/d)*	−31	−1.0***	−15
Morning PEFR (L/min)	6	15.0	2
Evening PEFR (L/min)	4	16.0	0
Office visit FEB_1 (L)	11	0.23**	1

*$p \leq 0.05$ for linear trend with dose analysis; **$p \leq 0.01$ compared with placebo; ***$p \leq 0.05$ compared with placebo. (Adapted and reprinted with permission from Ref. 29.)

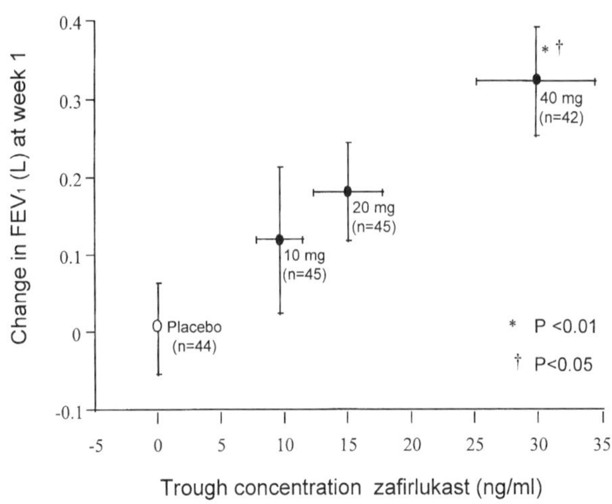

Figure 7 Relationship between change in FEV_1 and plasma concentration of zafirlukast and placebo after 4 weeks of treatment. *$p < 0.01$ for the difference in change in FEV_1 for zafirlukast and placebo. *$p < 0.05$ for linear trend with dose of zafirlukast. (Reprinted with permission from Ref. 29.)

Townley et al. (28) evaluated the clinical efficacy of zafirlukast in a dose-escalation study. After a 14-day run-in period patients with mild to moderate asthma were given zafirlukast 5 mg twice daily or placebo for 2 weeks; after this the dose was increased to 20 mg twice daily for 2 weeks, and at the end of this period the dose was increased again to 40 mg twice daily for 2 more weeks.

Two weeks of treatment with zafirlukast 5 mg twice daily decreased the mean daytime asthma symptoms score (−0.24/day), nighttime awakenings (−1.3/week), first morning asthma (−1.2/week), and β_2-agonist use (−0.6 puffs/day) compared with placebo (all $p < 0.05$). Modest additional improvements in these measures were seen during treatment with higher doses of zafirlukast. Compared with placebo, FEV_1 and morning and evening PEFR increased (+0.2 L, +18 L/min, and +22 L/min, respectively) after 2 weeks at the 5-mg twice-daily dosage of zafirlukast. These increases persisted to week 6 of the study.

Spector and colleagues (29) compared doses of zafirlukast ranging from 4 to 80 mg twice daily with placebo given for 13 weeks to 331 patients with mild-to-moderate asthma ($FEV_1 \geq 55\%$ predicted at trial entry). Two hundred and sixty-eight patients completed the 13-week trial. In this randomized double-blind study, prebronchodilator AM PEFR increased ($p < 0.05$) and as-needed β_2-agonist use decreased ($p < 0.05$) with increasing dose of zafirlukast. At the highest dose (80 mg twice daily), the improvement over baseline in morning PEFR was 10.7% ($p = 0.008$) compared with 3.2% in the lowest dose group (4 mg twice daily) and 4.3% in the placebo group.

Considered together, dose-response studies indicate that the minimum dosage of zafirlukast likely to provide consistent efficacy is 20 mg twice daily.

In a trial reported by Fish et al. (30), 762 nonsmoking patients (440 males) aged 12–76 years with mild-to-moderate asthma ($FEV_1 \geq 55\%$ predicted at trial entry, daytime asthma symptoms score ≥8 over 7 consecutive days) were randomized to treatment with zafirlukast 20 mg twice daily or placebo for 13 weeks. Randomized, double-blinded treatment was preceded by a single-blind run-in period of 7–14 days.

Six hundred and twenty-eight patients completed the study. At the end of 13 weeks of treatment, pulmonary function, as assessed by morning PEFR, office-visit FEV_1, and percent predicted FEV_1, were all significantly improved by zafirlukast (all $p < 0.05$). FEV_1 increased to >80% predicted in significantly more zafirlukast-treated patients than the placebo group ($p < 0.01$). The frequency of β_2-agonist use was also reduced by zafirlukast treatment ($p < 0.01$). The zafirlukast-treated group showed significant improvements compared with the group randomized to placebo with regard to nighttime awakenings and daytime symptom scores ($p < 0.05$), and zafirlukast treatment also produced a reduction in the number of mornings with asthma on awakening ($p < 0.01$). The overall changes noted from baseline in this study are depicted in Figure 8.

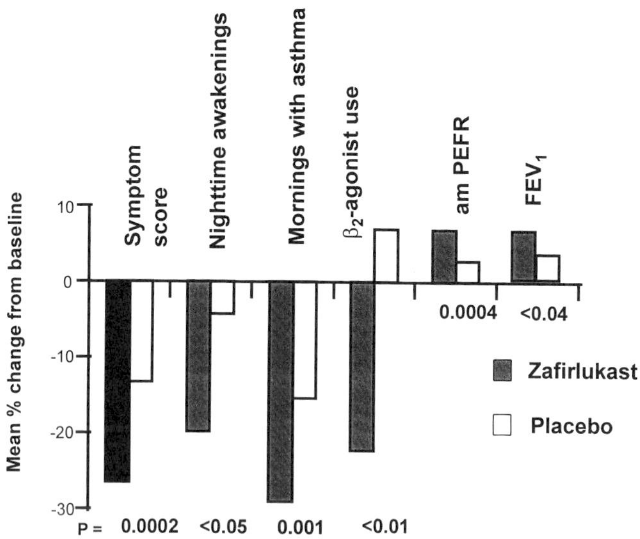

Figure 8 Percentage change from baseline for lung function and symptom assessments after 13 weeks of treatment with zafirlukast 20 mg twice daily or placebo.

Health economic aspects of the use of zafirlukast were reported for a subset of 146 patients from this trial (31). Patients on zafirlukast had 89% more days per month without symptoms, 89% more days without β_2-agonist use, and 98% more days without asthma episodes. They had 55% fewer contacts with health care personnel and days of absenteeism from work or school, used 17% fewer canisters of inhaled β_2-agonists, and 19% fewer nonasthma medications. The clinical and economic effectiveness of zafirlukast demonstrated in this study confirms the appropriateness of this medication as regular "preventive" therapy for patients with mild to moderate asthma.

An additional subprotocol of this 13-week efficacy trial assessed the bronchial hyperresponsiveness to methacholine in 36 patients randomized to zafirlukast and 12 patients randomized to placebo (32). The $PD_{20}FEV_1$ for methacholine inhalation challenge was determined at week 2 (evaluable data in 24 zafirlukast and 8 placebo patients) and at week 10 (21 zafirlukast and 7 placebo patients) of the study. Geometric means of 2.4 and 2.5 at weeks 2 and 10, respectively, indicated that $PD_{20}FEV_1$ during zafirlukast treatment was on average 2.5 times higher than during placebo, indicating that bronchial hyperresponsiveness was attenuated following 2 weeks of twice-daily dosing with zafirlukast.

Evidence of an early response to zafirlukast was noted at both the earliest diary (week 1) and spirometry (week 2) assessments in this trial (33). The beneficial effects were maintained throughout the 13 weeks of the trial. Daytime asthma symptoms scores, mornings with asthma, β_2-agonist use, and morning PEFR

Table 3 Comparison of Diary Card Assessments (means) for Week 2 and Week 13 of Zafirlukast Treatment

Assessment	Baseline	Week 2	% of Week 13
Daytime symptoms score	1.46	1.30	48
Nighttime awakenings (*n*)	0.44	0.38	35
Mornings with asthma (fraction of patients reporting)	0.61	0.52	53
Morning PEFR (L/min)	400	414	56
Evening PEFR (L/min)	434	445	73
β_2-Agonist use (puffs/day)	3.95	3.48	58

(measured before taking bronchodilator) were all significantly improved ($p < 0.05$) at day 3 of treatment for those who received zafirlukast. Morning and evening PEFR values increased by 14 and 11 L/min, respectively, on zafirlukast. Evening PEFR showed a trend in favor of zafirlukast, but this did not achieve statistical significance. By the second week of treatment at least 35% of the beneficial effects seen at week 13 had been achieved (Table 3).

B. Rapid Onset of Action of Zafirlukast—An Early Bronchodilator Effect

In a double-blind study reported by Hui and Barnes (34), 10 asthmatic patients with FEV_1 50–80% of predicted received a single dose of 40 mg oral zafirlukast and placebo in random order on 2 days at least 1 week apart. FEV_1 and specific airway conductance (SGaw) was measured every 30 minutes for 4 hours; after 4 hours, salbutamol was given by nebulization and FEV_1, and SGaw were measured 15 minutes later. FEV_1 increased significantly from baseline on the active treatment day in comparison with the placebo treatment day (Fig. 9), with a maximum increase of 8% (2–14%) above baseline at 3–5 hours. FEV_1 after salbutamol was greater on active treatment than on placebo (26 versus 18% above baseline). The differences in FEV_1 and SGaw after nebulized salbutamol between zafirlukast and placebo days were similar to those seen at 4 hours just before salbutamol.

This first-dose effect was confirmed in a trial reported by Nathan et al. (35). Two hundred and eighty-seven patients with asthma (aged 12–71 years) received 20 mg zafirlukast twice daily or 2 puffs of cromolyn sodium four times a day in a 13-week, multicenter, placebo-controlled, double-blind, double-dummy, parallel-group trial. Patients had cumulative daytime asthma symptoms scores of at least 8 over 7 consecutive days. FEV_1 measurements were taken every 30 minutes for the first 2 hours after treatment. At 2 hours after dosing, FEV_1 increased significantly from baseline for both active treatments compared with pla-

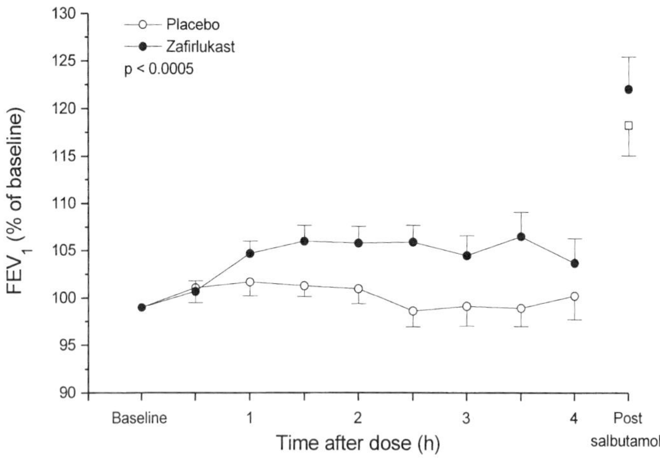

Figure 9 FEV_1 4 hours after zafirlukast or placebo and after nebulized β_2-agonist (albuterol/salbutamol). (Reprinted with permission from Ref. 34.)

cebo ($p < 0.02$). This first-dose effect size was doubled for patients with moderate to severe airway obstruction ($FEV_1 \leq 65\%$ predicted after zafirlukast, increasing by 0.35 L (16%) compared with 0.17 L (8%) and 0.04 L (2%) for cromolyn and placebo, respectively.

The rapid onset of action of zafirlukast has been confirmed in a study comparing 2 weeks of treatment in symptomatic asthmatic patients treated only with β_2-agonist given as required (36). One hundred and ninety-eight patients (FEV_1 50–75% predicted and ≥15% reversibility) were randomly assigned to treatment with placebo or zafirlukast 20 or 160 mg twice daily. Clinic PEFR measured 2 hours after the first dose of trial medication was significantly improved over baseline compared with placebo. Patients receiving zafirlukast showed improvements in morning PEFR after week 1, which were maintained at week 2 (Table 4). These data suggest that zafirlukast has an acute antibronchoconstrictor effect and results in sustained improvement of asthma. These results also confirm the role of leukotrienes in the maintenance of airflow obstruction in chronic asthma.

C. Efficacy Versus Placebo in Steroid-Treated Patients

The efficacy of 6 weeks of oral treatment with zafirlukast has been compared with that of placebo in 368 asthmatic patients who remained symptomatic despite treatment with high doses of inhaled corticosteroids (mean dose 1600 μg/day beclomethasone or equivalent) (37). Patients with FEV_1 50–75% predicted and

Table 4 Mean Changes in PEFR in Patients Treated with Placebo or Zafirlukast

Treatment	Morning PEFR (L/min) (week 1)	Morning PEFR (L/min) (week 2)	Clinic PEFR (L/min) (2 h after first dose)
Placebo	2.8	5.6	19.8
Zafirlukast 20 mg	22.2*	25.5*	37.9**
Zafirlukast 160 mg	30.0*	32.6*	45.3*

See text for details.
$*p < 0.05$; $**p < 0.06$ compared to placebo.

≥15% reversibility after β_2-agonist were randomized to either zafirlukast 80 mg twice daily or placebo in addition to their usual therapy.

Zafirlukast treatment significantly increased morning PEFR from baseline by 18.7 L/min compared with 1.5 L/min for placebo ($p < 0.001$). Other measures of lung function (FEV_1 and evening PEFR) and asthma symptom assessments (daytime asthma symptoms score, β_2-agonist use, and first morning asthma) also showed a significant benefit (all $p < 0.05$) from treatment with zafirlukast. Furthermore, fewer patients treated with zafirlukast experienced worsening asthma that required a change in treatment (8 vs. 15% for zafirlukast and placebo, respectively). The results of this study show that the use of zafirlukast produces clinical benefits in a typically difficult-to-manage patient population for whom additional treatment options are limited.

D. Effect on Asthma Exacerbations

An analysis of data pooled from double-blind comparisons of zafirlukast (4–80 mg twice daily) with placebo in trials ≥13 weeks duration has been reported (38). In these studies withdrawal criteria specified that patients requiring additional asthma therapy, hospitalization, or visit to an emergency department should discontinue trial therapy. Data from a total of five multinational trials encompassing a total of 1676 patients (1129 on zafirlukast and 547 on placebo) with mild to moderate asthma were considered. Withdrawals from the studies due to an exacerbation of asthma requiring a change in double-blind therapy were consistently less in the zafirlukast-treated group, and the difference between zafirlukast and placebo treatments was significant ($p = 0.008$). The risk of an asthma exacerbation on zafirlukast was about 50% that of the risk on placebo treatment (odds ratio = 0.51; 95% C.I. 0.34–0.84) ($p < 0.0001$).

Klim et al. estimated the possible cost-impact of these data across the same five multinational trials (39). Calculations based on the number of exacerbations per 1000 patients per year indicate that patients treated with zafirlukast are likely to incur costs of approximately £26,000 ($39,000) compared with £48,000 ($72,000) for patients randomized to the placebo group. This evaluation of the potential cost-impact of treatment failures does not consider efficacy benefits nor direct or indirect costs incurred by patients who successfully completed these studies.

E. Comparator Studies

The efficacy of zafirlukast, placebo, and cromolyn sodium has been compared. Nathan et al. reported on a randomized, double-blind, placebo-controlled, parallel-group multicenter study recruited 287 patients with mild to moderate asthma (FEV_1 74% predicted) (40). Thirteen weeks of randomized treatment with either zafirlukast 20 mg twice daily orally or inhaled cromolyn sodium 1600 μg four times daily [the maximum recommended dosage in the United States (41)] or placebo was preceded by a single-blind placebo run-in period of 7–14 days. Patients taking theophylline preparations before the study were weaned off before and during the placebo run-in period.

There were no consistent differences between the two active treatments with regard to efficacy assessments. Greater proportions of patients in both active therapy groups than in the placebo group responded to treatment by the end of the trial ($p < 0.05$ between active treatments and placebo). Both active treatments produced a similar rate of response to treatment (zafirlukast 64% and cromolyn sodium 68%).

VI. Safety of Zafirlukast

Zafirlukast has been well tolerated in clinical trials of more than 4000 patients worldwide. This includes more than 600 patients with asthma who have received zafirlukast at the recommended starting dosage of 20 mg b.i.d. for at least 1 year and up to 3 years. Longer-term safety information for doses of zafirlukast higher than the recommended starting dose of 20 mg b.i.d. is not available.

For all doses of zafirlukast studied, the most common adverse events reported with a frequency in excess of that observed on placebo have been headache, nausea, and infection (12.95 vs. 11.7%, 3.5 vs. 3.4%, and 3.1 vs. 2.0% for zafirlukast and placebo, respectively) (42). Abnormal laboratory findings have been rare; in particular, the frequency of hepatic transaminase elevations have been comparable between zafirlukast and placebo-treated patients. Rare cases of symptomatic hepatitis and hyperbilirubinemia, without attributable cause, were noted in the U.S. prescribing information for zafirlukast (42).

In dose-ranging trials of up to 13 weeks duration, higher doses of zafirlukast improved asthma symptoms, reduced β_2-agonist use, and improved pulmonary function with no increase in the number or severity of adverse events (27,29).

In the year following the introduction of zafirlukast in the U.S., approximately 750,000 patients received this medication. As part of the ongoing safety monitoring process it was noted that, in rare cases, patients on zafirlukast therapy may present with systemic eosinophilia, sometimes with clinical features of vasculitis consistent with Churg-Strauss syndrome (CSS), which is often treated with oral corticosteroid therapy. These events usually, but not always, have been associated with a reduction in oral corticosteroid therapy. Although a causal relationship with zafirlukast has not been established, caution is required when oral corticosteroid reduction is being considered (42). Wechsler and colleagues reported a case series involving eight adult patients with corticosteroid-dependent asthma who received zafirlukast, finding that these patients developed a clinical syndrome characterized by pulmonary infiltrates, eosinophilia, and acute dilated cardiomyopathy (atypical of CSS) from 3 days to 3 months after corticosteroid withdrawal (43). Although the exact pathogenesis for these clinical findings remains unclear, the authors speculated that these patients suffered from a primary eosinophilic infiltrative disorder that presented as moderate-to-severe asthma, which was suppressed by oral corticosteroid therapy and subsequently unmasked following corticosteroid withdrawal facilitated by zafirlukast.

VII. Summary

Considered together, the data currently available for zafirlukast indicate that in patients with asthma requiring chronic preventive therapy, zafirlukast at dosages of 20 up to 80 mg twice daily improves symptoms and pulmonary function, reduces the use of rescue (bronchodilator) medication, and reduces the likelihood of asthma exacerbation. A rapid onset of action following the first dose can be discerned, with considerable clinical benefit being obtained within 2 weeks of starting treatment. The drug appears to have efficacy similar to other asthma preventer drugs, and preliminary data in humans indicate that the drug suppresses infiltration and activation of inflammatory cells in the airway. Zafirlukast has been well tolerated in controlled clinical trials, with an adverse event profile similar to that of placebo.

Acknowledgment

The authors thank Gregg Truitt for his editorial assistance with this chapter.

References

1. Krell RD, Aharony D, Buckner CK, Keith RA, Kusner EJ, Snyder DW, Bernstein PR, Matassa VG, Yee YK, Brown FJ, Hesp B, Giles RE. The preclinical pharmacol-

ogy of ICI 204,219. A peptide leukotriene antagonist. Am Rev Respir Dis 1990; 141:978–987.

2. Snyder DW, Krell RD. Pharmacological evidence for a distinct leukotriene C_4 receptor in guinea pig trachea. J Pharmacol Exp Ther 1984; 231:616–622.
3. Krell RD, Tsai T-S, Berdoulay A, Barone M, Giles RE. Heterogeneity of peptide leukotriene receptors in guinea pig trachea. Prostaglandins 1983; 25:171–178.
4. Krell RD, Giles RE, Yee YK, Snyder DW. In vivo pharmacology of ICI 198,615: a novel, potent and selective peptide leukotriene antagonist. J Pharmacol Exp Ther 1987; 243:557–564.
5. Krell RD, Dehaas CJ, Lengel DJ, Kusner EJ, Williams JC, Buckner CK. Preclinical exploration of the potential antiinflammatory properties of the peptide leukotriene antagonist ICI 204,219 ('Accolate'). Ann NY Acad Sci 1994; 744:289–298.
6. Spreen RC, Bui KH, Savidge RD, Raybuck DL, Birmingham BK. Direct analysis of ICI 204,219 metabolites in biological samples by HPLC/electrospray MS and HPLC/MS/MS with radioactivity detection. Proceedings of the 42nd ASMS Conference on Mass Spectrometry and Allied Topics, Chicago, May 1994:360.
7. Floreani A, Robbins R, Melson J, Rennard S. Inhibitory effect of LTD_4 receptor antagonist 'Accolate' on agonist-induced bronchoconstriction in asthmatic subjects. Ann Allergy Asthma Immunol 1995; 76:98 Abs P33.
8. Smith LJ, Geller S, Ebright L, Glass M, Thyrum PT. Inhibition of leukotriene D_4-induced bronchoconstriction in normal subjects by the oral LTD_4 receptor antagonist ICI 204219. Am Rev Respir Dis 1990; 141:988–992.
9. Smith LJ, Glass M, Minkwitz MC. Inhibition of leukotriene D_4-induced bronchoconstriction in subjects with asthma: A concentration-effect study of ICI 204,219. Clin Pharmacol Ther 1993; 54:430–436.
10. Smith LJ, Glass M, Minkwitz MC. Dose response for 'Accolate' (zafirlukast) versus LTD_4-induced bronchoconstriction in patients with asthma. Am J Respir Crit Care Med 1995; 151 (4 pt 2):A378.
11. Smith LJ, Glass M, Miller CJ. Effect of oral 'Accolate' (zafirlukast) on leukotriene D_4-induced bronchoconstriction in patients with asthma. Am J Respir Crit Care Med 1995; 151 (4 pt 2):A378
12. Smith LJ, Cohn J, Minkwitz MC, Hanby LA. Effect of zafirlukast ('Accolate') on leukotriene D_4 (LTD_4)-induced bronchoconstriction in asthmatic patients receiving inhaled corticosteroids. Am J Respir Crit Care Med 1996; 153 (4 part 2): A803.
13. Dahlén B, Zetterstroem O, Bjoerck T, Dahlen SE. The leukotriene-antagonist ICI-204,219 inhibits the early airway reaction to cumulative bronchial challenge with allergen in atopic asthmatics. Eur Respir J 1994; 7:324–331.
14. Taylor IK, O'Shaughnessy KM, Fuller RW, Dollery CT. Effect of cysteinyl-leukotriene receptor antagonist ICI 204,219 on allergen-induced bronchoconstriction and airway hyperreactivity in atopic subjects. Lancet 1991; 337:690–694.
15. Findlay SR, Barden JM, Easley CB, Glass M. Effect of the oral leukotriene antagonist, ICI 204,219, on antigen-induced bronchoconstriction in subjects with asthma. J Allergy Clin Immunol 1992; 89:1040–1045.
16. O'Shaughnessy KM, Taylor IK, O'Connor B, O'Connell F, Dollery CT. Potent leukotriene D_4 receptor antagonist ICI 204,219 given by the inhaled route inhibits the

early but not the late phase of allergen-induced bronchoconstriction. Am Rev Respir Dis 1993; 147:1431–1435.
17. Nathan RA, Glass M, Minkwitz MC. Inhaled ICI 204,219 blocks antigen-induced bronchoconstriction in subjects with bronchial asthma. Chest 1994; 105:483–488.
18. Nathan RA, Storms WW, Bodman SF, Minkwitz MC, Glass M. Inhibition by aerosolized ICI 204,219, LTD_4 receptor antagonist, of allergen-induced bronchoconstriction. J Allergy Clin Immunol 1991; 87 (Part 2):256 Abs 465.
19. Calhoun WJ, Lavins BJ, Minkwitz MC, Evans, R, Gleich GJ, Cohn J. Effect of zafirlukast (ACCOLATE®) on cellular mediators of inflammation: bronchoalveolar lavage fluid findings after segmental antigen challenge. Am J Respir Crit Care Med. In press.
20. Finnerty JP, Wood-Baker R, Thomson H, Holgate ST. Role of leukotrienes in exercise-induced asthma. Inhibitory effect of ICI 204,219, a potent leukotriene D_4 receptor antagonist. Am Rev Respir Dis 1992; 145:746–749.
21. Makker HK, Lau LC, Thomson HW, Binks SM, Holgate ST. The protective effect of inhaled leukotriene D_4 receptor antagonist ICI 204,219 against exercise-induced asthma. Am Rev Respir Dis 1993; 147:1413–1418.
22. Boulet LP, Bai TR, Miller CJ, Lavins BJ, Cohn J, Turcotte H, Atton L. Effect of zafirlukast on cold-air-induced bronchoconstriction in patients with asthma. Eur Respir J 1996; 9 (suppl 23):273S Abs 1732.
23. Israel E, Lavins BJ, Miller CJ, Cohn J. Effect of zafirlukast (20 and 40 mg) on cold-air-induced bronchoconstriction in patients with bronchial asthma. Eur Respir J 1996; 9 (suppl 23):51S Abs P0381.
24. Glass M, Snader LA, Israel E. Effect of the inhaled LTD_4-receptor antagonist, ICI 204,219, on cold-air-induced bronchoconstriction in patients with asthma. J Allergy Clin Immunol 1994; 93 (1 pt 2):295 Abs 794.
25. Lazarus SC, Wong HH, Watts MJ, Boushey HA, Lavins BJ, Minkwitz MC. The leukotriene receptor antagonist zafirlukast inhibits sulfur-dioxide-induced bronchoconstriction in patients with asthma. Am J Respir Crit Care Med 1997; 156(6):1725–1730.
26. Kidney JC, Ridge SM, Chung KF, Barnes PJ. Inhibition of platelet-activating factor-induced bronchoconstriction by the leukotriene D_4 receptor antagonist ICI 204,219. Am Rev Respir Dis 1993; 147:215–217.
27. Spector SL, Smith LJ, Glass M, Accolate™ asthma trialists. Effects of 6 weeks of therapy with oral doses of ICI 204,219, a leukotriene D_4 receptor antagonist, in subjects with bronchial asthma. Am J Respir Crit Care Med 1994; 150:618–623.
28. Townley R, Glass M, Minkwitz MC. Six week dose escalation study with 'Accolate' (zafirlukast) in patients with mild to moderate asthma. Am J Respir Crit Care Med 1995; 151 (4 pt 2):A379.
29. Spector S, Miller CJ, Glass M. Thirteen week dose response study with 'Accolate' (zafirlukast) in patients with mild to moderate asthma. Am J Respir Crit Care Med 1995; 151 (4 pt 2):A379.
30. Fish JE, Kemp JP, Lockey RF, Glass M, Hanby LA, Bonuccelli CM, Zafirlukast Trialists Group. Zafirlukast for symptomatic mild-to-moderate asthma: A 13-week multicenter study. Clin Ther 1997;19(4):675–690.
31. Suissa S, Dennis RJ, Ernst P, Sheehy O, Wood-Dauphinee S. Effectiveness of the

leukotriene receptor antagonist zafirlukast for mild-to-moderate asthma. Ann Int Med 1997; 126:177–183.
32. Rosenthal RR, Lavins BJ, Hanby LA. Effect of treatment with zafirlukast ('Accolate') on bronchial hyperresponsiveness in patients with mild-to-moderate asthma. J Allergy Clin Immunol 1996; 97 (1 part 3):250 Abs 270.
33. Kemp JP, Glass M, Minkwitz MC. Onset of action of the leukotriene-receptor antagonist, zafirlukast ('Accolate') in patients with asthma. J Allergy Clin Immunol 1995; 95 (1 pt 2):351 Abs 844.
34. Hui KP, Barnes NC. Lung function improvement in asthma with a cysteinyl-leukotriene receptor antagonist. Lancet 1991; 337:1062–1063.
35. Nathan RA, Cohn J, Minkwitz MC. First dose effect of 'Accolate' (zafirlukast) in patients with asthma. Ann Allergy Asthma Immunol 1996; 76:91 Abs P6.
36. Bateman ED, Aitchison JA, Summerton L, Harris A. The early onset of action of zafirlukast (Accolate™) in patients with asthma. Am J Respir Crit Care Med 1997; 155 (4 part 2):A663.
37. Virchow J Chr, Hassall SM, Summerton L, Harris A. Improved asthma control over 6 weeks with Accolate® (zafirlukast) in patients on high-dose inhaled corticosteroids. J Invest Med 1997; 45(3):286A.
38. Barnes NC, Black B, Syrett N, Cohn JN. Reduction of exacerbations of asthma in multinational clinical trials with zafirlukast ('Accolate'). Allergy 1996; 51 (suppl 30):84 Abs.
39. Klim JB, Brown J, Syrett N, Cohn J. Cost impact of reducing exacerbations of asthma in multinational clinical trials with zafirlukast. Eur Respir J 1996; 9 (suppl 23):52S Abs P0382.
40. Nathan RA, Glass M, Snader L. Effects of 13 weeks of treatment with ICI 204,219 ('Accolate') or cromolyn sodium ('Intal') in patients with mild to moderate asthma. J Allergy Clin Immunol 1995; 95 (1 part 2):388 Abs 990.
41. Cromolyn sodium prescribing information. Physicians' Desk Reference. 52nd Ed. Medical Economics Company, 1998:2367–2368.
42. Zafirlukast prescribing information. Physicians' Desk Reference. 52nd Ed. Medical Economics Company, 1998:3148–3149.
43. Wechsler ME, Garpestad E, Flier SR, Kocher O, Weiland DA, Polito AJ, Klinek MM, Bigby TD, Wong GA, Helmers RA, Drazen JM. Pulmonary infiltrates, eosinophilia, and cardiomyopathy following corticosteroid withdrawal in patients with asthma receiving zafirlukast. JAMA 1998;279(6):455–457.

17

Zileuton: The First Leukotriene Synthesis Inhibitor for Use in the Management of Chronic Asthma

LOUISE M. DUBÉ, LINDA J. SWANSON, WALID M. AWNI, RANDY L. BELL, and GEORGE W. CARTER

Abbott Laboratories
Abbott Park, Illinois

RACHEL F. OCHS

Northwestern University Medical School
Chicago, Illinois

I. Introduction

Products of the 5-lipoxygenase pathway have long been postulated to play an important role in the pathogenesis of asthma (1). This hypothesis was based on evidence that 5-lipoxygenase products are synthesized and released by human lung during asthmatic reactions and have the ability to produce airway constriction and inflammation (2–7). Controlled clinical studies with 5-lipoxygenase inhibitors and leukotriene receptor antagonists have now established the importance of 5-lipoxygenase products in the asthmatic response and have demonstrated the utility of inhibitors of 5-lipoxygenase in the therapy of asthma.

Leukotrienes are a family of potent biological substances formed from arachidonic acid by the enzyme 5-lipoxygenase (8,9). These lipid mediators form two structural classes: the cysteinyl leukotrienes (leukotriene (LT) C_4, D_4, and E_4) and the dihydroxy leukotriene (LTB_4). The most notable biological activity of the cysteinyl leukotrienes is potent airway constriction, whereas LTB_4 has powerful chemoattractant effects on neutrophils and eosinophils (10).

The enzyme 5-lipoxygenase catalyzes the first, rate-limiting step in the biosynthetic pathway leading to leukotriene formation. This enzyme has a rather limited distribution and is found mainly in cells known to participate in inflammatory reactions (e.g., neutrophils, eosinophils, monocytes, macrophages, and mast cells). Since leukotrienes are not stored in cells, their extracellular release requires de novo synthesis. Therefore, inhibition of 5-lipoxygenase prevents the formation of all leukotrienes, as well as other biologically active 5-lipoxygenase products.

II. Preclinical Information on Zileuton

A. Discovery of Zileuton

Zileuton (Zyflo®) is the first specific inhibitor of 5-lipoxygenase approved for the treatment of chronic asthma. The discovery of zileuton began at Abbott Laboratories in the early 1980s. At that time, although growing evidence suggested that excessive production of 5-lipoxygenase products played an important role in asthma, suitable inhibitors to test this hypothesis had not been discovered. Since no structural information existed for 5-lipoxygenase, several different strategies to design an inhibitor were undertaken. The approach that ultimately succeeded was based on the hypothesis that 5-lipoxygenase, like soybean lipoxygenase, contained a catalytically important iron atom. Potent inhibitors of the enzyme were quickly identified when inhibitors were designed that contained pharmacophores that bound tightly to the active-site iron of 5-lipoxygenase. Although the initial compounds lacked activity in experimental animals due to their rapid metabolism, extensive structure-activity analysis, combined with the prudent usage of in vitro and in vivo biological assays, culminated in the discovery of zileuton (11).

B. 5-Lipoxygenase Inhibitor Activity

Zileuton is a highly effective and selective inhibitor of 5-lipoxygenase (12). Zileuton produced a concentration-dependent inhibition of 5-lipoxygenase from rat basophilic leukemia cells (RBL) supernatants, with an IC_{50} of 500 nM (12). Inhibition of RBL 5-lipoxygenase by zileuton is dependent on substrate concentration (arachidonic acid) and is readily reversible, findings expected with a competitive active-site inhibitor. In addition to inhibition of 5-lipoxygenase in cellular supernatants, zileuton is highly effective in preventing the formation of 5-lipoxygenase products (5-HETE and LTB_4) from intact cells. Zileuton inhibits 5-lipoxygenase product formation from both human and rat neutrophils with IC_{50} values in the 300–600 nM range (12). This inhibition is removed by a simple wash procedure, consistent with the reversible inhibition by zileuton. At comparable concentrations, zileuton prevents leukotriene formation by a wide variety of other cell types, including mast cells and eosinophils (13). The similar inhibitory potency of zileuton in broken cell preparations of 5-lipoxygenase compared to its inhibitory activity against leukotriene formation in intact cells suggests that zileuton readily penetrates cells and interacts with the enzyme in its intracellular environment. Zileuton produced little or no inhibition of related enzymes such as 12-lipoxygenase, 15-lipoxygenase, and cyclooxygenase at concentrations up to 100 μM. These and other studies have consistently demonstrated that zileuton selectively inhibits 5-lipoxygenase (13).

Numerous studies have demonstrated that zileuton effectively inhibits leukotriene formation in experimental animals following oral administration. Zileuton prevents leukotriene formation in the rat peritoneal cavity triggered by an antigen-antibody reaction with an ED_{50} of 3 mg/kg. In this model a 70 mg/kg dose of zileuton failed to significantly inhibit the formation of the cyclooxygenase product thromboxane B_2 (TxB_2), demonstrating the in vivo selectivity of zileuton for leukotriene inhibition. Oral doses of zileuton also inhibited ex vivo blood LTB_4 biosynthesis in the rat, dog, monkey, and sheep (13). In the dog, an oral dose of 5 mg/kg provided complete inhibition of ex vivo leukotriene formation for at least 24 hours.

C. Inhibition of Bronchoconstriction and Pulmonary Inflammation

Zileuton is also effective in animal models of bronchoconstriction. Co-administered with an antihistamine, zileuton completely inhibited the bronchoconstriction induced by aerosolized antigen in sensitized animals (14). A single oral dose of zileuton inhibited the pulmonary changes elicited by antigen for 12 hours. Zileuton alone was also very effective against early- and late-phase bronchoconstriction in naturally antigen-sensitive conscious sheep (15,16). The pulmonary changes in both species appear to be due to the inhibition of leukotrienes, since the compound does not inhibit smooth muscle contraction induced by a variety of agonists in vitro. Recently we have shown (17) that inhibition of 5-lipoxygenase could partially reverse an ongoing antigen-induced bronchospasm in the guinea pig.

The effect of zileuton on antigen-induced bronchospasm was predicted by the smooth muscle–contracting activity of cysteinyl leukotrienes (1). An effect on inflammatory cell influx into tissue was also predicted from the activities of LTB_4 (1). A number of studies have shown the effectiveness of zileuton in blocking inflammatory cell influx (12,13). In particular, eosinophilia appears to be inhibited by the compound. In the studies done by Abraham et al. (15) in antigen-challenged sheep, eosinophil influx as measured by lavage content 24 hours after challenge was significantly inhibited. Consistent with the hypothesis that airway inflammation contributes to airway hypersensitivity, airway hyperresponsiveness was also dampened. In addition, in a rat model of lung inflammation zileuton was quite effective in blocking the migration of eosinophils into the lungs following a challenge with sephadex particles (Fig. 1) (18). In this model, an increase in bronchial lavage cysteinyl leukotrienes preceded a marked increase in eosinophils both in lavage fluids and in lung tissue. Inhibition of this response was seen with zileuton but not with the LTD_4 antagonists MK476 or zafirlukast (18). Finally, Henderson et al. (19) showed that zileuton inhibited

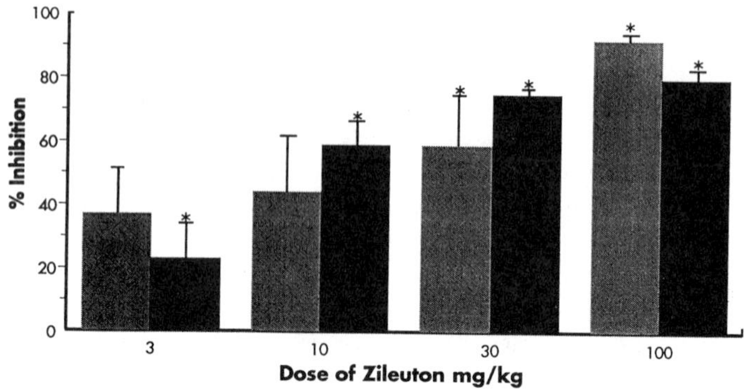

Figure 1 Inhibition of eosinophil influx and cysteinyl leukotriene formation following oral administration of zileuton. Results expressed as mean ± SEM of eight animals. Degree of inhibition of eosinophil influx shown in shaded bars and blockade of cysteinyl leukotriene formation shown in black bars. $*p \leq 0.05$ compared to baseline.

eosinophilia and mucus release in an antigen-driven mouse model of pulmonary inflammation (Fig. 2). As shown, eosinophils were nearly completely blocked from entering the lungs after zileuton dosing. Mucus production was also significantly blocked (>60%) by the inhibitor. These studies provided a framework of optimism that zileuton would provide effective anti-inflammatory therapy in the clinical setting.

III. Clinical Pharmacokinetics and Pharmacodynamics of Zileuton

A. Pharmacokinetics of Zileuton

In humans, zileuton is rapidly absorbed after oral administration with a mean ± SD T_{max} of 1.7 ± 0.9 hours and a mean zileuton peak level (C_{max}) of 5.0 ± 2.0 μg/ml for the 600-mg qid dose (20–23). After single and multiple doses, the mean area under the curve (AUC) following 600 mg zileuton administration is 19.2 ± 5.6 μg·h/ml. Plasma concentrations of zileuton are proportional to dose, and steady-state levels are predictable from single-dose data (20–22), indicating no unusual accumulation of the drug following qid dosing. The average apparent oral clearance of zileuton is approximately 7.0 ml/min/kg (22). The apparent volume of distribution of zileuton is approximately 1.2 L/kg (22). Zileuton is 93% bound to plasma proteins with albumin as the primary plasma binding protein (88% bound) and α_1-acid glycoprotein as a more minor binding protein (34% bound) (24). Administration of zileuton with food resulted in a small, but statisti-

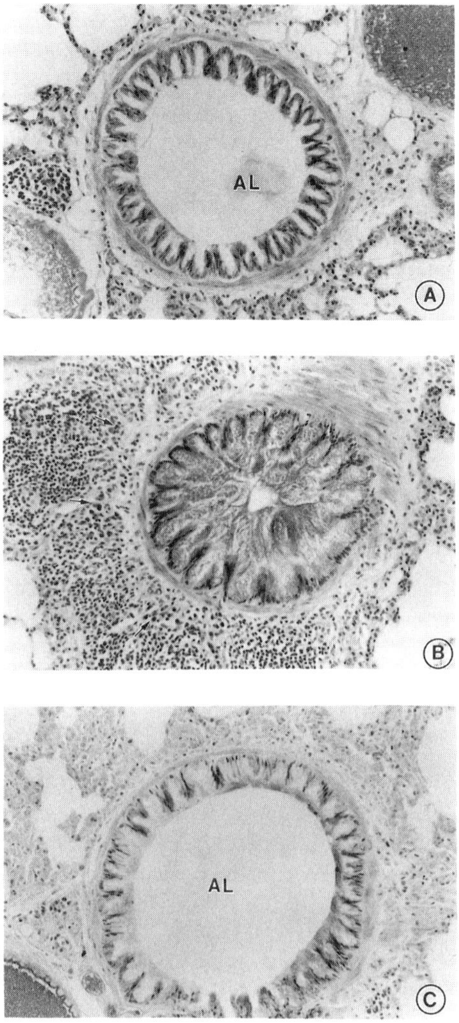

Figure 2 Histologic evidence of airway inflammation in ovalbumin-treated and control mice: effect of 5-lipoxygenase inhibition. Lung tissue was obtained from sham-sensitized and saline-challenged mice (A), and ovalbumin immunized/challenged mice in the absence (B) or presence (C) of zileuton treatment. Lung sections were stained in Discombe's solution, counterstained with methylene blue, and examined by light microscopy. Airway mucus release in the airway lumen (AL) is markedly reduced when zileuton is given before intranasal ovalbumin. The infiltration of the interstitial tissue by eosinophils is also reduced after zileuton treatment compared to ovalbumin challenge alone (B). Copyright permission from Rockefeller University Press. (From Ref. 19.)

cally significant, increase (27%) in zileuton C_{max} without significant changes in AUC or T_{max}. Therefore, zileuton can be administered with or without food (23).

Elimination of zileuton is predominantly via metabolism with a mean terminal half-life of 2.5 hours (20–22,25). The activity of zileuton is primarily due to the parent drug. Studies with radiolabeled drug in healthy volunteers have demonstrated that 94.5 and 2.2% of the radiolabeled dose is recovered in urine and feces, respectively (25). Several zileuton metabolites, including two diastereomeric *O*-glucuronide conjugates and an *N*-dehydroxylated metabolite, have been identified in humans (20,21,25). The major urinary metabolites in humans (approximately 80–90% of the dose) are the zileuton glucuronides (20,21,25). The urinary excretion of the inactive *N*-dehydroxylated metabolite and unchanged zileuton each accounted for less than 0.5% of the dose (20,21,25). In vitro studies utilizing human liver microsomes have shown that zileuton and its *N*-dehydroxylated metabolite can also be oxidatively metabolized by the cytochrome P450 isoenzymes CYP1A2, CYP3A, and CYP2C9 (26).

The pharmacokinetics of zileuton are essentially the same in healthy elderly subjects (>65 years) as in healthy younger adults (18–40 years) and in males compared to females, after adjustments for body weight. The pharmacokinetics are independent of the subject's race (27–29). The pharmacokinetics of zileuton in children (9–12 years) are similar to those in adults after adjustment for body weight or body surface area (30). The pharmacokinetics of zileuton were also similar between healthy volunteers and in patients with either mild to moderate asthma or rheumatoid arthritis (28,29). The pharmacokinetics of zileuton were similar in healthy subjects and in subjects with mild, moderate, and severe renal insufficiency (31). In subjects with renal failure who required hemodialysis, pharmacokinetics of zileuton were not altered by hemodialysis. A very small percentage of the administered zileuton dose (<0.5%) was removed by hemodialysis (31). Hence, dosing adjustment is not necessary in patients with renal dysfunction or in those undergoing hemodialysis.

B. Pharmacodynamics of Zileuton

Various indicators of zileuton-induced suppression of 5-lipoxygenase product formation, including LTB_4 from ex vivo stimulated whole blood, urinary LTE_4, bronchoalveolar lavage (BAL) fluid LTB_4 and cysteinyl leukotrienes, and nasal lavage fluid eicosanoids were measured during the course of several studies. In addition, the specificity of zileuton in inhibiting the products of the 5-lipoxygenase pathway was assessed by measuring cyclooxygenase products, including TxB_2 and prostaglandin D_2 (PGD_2).

The ex vivo percent inhibition of LTB_4 biosynthesis in whole blood after stimulation with calcium ionophore is directly related to the concentration of zileuton in plasma (28,32,33). The zileuton plasma concentration required to pro-

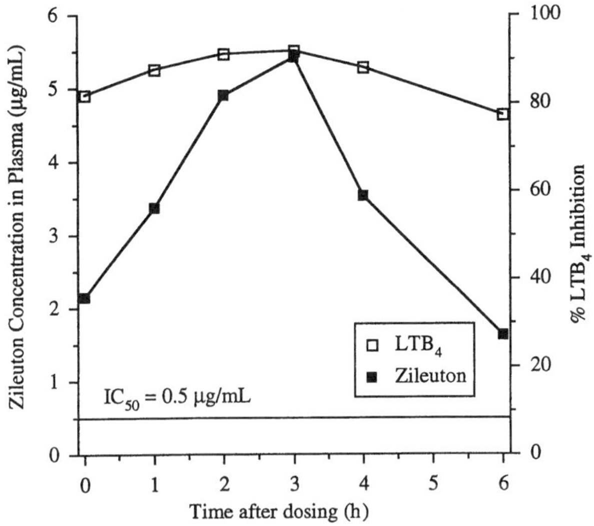

Figure 3 Mean zileuton concentration in plasma and simulated percent inhibition of LTB_4 biosynthesis at steady state after administration of 600 mg zileuton qid to healthy subjects. Zileuton levels shown with solid squares, percent LTB_4 inhibition with open squares.

duce 50% of the maximum inhibition of the LTB_4 biosynthesis in whole blood (IC_{50}) is approximately 0.5 µg/ml (28,32,33). The IC_{50} is similar in healthy volunteers and in children and adult patients with asthma. The mean zileuton concentration in plasma and simulated percent inhibition of LTB_4 biosynthesis at steady state after administration of 600 mg zileuton qid to healthy subjects are shown in Figure 3. While the ex vivo inhibition of LTB_4 production in whole blood is directly related to the plasma concentration of zileuton, no such correlation has been observed between ex vivo LTB_4 inhibition and the magnitude of improvement in pulmonary function in patients with asthma (28).

In a cold air challenge study ex vivo LTB_4 production in whole blood was reduced by 74% ($p \leq 0.001$) following a single 800-mg dose of zileuton (34). In contrast, TxB_2 production by the cyclooxygenase pathway was not affected by zileuton. In another bronchoprovocation study in aspirin-sensitive asthmatics, zileuton 600 mg qid for 1 week decreased the baseline urinary LTE_4 excretion by 71% ($p < 0.02$) and significantly blunted the maximum increase in urinary LTE_4 after aspirin ingestion by 68% ($p < 0.01$) (35).

The in vivo activity of zileuton was also examined in 10 patients by measuring LTE_4 in urine and BAL fluid following segmental allergen challenge. Urinary

LTE_4 was reduced by 86% compared to placebo ($p < 0.05$) 4 hours postchallenge (36). BAL LTE_4 was similarly reduced by 72% compared to placebo 24 hours after challenge (37). In patients with nocturnal asthma, LTB_4 and cysteinyl leukotrienes in BAL fluid were significantly reduced by 38.5 and 67%, respectively, after 1 week of zileuton treatment. Nocturnal urinary LTE_4 levels were reduced by 76% compared to placebo (38).

The effectiveness of 5-lipoxygenase inhibition was also assessed in chronic bronchial asthma patients receiving either zileuton 1.6 or 2.4 g/day for 4 weeks. In that study, urinary LTE_4 was reduced by 26 and 39% compared to baseline in patients receiving 1.6 or 2.4 g/day, respectively ($p < 0.01$), while no change was noted in the group receiving placebo (39).

Finally, the inhibitory effect of zileuton on leukotriene production in vivo was examined in nasal lavage fluid following antigen challenge in nine allergic rhinitis patients. A single 800-mg dose of zileuton suppressed LTB_4 production in nasal lavage fluid by 90% immediately following allergen challenge ($p < 0.01$). 5-HETE synthesis was also reduced by 74% ($p < 0.02$), while PGD_2 and histamine release were not significantly affected. Zileuton also inhibited LTB_4 release in whole blood stimulated with calcium ionophore ex vivo by 92% ($p < 0.01$). In contrast, zileuton did not affect the release of products of the cyclooxygenase (TxB_2) or 12-lipoxygenase pathway (40).

Overall, the results of these studies indicate that zileuton is a specific inhibitor of 5-lipoxygenase and that inhibition of the 5-lipoxygenase pathway does not result in shunting of arachidonic acid to the cyclooxygenase pathway.

IV. Effects of Zileuton on Asthma Induced by Provocatory Stimuli

A number of studies have been performed with zileuton to determine the action of zileuton on the bronchoconstrictor response or airway reactivity following exposure to various bronchoactive stimuli. Bronchoprovocation models were chosen to explore the effectiveness of zileuton following typical provocative stimuli that act as known triggers of bronchoconstriction in asthma patients, including cold air (34,41,42), exercise (43–45), allergen (46–48), and aspirin (35,49–51).

A. Cold Air–Challenge Model

Hyperventilation of cold, dry air is a naturally occurring stimulus that is known to induce bronchoconstriction in the majority of patients with asthma (41,42,52).

In a randomized, double-blind, placebo-controlled, crossover trial, the effect of a single dose of 800 mg of zileuton on bronchoconstriction induced by

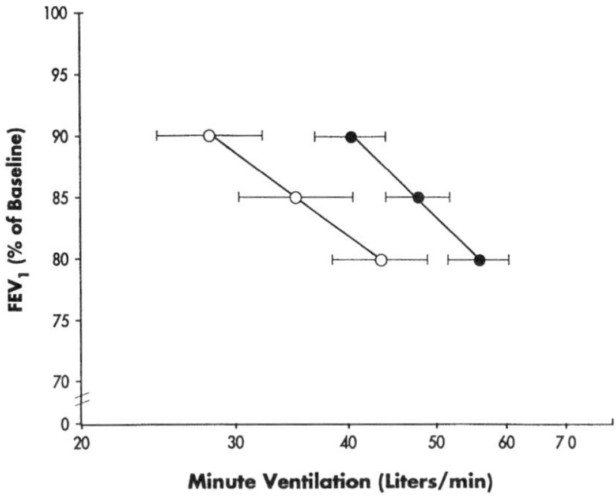

Figure 4 Composite dose-response curves illustrating the decrease in FEV_1 in relation to minute ventilation after subjects received placebo (open circles) or zileuton (closed circles). The minute ventilation is plotted on a log proportional scale. The differences in the PD_{10} FEV_1 (90% of baseline values), PD_{15} FEV_1 (85% of baseline values), and PD_{20} FEV_1 (80% of baseline values) between placebo and zileuton were all significant ($p \leq 0.005$, $p \leq 0.005$, and $p \leq 0.02$, respectively). Values are means ± SEM. (From Ref. 34.)

cold, dry air was examined in 13 patients with asthma (34). Patients who participated in this trial were 18–55 years of age, had a confirmed diagnosis of asthma, and had a known cold air–induced 20% drop in forced expiratory volume in 1 second (FEV_1).

The results of this study demonstrated that a single oral dose of zileuton inhibited formation of 5-lipoxygenase–derived leukotrienes, and this inhibition was accompanied by a significant blunting of the bronchoconstriction induced by cold, dry air. The amount of cold, dry air (calculated as a function of respiratory heat exchange) required to reduce the FEV_1 by 10% (PD_{10}) was increased by 47% after a single dose of zileuton ($p < 0.002$ compared to placebo). Zileuton, 800 mg, also produced a significantly greater increase (39 and 26%) in PD_{15}, PD_{20} than did placebo ($p < 0.005$ and $p < 0.02$, respectively). Zileuton produced differences of similar magnitude and significance when reactivity to cold, dry air was expressed as a function of minute ventilation. There was a 45, 38, and 28% increase in minute ventilation (L/min) for PD_{10}, PD_{15}, and PD_{20}, respectively ($p < 0.05$ compared to placebo) (Fig. 4).

Zileuton treatment, decreased ex vivo, stimulated synthesis of LTB_4 by

74% ($p < 0.001$), whereas there was no change in LTB_4 levels in patients treated with placebo. Synthesis of TxB_2, a product of the cyclooxygenase pathway, was unaffected by zileuton.

The results of this study suggest that leukotrienes play a definite role in the airway narrowing caused by a common stimulus of asthmatic bronchoconstriction—hyperventilation of dry cold air. In this model of asthmatic obstruction, zileuton compares favorably to other agents currently used in the treatment of asthma (41,53,54).

B. Exercise-Induced Asthma

In a randomized, double-blind, placebo-controlled, crossover study, zileuton, 600 mg qid, was administered for 2 days (a total of nine doses) prior to exercise challenge in 24 patients with exercise-induced asthma aged 21–45 years (45). Bronchoconstriction was less severe and of shorter duration following treatment with zileuton than with placebo. Zileuton pretreatment resulted in a 40 ± 7.1% reduction in exercise-induced bronchospasm (maximum change: 15.6% decrease from baseline with zileuton vs. 28.1% with placebo; $p < 0.01$). Five minutes postexercise, the FEV_1 in zileuton-treated patients was 85.7 ± 2.8%, while that for the placebo patients was 75.9 ± 3.0% of baseline ($p < 0.01$). The differences between the two groups remained significant for 45 minutes following exercise challenge (Fig. 5).

The effect of zileuton on exercise-induced bronchoconstriction supports the role of leukotrienes in the pathogenesis of exercise-induced asthma and suggests a possible therapeutic role of 5-lipoxygenase inhibitors in this disorder.

C. Aspirin-Sensitive Asthma

Aspirin-sensitive asthma is characterized by bronchoconstriction, and naso-ocular, gastrointestinal and/or dermal reactions that occur after ingestion of aspirin (ASA) or agents that inhibit cyclooxygenase (49–51). Leukotrienes have been implicated as mediators of this syndrome (35,55–58).

Eight aspirin-sensitive asthmatic patients were challenged with predetermined sub-threshold and then threshold doses of aspirin known to elicit a ≥15% drop in FEV_1 in a randomized, double-blind, placebo-controlled, crossover trial (35,59). Patients received zileuton 600 mg qid for 1 week prior to the challenge. Zileuton prevented the decline in FEV_1 in response to aspirin (Fig. 6) (mean minimal FEV_1 placebo period = 2.7 ± 0.2 L; 18.6% decrease and zileuton period = 3.3 ± 0.2 L; 4.4% decrease; $p \leq 0.014$). In addition, zileuton blocked the nasal, gastrointestinal, and dermal responses to aspirin administration. Zileuton prevented the increase in nasal symptoms after aspirin challenge (59), whereas during placebo treatment nasal symptoms increased more than twofold ($p <$ 0.006). Zileuton also decreased baseline urinary LTE_4 excretion (from 469 ±

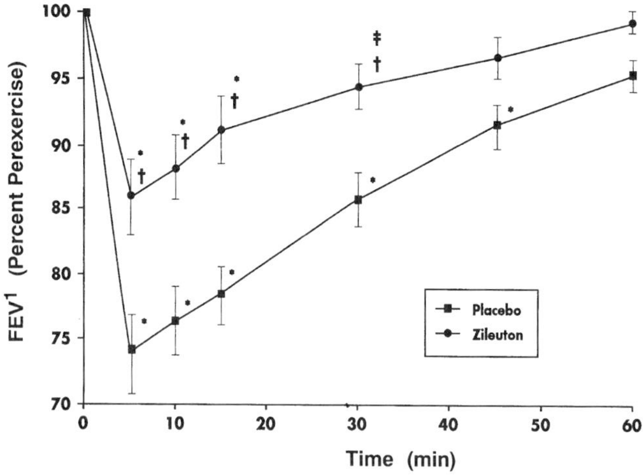

Figure 5 Effects of zileuton 600 mg (four times daily) on FEV_1 after exercise challenge. The percent change in FEV_1 from the preexercise value is measured in the 60-minute period following the completion of exercise. $^*p \leq 0.01$ compared with preexercise; $^\dagger p \leq 0.01$ zileuton compared with placebo; $^\ddagger p \leq 0.05$ compared with preexercise. (From Ref. 45.)

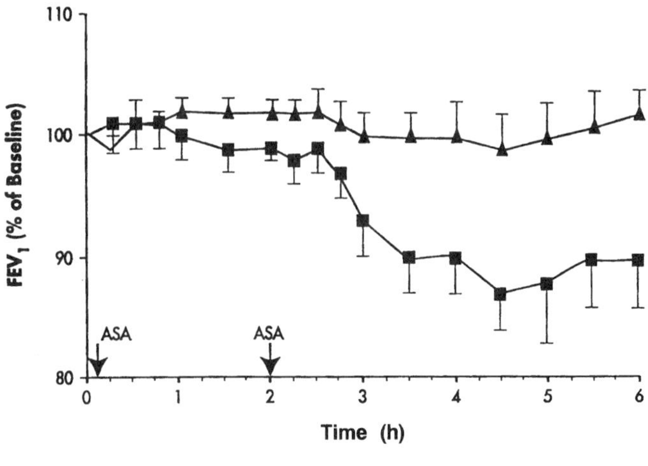

Figure 6 Effect of zileuton on change in FEV_1 after ASA challenge (closed triangles indicate zileuton, closed squares indicate placebo). The FEV_1 expressed as mean percentage of baseline (± SEM) for all eight patients is plotted versus time after dosing. Mean minimal FEV_1 was significantly different between treatments post–aspirin challenge ($p < 0.014$ zileuton vs. placebo). (From Ref. 35.)

141 pg/mg creatinine to 147 ± 69 pg/mg creatinine; $p < 0.02$) and blunted the maximum increase in urinary LTE_4 after aspirin challenge (3539 ± 826 pg/mg creatinine vs. 1120 ± 316 pg/mg creatinine; $p < 0.01$) (35). Finally, zileuton blocked the rise in nasal tryptase ($p = 0.011$) and nasal leukotriene ($p < 0.05$) levels after aspirin challenge (59).

A second trial (randomized, double-blind, placebo-controlled, crossover design) examined the effect of adjunctive zileuton therapy, 600 mg qid, for 6 weeks on changes in symptoms and hyperresponsiveness to histamine in 40 patients with documented aspirin intolerance (60). Two 6-week treatment periods were separated by a 4-week wash-out period. All but one patient received concomitant inhaled, nasal or systemic corticosteroids, and all were treated with some type of additional asthma medication (60). Prior to treatment patients had a baseline percent predicted FEV_1 of 80%.

After 6 weeks of treatment with zileuton 600 mg qid as add-on therapy, patients demonstrated a 7% (0.14 L) improvement in FEV_1 compared to the placebo period (−0.1% [−0.04 L]; $p < 0.05$) (60). These patients also demonstrated a significant increase in the PD_{20} to histamine compared to placebo ($p < 0.05$) (60). During zileuton treatment, patients experienced reduced nasal symptom scores ($p < 0.01$ vs. placebo period) (60) and a marked return of the sense of smell ($p < 0.001$ vs. placebo period) (data on file Abbott Laboratories). Urinary LTE_4 levels, known to be elevated in aspirin-sensitive asthmatics (57,58), were significantly reduced by zileuton (to 67 ng/mmol creatinine; CI 58–76) compared to placebo treatment (95 ng/mmol creatinine; CI 75–115; $p < 0.001$).

These findings further support the hypothesis that leukotrienes contribute significantly to the clinical picture of aspirin-sensitive asthma, particularly since patients in this trial continued to receive treatment with existing antiasthma agents, including inhaled and/or systemic corticosteroids.

D. Summary of Bronchoprovocation Studies

Overall, the results of the bronchoprovocation studies have clearly demonstrated that zileuton significantly reduced the airway responses to cold air, exercise, and aspirin. The efficacy of zileuton in reducing the bronchospasm caused by various stimuli was apparent after 1–7 days of treatment, but it may have been effective earlier than the time of the first measurement in these studies. The total inhibition of the response in the aspirin-intolerant asthmatics indicates that 5-lipoxygenase products may be virtually the sole mediators in this type of asthma. In other models of induced asthma, such as cold air and exercise, partial inhibition of the response by zileuton suggests that 5-lipoxygenase products play an important role, but that other mediators also contribute to the responses elicited by these stimuli.

V. Anti-Inflammatory Properties of Zileuton

Based on proinflammatory effects of leukotrienes and evidence that 5-lipoxygenase products are generated during asthmatic reactions, the effect of zileuton on the inflammatory response was examined in BAL fluid following segmental bronchoscopic antigen challenge in allergic patients and in patients with nocturnal asthma.

The effect of zileuton on inflammation produced by segmental allergen challenge, as assessed by eosinophils in BAL fluid, was evaluated in 10 subjects who were allergic to ragweed in a double-blind, placebo-controlled, crossover trial. The patients received zileuton 600 mg qid or placebo for 1 week and underwent bronchoscopy with BAL both before and 24 hours after an endobronchial allergen (ragweed) challenge. A statistically significant increase in eosinophils was found after antigen challenge ($0.6 \pm 0.2 \times 10^4$ eosinophils/ml increasing to $49.0 \pm 25.0 \times 10^4$) when subjects were treated with placebo, while the influx of eosinophils when subjects were treated with zileuton was not statistically different from baseline ($1.1 \pm 0.7 \times 10^4$ eosinophils/ml increasing to $16.5 \pm 4.1 \times 10^4$) (36). In addition, zileuton significantly reduced urinary LTE_4 concentrations by approximately 86% 4 hours after the challenge. Similar inhibition was noted in BAL fluid 24 hours after challenge; BAL LTE_4 levels following the zileuton treatment period were inhibited by 72% compared to placebo (37).

In a double-blind, randomized, placebo-controlled, crossover trial designed to examine airway inflammation in nocturnal asthma, Wenzel et al. (38) studied 12 asthmatic patients and 6 normal control subjects treated with zileuton 600 mg qid or placebo medication for 7 days. Airway inflammation was assessed by measuring eicosanoid levels and the numbers of cells obtained in BAL fluid. Pulmonary function testing and bronchoscopy (to measure cell counts and leukotriene and thromboxane levels in BAL fluid) were performed at 4:00 p.m. and 4:00 a.m. Urine was collected to measure urinary leukotriene levels. At 4:00 a.m. BAL LTB_4 and the cysteinyl leukotriene levels were increased and were significantly greater in asthmatic patients (13 ± 3 pg/ml and 36 ± 12 pg/ml, respectively) compared with those of normal control subjects (4 ± 1 pg/ml and 6 ± 2 pg/ml, respectively). Thromboxane levels were also higher at 4:00 a.m. in the asthmatic patients than in the normal controls ($p = 0.0019$). The increased LTB_4 levels were significantly correlated with the nocturnal fall in FEV_1 ($r = -0.66$, $p < 0.0001$). Urinary LTE_4 levels in the nocturnal asthmatics were also significantly higher than those observed in the control subjects ($p = 0.05$).

When patients were treated with zileuton, BAL fluid LTB_4 at 4:00 a.m. and nocturnal urinary LTE_4 concentrations were reduced from 13 ± 3 to 8 ± 2 pg/ml, $p = 0.01$, and 131 ± 25 to 32 ± 5 pg/mg creatinine, $p = 0.01$, respectively, with a trend toward an improvement in nocturnal FEV_1 (percent fall pla-

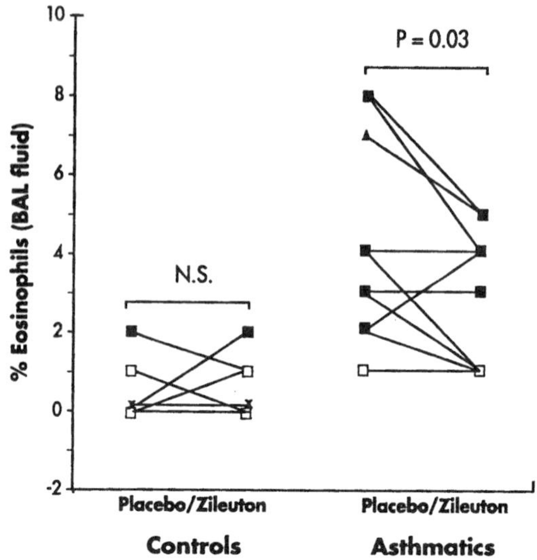

Figure 7 Eosinophil percentages in BAL fluid. Each line represents an individual patient. (From Ref. 38.)

cebo period: 27.9 ± 4.2%; zileuton period: 19.5 ± 4.0%; p = 0.086). These changes were associated with significant reductions in eosinophils in blood and BAL fluid at 4:00 a.m. compared to placebo ($p = 0.02$ and $p = 0.03$, respectively) (Fig. 7).

Results from this study demonstrate the importance of leukotrienes in both the inflammation and pathophysiology of nocturnal asthma. The results also indicate that by reducing the production of leukotrienes, zileuton attenuated the cellular influx into the airways. Taken together, the results of these two studies suggest that zileuton has antiinflammatory effects at both the mediator and cellular levels.

VI. Effects of Zileuton on Chronic Asthma

Results from a variety of clinical trials have demonstrated the efficacy of zileuton in the treatment of asthma.

A. Placebo-Controlled Trials

Three double-blind, randomized, placebo-controlled trials have been conducted to evaluate the efficacy of zileuton in the treatment of patients requiring daily inhaled β-agonists but not treated with inhaled corticosteroids. An early placebo-controlled, one-month trial demonstrated statistically significant improvements in patients with mild to moderate asthma treated with zileuton, either 600 mg qid or 800 mg bid, compared to placebo (39). After 4 weeks of zileuton therapy, both pulmonary function and subjective symptoms improved, with the greatest improvement in the 600 mg qid group. Rapid improvements in FEV_1 occurred, with a 14.6% increase within 1 hour of zileuton (600 mg) administration ($p <$ 0.001 versus placebo). Furthermore, patients treated with 600 mg qid demonstrated an increase in FEV_1 of 13.4% (0.32 L) after 4 weeks of treatment, compared to a 0.05 L increase in placebo-treated patients ($p = 0.02$ vs. placebo). Significant improvements also occurred in symptom scores (37% for zileuton 600 mg qid vs. 17% for placebo; $p = 0.02$). In addition, at the end of 1 month of therapy patients treated with zileuton decreased their β-agonist use by 24% compared to a 7% decrease in placebo-treated patients ($p = 0.03$). While improvements in subjective and objective parameters were observed with zileuton, 800 mg bid, these improvements were usually not significantly different from those seen with placebo medication. These clinical findings were supported by a significant decrease from baseline in mean urinary LTE_4 levels in patients receiving zileuton 800 mg bid (26%) or 600 mg qid (39%), which contrasted with a slight increase in LTE_4 levels in placebo patients ($p = 0.05$ and $p = 0.007$, respectively). The decrease in LTE_4 levels substantiated the inhibition of 5-lipoxygenase by zileuton.

This trial demonstrated that inhibition of 5-lipoxygenase with zileuton provided effective treatment of mild to moderate chronic asthma, showing improved airway function, decreased symptoms, and a reduction in bronchodilator use. These improvements were comparable to those observed following treatment with other therapeutic agents for asthma, including theophylline (61) and inhaled corticosteroids (62–64). In addition to the initial, acute bronchodilator effect, there was progressive improvement in airway function during the 4 weeks of treatment, which appears to occur via a mechanism that differs from β-agonist–induced relaxation of bronchial smooth muscle.

Subsequently, the results from two (one 3- and one 6-month) randomized, placebo-controlled trials in asthma patients treated with zileuton 400 or 600 mg qid or placebo confirmed these early findings (65,66). Approximately 750 patients at 34 and 36 centers in the United States entered the two trials combined. Entry criteria included an FEV_1 of 40–80% of the predicted normal value, reversible airway obstruction, and symptomatic asthma with treatment limited to daily inhaled β-agonist. The results of the two trials were similar, and observed improvements were maintained for at least 6 months. The results from 3 months of treatment for the two trials were combined for analysis, since the study designs were identical and no confounding factors precluded combination of the data. The remaining 3 months from the 6 month trial were not included in the analysis.

The combined data included approximately 255 patients per treatment arm.

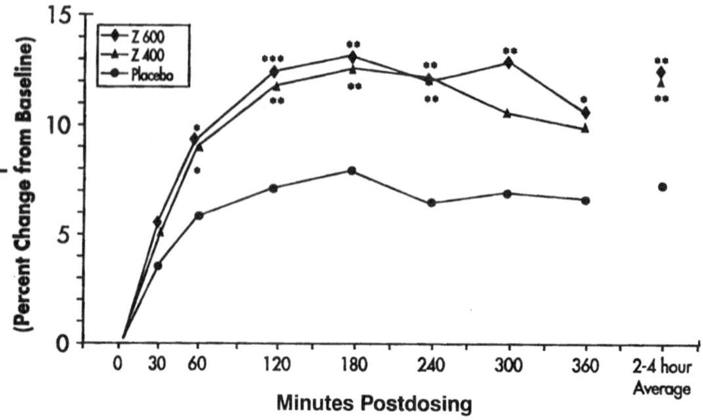

Figure 8 Mean percent change in FEV_1 from baseline over a 6-hour period following the initial dose of study medication. The 2- to 4-hour average represents the time period of peak plasma levels of zileuton. Solid diamonds represent zileuton, 600 mg qid; solid triangles represent zileuton, 400 mg qid; and solid circles represent placebo medication. $*p \leq 0.05$, $**p \leq 0.01$, and $***p \leq 0.001$; zileuton versus placebo.

Patients ranged in age from 18 to 62 years (mean 33 years) and were predominantly female (51–58%) and Caucasian (84–91%). Baseline FEV_1 was approximately 2.3 L, or 61% of the predicted normal value, and did not differ among the three treatment groups. Patients used approximately six puffs of β-agonist per day (67).

Patients showed a significant improvement in FEV_1 (9.3% increase, compared to 5.7% in the placebo group; $p \leq 0.05$) within 60 minutes of receiving the initial dose of zileuton (600 mg). A maximum increase in FEV_1 of 13.2% was observed 180 minutes postdosing (placebo = 7.9%; $p \leq 0.01$). The results are shown in Figure 8. Although this first dose-response was not as marked as that observed following β-agonist use, it is greater than that seen with other drugs with predominantly anti-inflammatory effects (62–64,66).

FEV_1 measurements were obtained prior to dosing on each visit day to evaluate chronic "trough" FEV_1 (prior to the morning dose; 8 hours post–previous evening's dose). Significant improvements in chronic FEV_1 (11.2%), observed within 8 days of initiating treatment ($p \leq 0.001$ vs. placebo), were maintained during 3 months of treatment with zileuton 600 mg qid (15.1% vs. 5.8% for placebo; $p \leq 0.001$;) (Fig. 9). Similar findings were sustained during 6 months of zileuton treatment in the 6-month trial (66,67).

Improvements in FEV_1 following zileuton treatment were most marked in patients who had the lowest percent predicted FEV_1 values at baseline. In fact,

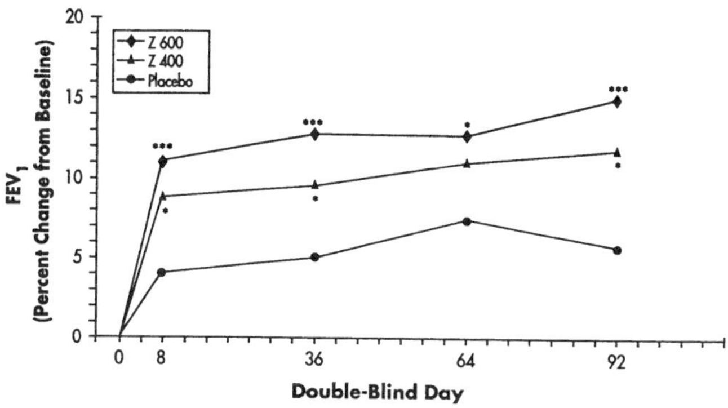

Figure 9 Mean percent change in FEV$_1$ from predrug baseline to predosing at each of 4 study days: 8, 36, 64, and 92. Solid diamonds represent zileuton, 600 mg qid; solid triangles represent zileuton, 400 mg qid; and solid circles represent placebo medication. $*p \leq 0.05$ and $***p \leq 0.001$; zileuton versus placebo.

patients with an FEV$_1$ of ≤50% of the predicted normal value demonstrated a 37% improvement in FEV$_1$ over 3 months of treatment ($p < 0.001$ vs. placebo; data on file, Abbott Laboratories).

In conjunction with the observed changes in FEV$_1$, patients treated with zileuton 600 mg qid had significant increases in their morning and evening peak expiratory flow rates (PEFR), which were evident within the first 2–22 days of treatment. They showed a 23 L/min increase in mean a.m. PEFR for the last month's interval (days 79–106) compared to a 6 L/min increase in the placebo group ($p \leq 0.001$) (Fig. 10); evening PEFR results were comparable. The results of the 6-month trial showed continued improvement in morning PEFR with an approximately 30 L/min improvement after 6 months ($p < 0.01$ vs. placebo) (66).

Zileuton treatment also resulted in a reduction in the need for concomitant therapy (β-agonist or systemic corticosteroid use for the treatment of an asthma exacerbation). Patients experienced a 26% reduction in the number of puffs of β-agonist per day after 3 months of treatment (combined data) with zileuton 600 mg qid ($p \leq 0.001$ vs. placebo) (67). β-Agonist use decreased significantly within the first 2–3 weeks of treatment, and this reduction was maintained throughout the 3-month treatment period (Fig. 11). Similar reductions were sustained during 6 months of treatment in the longer trial (66). Even with the reduction in β-agonist use, patients treated with zileuton 600 mg qid required fewer corticosteroid rescue treatments (6.6%) for an acute asthma exacerbation than did those treated with placebo medication (17.1%; $p \leq 0.001$) (67). The results for the 3-month treatment period represent a 61% reduction in the number of patients who required

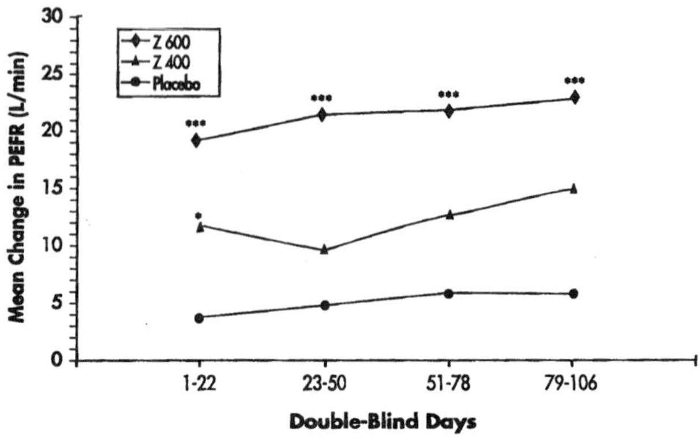

Figure 10 Mean change from predrug baseline (average of approximately 10 days) in morning peak expiratory flow rates. Daily rates were averaged over the intervals shown. Solid diamonds represent zileuton, 600 mg qid; solid triangles represent zileuton, 400 mg qid; and solid circles represent placebo medication. $*p \leq 0.05$ and $***p \leq 0.001$; zileuton versus placebo.

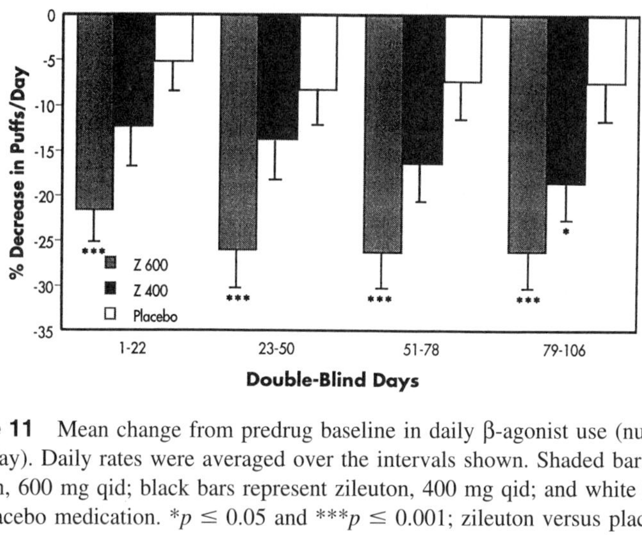

Figure 11 Mean change from predrug baseline in daily β-agonist use (number of puffs/day). Daily rates were averaged over the intervals shown. Shaded bars represent zileuton, 600 mg qid; black bars represent zileuton, 400 mg qid; and white bars represent placebo medication. $*p \leq 0.05$ and $***p \leq 0.001$; zileuton versus placebo.

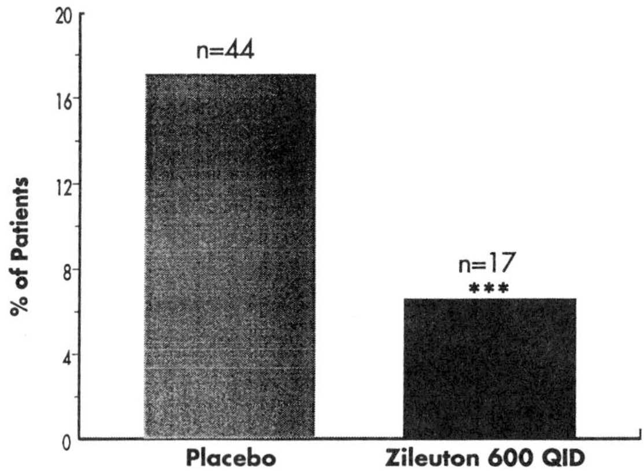

Figure 12 Percentage of patients receiving systemic corticosteroid rescue treatment for an acute exacerbation. Numbers (n) shown at top of bars are numbers of patients experiencing such exacerbations. ***$p \leq 0.001$; zileuton versus placebo.

corticosteroid rescue following zileuton treatment compared to placebo (Fig. 12). Similar results were observed in the 6-month trial (66). This ''steroid-sparing effect'' was most evident in those patients with more severe airway obstruction ($FEV_1 \leq 50\%$ of predicted). In those patients, the relative risk of an asthma exacerbation that required systemic corticosteroid treatment was approximately sixfold greater in the placebo group (36%) than in the 600 mg qid zileuton group (6%; $p \leq 0.001$). Reducing the need for corticosteroid rescues is beneficial because it suggests a decreased frequency and severity of exacerbations during chronic treatment with zileuton.

In addition to improvements in objectively measured pulmonary function, patients reported rapid and sustained improvements in their daytime and nighttime symptoms, which translated into improvements in their overall quality of life after treatment with zileuton, compared to placebo treatment. Patients recorded the severity of their symptoms every morning and evening using a graded scale (0–3); data were analyzed at 3- to 4-week intervals. Significant improvements (decreases in the score of approximately 20%) were observed in both daytime and nighttime symptoms during the first interval (days 1–22; $p \leq 0.001$ and $p \leq 0.01$, respectively, vs. placebo), and patients continued to improve throughout the study. After 3 months, patients experienced a 33% and a 30% improvement (decrease) in daytime and nighttime symptoms (Fig. 13), respectively ($p \leq 0.001$ and $p \leq 0.01$, respectively, vs. placebo). These improvements were sustained during the 6-month trial (66).

Patients also evaluated their quality of life in the 3-month trial using a

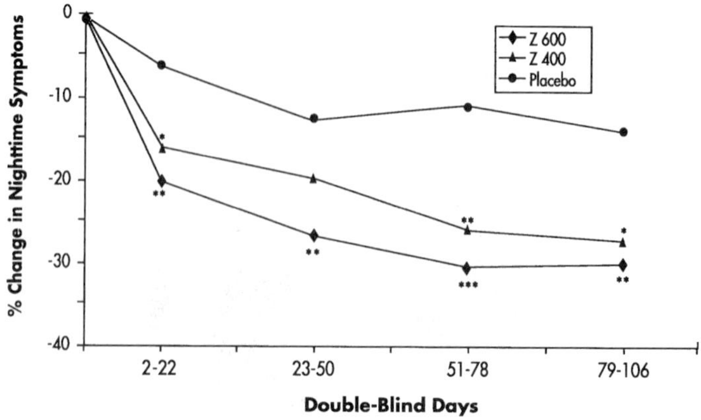

Figure 13 Mean percent change from prestudy baseline (approximately 10 days) in nighttime symptom scores. Scores were averaged over the intervals shown. Solid diamonds represent zileuton, 600 mg qid; solid triangles represent zileuton, 400 mg qid; and solid circles represent placebo medication. $*p \leq 0.05$, $**p \leq 0.01$, and $***p \leq 0.001$; zileuton versus placebo.

validated Asthma Quality-of-Life Questionnaire (68). The questionnaire used a seven-point scale to examine four domains of the patient's disease (symptoms, activities, emotions, and environment); these values were also combined to provide an overall score. A minimal important difference (MID) in this validated instrument is defined as a 0.5 point change: ''the smallest difference in score . . . which patients would perceive as beneficial and which would mandate, in the absence of troublesome side effects and excessive cost, a change in the patient's management'' (69). Patients treated with zileuton, 600 mg qid, reported improvements that exceeded the MID in both their overall quality of life (0.78) and in all four domains (range 0.65–0.89). Differences from placebo were significant for all five measures. In contrast, none of the scores observed in the placebo group reached the level of the MID (range 0.28–0.49).

While improvements were observed in some variables with zileuton, 400 mg qid, the results were not consistent. The results of the placebo-controlled trials demonstrated that zileuton 600 mg qid was the only dosing regimen consistently significantly superior to placebo in improving subjective and objective measures of response. The results of the trials indicated a dose-response relationship between the two regimens and demonstrated that zileuton 600 mg qid was the optimum regimen.

B. Comparison of Zileuton and Theophylline Treatments

A large proportion of patients are still treated with theophylline, although its use has been declining. A study was conducted to evaluate the efficacy and safety of zileuton as a possible alternative therapy to theophylline. Zileuton 600 and 400 mg qid was compared to a titrated dose of long-acting theophylline (SLO-BID®) in a 3-month, multicenter, randomized, double-blind, parallel trial (61,70). An initial, open phase (2–71 days), during which theophylline was titrated to therapeutic levels (8–15 μg/ml), was followed by a 4-day washout and a one-week placebo lead-in period. The subsequent double-blind treatment period lasted 3 months (13 weeks). As in the placebo-controlled trials, entry criteria included symptomatic asthma patients with an FEV_1 of 40–80% of the predicted normal value and 15% reversibility of FEV_1 in response to inhaled β-agonists.

Asthma treatment was restricted to inhaled β-agonists, which patients used on a daily basis. Approximately 125 patients were enrolled in each of the three treatment arms. Among the treatment groups, patients were similar in age (approximately 35 years), were slightly predominantly female (56–61%), and predominantly Caucasian (85–91%) (61). Since zileuton 600 mg qid has been established as the effective dose, results from the 400 mg qid regimen will not be discussed here.

Significant improvements in FEV_1 were found within 30 minutes after the first dose of both zileuton 600 mg and theophylline (approximately 10%). This improvement continued, and by 120 minutes FEV_1 values improved over baseline by 18% in the zileuton and 17% in the theophylline group (NS) and were sustained over a 6-hour observation period (61,70). In addition, improvements in FEV_1 following treatment with both zileuton 600 mg qid and theophylline continued throughout this 3-month study. Between 30 and 360 minutes following the morning dose of study drug on day 36, improvements in FEV_1 for both dose groups ranged between 18 and 24% (61).

Comparisons of maximum percent changes from baseline in FEV_1 between 0 and 6 hours postdosing, when levels were optimum for both drugs, showed no significant difference in FEV_1 between the zileuton 600 mg qid group and the theophylline group on either day 36 or 92; both showed an approximate 30% improvement (Fig. 14) (61).

As in the placebo-controlled trials, patients also recorded subjective improvement in their symptoms. By the end of the 3-month trial, β-agonist use was reduced by 26–30% and daily and nocturnal symptom scores had decreased (improved) by 28–41% in both the zileuton 600 mg qid and theophylline groups. No significant differences were noted between the two treatment groups (61). In addition, no significant difference in corticosteroid rescue was noted between zileuton 600 mg qid (10.4%) and theophylline (14.5%) (70).

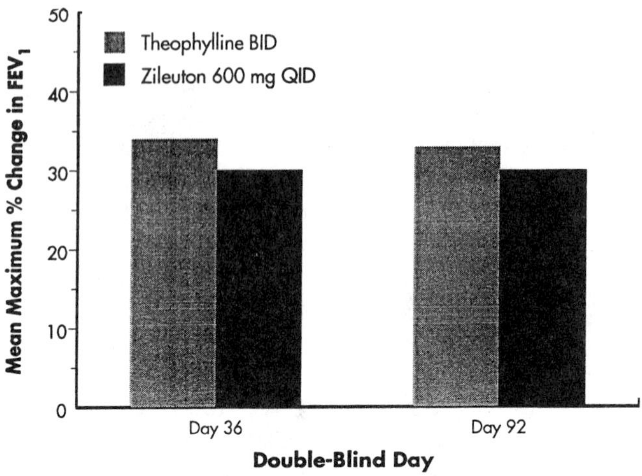

Figure 14 Mean percent change from predrug baseline in 0- to 6-hour maximum FEV_1 on days 36 and 92. Black bars represent zileuton 600 mg qid–treated patients, and shaded bars represent those treated with theophylline. Copyright 1998, American Medical Association. (From Ref. 61.)

The results of this comparative study indicate that zileuton is as effective as theophylline in the management of patients with moderate asthma. In addition, the response of patients to zileuton for both objective and subjective measures was comparable to that observed in the 3- and 6-month trials described above.

C. Zileuton as Adjunctive Therapy to Low Doses of Inhaled Beclomethasone

A clinical trial was designed to evaluate the additive benefit of zileuton to a low dose of inhaled beclomethasone compared to the added benefit of doubling the dose of beclomethasone (71). Entry criteria were similar to those described for the placebo-controlled trials (65,66). However, patients could have been treated with low doses of inhaled corticosteroids (≤300 μg bid) prior to the lead-in phase.

This randomized, double-blind, multicenter trial included a 2-week, single-blind, lead-in phase during which patients already treated with inhaled corticosteroids received a fixed dose of 200 μg bid inhaled beclomethasone. This was followed by a 13-week (3-month) double-blind phase during which patients were treated with zileuton 400 or 600 mg qid added to 200 μg bid beclomethasone (400 μg daily), or a doubling dose of 400 μg bid (800 μg daily) beclomethasone. To qualify for the double-blind randomized period, patients had to have an FEV_1 of ≤80% of the predicted normal value while on a fixed low dose of inhaled beclomethasone. A total of 320 patients were studied, approximately 105 in each of the three treatment arms. Mean baseline FEV_1 values obtained after 2 weeks of treatment with 200 μg bid beclomethasone, but prior to randomization, ranged from 62 to 64% of the predicted normal value among treatment groups. Patients in the study were mildly symptomatic and used an average of three puffs of β-agonist per day. They were predominantly male (51–66%), and most were Caucasian (92–99%). Since 600 mg qid has been shown to be the effective dose of zileuton, results from the 400 mg qid plus 400 μg daily beclomethasone regimen will not be discussed here.

FEV_1 measurements were performed following the first daily dose of study medications at each visit. By day 15 significant improvements over the pretreatment baseline were observed for all three treatment groups with no significant differences among the groups. The improvements were maintained over the 3 months of the trial. Maximum mean changes in FEV_1 in patients treated with zileuton 600 mg qid plus 400 μg daily beclomethasone (10.25%) were comparable to those observed in the patients treated with the higher dose of beclomethasone, 800 μg/day (10.89%) (71).

There were significant improvements from baseline in morning PEFR, and, in general, the improvements did not differ between treatment groups. However, during study days 30–57 there was significantly greater improvement in the mean percent change in morning PEFR in the zileuton 600 mg qid plus beclomethasone group compared to the beclomethasone group (21.5 L/min vs. 7.8 L/min, respectively, and 8.4 vs. 2.4%, respectively, $p \leq 0.05$) (71). The results for evening PEFR were comparable to those observed for morning PEFR.

In addition to these objective findings, patients in both groups noted significant changes in subjective parameters, improvements in daily and nocturnal symptom scores, and reductions in both acute asthma exacerbations and β-agonist use, all of which were similar among treatment groups. Daily symptoms improved (decreased) by approximately 30%, and daily β-agonist use was reduced by about 15% in both groups over the 3 months of double-blind treatment (71).

The results of this study provide evidence that the concomitant administration of 600 mg qid zileuton with low doses of inhaled beclomethasone is an alternative to higher doses of inhaled corticosteroids. Asthma control was demonstrated in the study by improved pulmonary function, improved (decreased) symptoms, reductions in β-agonist use, and similar rates of prevention of asthma exacerbations in both treatment groups.

D. Zileuton as Adjunctive Therapy to Usual Asthma Care—Long-Term Surveillance Trial

This one-year, randomized, open trial evaluated the safety of zileuton 600 mg qid plus usual asthma care (UC) compared to usual asthma care alone (72). While the trial was designed to characterize changes in ALT abnormalities (to be discussed), selected clinical outcomes were also measured including the percentage of patients who had an acute asthma exacerbation and those who required steroid rescue, an emergency room (ER) visit, or hospitalization (72). For the purposes of this trial, a determination of acute exacerbation was made by the investigator if the patient presented (or contacted the investigator) with worsened asthma symptoms which required significant additional and/or alternate therapy and/or an emergency room visit and/or hospitalization.

A total of 2458 patients received zileuton 600 mg qid plus their UC, while 489 received their UC alone. Approximately 1400 patients on zileuton plus UC remained in the trial after one year. Concomitant medications used by both groups during the trial included β-agonist (95%), inhaled corticosteroids (56%), theophylline (30%), and cromolyn (11%). Unlike the placebo-controlled studies, patients in this study had more severe asthma since they required a variety of additional asthma medications not permitted during the placebo-controlled trials. Despite the additional medications, both groups demonstrated a baseline mean percent predicted FEV_1 of about 64% prior to study onset (72), values similar to those observed in prior placebo-controlled trials (65,66).

The percentage of patients who had an acute asthma exacerbation when treated with zileuton compared to UC did not differ (45.1 vs. 49.4%, respectively). However, significantly fewer zileuton-treated patients compared to UC patients required at least one systemic corticosteroid rescue for an acute exacerbation (23.0 vs. 30.3%, respectively; $p < 0.001$) or an ER visit (7.7% for zileuton vs. 11.5% for UC; $p < 0.05$) during the study. In addition, there were fewer hospitalizations in patients treated with zileuton plus usual care compared to those treated with usual care alone (3.2% for zileuton vs. 4.1% for UC; $p > 0.10$). The lack of change in the rate of asthma exacerbations is consistent with the mechanisms for triggering an exacerbation, i.e., acute viral infections or exposure to allergens, which would not be affected by a 5-lipoxygenase inhibitor. However, the more serious sequelae of an exacerbation, such as corticosteroid rescue or emergency room visits, often result from a marked inflammatory response. This response may be more dependent upon the presence of leukotrienes, which are inhibited by zileuton, than are the initial symptoms of an exacerbation following exposure to a virus or allergen.

A reduction in costly ER visits and hospitalizations may have a profound impact on the cost of treating asthma in the future.

E. Reduction in Dosage Regimen of Zileuton

This study evaluated the effect of a reduction in the dose and/or frequency of dosing on asthma control following initial treatment with zileuton 600 mg qid. The rationale for this study was based on an hypothesized reduction in the patient's chronic inflammation following initial treatment with more frequent administration of zileuton. This would allow patients to lower their doses after achieving better asthma control and to maintain improved control with maintenance doses of zileuton. Similar reductions in dose have been used with other anti-inflammatory asthma drugs, such as nedocromil sodium (73) and triamcinolone acetonide (74).

This randomized, double-blind, multicenter study was designed to explore dose reduction for patients using zileuton. Patients were treated with zileuton 600 mg qid during an 8-week, open label phase, followed by an 8-week double-blind phase during which patients received a reduced dose/frequency of zileuton, either 600 ($N = 72$) or 800 mg ($N = 67$) tid. Subsequently, during an additional 8-week double-blind phase, the zileuton dose/frequency was further reduced to either 600 ($N = 53$) or 800 mg ($N = 60$) bid (75,76). Patients had to demonstrate an improvement of at least 10% from baseline in FEV_1 at the end of both months 1 and 2 of qid treatment in order to qualify for entry into the tid phase of the trial. Entry criteria also stipulated that patients used only β-agonist to treat their asthma.

A total of 278 patients were enrolled in the initial phase of the trial; of those, 139 met the required criterion for improvement in FEV_1 during the qid phase and entered the tid period. One hundred and five patients completed both the tid and bid periods (75,76).

Study results showed a mean percent increase from prestudy baseline in FEV_1 of approximately 37% (0.72 L) among the patients who qualified based on their FEV_1 response at months 1 and 2 of the qid phase and entered the tid period (76). After 8 weeks of treatment with zileuton 600 or 800 mg tid, patients experienced a slight decrease in FEV_1, compared to the final qid baseline value (5.1%; $p \leq 0.01$, and 0.21%, NS, respectively) (Fig. 15). Similarly, during bid treatment with zileuton (600 or 800 mg) patients experienced decreases in FEV_1 of 4.75% ($p \leq 0.05$) and 8.53% ($p \leq 0.001$) (Fig. 15), respectively, compared to the final value from the qid period (76). These reductions during the tid and bid periods were not considered clinically meaningful, because improvements from the prestudy FEV_1 values to those obtained at the end of the qid, tid, and bid periods still ranged from 25 to 39% (76).

Several outcome variables were not measured at baseline. Therefore, instead of measuring overall improvement, changes from the improvements found at the end of the qid dosing period were compared with findings from the tid and bid periods. Therefore, the lack of a significant change shows that patients did not deteriorate when their zileuton dose was changed from qid to tid and finally to bid. For example, PEFR and daytime and nighttime symptoms did not change significantly from the end of qid to the end of tid and bid dosing. Daily β-agonist usage continued to decrease during the tid period ($p < 0.05$ for 600 mg tid) and increased only slightly during the bid period (NS) (Fig. 16) (76). In addition, the reduction in dosage did not lead to an increase in acute asthma

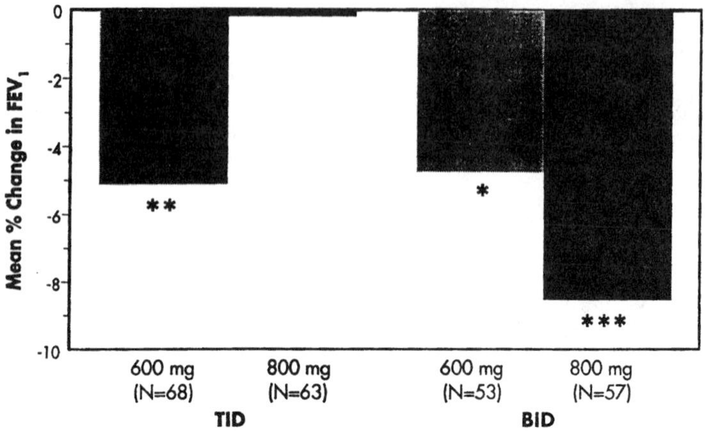

Figure 15 Mean percent change in FEV_1 from the end of the qid period to the end of each reduced dosing period: tid and bid. Shaded bars represent 600 mg, black bars represent 800 mg. $*p \leq 0.05$, $**p \leq 0.01$, and $***p \leq 0.001$ compared to baseline values.

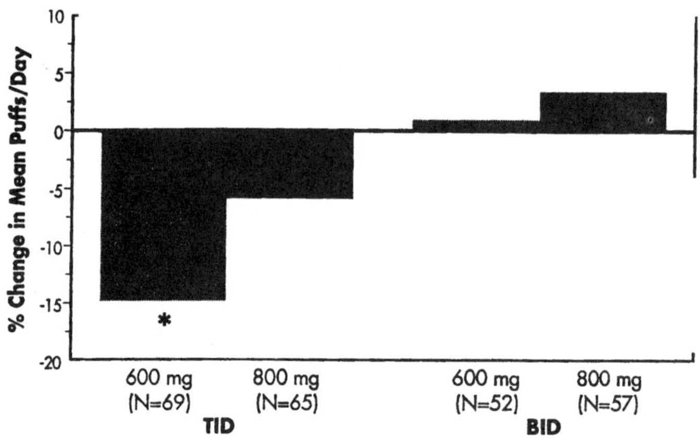

Figure 16 Percent change in β-agonist use from the end of the qid period to the end of each reduced dosing period: tid and bid. The average of the daily values for the last 4 weeks of qid treatment was used as the baseline. Shaded bars represent 600 mg, black bars represent 800 mg. $*p \leq 0.05$ compared to baseline values. (From Ref. 76.)

exacerbations or systemic corticosteroid rescue treatments during the tid and bid periods.

Therefore, patients who demonstrate improved pulmonary function following treatment with zileuton 600 mg qid may be able to maintain a comparable level of improved lung function, symptom control, reduced β-agonist use, and fewer systemic corticosteroid rescue treatments on a lower dose and/or frequency of zileuton administration.

F. Summary of Studies in Chronic Asthma

Zileuton improved airway function and asthma symptoms and reduced the need for concomitant medication in patients with asthma in a variety of multicenter, parallel clinical trials. In an additional study, zileuton was as effective as theophylline in the management of patients with asthma. Another clinical trial demonstrated that the addition of zileuton to low-dose inhaled beclomethasone produced efficacy comparable to a higher dose of beclomethasone. In another study, patients who demonstrated improvements in pulmonary function following treatment with zileuton 600 mg qid maintained comparable asthma control with reduced dosage and frequency of zileuton treatment using a tid or bid regimen. Most importantly, a large one-year surveillance trial provided evidence that the combination of zileuton to a patient's usual asthma care resulted in significant reductions in the need for systemic corticosteroid rescue for an acute exacerbation and in emergency room visits. These reductions could lead to marked decreases in health care costs for asthma in the future.

VII. Safety

A. Tolerability

More than 5000 patients have been exposed to zileuton in clinical trials—more than 2000 for longer than 6 months and almost 1000 for 1 year or more. Generally, zileuton is well tolerated at its recommended dosage of 600 mg qid. There was no evidence of a dose relationship for the incidence of adverse events. Most adverse events were reported in similar frequency between zileuton groups and the control groups. In placebo-controlled trials, the most common adverse events were headache and infection (Table 1) (39,65,66). The only adverse event for which the incidence differed significantly between zileuton and placebo patients was dyspepsia, observed in 8.2% of zileuton-treated patients versus 2.9% of placebo patients (77). In most patients, adverse events were mild to moderate in severity, and very few resulted in premature termination from studies. The overall rate of premature termination due to an adverse event was similar between zileuton (9.7%) and placebo-treated (8.4%) groups. In general, the onset of most adverse events occurred during the first 2 weeks of dosing and frequently resolved

Table 1 Incidence (>3%) of Adverse Events in Placebo-Controlled Asthma Studies

Body system/event	Zileuton 600 mg qid (n = 475) %	Placebo (n = 491) %
Body as a whole		
Headache	24.6	24.0
Infection	21.1	21.6
Pain	7.8	5.3
Abdominal pain	4.6	2.4
Asthenia	3.8	2.4
Accidental injury	3.4	2.0
Digestive system		
Dyspepsia	8.2[a]	2.9
Nausea	5.5	3.7
Musculoskeletal		
Myalgia	3.2	2.9

[a] $p < 0.05$ vs. placebo.
Source: Ref. 78.

upon continued dosing. Overall, the safety profile was not related to the patients' age, race, or gender. No clinically significant changes in vital sign parameters, physical examination observations, or ECG findings were observed.

Except for liver function tests, clinical laboratory results revealed no relevant adverse changes in renal and electrolyte, metabolic, nutritional, endocrine, or hematology parameters. The only clinically significant trend in hematology parameters was a greater reduction in eosinophils in zileuton patients compared to placebo (66). This observation may reflect changes in the underlying disease of asthma following treatment-induced anti-inflammatory effects of zileuton.

Zileuton caused elevations in one or more liver function tests in a small percentage of patients. The ALT (SGPT) test is considered the most sensitive indicator of liver injury. In placebo-controlled trials, the frequency of ALT elevations greater than or equal to three times the upper limit of normal (3 × ULN) was 1.9% for zileuton-treated patients compared to 0.2% for placebo-treated patients (77). In a long-term surveillance trial (described above) designed primarily to characterize liver test abnormalities, 2458 patients received zileuton in addition to their usual asthma care (UC) and 489 patients received their UC. In patients treated for up to 12 months with zileuton in addition to their UC, 4.6% developed an ALT of at least 3 × ULN, compared with 1.1% of patients who received only UC (72). Typically, patients developed their liver test abnormalities within the first 3 months. The monthly risk of an elevation of ALT of 3 × ULN in the zileuton group was 2.05% for the first month, decreasing to 1.29% for the second month and to 0.35% for the third month. After the third month there was no significant difference between the risk of an elevation of ALT of 3 × ULN on zileuton (0.19–0.49%) and that on UC only (0.18–0.25%). The magnitude of elevation was independent of the duration of zileuton exposure. The pattern of liver abnormalities is predominantly hepatocellular with no associated elevation of alkaline phosphatase or bilirubin and is usually asymptomatic. In subset analyses, females over the age of 65 appeared to be at an increased risk for ALT elevations. Spontaneous resolution of the elevations was observed in 52% of patients who had an ALT elevation between 3 × ULN and 5 × ULN and still continued to receive zileuton. All other cases of ALT elevations resolved within a mean time of 4 weeks upon cessation of therapy (77). It is recommended that ALT be monitored before initiation of zileuton therapy once a month for the first 3 months, every 2 to 3 months for the remainder of the first year, and periodically thereafter. Zileuton should be discontinued if any signs and/or symptoms of liver dysfunction (e.g., nausea, fatigue, lethargy, pruritis, jaundice, and "flulike" symptoms) or ALT elevations greater than five times the ULN occur (77). It should be noted, however, that the majority of patients are asymptomatic and do not present with the usual signs and symptoms of liver dysfunction.

Overall, more than 5000 patients have been treated with zileuton in clinical trials. Only one patient developed symptomatic hepatitis with jaundice, which totally resolved upon discontinuation of therapy. No deaths have been associated with liver injury. The profile of liver test abnormalities observed to date strongly support a mechanism of liver injury related to a metabolic idiosyncrasy similar to that reported with other compounds such as nonsteroidal anti-inflammatory agents (78–80) and cholesterol-lowering agents in the HMG CoA reductase inhibitor class (81). No systemic features of rash, fever, and severe eosinophilia expected with an immune response have been reported.

B. Drug Interactions

Zileuton is primarily eliminated in humans by metabolism to zileuton glucuronides (approximately 80–90% of the dose), (20,21,25). However, in vitro studies utilizing human liver microsomes have shown that zileuton can also be oxidatively metabolized by the cytochrome P450 isoenzymes CYP1A2, CYP3A, and CYP2C9 (26). Several drug-drug interaction studies were conducted with zileuton. These results suggest that the primary mechanism for interaction between zileuton and other drugs is through inhibition of the CYP1A2 isoenzyme by zileuton.

Co-administration of zileuton and theophylline resulted in an approximate doubling of theophylline AUC, an increase in theophylline C_{max} (by 73%), and an increase in theophylline half-life (by 24%) (82). Theophylline is primarily metabolized in humans by the CYP1A2 isoenzyme (83). Thus, the theophylline dose should be reduced by approximately one half and plasma theophylline concentrations monitored when theophylline is co-administered with zileuton. To date, this recommended reduction in theophylline dosage when co-administered with zileuton has been used successfully in hundreds of patients.

Concomitant administration of zileuton and warfarin resulted in a 15% decrease in R-warfarin clearance and an increase in AUC of 22% (84). The pharmacokinetics of S-warfarin were not affected. R-warfarin is metabolized primarily by CYP1A2, and S-warfarin is metabolized mainly CYP2C9 (85). Monitoring of prothrombin time, or other suitable coagulation tests, with the appropriate dose titration of warfarin is recommended in patients receiving concomitant zileuton and warfarin therapy.

Co-administration of zileuton and propranolol results in an increase in propranolol C_{max}, AUC, and elimination half-life by 52, 104, and 25%, respectively (Abbott Laboratories, data on file). Propranolol is primarily metabolized in humans by the CYP1A2 and CYP2D6 isoenzymes (86). However, even though propranolol and other β-blockers are contraindicated in bronchial asthma, patients on zileuton and propranolol should be closely monitored and the dose of propranolol reduced as necessary.

Co-administration of terfenadine and zileuton resulted in a statistically significant increase in mean AUC and C_{max} of terfenadine of approximately 35% (87). This increase in terfenadine plasma concentration in the presence of zileuton was not associated with a significant prolongation of the QTc interval. There was also no change in morphology of the TU complex. Terfenadine is primarily metabolized in humans by the CYP3A isoenzyme, but other isozymes may also make some contribution to the metabolism of terfenadine (88). Of the other isozymes, 1A2 had the highest correlation with the rate of terfenadine metabolism in human liver microsomes (88). The effect of zileuton on terfenadine pharmacokinetics appears to be different and much smaller than that of ketoconazole, erythromycin, or even grapefruit juice (87). Nevertheless, given the high interindividual pharmacokinetic variability of terfenadine, co-administration of zileuton and terfenadine is not recommended.

Drug-drug interaction studies between zileuton and prednisone (89) and ethinyl estradiol (oral contraceptive, Abbott Laboratories, data on file), drugs known to be metabolized by the P450 3A4 (CYP 3A4) isoenzyme, have shown no significant interaction. Other drug-drug interaction studies showed no significant interaction between zileuton and digoxin (90), phenytoin (91), sulfasalazine (92), or naproxen (93).

In the large surveillance study, patients were allowed to continue other asthma medications (inhaled steroids, nedocromil, reduced dose of theophylline), as well as other types of drugs (antihypertensives, oral contraceptives, lipid-lowering agents) on a case-by-case basis. Despite the variety of concomitant medications allowed in this trial, the safety profile of this study did not differ from that of the placebo-controlled trials.

VIII. Discussion of Treatment of Asthma with Zileuton

Zileuton, a member of a new class of drugs, presents a novel therapeutic option for the effective treatment of patients with bronchial asthma. Clinical efficacy has been demonstrated in patients requiring daily β-agonists. In those patients, zileuton significantly improved pulmonary function (peak flows and spirometry), reduced daily and nocturnal symptoms, and still decreased β-agonist usage (65,66). Most of these improvements occurred within the first 2–4 weeks after the initiation of therapy and were sustained throughout treatment. Furthermore, the reduced need for steroid rescue for asthma exacerbation represents a significant benefit to the patient, indicative of a better control of their asthma. Current management guidelines suggest that reductions in such episodes are a major goal of asthma therapy (94).

Zileuton has also produced clinical benefit when used as adjunctive therapy to low-dose inhaled corticosteroids (400 μg beclomethasone) (71). Results have demonstrated that zileuton 600 mg qid added to low-dose inhaled corticosteroid improved both objective and subjective parameters. The magnitude of improvement was similar to doubling of the inhaled corticosteroid dose (800 μg beclomethasone) (71). The clinical benefit of zileuton as adjunctive therapy was also demonstrated in aspirin-sensitive patients treated with high doses of inhaled steroids and/or oral steroids. In those patients, the addition of zileuton to their usual asthma care resulted in further improvements in pulmonary function, a reduction in reactivity to histamine (60), and a marked return of the sense of smell. The clinical benefit of zileuton for improved asthma control is also demonstrated by the results of the long-term surveillance trial. In patients already treated with inhaled corticosteroids (60%) and/or theophylline (35%), the addition of zileuton to patients' usual asthma care resulted in a decrease in ER visits and hospitalizations when compared to UC alone (72). Reductions in ER visits and hospitalizations may have a profound impact on the cost of treating asthma, since these events represent a significant expenditure of health care resources.

Zileuton exerts its effect by inhibiting the synthesis of leukotrienes. Wenzel et al. (38) and Kane et al. (36,37) demonstrated that zileuton can reduce the numbers of inflammatory cells in BAL fluid, suggesting that it possesses anti-inflammatory properties. The results of studies of commonly used provocative stimuli such as aspirin (35), cold air (34), and exercise (45) suggest that zileuton, in addition to its benefits in the treatment of chronic asthma, may prevent bronchoconstriction induced by various stimuli.

Zileuton was well tolerated by patients in clinical trials. The most clinically important risk identified with zileuton is potential elevated liver tests in a small percentage of patients. Overall, the rate of ALT elevations among 5000 treated patients was 3.2%. However, elevations usually developed within the first 2–3 months and either resolved spontaneously while patients continue receiving zileuton or upon discontinuation of the drug. To minimize the risk of severe liver abnormalities and to ensure safe usage of zileuton until more extensive data are available, ALT levels should be measured once per month for the first 3 months, every 2–3 months for the remainder of the first year, and periodically thereafter.

Zileuton is also known to inhibit the metabolism of certain drugs metabolized by cytochrome P450 isozymes, but the clinical relevance of these drug interactions was mostly apparent with theophylline (82). Therefore, the theophylline dose should be reduced by half when both drugs are required and plasma theophylline levels monitored. In the surveillance trial, 772 patients received a reduced dose of theophylline in addition to zileuton, were monitored, and did not have any significant adverse events due to the combination of the drugs.

Since zileuton has a relatively rapid onset of efficacy, patients only need to remain on therapy for 2–4 weeks before the physician can determine whether or not the drug has a beneficial effect. Thus, patients who do not benefit from zileuton should only receive the drug for a short time and will incur little risk of elevated liver enzymes. For patients who show clear benefit and continue zileuton therapy, the risk can be minimized by liver test monitoring.

Once asthma control is achieved using zileuton 600 mg qid, clinical benefit may be maintained with a reduced dose or frequency of administration (76). Patients who demonstrated improved pulmonary function with zileuton 600 mg qid maintained a comparable level of lung function, symptom control, and reduced concomitant asthma treatment when they received a lower dose and/or frequency of zileuton. Similar reductions in dose subsequent to establishing asthma control have been used successfully with other asthma drugs with anti-inflammatory mechanisms.

In conclusion, zileuton is the first 5-lipoxygenase pathway inhibitor to prove effective in the treatment of asthma. Furthermore, zileuton is well tolerated with monitoring of liver function. When added to low doses of inhaled corticosteroids, zileuton can prevent the need for an increased steroid dose. Most importantly, zileuton reduced the need for corticosteroid rescue, emergency room visits, and/or hospitalizations following acute asthma exacerbations.

References

1. Samuelsson B. Leukotrienes: mediators of immediate hypersensitivity reactions and inflammation. Science 1983; 220:568–575.

2. Bel EH, Vander Veen H, Kramps JA, Dijkman JH, Sterk PJ. Maximal airway narrowing to inhaled leukotriene D_4 in normal subjects. Am Rev Respir Dis 1987; 136: 979–984.
3. Drazen JM, Austen KF. Leukotrienes and airway responses. Am Rev Respir Dis 1987; 136:985–998.
4. Henderson WR Jr. Role of leukotrienes in asthma. Ann Allergy 1994; 72:272–278.
5. Piper PJ, Conroy DM, Costello JF, Evans JM, Green CP, Price JF, Sampson AP, Spencer DA. Leukotrienes and inflammatory lung disease. Ann NY Acad Sci 1991; 629:112–119.
6. Taylor GW, Taylor I, Black P, Maltby NH, Turner N, Fuller RW, Dollery CT. Urinary leukotriene E_4 after antigen challenge and in acute asthma and allergic rhinitis. Lancet 1989; 8638:584–588.
7. Wenzel SE. Asthma as an inflammatory disease. Ann Allergy 1994; 72:261–271.
8. Samuelsson B, Hammarstrom S, Murphy RC, Borgeat P. Leukotrienes and slow reacting substance of anaphylaxis (SRS-A). Allergy 1980; 35(5):375–381.
9. Murphy RC, Hammarstrom S, Samuelsson B. Leukotriene C: a slow-reacting substance from murine mastocytoma cells. Proc Natl Acad Sci 1979; 76(9):4275–4279.
10. Lewis RA, Austen KF, Soberman RJ. Leukotrienes and other products of the 5-lipoxygenase pathway. Biochemistry and relation to pathobiology in human diseases. N Engl J Med 1990; 323:645–655.
11. Brooks CD, Carter GW. The discovery of zileuton (Leutrol). In: Merluzzi VJ, Adams J, eds. The Search for Anti-inflammatory Drugs. Boston: Birkhauser, 1996: 130–160.
12. Carter GW, Young PR, Albert DH, Bouska J, Dyer R, Bell RL, Summers JB, Brooks DW. 5-Lipoxygenase inhibitory activity of zileuton. J Pharmacol Exp Ther 1991; 256:929–937.
13. Bell RL, Young PR, Albert D, Lanni C, Summers JB, Brooks DW, Rubin P, Carter GW. The discovery and development of zileuton: an orally active 5-lipoxygenase inhibitor. Int J Immunopharmacol 1992; 14:505–510.
14. Malo P, Bell R, Shaughnessy T, Summers J, Brooks D, Carter G. The 5-lipoxygenase inhibitory activity of zileuton in in vitro and in vivo models of antigen-induced airway anaphylaxis. Pulmonary Pharmacol 1994; 7:73–79.
15. Abraham WM, Ahmed A, Cortes A, Sielczak MW, Hinz W, Bouska J, Lanni C, Bell RL. The 5-lipoxygenase inhibitor zileuton blocks antigen-induced late airway responses, inflammation and airway hyperresponsiveness in allergic sheep. Eur J Pharmacol 1992; 217:119–126.
16. Scuri M, Allegra L, Abraham ML. The effect of multiple dosing with zileuton on early and late bronchial responses to inhaled allergen in sheep. Eur Respir J 1995; 8(suppl 19):432S.
17. Bell RL, Harris RR, Malo PE, Bouska JB, Shaughnessy TK, Hulkower KI, Brooks CDW, Carter GW. ABT-761 attenuates bronchoconstriction and pulmonary inflammation in rodents. J Pharm Exp Ther 1997; 280:1366–1373.
18. Namovic MT, Walsh RE, Goodfellow C, Harris RR, Carter GW, Bell RL. Pharmacological modulation of eosinophil influx into the lungs of Brown Norway rats. Eur J Pharmacol 1996; 315:81–88.
19. Henderson WR, Lewis DB, Albert RK, Zhang Y, Lamm WJE, Eriksen P, Jonas M,

Chi EY. The importance of leukotrienes in airway inflammation in a mouse model of asthma. J Exp Med 1996; 184(4):1483–1494.

20. Awni WM, Braeckman RA, Granneman GR, Witt G, Dubé LM. Pharmacokinetics and pharmacodynamics of zileuton after oral administration of single and multiple dose regimens of zileuton 600 mg in healthy volunteers. Clin Pharmacokin 1995; 29(suppl 2):22–33.
21. Wong SL, Awni WM, Cavanaugh JH, El-Shourbagy T, Locke C, Dubé LM. The pharmacokinetics of single oral doses of zileuton 200 to 800 mg, its enantiomers, and its metabolites, in normal health volunteers. Clin Pharmacokin 1995; 29(suppl 2):9–21.
22. Awni WM, Locke CS, Dubé LM, Cavanaugh JH. Evaluation of the diurnal variation in the pharmacokinetics of zileuton in normal healthy volunteers. J Clin Pharmacol 1997; 37:388–394.
23. Awni WM, Cavanaugh JH, Witt G, Granneman GR, Dubé LM. The effect of food on the pharmacokinetics of zileuton. Clin Pharmacokin 1995; 29(suppl. 2): 62–66.
24. Machinist JM, Kukulka MJ, Bopp BA. In vitro plasma protein binding of zileuton and its N-dehydroxylated metabolite. Clin Pharmacokin 1995; 29(suppl. 2):34–41.
25. Mayer MD, Kukulka MJ, Amann MT, Machinist JM. Human in vivo and in vitro metabolism of zileuton (abstr). Proc 7th North Am ISSX Meeting 1996; 10:315.
26. Machinist JM, Mayer MD, Shet MS, Ferrero JL, Rodrigues AD. Identification of the human liver cytochrome P450 enzymes involved in the metabolism of zileuton (ABT-077) and its N-dehydroxylated metabolite, Abbott-66193. Drug Metab Dispos 1995; 23:1163–1174.
27. Braeckman RA, Granneman GR, Locke CS, Machinist JM, Cavanaugh JH, Awni WM. The pharmacokinetics of zileuton in healthy young and elderly volunteers. Clin Pharmacokin 1995; 29(suppl 2):42–48.
28. Awni WM, Cohn J, Lanni C, Dubé L, Leutrol Study Group. The relationship of zileuton pharmacokinetics and pharmacodynamics as assessed by inhibition of leukotriene B_4 biosynthesis and improvement in pulmonary function in patients with moderate asthma (abstr). Eur Respir J 1994; 7(suppl 18):152s.
29. Awni WM, Granneman GR, Locke C, Brandwein SR, Dubé LM. Population pharmacokinetics of zileuton, a selective 5-lipoxygenase inhibitor, in patients with rheumatoid arthritis. Eur J Clin Pharm 1995; 48:155–160.
30. Coleman D, Awni W, Kelly HW, McWilliams BC, Bialek-Smith S, Dubé L. Initial pharmacokinetics evaluation of zileuton in asthmatic children (abstr). Am J Respir Crit Care Med 1995; 151(4, suppl):A377.
31. Awni WM, Wong W, Chu S-Y, Patterson K, Hansen R, Machinist JM, Drajesk J, Keane WF, Halstenson CE. Pharmacokinetics of zileuton and its metabolites in subjects with renal impairment. J Clin Pharmacol 1997; 37:395–404.
32. Awni W, Cao G, Locke C. Population modeling of leukotriene B_4 (LTB_4) inhibition by zileuton in asthmatic children (abstr). Pharm Res 1995; 12(suppl 9):S-362.
33. Wong SL, Locke C, Dubé L, Granneman GR, Awni WM. Meta-analysis of the pharmacodynamic relationship between the ex vivo LTB_4 inhibition in whole blood and zileuton plasma concentrations from Phase I studies in normal volunteers using NONMEM approach (abstr). Pharm Res 1994; 11(suppl 10):S-434.

34. Israel E, Dermarkarian R, Rosenberg M, Sperling R, Taylor G, Rubin P, Drazen JM. The effects of a 5-lipoxygenase inhibitor on asthma induced by cold, dry air. N Engl J Med 1990; 323:1740–1744.
35. Israel E, Fischer AR, Rosenberg MA, Lilly CM, Callery JC, Shapiro J, Cohn J, Rubin P, Drazen JM. The pivotal role of 5-lipoxygenase products in the reaction of aspirin-sensitive asthmatics to aspirin. Am Rev Respir Dis 1993; 148:1447–1451.
36. Kane GC, Pollice M, Kim C-J, Cohn J, Dworski RT, Murray JJ, Sheller JR, Fish JE, Peters SP. A controlled trial of the effect of the 5-lipoxygenase inhibitor, zileuton, on lung inflammation produced by segmental antigen challenge in human beings. J Allergy Clin Immunol 1996; 97:646–654.
37. Kane GC, Tollino M, Pollice M, Kim C-J, Cohn J, Murray JJ, Dworski R, Sheller J, Fish JE, Peters SP. Insights into IgE-mediated lung inflammation derived from a study employing a 5-lipoxygenase inhibitor. Prostaglandins 1995; 50:1–18.
38. Wenzel SE, Trudeau JB, Kaminsky DA, Cohn J, Martin RJ, Westcott JY. Effect of 5-lipoxygenase inhibition on bronchoconstriction and airway inflammation in nocturnal asthma. Am J Respir Crit Care Med 1995; 152:897–905.
39. Israel E, Rubin P, Kemp JP, Grossman J, Pierson W, Siegel SC, Tinkelman D, Murray JJ, Busse W, Segal AT, Fish J, Kaiser HB, Ledford D, Wenzel S, Rosenthal R, Cohn J, Lanni C, Pearlman H, Karahalios P, Drazen JM. The effect of inhibition of 5-lipoxygenase by zileuton in mild-to-moderate asthma. Ann Intern Med 1993; 119: 1059–1066.
40. Knapp HR. Reduced allergen-induced nasal congestion and leukotriene synthesis with an orally active 5-lipoxygenase inhibitor. N Engl J Med 1990; 323:1745–1748.
41. Latimer KM, O'Byrne PM, Morris MM, Roberts R, Hargreave FE. Bronchoconstriction stimulated by airway cooling. Am Rev Respir Dis 1983; 128:440–443.
42. Deal EC Jr, McFadden ER Jr, Ingram RH Jr, Breslin FJ, Jaeger JJ. Airway responsiveness to cold air and hyperpnea in normal subjects and those with hay fever and asthma. Am Rev Respir Dis 1980; 121:621–628.
43. Manning PJ, Watson RM, Margolskee DJ, Williams VC, Schwartz JI, O'Byrne PM. Inhibition of exercise-induced bronchoconstriction by MK-571; a potent leukotriene D_4-receptor antagonist. N Engl J Med 1990; 323:1736–1739.
44. Finnerty JP, Wood-Baker R, Thomson H, Holgate ST. Role of leukotrienes in exercise-induced asthma. Inhibitory effect of ICI 204219, a potent leukotriene D_4 antagonist. Am Rev Respir Dis 1992; 145:746–749.
45. Meltzer SS, Hasday JD, Cohn J, Bleecker ER. Inhibition of exercise-induced bronchospasm by zileuton: a 5-lipoxygenase inhibitor. Am J Respir Crit Care Med 1996; 153:931–935.
46. Dahlén S-E, Hansson G, Hedqvist P, Bjorck T, Granstrom E, Dahlén B. Allergen challenge of lung tissue from asthmatics elicits bronchial contraction that correlates with the release of leukotrienes C_4, D_4 and E_4. Proc Natl Acad Sci 1983; 80:1712–1716.
47. Taylor IK, O'Shaughnessy KM, Fuller RW, Dollery CT. Effect of the cysteinyl-leukotriene receptor antagonist ICI 204, 219 on allergen-induced bronchoconstriction and airway hyperreactivity in atopic subjects. Lancet 1991; 337:690–694.
48. Liu MC, Hubbard WC, Proud D, Stealey BA, Galli SJ, Kagey-Sobotka A, Bleecker ER, Lichtenstein LM. Immediate and late inflammatory responses to ragweed anti-

gen challenge of the peripheral airways in allergic asthmatics. Am Rev Respir Dis 1991; 144:51–58.

49. Spector SL, Wangaard CH, Farr RS. Aspirin and concomitant idiosyncrasies in adult asthmatic patients. J Allergy Clin Immunol 1979; 64(6):500–506.
50. Samter M, Beers RF. Intolerance to aspirin. Clinical studies and consideration of its pathogenesis. Ann Intern Med 1968; 68:975–983.
51. McDonald JR, Mathison DA, Stevenson DD. Aspirin intolerance in asthma. Detection by oral challenge. J Allergy Clin Immunol 1972; 50(4):198–207.
52. McFadden ER Jr. Respiratory heat and water exchange: physiological and clinical implications. J Appl Physiol 1983; 54:331–361.
53. O'Byrne PM, Thomson NC, Morris M, Roberts RS, Daniel EE, Hargreave FE. The protective effect of inhaled chlorpheniramine and atropine on bronchoconstriction induced by airway cooling. Am Rev Respir Dis 1983; 128:611–617.
54. Merland N, Cartier A, L'Archeveque J, Ghezzo H, Malo JL. Theophylline minimally inhibits bronchoconstriction induced by dry cold air inhalation in asthmatic subjects. Am Rev Respir Dis 1988; 137:1304–1308.
55. Christie PE, Tagari P, Ford-Hutchinson AW, Charlesson S, Chee P, Arm JP, Lee TH. Urinary leukotriene E_4 concentrations increase after aspirin challenge in aspirin-sensitive asthmatic subjects. Am Rev Respir Dis 1991; 143:1025–1029.
56. Kumlin M, Dahlén B, Björck T, Zetterström O, Granström E, Dahlén S-E. Urinary excretion of leukotriene E_4 and 11-dehydro-thromboxane B_2 in response to bronchial provocations with allergen, aspirin, leukotriene D_4 and histamine in asthmatics. Am Rev Respir Dis 1992; 146:96–103.
57. Knapp HR, Sladek K, Fitzgerald GA. Increased excretion of leukotriene E_4 during aspirin-induced asthma. J Lab Clin Med 1992; 119:48–51.
58. Sladek K, Szczeklik A. Cysteinyl leukotriene overproduction and mast cell activation in aspirin-provoked bronchospasm in asthma. Eur Respir J 1993;6: 391–399.
59. Fischer AR, Rosenberg MA, Lilly CM, Callery JC, Rubin P, Cohn J, White MV, Igarashi Y, Kaliner MA, Drazen JM, Israel E. Direct evidence for a role of the mast cell in the nasal response to aspirin in aspirin-sensitive asthma. J Allergy Clin Immunol 1994; 94:1046–1056.
60. Dahlén S-E, Nizankowska E, Dahlén B, Bocheneki G, Kumlin M, Mastalerz L, Blomqvist H, Pinis G, Rasberg B, Swanson L, Larsson L, Dubé L, Stensvad F, Zetterström O, Szczeklik A. The Swedish-Polish treatment study with the 5-lipoxygenase inhibitor, zileuton, in aspirin-intolerant asthmatics. Am J Respir Crit Care Med 1995; 151,4(2):A376.
61. Schwartz HJ, Petty T, Dubé LM, Swanson LJ, Lancaster JF, Zileuton Study Group. A randomized controlled trial comparing zileuton with theophylline in moderate asthma. Arch Intern Med 1998; 158(2):141–148.
62. Bergmann K-Ch, Bauer C-P, Overlak A. A placebo-controlled, blind comparison of nedocromil sodium and beclomethasone dipropionate in bronchial asthma. Curr Med Res Opin 1989; 11:533–542.
63. Haahtela T, Alanko K, Muittari A, Lahdensuo A, Sahlström K, Vilkka V. The superiority of combination beclomethasone and salbutamol over standard dosing of salbutamol in the treatment of chronic asthma. Ann Allergy 1989; 62:63–66.

64. Molema J, Lammers J-WJ, van Herwaarden CLA, Folgering HThM. Effects of inhaled beclomethasone dipropionate on beta$_2$-receptor function in the airways and adrenal responsiveness in bronchial asthma. Eur J Clin Pharmacol 1988; 34:577–583.
65. Israel E, Cohn J, Dubé L, Drazen JM, Zileuton Clinical Trial Group. Effect of treatment with zileuton, a 5-lipoxygenase inhibitor, in patients with asthma, a randomized controlled trial. JAMA 1996; 275:931–936.
66. Liu MC, Dubé LM, Lancaster J, Zileuton Study Group. Acute and chronic effects of a 5-lipoxygenase inhibitor in asthma: a 6-month randomized multicenter trial. J Allergy Clin Immunol 1996; 98:859–871.
67. Drazen JM, Israel E, Cohn J, Dubé L, Zileuton Study Group. The efficacy of zileuton in the treatment of asthma: results of combined double-blind, placebo-controlled trials. J Allergy Clin Immunol 1995; 95(Part 2):388.
68. Juniper EF, Guyatt GH, Ferrie PJ, Griffith LE. Measuring quality of life in asthma. Am Rev Respir Dis 1993; 147:832–838.
69. Juniper EF, Guyatt GH, Willan A, Griffith LE. Determining a minimal important change in a disease-specific quality of life questionnaire. J Clin Epidemiol 1994; 47: 81–87.
70. Schwartz HJ, Petty T, Reed R, Dubé LM, Swanson LJ, Zileuton Study Group. The comparative effects of zileuton, a 5-lipoxygenase inhibitor, vs. theophylline in patients with moderate asthma: results from a 13-week, multicenter trial. Am J Respir Crit Care Med 1995; 151:A376.
71. O'Connor BJ, Godard P, Dubé LM, Swanson LJ, Rountree LV, for the European Zileuton Study Group. The effect of zileuton, a 5-lipoxygenase inhibitor, plus low-dose inhaled beclomethasone, compared to higher dose beclomethasone alone in patients with asthma. Eur Respir 1996; 9:273S. Abstract 1737.
72. Lazarus SC, Lee TM, Wright S, Sarocco P, Rosenstein L, Bialek-Smith S, Dubé L, Zileuton Safety Trial Study Group. Secondary outcomes analysis of zileuton plus usual care vs. usual care alone in the treatment of patients with asthma. Annual meeting of the American College of Allergy, Asthma, and Immunology, Boston, November 8–13, 1996. Abstract 50.
73. Arky R. Physician's Desk Reference. 50th ed. Montvale, NJ: Medical Economics Co., 1996:996–998.
74. Arky R. Physician's Desk Reference. 50th ed. Montvale, NJ: Medical Economics Co., 1996:2011–2012.
75. Du Buske LM, Grossman J, Carpentier PJ, Dubé LM, Zileuton Study Group. The effect of reducing zileuton 600 mg QID in patients with moderate asthma. Annual meeting of the American College of Allergy, Asthma, and Immunology, Boston, November 8–13, 1996. Abstract P42.
76. Du Buske LM, Grossman J, Swanson LJ, Dubé LM, Lancaster JF, Zileuton Study Group. Randomized trial of zileuton in patients with moderate asthma: effect of reduced dosing frequency and amounts on pulmonary function and asthma symptoms. Am J Managed Care 1997; 3(4):633–640.
77. Zyflo Package Insert, Abbott Laboratories, North Chicago, IL, 1998.
78. Zimmerman HJ, Maddrey WC. Toxic and drug-induced hepatitis. In: Schiff L, Schiff ER, eds. Diseases of the liver. 7th ed. Philadelphia: JB Lippincott, 1993:707–783.

79. Zimmermam HJ. Hepatotoxicity: The Adverse Effects of Drugs and Other Chemicals on the Liver. New York: Appleton Century Crofts, 1978.
80. Lewis JH. Hepatic toxicity of nonsteroidal antiinflammatory drugs. Clin Pharm 1984; 3:128–138.
81. Tobert J, Shear CL, Chramos AN, Mantell GE. Clinical experience with lovostatin. Am J Cardiol 1990; 65:23F.
82. Granneman GR, Braeckman RA, Locke CS, Cavanaugh JH, Dubé LM, Awni WM. Effect of zileuton on theophylline pharmacokinetics. Clin Pharmacokin 1995; 29(suppl 2):77–83.
83. Sarker MA, Jackson BJ. Theophylline N-demethylations as probes for P450 1A1 and P450 1A2. Drug Metab Dispos 1994; 22:827–834.
84. Awni WM, Hussein Z, Granneman GR, Patterson KJ, Dubé LM, Cavanaugh JH. Pharmacodynamic and stereoselective pharmacokinetic interactions between zileuton and warfarin in humans. Clin Pharmacokin 1995; 29(suppl 2):67–76.
85. Rettie AE, Korzekwa KR, Kunze KL, Lawrence RF, Eddy AC, Aoyama T, Gelboin HV, Gonzalez FJ, Trager WF. Hydroxylation of warfarin by human cDNA expressed cytochrome P-450: a role for P-4502C9 in the etiology of (S)-warfarin drug interaction. Chem Res Toxicol 1992; 5:54–59.
86. Yoshimoto K, Echizen H, Chiba K, Tani M, Ishizaki T. Identification of the human CYP isoforms involved in the metabolism of propranolol enantiomers-N-desisopropylation is mediated mainly by CYP1A2. Br J Clin Pharmacol 1995; 39:421–431.
87. Awni WM, Cavanaugh JH, Leese P, Kaiser JF, Cao G, Locke CS, Dubé LM. The pharmacokinetic and pharmacodynamic interaction between zileuton and terfenadine. Eur J Clin Pharmacol 1997; 52:49–54.
88. Yun C-H, Okerholm RA, Guengerich FP. Oxidation of the antihistaminic drug terfenadine in human liver microsomes. Drug Metab Dispos 1993; 21:403–407.
89. Awni WM, Cavanaugh JH, Tzeng T-B, Witt G, Granneman GR, Dubé LM. Pharmacokinetic interactions between zileuton and prednisone. Clin Pharmacokin 1995; 29(suppl 2):105–111.
90. Awni WM, Hussein Z, Cavanaugh JH, Granneman GR, Dubé LM. Assessment of the pharmacokinetic interaction between zileuton and digoxin in humans. Clin Pharmacokin 1995; 29(suppl 2):92–97.
91. Samara E, Cavanaugh JH, Mukherjee D, Granneman GR. Lack of pharmacokinetic interaction between zileuton and phenytoin in humans. Clin Pharmacokin 1995; 29(suppl 2):84–91.
92. Awni WM, Braeckman RA, Locke CS, Dubé LM, Granneman GR. The influence of multiple oral doses of zileuton on the steady state pharmacokinetics of sulfasalazine and its metabolities, sulfapyridine and N-acetylsulfapyridine. Clin Pharmacokin 1995; 29(suppl 2):98–104.
93. Awni WM, Braeckman RA, Cavanaugh JH, Locke CS, Linnen PJ, Granneman GR, Dubé LM. The pharmacokinetic and pharmacodynamic interactions between the 5-lipoxygenase inhibitor zileuton and the cyclo-oxygenase inhibitor naproxen in human volunteers. Clin Pharmacokin 1995; 29(suppl 2):112–124.
94. National Heart, Lung, and Blood Institute, National Asthma Education Program, Expert Panel Report. Guidelines for the diagnosis and management of asthma. J Allergy Clin Immunol 1991; 88:425–534.

18

Antileukotrienes in the Management of Asthma

PAUL M. O'BYRNE

McMaster University
Hamilton, Ontario, Canada

I. Introduction

Asthma is a disease characterized by the presence of symptoms such as dyspnea, wheezing, chest tightness, and cough. These symptoms are usually caused by airflow obstruction, which is characteristically variable. Asthmatics are also known to have airway hyperresponsiveness to a variety of chemical bronchoconstrictor stimuli and physical stimuli such as exercise and hyperventilation of cold dry air (1). More recently, it has been recognized that asthma symptoms, variable airflow obstruction, and airway hyperresponsiveness occur as a consequence of a characteristic form of cellular inflammation and structural changes in the airway wall (2). The inflammation consists of the presence of activated eosinophils, lymphocytes, and an increased number of mast cells. Also, the structural changes described in asthmatic airways appear to be characteristic of the disease and are likely caused by persisting airway inflammation.

The identification of the mediators that cause the persisting airway inflammation of asthma, as well as those that are released from activated inflammatory cells to cause the physiological abnormalities of asthma, has been partially elucidated. It is likely that proinflammatory cytokines and chemokines, which are important in the development of eosinophils in the bone marrow, or their recruitment, activation, and prolonged survival in the airways, such as granulocyte macrophage-colony stimulating factor (GM-CSF) (3,4), interleukin (IL)-5 (5), and eotaxin (6), are involved in the eosinophilic inflammation of asthma. IL-3 may be responsible for the increases in mast cell numbers (7). Both activated eosinophils and mast cells produce and release the cysteinyl leukotriene (LT) C_4 from the cytosol to the extracellular microenvironment, where it is metabolized to form LTD_4. Further metabolism by a variety of dipeptidases results in the formation of the stable excretory product LTE_4. The cysteinyl leukotrienes have been demonstrated in a number of different studies to be the most important mediators of asthmatic bronchoconstriction (8–11). They also cause airway edema and mucus secretion, which contributes to airway narrowing in asthmatics. A variety of antileukotriene drugs have been developed and studied in patients with asthma. The purpose of this review is to consider the efficacy of these anti-leukotrienes in asthma management.

II. Objectives of Asthma Management

There have been published consensus statements from a variety of countries on asthma management (12–14) . These documents have been remarkably consistent in identifying the goals and objectives of asthma treatment, which are:

1. To minimize or eliminate asthma symptoms.
2. To achieve the best possible lung function.
3. To prevent asthma exacerbations.
4. To do the above with the least possible medications.
5. To educate the patient about the disease and the goals of management.

One objective that is implied, but not explicitly stated, is the prevention of the decline in lung function and the development of fixed airflow obstruction that occurs in some asthmatic patients.

In addition to these goals and objectives, each of these documents has identified what is meant by the term "asthma control." This includes the above objectives of minimal or no symptoms and best lung function, but also includes minimizing the need for rescue medications, such as inhaled β_2-agonists, to less than daily use, minimizing the variability of flow rates that is characteristic of asthma, as well as having normal activities of daily living. Achieving this level of asthma control should be an objective from the very first visit of the patient to the treating physician. Unfortunately, many studies suggest that this does not happen. This may be, in part, because the patient has learned to live with daily asthma symptoms and limitations in their daily activities and minimizes these to the physician. Alternatively, the idea of asthma control may not be widely accepted or understood by many physicians who see patients with asthma. This means that many (perhaps even most) patients with diagnosed asthma are not optimally controlled.

III. Current Asthma Treatment

The most recent consensus statement on asthma management (14) has divided asthmatic patients into four groups for the purposes of deciding on asthma treatment (Fig. 1):

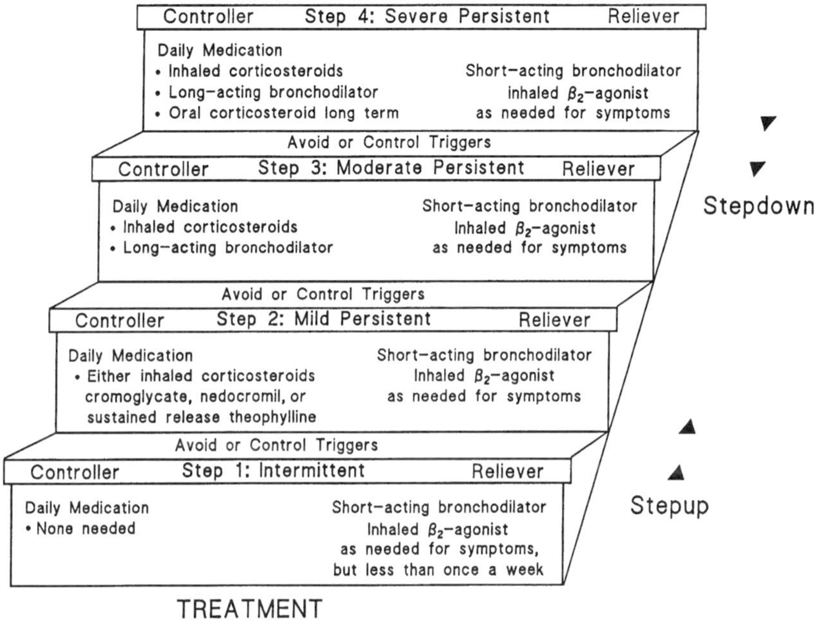

Figure 1 Asthma-management guidelines adapted from the Global Initiative for Asthma. (From Ref. 14.)

1. Mild intermittent asthma: patients with infrequent symptoms, normal lung function most of the time, and no limitation in their activities of daily living. These patients should be treated with short-acting inhaled β_2-agonists when needed for symptom relief—at most two or three times each week.
2. Mild persistent asthma: patients with symptoms more frequently than two or three times each week, indeed, often every day, but who have normal lung function most of the time and no limitation in their activities of daily living. These patients require regular treatment to prevent the development of symptoms, as well as with short-acting inhaled β_2-agonists when needed for symptom relief. In adult patients, low doses of inhaled corticosteroids (400–500 μg of beclomethasone dipropionate or budesonide) are the most effective treatment, but inhaled cromones, such as sodium cromoglycate or nedocromil, are often used in children.
3. Moderate persistent asthma: patients with daily symptoms, with nocturnal symptoms, with variable airflow obstruction, and with some lim-

itation of their activities of daily living. These patients are usually using inhaled β_2-agonists several times each day and often at night. Inhaled corticosteroids are the mainstay of treatment in these patients, who often need higher doses (800–2000 μg/day). However, the addition of inhaled long-acting β_2-agonists, such as salmeterol or formoterol, may provide better asthma control than increasing the doses of inhaled corticosteroids in these patients (15). Also, in some patients, oral theophylline may be effective if added to inhaled corticosteroids, but inhaled long-acting β_2-agonists are likely to be as or more effective and easier to use. Asthma exacerbations need to be treated with short courses of oral corticosteroids.

4. Severe persistent asthma: patients with frequent daily and nocturnal symptoms, usually abnormal lung function, and limitation of their activities of daily living. These patients are usually using inhaled β_2-agonists many times each day, and frequently at night. High doses of inhaled corticosteroids remain the mainstay of treatment in these patients, together with inhaled long-acting β_2-agonists or theophylline. These patients often need daily or alternate daily oral corticosteroids in an effort to control asthma.

While there is little debate in the literature that corticosteroids are the most effective treatment for asthma (16) and that the inhaled route is preferable to minimize unwanted effects, there is considerable debate over the early use of inhaled corticosteroids in the asthmatic patient considered to have mild asthma (17). Such patients are usually treated with drugs considered to be less effective than inhaled corticosteroids. Some recent studies have evaluated which treatment approaches achieve the best asthma control in patients, who, although considered to have mild asthma, have persistent symptoms. One option is to use regular, rather than intermittent, inhaled β_2-agonists. In patients with more severe disease, the regular use of the inhaled β_2-agonist fenoterol was shown to worsen asthma control (18), and regular use of this and other β_2-agonists was associated with increased asthma mortality (19). In another study in patients with mild persistent asthma, the regular use of the inhaled β_2-agonist albuterol caused a slight, but not significant, deterioration in most indices of asthma control measured (20). There was, however, no increase in asthma exacerbations with regular inhaled albuterol and no obvious advantage or clinically important disadvantage to the regular use of inhaled β_2-agonists.

In contrast to these results, a study of patients considered by their family physicians to have such mild asthma that they would not receive any clinical benefit from the use of inhaled corticosteroids demonstrated marked improvements in both symptom control and airway obstruction, associated with a reduction in asthma exacerbations, when treated with low doses of inhaled corticoste-

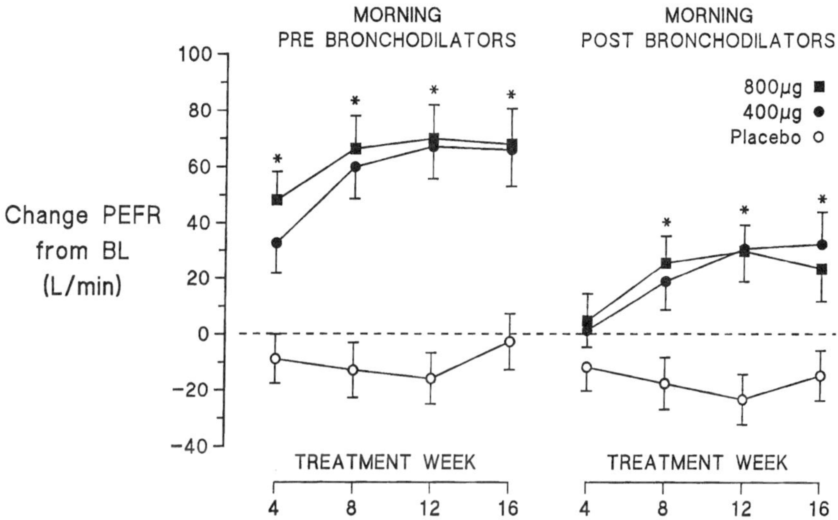

Figure 2 Changes in PEFR from baseline measured in the morning upon waking both before and after inhaled bronchodilator for weeks 4–16 for patients with mild persistent asthma treated with placebo (open circles), budesonide 400 μg/day (closed circles) or 800 μg/day (closed squares). $^{**}p < 0.01$; $^{***}p < 0.001$. (From Ref. 21.)

roids (21). Indeed, the magnitude of the improvements in peak expired flows (PEF) obtained in these patients (mean improvement of morning PEF of 70 L/min) (Fig. 2) is one of the largest described in placebo-controlled studies of asthmatic patients. This study demonstrated that some asthmatic patients considered to have mild intermittent asthma, have, in fact, much more persisting disease, which is benefited by the use of low doses of inhaled corticosteroids. It is troubling that neither the physician nor the patient had identified that asthma control was not optimal, requiring a step-up in treatment.

Asthmatics lose lung function more rapidly than nonasthmatics, although less rapidly than cigarette smokers. Infrequently, this leads to severe, permanent, fixed airflow obstruction, with all of the attendant disability and handicap associated with this condition. A number of recent studies in both adults (22) and children (23) have demonstrated that inhaled steroids provide a protective effect against the deterioration in lung function seen with prolonged regular use of inhaled bronchodilator therapy alone. These studies taken together indicate that inhaled corticosteroids can diminish the decline in lung function that occurs in asthmatics and suggest that early intervention with inhaled corticosteroids can optimize lung function in asthmatics.

IV. Antileukotriene Drugs

A variety of antileukotriene drugs have been developed for asthma treatment. It is theoretically possible to inhibit the production of the leukotrienes by inhibition of any of the enzymes in their biosynthetic pathway. However, at this point the only enzyme that has been selectively inhibited is 5-LO (5-LO inhibitors) (24). An example of this class is zileuton. It has also been possible to interrupt leukotriene formation by preventing the binding of arachidonic acid to the enzyme 5-lipoxygenase–activating protein (FLAP-antagonists) (25). An example of this class is Bay X 1005. Finally, drugs have been developed that antagonize the specific receptor in human airways on which the cysteinyl leukotrienes act, the $CysLT_1$ (leukotriene receptor antagonists) (26). Examples of this class are zafirleukast, pranleukast, or monteleukast.

V. Place of Antileukotriene Drugs in Asthma Management

The studies described elsewhere in this book that have documented the efficacy of the antileukotrienes used study designs required to obtain registration of the drugs to allow them to be available for prescription. These studies have demonstrated that antileukotrienes improve asthma control in patients with moderate to severe asthma (27,28) but have not yet clearly shown how they will fit into asthma-management schemes. This is because there are, as yet, no peer-reviewed published reports of the *comparative* efficacy against already well-established antiasthma drugs, particularly inhaled corticosteroids, in overall asthma management. The only comparative study as yet reported has suggested that a receptor antagonist, SKF 104353, is equally effective as cromoglycate in protecting against exercise-induced bronchoconstriction (29). Finally, no published studies have focused on patients considered to have mild asthma only.

Despite the absence of comparative studies, particularly with inhaled corticosteroids, the published studies do already support two indications for the use of antileukotrienes. One of these is in patients with aspirin-sensitive asthma, where these drugs are completely effective in blocking aspirin-induced asthmatic responses (10), which can be life-threatening and are not prevented by any other currently available antiasthma treatment. Thus, antileukotrienes should be used in all patients with aspirin-induced asthma, together with other antiasthma treatment needed to control other manifestations of their asthma. The second indication is in patients taking regular inhaled β_2-agonists and who have exercise-induced bronchoconstriction. In these patients, the regular use of inhaled β_2-agonists will reduce their ability to protect against exercise-induced bronchoconstriction (30,31), and, while no direct evaluation has been made, it is likely that antileukotrienes will be effective in this setting because antileukotrienes are effective in

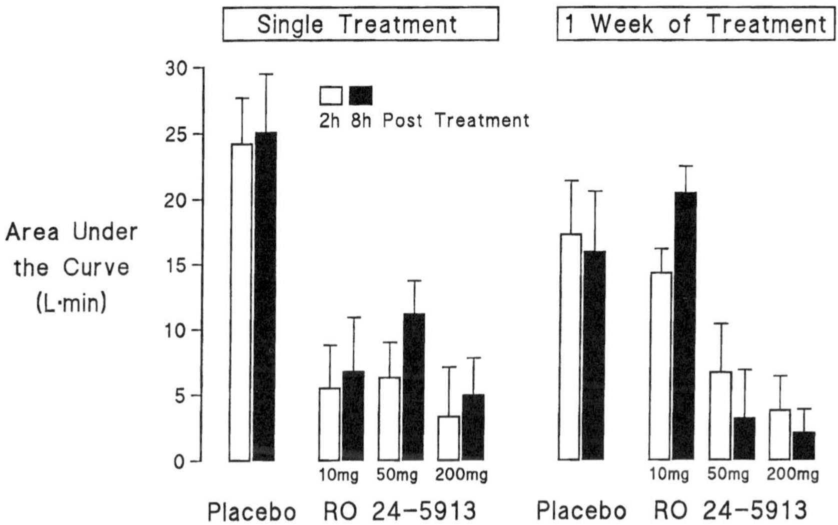

Figure 3 Protection against exercise-induced bronchoconstriction for more than 8 hours achieved with three doses of the leukotriene receptor antagonist cinalukast. The response is expressed as the area under the time-response curve. The protection achieved with the highest dose was lost after 1 week of regular treatment, but persisted for the two higher doses. (From Ref. 33.)

attenuating exercise-induced bronchoconstriction (8,32) and in some patients the attenuation is complete. Also, a recent study has demonstrated that one antileukotriene can provide protection for at least 8 hours, and at higher doses of the drug no loss of this protection was seen with regular dosing for 1 week (33) (Fig. 3).

There does not appear to be any indication for the use of antileukotrienes in patients with very mild, intermittent asthma in whom infrequent inhaled β_2-agonist use is adequate to control symptoms. In patients with more persisting symptoms in whom another treatment is needed, the currently available consensus guidelines on asthma management suggest that inhaled corticosteroids or cromones be considered (14). The available studies suggest that the antileukotrienes will be effective in some—perhaps up to 50%—of these patients. If an antileukotriene is chosen as the next line of treatment, a therapeutic trial of 6–8 weeks will allow a decision to be made about the efficacy of the treatment. If the treatment is not effective, there is no currently available evidence that it should be continued beyond this time. Obviously, direct comparative studies of the antileukotrienes with more established antiasthma therapy are eagerly awaited.

There is some preliminary evidence that the antileukotrienes may be even more effective in patients with more severe asthma. Their additive effect to the bronchodilation achieved even with high doses of inhaled β_2-agonists (11,34) suggests that they may have a place in the treatment of the severe bronchoconstriction associated with acute severe asthma. Also, clinical benefit has been demonstrated with their addition to the treatment of patients with poor asthma control already taking high doses of inhaled corticosteroids (35). There is, however, no evidence yet published in the archival literature that they can reduce the doses of inhaled or ingested corticosteroids required for asthma control.

When considering the available asthma-treatment guidelines, it is clear that antileukotrienes will have a place in treating some patients with moderate and severe persistent asthma. These patients are usually not optimally controlled on low doses of inhaled corticosteroids. It is also likely that the antileukotrienes will be effective in some patients with mild persistent asthma; however, as low doses of inhaled corticosteroids, which are free of systemic unwanted effects, are very effective in this patient population, the use of antileukotrienes cannot be recommended until comparative studies with low doses of inhaled corticosteroids have been performed.

VI. Conclusions

Antileukotrienes are the first novel class of asthma therapy that has been developed over the past 25 years. Currently available data indicate that inhibition of leukotriene synthesis or action has a beneficial effect in the treatment of both induced and spontaneously occurring asthma. Although encouraging results have been obtained from clinical trials of the antileukotrienes, the results do not yet provide guidelines for the optimal clinical use of antileukotrienes in asthma treatment; such recommendations await further comparative studies with other effective antiasthma treatment, particularly inhaled corticosteroids.

References

1. O'Byrne PM. Airway hyperresponsiveness. In: Middleton E, Adkinson NF, Busse WW, Ellis EF, Reed CE, eds. Allergy: Principals and Practice. St. Louis, MO: Mosby Year Books Inc., 1993: 1203–1214.
2. Adelroth E, O'Byrne PM. Inflammatory mechanisms in airway hyperresponsiveness. In: Holgate ST, Busse WW, eds. Asthma and Rhinitis. Boston: Blackwell Scientific Publications, 1994: 1067–1074.
3. Woolley KL, Adelroth E, Woolley MJ, Ellis R, Jordana M, O'Byrne PM. Granulocyte-macrophage colony-stimulating factor, eosinophils and eosinophil cationic protein in subjects with and without mild, stable, atopic asthma. Eur Respir J 1994; 7: 1576–1584.

4. Woolley KL, Adelroth E, Woolley MJ, Ellis R, Jordana M, O'Byrne PM. Effects of allergen challenge on eosinophils, eosinophil cationic protein, and granulocyte-macrophage colony-stimulating factor in mild asthma. Am J Respir Crit Care Med 1995; 151:1915–1924.
5. Ohnishi T, Kita H, Weiler D, et al. IL-5 is the predominant eosinophil-active cytokine in the antigen-induced pulmonary late-phase reaction. Am Rev Respir Dis 1993; 147:901–907.
6. Humbles AA, Conroy DM, Marleau S, et al. Generation and action of an eosinophil-selective chemoattractant, eotaxin, in vivo. Am J Respir Crit Care Med 1996; 153: A219.
7. Woolley KL, Adelroth E, Woolley MJ, et al. Interleukin-3 in bronchial biopsies from nonasthmatics and patients with mild and allergen-induced asthma. Am J Respir Crit Care Med 1996; 153:350–355.
8. Manning PJ, Watson RM, Margolskee DJ, Williams VC, Schwartz JI, O'Byrne PM. Inhibition of exercise-induced bronchoconstriction by MK-571, a potent-leukotriene D4-receptor antagonist. N Engl J Med 1990; 323:1736–1739.
9. Taylor IK, O'Shaughnessy KM, Fuller RW, Dollery CT. Effect of a cysteinyl leukotriene receptor antagonist, ICI 204-219 on allergen-induced bronchoconstriction and airway hyperactivity in atopic subjects. Lancet 1991; 337:690–694.
10. Israel E, Fischer AR, Rosenburg MA, et al. The pivotal role of 5-lipoxygenase products in the reaction of aspirin-sensitive asthmatics to aspirin. Am Rev Respir Dis 1993; 148:1447–1451.
11. Gaddy JN, Margolskee DJ, Bush RK, Williams VC, Busse WW. Bronchodilation with a potent and selective leukotriene D4 (LTD4) antagonist (MK-571) in patients with asthma. Am Rev Respir Dis 1992; 146:358–363.
12. Woolcock AJ, Rubinfeld A, Seale P. The Australian asthma management plan. Med J Aust 1989; 151:650–653.
13. Sheffer AL, Bartal M, Bousquet J, Carrasco E, et al. Global strategy for asthma management and prevention. Natl Inst Health 1995; 95-3659:70–114.
14. Global initiative for asthma. National Heart, Lung and Blood Institute Publication 95-3659. Bethesda, MD: U.S. Department of Health and Human Services, 1995.
15. Greening AP, Ind PW, Northfield M, Shaw G. Added salmeterol versus higher-dose corticosteroid in asthma patients with symptoms on existing inhaled corticosteroid. Lancet 1994; 344:219–224.
16. Barnes PJ, Pedersen S. Efficacy and safety of inhaled corticosteroids in asthma. Am Rev Respir Dis 1993; 148:S1–26.
17. Drazen J, Israel E. Treating mild asthma, when are inhaled steroids indicated? N Engl J Med 1994; 331:737–738.
18. Sears MR, Taylor DR, Print CG, et al. Regular inhaled beta-agonist treatment in bronchial asthma. Lancet 1990; 336:1391–1396.
19. Spitzer WO, Suissa S, Ernst P, et al. The use of beta-agonists and the risk of death and near death from asthma. N Engl J Med 1992; 326:501–506.
20. Drazen JM, Israel E. Comparison of regularly scheduled with "as needed only" use of albuterol in mild asthma. N Engl J Med 1996; 335:841–847.

21. O'Byrne PM, Cuddy L, Taylor DW, Birch S, Morris J, Syrotiuk J. The clinical efficacy and cost benefit of inhaled corticosteroids as therapy in patients with mild asthma in primary care practice. Can Respir J 1996; 3:169–175.
22. Haahtela T, Jarvinen M, Kava T, et. al. Effects of reducing or discontinuing inhaled budesonide in patients with mild asthma. N Engl J Med 1994; 331:700–705.
23. Agertoft L, Pedersen S. Effects of long-term treatment with an inhaled corticosteroid on growth and pulmonary function in asthmatic children. Respir Med 1994; 88:373–381.
24. Carter GW, Young PR, Albert DH, et al. 5-Lipoxygenase inhibitory activity of zileuton. Pharmacol Exp Ther 1991; 256:929–937.
25. Ford-Hutchinson AW. FLAP: a novel drug target for inhibiting the synthesis of leukotrienes. TIPS 1991; 12:68–70.
26. Coleman RA, Eglen RM, Jones RL, et al. Prostanoid and leukotriene receptors: a progress report from the IUPHAR working parties on classification and nomenclature. Prostaglandins Rel Compounds 1996; 23:280–285.
27. Israel E, Rubin P, Kemp JP, et al. The effect of inhibition of 5-lipoxygenase by zileuton in mild-to-moderate asthma. Ann Intern Med 1993; 119:1059–1066.
28. Spector SL, Glass M, Birmingham BK, et al. Effects of 6 weeks of therapy with oral doses of ICI 204,219 a leukotriene D4 receptor antagonist, in subjects with bronchial asthma. Am J Respir Crit Care Med 1994; 150:618–623.
29. Robuschi M, Riva E, Fuccella LM, et al. Prevention of exercise-induced bronchoconstriction by a new leukotriene antagonist (SKF 104353). A double-blind study versus disodium cromoglycate and placebo. Am Rev Respir Dis 1992; 145:1285–1288.
30. Inman M, O'Byrne PM. The effect of regular inhaled albuterol on exercise-induced bronchoconstriction. Am J Respir Crit Care Med 1996; 153:65–69.
31. Ramage L, Lipworth BJ, Ingram CG, Cree IA, Dhillon DP. Reduced protection against exercise induced bronchoconstriction after chronic dosing with salmeterol. Respir Med 1994; 88:363–368.
32. Finnerty JP, Wood-Baker R, Thomson H, Holgate ST. Role of leukotrienes in exercise-induced asthma. Inhibitory effect of ICI 204219, a potent leukotriene D4 receptor antagonist. Am Rev Respir Dis 1992; 145:746–749.
33. Adelroth E, Inman MD, Summers E, Pace D, Modi M, O'Byrne PM. Prolonged protection against exercise-induced bronchoconstriction by the leukotriene D4-receptor antagonist Cinalukast. J Allergy Clin Immunol 1997; 99:210–215.
34. Hui KP, Barnes NC. Lung function improvement in asthma with a cysteinyl-leukotriene receptor antagonist. Lancet 1991; 337:1062–1063.
35. Chapman KR, Friedman BS, Shingo S, Heyse J, Reiss T, Spector R. The efficacy of an oral inhibitor of leukotriene synthesis (MK-0591) in asthmatics treated with inhaled steroids. Am J Respir Crit Care Med 1994; 149:A215

AUTHOR INDEX

Italic numbers give the page on which the complete reference is listed.

B

C

G

I

J

K

N

T

U

V

W

X

Y

SUBJECT INDEX

A

B

C

D

E

F

G

J

K

L

M

N

O

P

Q

R

U

V

W

Y

Z